Encyclopedia of Health Psychology

Encyclopedia of Health Psychology

Edited by

Alan J. Christensen
Departments of Psychology and Internal Medicine
The University of Iowa
Iowa City, Iowa

René Martin
College of Nursing
The University of Iowa
Iowa City, Iowa

and

Joshua Morrison Smyth
Department of Psychology
Syracuse University
Syracuse, New York

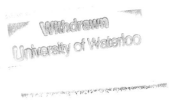
Kluwer Academic / Plenum Publishers
New York, Boston, London, Dordrecht, Moscow

Library of Congress Cataloging-in-Publication Data

Encyclopedia of health psychology / edited by Alan J. Christensen, René Martin, and Joshua Morrison Smyth.
    p.   cm.
Includes bibliographical references and index.
ISBN 0-306-48336-X
1. Clinical health psychology–Encyclopedias.   I. Christensen, Alan J.   II. Martin, René, 1960–   III. Smyth, Joshua M.
R726.7.E53 2004
616′.001′9–dc22
                      2003070328

ISBN 0-306-48336-X

© 2004 Kluwer Academic/Plenum Publishers, New York
233 Spring Street, New York, New York 10013

http://www.kluweronline.com

10 9 8 7 6 5 4 3 2 1

A C.I.P. record for this book is available from the Library of Congress.

Permissions for books published in Europe: permissions@wkap.nl
Permissions for books published in the United States of America: permissions@wkap.com

Printed in the United States of America

Preface

Over the last 25 years, interest in health psychology has grown at a rapid rate. With a focus on the promotion and the maintenance of both physical and mental health and an emphasis on the prevention as well as the treatment of disease, health psychology holds a unique place within the discipline of psychology. More broadly, health psychology draws on, and contributes to, the varied fields of psychology, medicine, nursing, sociology, anthropology, and many others. A variety of factors have contributed to this rapid growth and increased interest in health psychology. One central factor has been a shift in the very types of disease people live with and/or die from, from more acute or time-limited illnesses (e.g., infectious disease) toward more *chronic conditions* (e.g., diabetes, heart disease), which often require sustained attention over an entire lifetime. A second key factor has been the increasing recognition that *health practices and other behavioral factors* (e.g., smoking, diet, exercise) are major contributors to the development of many common and costly diseases. Third, enhanced recognition of the importance of *mind–body connections* (e.g., stress effects on physiological processes) in understanding health and illness has greatly increased interest in health psychology because of its unique focus on the interplay between psychological factors and physical disease. Finally, although human beings are living longer than ever before, with *increased life expectancy* has come an increase in the number of individuals living with disease for an extended period of time. This gives rise to a need for greater attention to issues of disease adaptation and rehabilitation, quality of life, patient adherence to medical interventions, and the impact of disease on the aging population.

The goal of this volume is a difficult one: to provide a relatively comprehensive and accessible overview of the central concepts, issues, conditions, and terms that comprise the broad discipline of health psychology. Clearly, no single book can exhaustively cover such a broad area. With more than 200 contributions by more than 150 of the leading researchers, educators, and practitioners in the field, however, we believe that *The Encyclopedia of Health Psychology* successfully covers most (though certainly not all) of the central topics in the field. The common goal of each of these entries is to provide an accessible introduction for the nonexpert reader, serve as a topical primer for undergraduate and graduate students studying the health and behavioral sciences, and provide a useful reference source for interested teachers, researchers, and health care providers.

There are many people to acknowledge whose combined efforts were essential in completing this encyclopedia. First and foremost we thank the more than 150 contributors who devoted considerable time, energy, expertise, and patience to this project. Above all else the contributors shared their excitement and enthusiasm for their field in a way that is sure to be both informative and contagious to the reader. Thanks to Sarah Williams, the Brain and Behavior Editor at Kluwer Academic/Plenum Publishers, for quickly and enthusiastically seeing the merits in this project, and for always being available to provide much-needed assistance as the book became a reality. Last but certainly not least, we thank our invaluable editorial assistant, Jamie Cvengros, who beautifully managed the difficult task of coordinating contacts, correspondence, and contributions from scores of busy contributors literally from around the world.

On behalf of all of our contributor colleagues, we hope you find *The Encyclopedia of Health Psychology* useful and informative, and we sincerely welcome your feedback about the volume.

ALAN J. CHRISTENSEN
RENÉ MARTIN
JOSHUA SMYTH

Aa

Accidents

Accidental injuries (also called unintentional injuries) are a significant public health problem in the United States. Unintentional injuries accounted for 97,860 deaths in 1999 and 40.4 million emergency department visits in 2000. By a very large margin, unintentional injuries are the leading cause of death for individuals between the ages of 1 and 34 years. In 1999, unintentional injuries accounted for 43 percent of deaths in the 1- to 24-year-old age group, with deaths from accidents peaking between 15 and 19 years of age. Males are more susceptible to unintentional injuries than are females. For males, unintentional injuries rank as the fourth leading cause of death, whereas for females, unintentional injuries are the seventh leading cause of death. Unintentional injuries are caused most commonly by motor vehicles, followed in number by falls, poisoning, drowning, suffocation (especially for infants), and fire/burns. Billions of dollars are spent each year in the United States dealing with the problem of unintentional injuries.

Despite the growing national concern over reducing unintentional injuries, the underlying behavioral causes of such injuries have received relatively little attention from injury researchers. However, without a clear understanding of the behaviors that lead to accidents, it is difficult to know who or what to target for intervention. For example, although all children would benefit from wearing bicycle helmets, it is particularly important to increase helmet use among children who routinely engage in behaviors that put them at risk for bicycling crashes. Thus, understanding the behavioral causes of unintentional injuries is critical for designing effective interventions.

PERSONALITY FACTORS AND INJURY PRONENESS

Personality traits are frequently implicated as a major contributor to injury risk, especially during childhood and adolescence. In the first investigation to examine links between children's personality traits and injury risk, researchers examined the records of San Francisco Bay area children aged 4 to 18 years who had been enrolled in a particular medical insurance plan. Using insurance records, they divided children into three groups of high, medium, or low annual injury rates. They found that children who experienced a high number of injuries were rated by their mothers as more hyperactive, impulsive, aggressive, extraverted, independent, curious, daring, and careless. Other research has also linked personality traits with more minor, everyday injuries. Specifically, 8-year-olds whose parents described them as highly active, impulsive, and undercontrolled had more severe day-to-day injuries.

Several studies following the same children over a long period of time have also found a link between personality traits and unintentional injuries. In one study, more than 10,000 children were tested at age 5 years and again at age 10 years. An important finding was that high activity and aggression levels were linked to higher injury rates. Likewise, a Finnish study that tested individuals at ages 8, 14, and 27 years revealed that boys who were aggressive at ages 8 and 14 years had experienced more injuries by age 27 years. Another study examined how impulsivity and self-control at age 4 years were related to injury risk at age 6 years. Children who were impulsive and undercontrolled at age 4 years had a history of injuries requiring medical attention at age 6 years. Thus, it appears that early manifestations of impulsivity, noncompliance, and high activity level are predictive of later injury risk.

Research on children with clinical diagnoses has yielded similar results and generally indicates that children with externalizing disorders such as Attention Deficit/Hyperactivity Disorder (ADHD), Oppositional Defiant Disorder (ODD), and Conduct Disorder (CD) are more at risk for injury. One study revealed that parents who described their children as hyperactive also described their children as more at risk for injury. An investigation of nearly 1,000 children from two hospitals in South Wales from birth through age 5 years revealed that children with serious discipline problems had more injuries. Another study found that children with ADHD anticipated less severe consequences following risky behaviors than did non-ADHD control children. Thus, clinical studies suggest that injury-prone children are more aggressive, overactive, and poorly disciplined.

Together, these studies suggest that impulsive and undercontrolled children are more at risk for injury. How might such traits put children at risk for injury? Certain personality characteristics may lead children to seek out some situations and avoid others. For example, highly active and approach-oriented children may seek out new and unfamiliar situations. Novel situations may lead to injuries because such situations force children to react to potentially unforeseen, dangerous problems. Thus, by seeking out some situations, children may put themselves at greater risk of injury.

COGNITIVE FACTORS AND INJURY PRONENESS

One cognitive factor that has been recently linked to injury risk is overestimation of physical ability. More specifically, errors in judging the relation between one's physical abilities and the demands of the situation may contribute to injury risk. For example, to bicycle across a road safely, children must evaluate their own level of bicycling skill in relation to the demands of the situation. In the case where cross-traffic does not stop, children must wait for a sufficient gap between vehicles before crossing. To determine whether the gap between two vehicles affords safe crossing, children must accurately judge the size of the gap in relation to the time it will take them to bicycle across the road. If children overestimate how quickly they can bicycle across the road, they may choose a gap that is too short for safe crossing. Such errors in judgment may lead to severe injury if the child is hit by an oncoming car.

Several studies have examined children's ability to judge traffic gaps. In one study, researchers developed a road-crossing task to assess age changes in children's ability to accurately judge whether traffic gaps afford safe crossing. Five- to 10-year-old children crossed a "pretend" road set up directly parallel to an actual road. Children watched the cars on the actual road and crossed the pretend road when they felt that they could safely

reach the other side. Although children generally were cautious, they occasionally accepted gaps that were too short. In addition, a higher proportion of younger than older children made such errors. These findings suggest that younger children are more likely to overestimate their ability to walk through traffic gaps.

The finding that children sometimes overestimate their ability to cross roads is consistent with other studies showing that children also overestimate other physical abilities. For example, one study found that 9- and 12-year-old boys overestimated the height of the stairs they could climb. Other studies have consistently shown that 6- and 8-year-olds overestimate their reaching and stepping abilities. Moreover, 6-year-olds who overestimate their physical abilities tend to have more unintentional injuries requiring medical attention. Thus, it appears that overestimation of ability may be a risk factor for unintentional injuries during childhood.

The role that overestimation of ability plays in unsafe behavior has also been investigated in studies of young automobile drivers. In one study, researchers found that young male drivers perceived their chances of having a collision to be significantly lower than those of both their male peers and older male drivers. Older male drivers, on the other hand, saw their chances of a collision as comparable to those of their male peers and less than those of younger male drivers. Another study revealed that young males rated their driving abilities as being the same as those of older males, but saw their peers as being at greater risk and having poorer driving abilities than themselves. The discrepancy between young drivers' perceived and actual driving ability may result in a misperception of danger, and hence a greater likelihood of automobile collisions.

Taken together, these results suggest that children and adolescents may perceive the boundary between actions that are within and beyond their ability as fuzzy. Moreover, when faced with uncertainty, children and adolescents are more likely to overestimate than underestimate their abilities. Thus, errors in judgment appear to be another risk factor for unintentional injury.

CONCLUSION

Unintentional injuries are the leading cause of death for individuals up to age 34 years. Understanding the behavioral factors that put people at risk for injury is critical for designing interventions to prevent such injuries. Recent studies show that both personality and cognitive factors lead to risky behaviors, particularly during childhood and adolescence. Targeting intervention efforts at individuals who are the most likely to engage in risky behaviors is one promising avenue for preventing unintentional injuries.

Related Entries: Prevention, Public Health

BIBLIOGRAPHY

Bijur, P., Golding, J., Haslum, M., & Kurzon, M. (1988). Behavioral predictors of injury in school-age children. *American Journal of Diseases of Children, 142*, 1307–1312.

Bijur, P. E., Stewart-Brown, S., & Butler, N. (1986). Child behavior and accidental injury in 11,966 preschool children. *American Journal of Diseases of Children, 140*, 487–492.

Davidson, L. L. (1987). Hyperactivity, antisocial behavior, and childhood injury: A critical analysis of the literature. *Developmental and Behavioral Pediatrics, 8*, 335–340.

Farmer, J. E., & Peterson, L. (1995). Injury risk factors in children with Attention Deficit Hyperactivity Disorder. *Health Psychology, 14*, 325–332.

Fingerhut, L. A., & Warner, M. (1997). *Injury Chartbook. Health, United States 1996–97.* Hyattsville, MD: National Center for Health Statistics.

Finn, P., & Bragg, B. W. (1986). Perception of the risk of an accident by young and older drivers. *Accident Analysis and Prevention, 18*, 289–298.

Gayton, W. G., Bailey, C., Wagner, A., & Hardesty, V. A. (1986). Relationship between childhood hyperactivity and accident proneness. *Perceptual and Motor Skills, 63*, 801–802.

Institute of Medicine. (1999). *Reducing the burden of injury.* Washington, DC: National Academy Press.

Lee, D. N., Young, D. S., & McLaughlin, C. M. (1984). A roadside simulation of road crossing for children. *Ergonomics, 12*, 1271–1281.

Mathews, M. L., & Moran, A. R. (1986). Age differences in male drivers' perception of accident risk. The role of perceived driving ability. *Accident Analysis and Prevention, 18*, 299–313.

Manheimer, D., & Mellinger, G. (1967). Personality characteristics of the child accident repeater. *Child Development, 38*, 491–514.

McKenzie, B. E., & Forbes, C. (1992). Does vision guide stair climbing? A developmental study. *Australian Journal of Psychology, 44*, 177–183.

National Center for Health Statistics. *Latest statistics on injuries in the United States.* Available from www.cdc.gov/nchs/.

Plumert, J. M. (1995). Relations between children's overestimation of their physical abilities and accident proneness. *Developmental Psychology, 31*, 866–876.

Plumert, J. M., & Schwebel, D. C. (1997). Social and temperamental influences on children's overestimation of their physical abilities: Links to accident proneness. *Journal of Experimental Child Psychology, 67*, 317–337.

Pulkkinen, L. (1995). Behavioral precursors to accidents and resulting physical impairment. *Child Development, 66*, 1660–1679.

Rivara, F. P., & Aitken, M. (1998). Prevention of injuries to children and adolescents. *Advances in Pediatrics, 45*, 37–72.

Schwebel, D. C., & Plumert, J. M. (1999). Longitudinal and concurrent relations between temperament, ability estimation, and injury proneness. *Child Development, 70*, 700–712.

JODIE M. PLUMERT

Activities of Daily Living

Activities of daily living (ADLs) are the everyday tasks that are necessary for maintaining optimal independent living and functioning. The ability to perform ADLs is an important contributor to both a person's level of function and his or her quality of life. ADLs encompass a wide variety of daily tasks, particularly activities that involve personal care, as well as activities that promote independent community living. Tasks that characterize ADLs include, but are not limited to, the following: toileting, hygiene, bathing, grooming, dressing, eating, homemaking, cleaning, shopping, personal health care, family care, work activities, managing finances, and using transportation. The ability or inability to perform specific ADLs is often used as an assessment criterion when determining whether an individual qualifies for special services or programs (e.g., interventions such as assisted living, hospice, or respite care).

Related Entry: Quality of Life

JENNIFER E. LEE-HOWARD

Acupuncture

Acupuncture is a Chinese medical technique that emphasizes mind–body holism, harmony with the environment, and restoration of balance. Ancient Chinese medical theories postulate that *qi* or "life energy" flows throughout a system of bodily channels called meridians (*Jing-luo*). When *qi* is blocked, dysfunctions occur. In order to unblock *qi*, fine acupuncture needles are inserted into specific locations under the human skin.

As a form of complementary and alternative medicine, acupuncture's wide practice in the U.S. mainstream was fostered by publicity since the normalization of Sino-American relations in the 1970s. In 1994, an estimated, 3,000 physicians and osteopaths and another 7,000 nonphysicians practiced acupuncture for a wide range of illnesses. Since 1995, the U.S. Food and Drug Administration has regarded acupuncture needles as medical devices not requiring "investigational" labeling. Acupuncture needles can be used with heat, water, electric current, or manual manipulation.

According to a National Institute of Health consensus statement in 1997, randomized clinical trials or double-blind experiments have shown promising results of acupuncture's efficacy in treating adult postoperative and chemotherapy nausea, vomiting, pregnancy-related nausea, and postoperative dental pain. The statement also summarized clinical findings and anecdotal studies suggesting acupuncture is an effective component of a comprehensive treatment for substance abuse and asthma. Many other reports have cited acupuncture's effectiveness in relaxation, stress reduction, analgesia, and treatment of other organic, musculoskeletal, and psychosomatic symptoms as well. However, the scientific community has often been skeptical about these reports, and has called for robust evidence to show acupuncture's efficacy in those areas.

Some acupuncture critics cite placebo and psychological factors as reasons for alleged positive outcomes, and claim that users are collectively deluded. Others attempt to explain acupuncture with neurobiological theories. Many in the Western biomedical community call for more randomized clinical trials to objectively demonstrate acupuncture's *efficacy*. In contrast, sympathetic acupuncture users and advocates support claims of acupuncture's *effectiveness* with largely anecdotal studies of varied scientific quality. They challenge total reliance on randomized clinical trials and the use of placebos for studying the outcomes of acupuncture. Instead, they call for high-quality anecdotal reports to document these results.

Despite such debates, there is a consensus regarding the need for single-use, disposable needles, adequate regulation of training, and acupuncture licensure in different U.S. jurisdictions and other parts of the world. Adverse effects of acupuncture are possible if practitioners are inexperienced, if other, concurrent treatments adversely interact with acupuncture, or if acupuncture veils pain symptoms that are indicative of a serious illness. Possible side effects include drowsiness, malaise, slight discomfort, pain, sweating, and numbness. National and U.S. state boards have regulated the process of training and certifying nonphysician acupuncturists. The World Health Organization has also encouraged and established safety guidelines for acupuncture treatments and training of acupuncturists for improving the world's health status.

BIBLIOGRAPHY

Kaptchuk, T. J. (2000). *The web that has no weaver: Understanding Chinese medicine* (rev. ed.). Chicago: Contemporary.

Klein, L. J., & Trachtenberg, A. I. (Comp.). (1997, October). Acupuncture: January 1970 through October 1997. *Current bibliographies in medicine*, 97–6. Bethesda, MD: National Library of Medicine. Retrieved July 11, 2003 from http://www.nlm.nih.gov/pubs/cbm/acupuncture.html

National Institutes of Health. (1997, November). *Acupuncture: NIH Consensus Statement, 15*(5), 1–34.

World Health Organization/Department of Essential Drugs and Medicines Policy. (1999). *Guidelines on Basic Training and Safety in Acupuncture* (WHO/EDM/TRM/99.1). Geneva: Author.

DOMINICUS W. SO

Acute Illness

Acute illnesses are those physical or mental conditions that are clearly time limited in course. Acute illnesses generally have a clear starting point and a clear ending point. They include common, less severe conditions (e.g., acute upper respiratory infections) as well as less common or more severe conditions (e.g., acute appendicitis). What is initially believed to be an acute illness can later become chronic or can take on a chronic form, as, for example, when an acute upper respiratory infection gives rise to a chronic respiratory infection. From a population perspective, acute illnesses cause less death and disability than do chronic conditions.

ALAN J. CHRISTENSEN

Addiction

Addiction (also called substance dependence) is a chronic, often progressive disease that occurs when a person consumes psychoactive substances to the point that he or she develops a number of physical and psychological symptoms and suffers negative social consequences. The four primary symptoms are craving, which is a strong urge to use the substance; loss of control, which is indicated by one's inability to discontinue substance use in the face of negative consequences; physical dependence, indicated by withdrawal symptoms such as nausea, sweating, shakiness, and anxiety when the substance intake is discontinued after a period of heavy use; and tolerance, which occurs when one needs to ingest increasing amounts of the substance to feel its effects or when one no longer feels the same effects from the consuming the same amount of the substance. It is difficult to estimate the prevalence of substance dependence, but one large-scale study estimates the lifetime prevalence of alcohol dependence and alcohol abuse, a less severe form of problem drinking, at 13.6 percent for the United States.

Substance dependence has a multifactorial etiology, which is not yet fully understood. However, it is clear that there are biological and environmental factors that interact. The primary biological cause of substance dependence is genetics. Evidence shows that addiction tends to run in families, and children of addicted parents have a greater chance of becoming substance dependent in adulthood than children from nonaddicted families. However, because not all children of substance-dependent parents have problems with drugs, other factors must influence one's risk for substance dependence. Environmental variables, such as the influence of friends, stress levels, and access to drugs, may influence the development of the disease.

The course of substance dependence is progressive and can even result in fatal consequences. It is characterized by either continuous or episodic use, with recovery and relapse to use a common pattern. The psychological, emotional, and physical changes that arise are often cumulative and may progress to premature death through overdose; from physical complications involving the brain, liver, heart, and other organs; and by contributing to suicide, accidents, motor vehicle crashes, and other traumatic events.

At this time, although there is no cure for substance dependence, there are effective treatments. Psychotherapy can reduce use of drugs, and there are a number of Food and Drug Administration-approved medications for the treatment of dependence on certain substances. For example, methadone and L-α-acetylmethadol are commonly used for the treatment of dependence on certain pain medications. Benzodiazepines, including Valium and Librium, are used to treat withdrawal symptoms in the first few days of sobriety. Finally, there is some evidence for the efficacy of a new drug, naltrexone, in the reduction of craving for drugs of abuse.

There is a growing body of literature to support the notion that certain behaviors can be addictive, such as gambling and Internet usage. Persons who develop a craving and loss of control (psychological addiction) over their gambling or Internet usage may experience the same physiological brain changes as those addicted to drugs. Psychotherapies are being developed to treat these types of addictions.

Related Entries: Alcoholics Anonymous, Alcoholism, Smoking Prevention

SARA L. DOLAN

Aging

DEMOGRAPHICS OF AGING

Older adults represent a large and growing segment of the population, both in the United States and worldwide. Recent population demographic estimates suggest that by the year 2030, 20 percent of the U.S. population will be 65 years old and older. Adults aged 85 years and older are the fastest growing segment of the population. These demographic shifts are due to many factors, including improved health care, greater longevity, and declining birth rates in industrialized countries. The projected population increase is substantial and will likely have a large impact on the health care system. In particular, there is expected to be growing demand for specialized clinicians and appropriately adapted interventions to provide health services for older adults. As psychologists have responded to these demographic trends, recent years have seen a growing research interest in

understanding behavioral changes that occur with age and how behavior affects the health and well-being of older adults.

PSYCHOLOGICAL CHANGES WITH AGE

Studies have found some areas of psychological change with age, whereas other dimensions demonstrate stability. Changes encompass positive aspects of development as well as declines in some areas of functioning. The slowing that occurs with greater age on all cognitive tasks where speed is required is a well-established finding. Fluid intelligence, which is usually measured by tasks that involve a timed component, shows clear evidence of change with developmental aging. Inferential reasoning (e.g., as measured by questions that ask what comes next in a series) is an aspect of fluid intelligence. However, crystallized intelligence, which includes intellectual capacities such as general fund of information and vocabulary, shows relatively little change as a result of the aging process. With the accumulation of experience, older adults have a considerable store of knowledge, especially in their individual areas of expertise, informed by a lifetime of work and family experiences.

Changes in memory with age have received much study. In particular, working memory has been found to decline with age. Working memory is the limited-capacity resource through which information must be processed before being registered in long-term memory. Although there are clearly increasing numbers of older adults suffering from dementia with each decade of advanced age, the practical impact of normal memory changes is less clear. Research suggests that differences between younger and older adults in memory performance are not large when the material is meaningful and relevant to the older adult and the older adult is motivated to learn. For those working with older adults in a clinical context, reduced capacity in working memory and speed of processing implies slower pace of speaking, with greater repetition of material, to ensure effective communication.

Personality and emotion have also been studied among older adults. Studies on personality development in adulthood and later life have found stability on the major personality dimensions introversion/extroversion, neuroticism, openness to experience, dependability, and agreeableness. Some researchers have argued that the accumulation of experience leads to more complex and less extreme emotional experiences in later life. Whereas previously, older adults were thought to become disengaged from others, more recent research has found that adults increasingly focus on emotionally close relationships as they get older, whereas casual relationships become less important.

Some psychological phenomena associated with age appear to put older adults at risk for maladaptive health behaviors. In particular, an inadequate sense of control over life circumstances (and low self-efficacy to effect change) may significantly interfere with health. Unfortunately, sense of control may decrease with age, especially if there are losses that limit the choices available to an older person (e.g., bereavement, illness, disability). Nursing home environments may encourage dependency and inhibit a healthy sense of self-efficacy. Older adults with a reduced sense of control may be less motivated to alter health-damaging behaviors, even after diagnosis with a chronic illness. For example, research has found that older adults who perceive less control over their disease engage in fewer healthy behaviors during the course of a serious and painful medical illness such as coronary heart disease even after suffering through coronary artery bypass graft surgery. Low self-efficacy has also been linked to depression and poor memory performance.

COHORT EFFECTS

In the study of aging, it is important to distinguish which psychological changes are due to the effects of getting older and which are due to generational effects or "cohort effects." Researchers have found that many of the differences between older and younger adults that society has attributed to the aging process are actually due to cohort effects. Cohort differences are explained by membership in a birth-year-defined group that is socialized into certain abilities, beliefs, attitudes, and personality dimensions that remain stable as it ages and that distinguish the cohort from those born earlier and later. For example, in the United States, later-born cohorts have more years of formal education than groups of individuals born earlier in the century. In terms of thinking skills, later-born cohorts tend to be superior in reasoning ability and spatial orientation, but some earlier-born cohorts (people who are now older) are superior in arithmetic ability and verbal fluency. These examples illustrate that the absence of developmental change (change due to aging) does not necessarily mean that today's older people are comparable to today's younger people. In addition, some differences between cohorts favor the older groups.

THE SOCIAL CONTEXT OF OLDER ADULTS

Professionals and lay people who work with older adults should be familiar with social aspects of aging. For example, research on older adults' social adaptation indicates that as adults age, they become more selective about the people with whom they interact. Thus, older adults tend to have small and close social networks. In the United States, the social context of older adults includes specific environments (community living, age-segregated housing, age-segregated social and recreational centers, the aging services network, long-term care facilities, etc.). Many localities also have community-based networks of aging services that are very useful for older adults. These services may include specialized transportation and medical and

counseling centers. Developing familiarity with these aspects of older adults' lives is very useful in providing optimal physical and mental health services.

On an individual level, many older adults face changes to familiar social resources and established social roles. For example, bereavement related to the loss of a spouse is very common. Likewise, the functional and emotional challenges to family members posed by dementing illnesses such as Alzheimer's disease are specific to later life. Caregiving for a loved one who is chronically ill, loss of long term friends to illness and death, retirement, and relocation to new living environments are additional significant life events that may pose particular challenges for older adults.

Other social contextual aspects include a number of specific laws and regulations that may significantly affect the lives of older adults. For example, Medicare, a national health insurance plan for older adults, has many regulations that may influence when and where older adults may receive clinical services. On both the state and the national level, legislation outlines the proper handling of identified elder abuse and conservatorship regulations for older adults who have become unable to take care of themselves or their finances.

DISORDERS ASSOCIATED WITH AGING

Estimates of the prevalence of adults over the age of 56 years with at least one chronic illness range from 50 to 86 percent. As a result, older adults are more likely than younger adults to have ongoing health problems and to take multiple medications in order to manage these illnesses. Individuals who work with the elderly should have substantial familiarity with chronic illnesses and their psychological impact, control of chronic pain, adherence to medical treatment, rehabilitation strategies, and assessment of behavioral signs of medication reactions. Fortunately, professionals skilled in health psychology are able to make substantial contributions to care for older adults with physical and psychological disorders.

A frequent component of working with chronically ill or disabled elders is addressing comorbid depression. Contrary to some stereotypes, physically healthy older adults in the general population do not suffer from depression at higher rates than younger adults. However, prevalence studies of depression among chronically ill elderly have found rates of depression up to 59 percent. Conversely, depression may actually increase vulnerability to physical health problems, and has been associated with increased disability, poorer rehabilitation, and greater risk of mortality. If depression is identified in a clinical setting, immediate treatment should be sought—depression in older people is highly treatable with either psychotherapy or medication, or a combination of these two interventions.

Problems in thinking and memory increase as people age, and among an increasing proportion of older adults, cognitive dysfunction and dementing conditions may interfere with community living and other activities. Prevalence of dementia, including Alzheimer's disease and vascular dementia, increases with age. Depression and dementia may present similar symptoms, such as problems in memory for recent events. As a result, older adults in clinical settings who are suspected of dementia should be screened for depression. To detect dementia, clinicians who work with older adults may routinely use a brief screening instrument such as the Folstein Mini Mental State Exam. If there is evidence of both depression and thinking problems during a brief assessment, a more extensive neuropsychological evaluation should be considered. If a dementing condition is present, early identification will allow medical treatment and long-term planning. For spouses and children providing care to an older adult suffering from dementia, psychological interventions such as support groups may help to reduce stress.

Chronic pain is a widespread problem among older adults. It is estimated that 25 to 50 percent of community-dwelling elderly suffer from chronic pain. Chronic pain is associated with rheumatoid arthritis and poor healing following injury. Although medication is frequently indicated to help relieve pain in older adults, there are medical risks associated with these medications that are amplified for the elderly. For this reason, it is fortunate that there are cognitive and behavioral treatments that are effective in helping older clients manage pain. These include methods such as distracting oneself from the pain, reinterpreting pain sensations, using pleasant imagery, using calming self-statements, and increasing daily pleasurable activities. Employment of these psychological techniques, all of which serve to increase a sense of control over the chronic pain symptoms, may help clients reduce dependence on medication to manage pain.

Insomnia is a frequent problem for older adults, and has adverse consequences for physical and emotional health. Between 12 and 25 percent of adults over the age of 65 years complain of chronic sleep difficulties. In sleep-maintenance insomnia, the individual may awaken in the middle of the night and be unable to get back to sleep. He or she may then take naps during the day to make up the sleep time lost, resulting in greater and greater time spent in bed to receive a normal amount of sleep. A combination of educational and behavioral interventions has been recommended in treating this type of insomnia in older adults. This combined intervention has been useful in reducing insomnia without use of drugs.

GENERAL TREATMENT ISSUES WITH OLDER ADULTS

Research has demonstrated that older adults benefit from psychological interventions to address a range of problems. However, older adults are faced with social, medical, and time constraints that can influence participation in formal psychotherapy. Therefore, several adaptations have been recommended. Treatments should be flexible with regard to structure, location, and presentation. Slower pace and simplified content of information presented to older adults may help to maximize effective communication. These adaptations help to ensure that older adults get the maximum benefit from the interventions offered them.

The complexity of older adults' health issues should be reflected in care models. For example, it is common for interventions to incorporate case management strategies, such as connecting patients with additional resources (e.g., medical referrals, housing and nutritional services, transportation, and respite care for patients who are also caregivers). In medical settings, one effective treatment strategy is an interdisciplinary team approach in which health professionals with different specialties in the same clinic (such as medicine, psychology, physical therapy, and social work) provide coordinated care for older patients. Because problems of older adults may be complex, clinicians should assess a broad range of outcomes including activity engagement, disability level, life satisfaction, and psychosocial functioning.

HEALTH BEHAVIORS

Health behaviors include actions that affect an individual's physical and psychological functioning. Smoking, drinking alcohol, and using caffeine are all health behaviors that may negatively affect health, particularly among physiologically vulnerable populations such as older adults. Other important health behaviors include screening for cancer, medication adherence, and safer sexual behavior. Poor medication adherence may also be a problem for older adults, who often are taking a complex regimen involving multiple medications. Cognitive changes such as worsening memory skills may also interfere with medication adherence. With regard to sexual activity and HIV risk, a sizable proportion of HIV infections have been diagnosed among older adults. Contrary to popular stereotype, many older adults are sexually active. Those individuals who report risk factors for HIV infection should be offered sexual health and safety interventions.

Lifestyle factors such as exercise, diet, and stress management have a significant impact on healthy aging. Moderate exercise has the potential to prevent obesity; improve physical strength, circulation, and cardiac health; and reduce depression. For these reasons, recent research has focused on the development of psychoeducational interventions to increase healthy behaviors (e.g., physical activity/exercise interventions) among older adults. These interventions focus on increasing knowledge about healthy behaviors, getting regular exercise, and maintaining adequate social support. Among older adults at risk for alcohol problems, brief interventions about the health dangers of excessive drinking have been effective in reducing consumption.

USE OF HEALTH SERVICES

Although older adults generally use health services more than younger adults, there are also age-associated factors that may negatively affect treatment access. Practical barriers to health service use among the elderly include the cost of services, the distance to sites providing services, and the availability of transportation. Access to mental health services has unique challenges. In addition to practical barriers, stigma associated with mental health problems is common in the current cohort of older adults and may negatively affect treatment seeking. Potential misunderstandings around psychological services may be reduced by clear explanation of the nature and the usefulness of the interventions offered. In addition, sociocultural factors also influence access to care. Ethnic minority elderly often have problems with access and engagement in the health system due to language difficulties, cost, and cultural beliefs about mental illness and caregiving. For example, many Asian cultures attach greater stigma to mental health problems than is typical of White American culture and have more reluctance to share problems with non-family members. Providers need to be sensitive to these barriers and their impact on access to health care.

Primary care settings are key settings for psychoeducational interventions focused on reducing unhealthy behaviors such as alcohol abuse and smoking among both healthy and medically ill older adult populations. Primary care health care providers also have the opportunity to identify depressed older adults who might benefit from mental health services and who are at risk for functional decline and/or suicide. Physical illness and depression are major risk factors for suicide among older adults. Studies have shown that older males have the highest rate of completed suicide in the United States. Therefore, suicide assessment is an important aspect of older adult mental health screening in primary care.

In addition to providing substantial benefit to individuals, connecting older adults to effective psychological services is desirable to reduce strain on the health care system. Older adults with mental illnesses such as depression or psychologically treatable medical disorders such as insomnia and chronic pain use primary care health services more frequently than healthy older adults. Older adults with dual diagnoses of substance abuse and other mental health problems are particularly heavy users of health services. Appropriate psychological intervention with these individuals therefore has the potential to reduce need for medical services. To assist individuals with the challenges associated with aging and to maximize the effective functioning of health care systems, providers of psychological interventions clearly have much to offer in health care settings serving older adults.

Related Entries: Dementia, Neuropsychology

BIBLIOGRAPHY

Bortz, W. M., & Bortz, S. S. (1996). Prevention, nutrition, and exercise in the aged. In L. L. Carstensen, B. A. Edelstein, & L. Dornbrand (Eds.). *The practical handbook of clinical gerontology* (pp. 36–53). Thousand Oaks, CA: Sage.

Carstensen, L. L. (1992). Social and emotional patterns in adulthood: Support for socioemotional selectivity theory. *Psychology and Aging, 7,* 331–338.

Costa, P. T., & McCrae, R. R. (1988). Personality in adulthood: A six-year longitudinal study of self-reports and spouse ratings on the NEO personality inventory. *Journal of Personality and Social Psychology, 54,* 853–863.

Folstein, M. F. (1975). Mini-Mental State: A practical method for grading the cognitive state of patients for the clinician. *Journal of Psychiatric Research, 12,* 189–198.

Gott, M. C. (1999). Sexual risk-taking in later life. *Reviews in Clinical Gerontology, 9,* 139–150.

Gump, B. B., Matthews, K. A., Scheier, M. F., Schulz, R., Bridges, M. W., & Magovern, G. J. (2001). Illness representations according to age and effects on health behaviors following coronary artery bypass surgery. *Journal of the American Geriatrics Society, 49,* 284–289.

Knight, B. G., & Satre, D. D. (1999). Cognitive behavioral psychotherapy with older adults. *Clinical Psychology: Science and Practice, 6,* 188–203. Knight,

Melding, P. S. (1995). How do older people respond to chronic pain? A review of coping with pain and illness in elders. *Pain Reviews, 2,* 65–75.

Salthouse, T. A. (1991). *Theoretical perspectives on cognitive aging.* Hillsdale, NJ: Erlbaum.

Satre, D. D. (2002). Psychosocial interventions for distressed caregivers. In S. Andrieu & J. P. Aquino (Eds.) *Research and practice in Alzheimer's Disease: Family and professional carers* (pp. 120–124). Paris: Serdi.

Schaie, K. W. (1996). Intellectual development in adulthood. In J. E. Birren & K. W. Schaie (Eds.), *Handbook of the psychology of aging* (4th ed., pp. 266–286). San Diego: Academic.

Van der Bij, A. K., Laurant, M. G. H., & Wensing, M. (2002). Effectiveness of physical activity interventions for older adults. *American Journal of Preventive Medicine, 22,* 120–133.

DEREK D. SATRE
BETH L. COOK

Alcoholics Anonymous

Alcoholics Anonymous (AA) is a fellowship of people who come together to support each other in sobriety. The only requirement for membership is a desire to abstain completely from alcohol. Membership and attendance at meetings is voluntary, and there are no dues or membership fees. It is estimated that approximately 2,000,000 people in over 150 countries are actively involved in AA.

AA was founded in 1935 by a New York stockbroker and an Ohio surgeon who considered themselves "hopeless" alcoholics. They formed AA to help each other stay sober and to help others who suffer from the disease of alcoholism.

The AA program is based on total abstinence from alcohol. Members are encouraged to stay away from one drink, "one day at a time." Support for sobriety is offered through attendance at group meetings where members share their experiences, strength, and hope for recovery. Sobriety is also supported through the tenets of the suggested Twelve Steps to recovery. These Twelve Steps incorporate faith, acceptance of the disease of alcoholism, and acknowledgment of the effects that drinking has had on the lives of self and others.

Anonymity is the foundation of the AA recovery program. It allows the fellowship, a society of peers, to be governed by principles rather than personalities. Anonymity also assures newcomers and other members that their participation will not be disclosed, making it a safe environment to share their experiences.

AA has spawned a number of related programs, such as Narcotics Anonymous (NA) to support the effort to maintain abstinence from cocaine and other narcotics, as well as support groups (Al-Anon and Alateen) for those with family or friends who struggle with addiction. There are also a number of other Twelve Step groups that have been formed to support people's efforts to abstain from behaviors like smoking and overeating.

Because anonymity is a core concept in AA, research done by non-AA members is discouraged, and empirical data on its effectiveness have been difficult to obtain. However, internal publications report an abstinence rate for those who commit to following the program's tenets of approximately 50 percent immediately after entering the program and 25 percent after a number of relapses. Other estimates are closer to 10 percent abstinence for all those who attempt the program.

Related Entries: Addiction, Alcoholism

SARA L. DOLAN

Alcoholism

According to recent national surveys, most noninstitutionalized individuals in the United States who are 12 years of age or older drink beverages containing alcohol. In the year 2000 national survey, more than 60 percent of the respondents said that they drank alcohol in the last year and more than 46 percent said that they used it in the past month. However, "alcoholism" usually refers broadly to the use of alcohol that is associated with problems of various kinds, including health, legal, family, social, employment, or psychological. In the United States (and the rest of the Western world), although widely used, "alcoholism" is not a formally defined term. Instead, the fourth edition of the *Diagnostic and Statistical Manual of Mental Disorders (DSM)*, (American Psychiatric Association, 1994), which is the psychiatric diagnostic system followed most commonly in the United States, defines two "alcohol use disorders": alcohol dependence and alcohol abuse. Most Americans who use alcohol do *not* meet the criteria for either of these disorders; in the United States, estimates of the prevalence of either current (last 12 months) alcohol abuse or alcohol dependence among adults who drink alcohol typically range around 10 percent, with the majority of diagnoses being alcohol abuse.

Alcohol dependence is most analogous to what traditionally has been called "alcoholism." The *DSM* lists seven criteria for alcohol dependence, three or more of which must be met to make the diagnosis. The criteria refer to tolerance to alcohol, evidence of physical dependence on it, and cognitive and behavioral features that accompany the procurement of alcohol and its consumption. There are four criteria for alcohol abuse, and one or more of them must be met to make the diagnosis. The criteria focus on the negative consequences of alcohol use in different areas of life functioning. According to the *DSM*, dependence and abuse are mutually exclusive diagnostic categories, and a diagnosis of dependence preempts assigning a diagnosis of abuse.

TOLERANCE TO AND DEPENDENCE ON ALCOHOL

Regular use of alcohol results in tolerance to it, which means that more alcohol must be consumed to experience an effect once reached with a lesser amount, or that a given dose of alcohol has less of an effect than it did earlier in the individual's drinking history. With chronic, heavy drinking, physical dependence on alcohol may develop. This means that with a decline in the amount of alcohol in the blood or with the complete cessation of drinking, a pattern of physical and psychological symptoms appears that is associated with the passage of time. Alcohol withdrawal can be severe and may be fatal if not managed with established medical treatment protocols. The full train of symptoms that define the alcohol withdrawal syndrome may take 5–7 days to run its course.

ACUTE EFFECTS OF ALCOHOL

"Acute effects" refer to the physical, psychological, and social consequences experienced upon consuming a given amount (dose) of a drug. Alcohol is a drug that has pervasive effects on the body and thus has a variety of acute effects. Generally, alcohol is classified as a depressant drug, based on its action on the central nervous system (brain and spinal cord), and its effects are proportional to the amount of alcohol in the blood. Therefore, as the dose of alcohol consumed increases, its acute effects tend to increase in number and intensity. For example, for the "average" drinker who is not highly tolerant to alcohol, having one or two drinks typically is associated with feelings of warmth, well-being, relaxation, and happiness. Following the consumption of three or four drinks, these same effects become more noticeable, and there often are more exaggerated changes in emotion, judgment (more impaired), and inhibitions (lowered). Consumption of higher amounts of alcohol is associated with evidence of slowed reaction time, impaired muscle coordination, and further impairment in judgment. In the United States, the legal level of intoxication is 0.08 percent in 24 states and the District of Columbia and 0.10 percent in 25 states (one state does not have a "per se" legal level of intoxication). For a reference, if a 160-lb man had about five drinks (each containing the equivalent of 0.6 ounces of pure alcohol) in a 2-hr period, he would be legally intoxicated according to the 0.10 percent criterion; it would take slightly less than four drinks to be legally intoxicated according to the 0.08 percent criterion. If an individual who weighs 160 lb drinks about 25 ounces of hard liquor (e.g., gin, scotch, or vodka) that is 40 percent alcohol in 1 hr, there is a 50 percent chance that death will result.

In discussing alcohol's acute effects, it is essential to comment on driving skills. The problem of driving while under the influence of alcohol has been a problem for many years, but it has been widely recognized in the United States as a major public health problem only in the last two decades. A strong case can be made that alcohol can be a causal factor in motor vehicle accidents; this becomes a major public health problem because fatal automobile crashes are the most common nonnatural cause of death among individuals aged 1–24 years. Although the rate of association of alcohol with fatal motor vehicle crashes has declined over the last two decades, it still approaches 40 percent. Indeed, in an individual who weighs 160 lb, driving skills may begin to show impairment after the consumption of about two drinks over a 2-hr period.

CHRONIC EFFECTS OF ALCOHOL

The effects of chronic, heavy drinking are the major reasons for the public's concern about the alcohol use disorders. It is well known that a relatively long history of heavy alcohol use is associated with often severe impairment in psychological and social functioning. Furthermore, because alcohol's effects on the body are so pervasive, chronic heavy alcohol use may have major damaging effects on a variety of body systems. Before

describing these effects, it is important to say that "chronic, heavy use" of alcohol is difficult to define. However, it can be said with confidence that the chronic effects on the body that will be described here often take years to develop, and that people vary considerably in their susceptibility to alcohol's chronic effects.

Chronic heavy alcohol use can affect the following body systems. *Central nervous system* functioning (reasoning, memory, judgment) may show specific and general impairments, which may be reversible, if there is no structural damage to the brain, with years of abstinence for alcohol. The *liver* is directly affected by alcohol because it is the primary site where the body metabolizes this drug. Damage to the liver may be reversible ("fatty" liver and alcohol hepatitis) or may be irreversible (cirrhosis, or scarring of the liver). The *cardiovascular system* may be affected, as there is increased mortality from coronary heart disease and increased risk for heart disease in general. Alcohol cardiomyopathy (alcohol-induced wasting of the heart muscle) also is a possible consequence. Alcohol can affect the *endocrine system* by altering the secretion of hormones in different hormone hierarchies or "axes." These include the hypothalamic–pituitary–adrenal axis and the hypothalamic–pituitary–gonadal axis. The latter axis influences sexual behavior and reproductive function. The *immune system* may be compromised by alcohol, so that the individual has increased susceptibility to various diseases. Alcohol may affect the *gastrointestinal system* and lead to the development of gastritis and increase the risk of contracting pancreatitis. Finally, alcohol is associated with higher risk of contracting various *cancers*, including oral cavity, tongue, pharynx, larynx, esophagus, stomach, liver, pancreas, colon, and rectum cancer.

Before leaving this section, it is important to cite a chronic alcohol effect that does not focus on a specific body system or the drinker. Rather, the focus is alcohol's effect on the fetus if the mother drinks during pregnancy. Because *fetal alcohol syndrome* has its own entry in this book, it is not discussed further here. However, it is essential to say that research has not established a "safe" level of alcohol consumption during pregnancy. As a result, the only guaranteed way to avoid fetal alcohol effects is not to use alcohol at all during pregnancy.

MODERATE DRINKING AND HEALTH

Despite the preponderance of evidence that drinking heavily over a long term can result in severe and sometimes fatal health consequences, there are data showing that a long-term pattern of "moderate" drinking is associated with better health. Here, "better health" has been defined as cardiovascular health, and "moderate" means one to three drinks a day. The association of moderate alcohol use and health has been researched fairly intensely for more than 10 years, and previously there was skepticism that the association is real. However, more recent, better-designed studies have provided support for the moderate alcohol use–cardiovascular health association. Alcohol appears to increase the production of high-density lipoproteins as well as alter other biological indicators of risk of cardiovascular disease.

ETIOLOGY OF ALCOHOL USE DISORDERS

Given the major cost of alcohol use disorders in both human and financial terms (over $166 billion in the United States in 1995), it is not surprising that numerous theories about their development (etiology) have been proposed. Traditionally, these theories have reflected only one set of factors, either biological, psychological, or social/environmental. The research that these theories helped to generate typically could provide some support for a given theory, but also left many questions unanswered.

More recent theories of the etiology of the alcohol use disorders have been consistent with other areas of health-related behaviors in taking a "multivariate approach." That is, research suggests that "single-factor" theories of the etiology of the alcohol use disorders are inadequate. Instead, biological, psychological, and social/environmental variables must be considered simultaneously if a theory that can explain the etiology of the alcohol use disorders is to be generated. For example, there is strong evidence that there is a genetic predisposition to some manifestations of alcohol use disorders, especially more severe types in males. However, whether such an inherited predisposition ("what" is inherited is a matter of considerable controversy and research) is expressed later as alcohol use disorder may depend on the existence of specific personality characteristics in the individual and the social environment's reaction to them. An overarching factor is the attitudes and norms regarding alcohol consumption in the society or subculture that the individual lives in.

TREATMENT OF ALCOHOL USE DISORDERS

Treatment of behavioral problems like the alcohol use disorders refers to systematic activities that are designed to change some pattern of behavior(s) of individuals or their families. In discussing the alcohol use disorders, the primary target of change is drinking behavior. However, because heavy alcohol use over a long period of time may affect an individual or his or her family in a number of areas of life functioning, treatment may target these other areas as well, depending on the individual's needs and goals.

If there is recognition that there is need for modification of an individual's drinking pattern, whether it comes from external pressures (such as an employer) or from within the individual

himself or herself, then change may occur in a variety of ways. For example, a considerable number of people modify their patterns of alcohol use on their own, without the use of any kind of treatment. This has been referred to as "spontaneous remission." In addition, people may attend peer self-help groups to help them change; probably Alcoholics Anonymous (AA) is the peer self-help group that is most widely known. Because there is a separate entry on AA in this book, it is not discussed further here. However, it does warrant mention that millions of people in the United States (and around the world) attend AA groups. It also is important to mention that, in recent years, alternative (to AA) self-help groups have become available to assist people in modifying their alcohol (or other drug) use. Some examples of these alternative groups include Women for Sobriety, Self-Management and Recovery Training (SMART), and Secular Organizations for Sobriety (SOS).

Before proceeding in this section, it should be mentioned that "modifying alcohol use" as a goal can mean stopping altogether (abstinence) or reducing alcohol use but not committing to abstinence. In the United States, by far the goal that is supported most in the professional and self-help (one exception is the self-help group called Moderation Management) treatment communities is abstinence. However, it is becoming more widely accepted in the United States that moderation to levels of use not associated with problems is a feasible goal for individuals who desire it, whose alcohol use disorder is not severe (e.g., abuse rather than dependence), and whose social life is relatively stable (employed, in a stable relationship, has a permanent residence). There also is support for a moderation treatment goal from those who follow a "harm reduction" model, which focuses on using treatment to reduce the negative consequences of alcohol use rather than targeting alcohol consumption. Typically, however, a focus of reducing negative consequences of use also means addressing amount of use because they are directly related. That is, as one increases, the other tends to as well.

The first consideration in professional treatment provision is whether the individual needs detoxification from alcohol, which is necessary if physical dependence is present. Established protocols are available to manage detoxification medically, and they may be delivered in some cases in the outpatient setting. If further professional treatment is sought, then the individual has a wide variety of options, depending on factors such as severity of his or her alcohol problem, presence of another psychiatric problem, such as depression or anxiety, desired level of treatment intensity or of treatment type, and financial resources. For example, treatment activities may occur in inpatient, outpatient, hospital, or residential settings, and may vary in their duration. By far the most common treatment setting is outpatient, as inpatient or residential settings typically are reserved for treatment of more severe problems. Treatment components may be "psychosocial" or pharmacological. Due to the number of areas of life functioning that may be affected in individuals with alcohol use disorder, psychosocial treatment components cover a wide variety of activities, and may be delivered in individual, couples/family, or group modalities. Professional treatment programs may also recommend self-help group attendance to complement their treatment services. Another option is the use of "brief interventions" for individuals whose problems are less severe. Pharmacological treatments involve the use of medication to help the individual abstain from alcohol use. The drug that has been used for the longest time in the treatment of alcohol use disorders and that is available in the United States is disulfiram (trade name Antabuse). The chemical action of disulfiram results in an increase in the blood level of acetaldehyde after alcohol consumption. The consequence of the heightened acetaldehyde depends on how much alcohol is drunk. For people on therapeutic doses of disulfiram, one or two drinks will produce flushing, tachycardia (excessively rapid heartbeat, usually a pulse rate of over 100 per min), tachypnea (excessively rapid respiration), sensations of warmth, heart palpitations, and shortness of breath. These effects usually last about 30 min and are not life threatening. However, if larger quantities of alcohol are consumed, the reaction may include intense palpitations, dyspnea (difficult or labored breathing), nausea, vomiting, and headache, all of which may last more than 90 min. The notion is that individuals will avoid alcohol to avoid these unpleasant consequences of drinking when a therapeutic level of disulfiram is in the blood.

In 1995, the Federal Drug Administration also approved the use of naltrexone in the treatment of alcohol use disorder. A considerable amount of research is in progress in the development or evaluation of additional medications. It is essential to note that medications are typically used in conjunction with psychosocial treatment components.

EFFECTIVENESS OF ALCOHOL TREATMENT

An important question concerns whether alcohol treatment is effective. Overall, research has not identified a psychosocial treatment that generally is effective for everyone, but it has shown that staying involved in treatment is associated with better outcomes than is dropping out. It also appears that there are several treatment approaches that have shown promising results in controlled clinical research, and these include motivational enhancement therapies. It also appears that "matching" selection of treatment setting or content to the individual's characteristics, such as marital or employment status or severity of co-occurring psychiatric problems, can be beneficial. Unfortunately, due to the principles of AA, particularly anonymity, it has proved extremely difficult to conduct controlled clinical trials of its effectiveness, so that no firm answers to that question are available.

Except for disulfiram, which has been available since the early 1950s, there are relatively little data on the effectiveness of pharmacotherapies. The findings on disulfiram's effectiveness have been inconsistent, perhaps in part because the relevant studies have not always been done well. However, it does seem that disulfiram's effectiveness can be enhanced considerably if part of the treatment consists of supervised administration of the required dose, say with the cooperation of the individual's spouse. Naltrexone, the other approved pharmacotherapy for alcohol use disorders in the United States, has shown modest effectiveness. Research on this drug continues. Finally, the use of medications designed for treating depression and anxiety also has shown promise in the treatment of alcohol use disorders. This is especially the case in individuals who present with symptoms of anxiety or depression along with alcohol problems.

RELAPSE

A major problem for clinicians who treat alcohol use disorders (or other addictions) is relapse, which broadly refers to the reappearance of a problem following some period of its (voluntary) resolution. Although relapse is an aspect of alcohol treatment that clinicians have struggled with for many years, it has been only recently (last 20 years) that systematic relapse prevention methods have been developed and applied on a wide scale in clinical settings. The problem of relapse is common; if a return to alcohol use after a period of abstinence of more than 1 year following treatment is defined as relapse (other definitions are possible), then it can be expected that about 80 percent of individuals will relapse. Theories of relapse have been generated, and most relapse prevention methods involve application of principles of learning theory and cognitive psychology. In fact, relapse prevention typically is part of alcohol treatment and is not a stand-alone intervention because it concerns sustaining any changes made in treatment over the longterm.

SUMMARY AND CONCLUSIONS

This entry has provided an extremely brief overview of alcohol use, its acute and chronic effects, alcohol use disorders, and their treatment. Alcohol is a drug that is used by most American adults, and for a small but significant percentage of them, such use is associated with problems for the individual, for his or her interpersonal relationships, or in larger social contexts such as employment or the legal system. However, in the last 25 years, research has considerably improved our knowledge about what causes alcohol use disorders and about ways to modify alcohol use and related behaviors so that individuals who choose to change their drinking patterns have effective ways of doing so available to them.

Related Entries: Addiction, Alcoholics Anonymous, Fetal Alcohol Syndrome

BIBLIOGRAPHY

American Psychiatric Association. (1994). *Diagnostic and statistical manual of mental disorders* (4th ed.). Washington, DC: Author.

Brands, B., Sproule, B., & Marshman, J. (1998). *Drugs and drug abuse* (3rd ed.). Toronto: Addiction Research Foundation.

Connors, G., Maisto, S., & Donovan, D. (1996). Conceptualizations of relapse: A summary of psychological and psychobiological models. *Addiction, 91*(Supplement), S5–S14.

Litten, R., & Allen, J. (1999). Medications for alcohol, illicit drug, and tobacco dependence: An update of research findings. *Journal of Substance Abuse Treatment, 16*, 105–112.

Maisto, S., Galizio, M., & Connors, G. (1999). *Drug use and abuse* (3rd ed.). Fort Worth, TX: Harcourt.

Marlatt, G. A., & Gordon, J. (1985). *Relapse prevention.* New York: Guilford.

National Institute on Alcohol Abuse and Alcoholism (2000). *Tenth special report to the U.S. Congress on alcohol and health.* Washington, DC: U.S. Department of Health and Human Services.

Rimm, E. (2000). Moderate alcohol intake and lower risk of coronary heart disease: Meta-analysis of effects on lipids and homeostatic factors. *Journal of the American Medical Association, 319*, 1523–1528.

Schneider Institute for Health Policy. (2001). *Substance abuse: The nation's number one health problem.* Waltham, MA: Heller Graduate School, Brandeis University.

Schukit, M. (1996). Recent developments in the pharmacotherapy of alcohol dependence. *Journal of Consulting and Clinical Psychology, 64*, 669–676.

Sobell, L., Sobell, M., Toneatto, T., & Leo, G. (1993). What triggers the resolution of alcohol problems without treatment? *Alcoholism: Clinical and Experimental Research, 17*, 217–224.

STEPHEN A. MAISTO

Allostatic Load

Allostasis refers to physiological changes designed to maintain homeostasis (i.e., the body's internal balance necessary for living). Allostatic systems adapt to environmental and psychosocial challenges with a broad range of bodily changes. The autonomic nervous system and endocrine system are typically involved, resulting in release of stress hormones (e.g., cortisol and adrenaline) and alteration of organ system activity (e.g., increased cardiovascular or immune system activation). Allostatic load pertains to the frequent fluctuations or chronic elevations of stress hormones and activity of organ systems across months or years that result from the failure of allostatic systems to shutoff. Chronic stress, repeated exposure to the same stress, allostatic systems not recovering after stress, and/or allostatic systems failing to counterregulate each other can evoke allostatic load. This load, then, can create bodily wear and tear, fostering

such sequelae as high blood pressure, persistent psychological distress, impaired memory function, adult-onset diabetes, and an acceleration of the aging process.

Related Entries: Cortisol, Endocrine System, Fight-or-Flight Response, Homeostasis, Immune System, Psychoneuroimmunology, Stressful Life Events

RANDALL S. JORGENSEN

American Psychological Association

The American Psychological Association (APA), headquartered in Washington, D.C., is the largest scientific and professional organization representing psychology in the United States, and is the world's largest association of psychologists. APA's membership includes more than 155,000 researchers, educators, clinicians, consultants, and students. Through its divisions in 53 subfields of psychology and affiliations with 60 state, territorial, and Canadian provincial associations, APA works to advance psychology a science, a profession, and a means of promoting human welfare.

Division 38, the division of Health Psychology of APA, was founded in 1978 to advance the contributions of psychology as a discipline to the understanding of health and illness. The Division was established to facilitate collaboration among psychologists and other health science and health care professionals interested in the behavioral aspects of physical and mental health. Division 38 supports the educational, scientific, and professional contributions of psychology to understanding the etiology, promotion, and maintenance of health; the prevention, diagnosis, treatment, and rehabilitation of physical and mental illness; the study of psychological, social, emotional, and behavioral factors in physical and mental illness; the improvement of the health care system; and the formulation of health policy.

The many areas of research and service delivery illustrate the richness of the field of health psychology. Reports by the Surgeon General's Office indicate that the leading causes of mortality in the United States have substantial behavioral components. These reports recommend that behavioral risk factors (e.g., drug and alcohol abuse, high-risk sexual behavior, smoking, diet, sedentary lifestyle, and stress) be the main focus of efforts in the area of health promotion and disease prevention. Division 38 is committed to asserting proactive advocacy for health psychology in research, practice, education, policy, and the public interest.

Health psychologists are conducting applied research on the development of healthy habits as well as the prevention or reduction of unhealthy behaviors. The impact of behavior on health as well as the influence of health and disease states on psychological factors are being explored. Psychosocial and physiological linkages in areas such as psychoneuroimmunology, cardiovascular disorders, and other chronic diseases are being defined. Ground-breaking work is being conducted in psychopharmacology as the neurological bases of behavior are being mapped.

This is a period of rapid change in health care delivery. Division 38, as part of the American Psychological Association, is working to build on established liaisons with legislators, researchers, and psychologist practitioners to ensure access to health psychologists as a part of quality health care and to become the recognized leader for health psychology, nationally and internationally.

Related Entries: American Psychosomatic Society, National Institutes of Health, Society of Behavioral Medicine

BARBARA A. KEETON

American Psychosomatic Society

The essential mission of the American Psychosomatic Society is to promote and advance the scientific understanding of the interrelationships among biological, psychological, social, and behavioral factors in human health and disease and the integration of the fields of science that separately examine each, and to foster the application of this understanding in education and improved health care.

PROFESSIONAL INTERESTS AND ACTIVITIES OF MEMBERS

The Society is a forum for the discussion of data from any discipline that may enhance our understanding of the complex relationships that have led to a new appreciation of how mind and body interact in the maintenance of health and the causation of disease. This includes basic studies of brain, behavior, and bodily disease relationships; basic and applied psychopharmacological studies; demographic, transcultural, and epidemiologic studies of the risk factors and natural history of disease; clinical studies of the risk factors and natural history of disease; and clinical studies derived from insights that emerge from the laboratory, all of which address the biopsychosocial and behavioral interactions that influence adaptive processes. Another important area for investigation is the multiplicity of factors that enter into the physician–patient relationship and their

potential significance. In summary, the Society is dedicated to psychosomatic research in various disciplines and the application of this new knowledge in the education of professionals and the care of patients.

HISTORY OF THE AMERICAN PSYCHOSOMATIC SOCIETY

Inception

The American Psychosomatic Society grew from a desire among several academicians, practitioners, and foundations to link developments in psychology and psychiatry to internal medicine, physiology, and other disciplines.

In 1936, Kate Macy Ladd, the philanthropist and founder of the Josiah Macy, Jr., Foundation, directed the Foundation to provide support for the fledgling field of psychosomatic investigation. The initial project, undertaken by the New York Academy of Medicine's joint committee on Religion and Medicine, was to assemble a bibliography of the "psychosomatic" medical literature, 1910–1933, together with publications examining the relationship of religion to health. The task was undertaken by Dr. Helen Flanders Dunbar, director of the joint committee. The first volume was published in 1935 as *Emotions and Bodily Changes*. Two further revisions brought the literature survey up to 1945.

Journal

With further financial assistance from the Macy Foundation, the National Research Council's Division of Anthropology and Psychology, Committee on Problems of Neurotic Behavior, began publication of the journal *Psychosomatic Medicine*, in an effort to encourage collaboration among the medical specialties, psychology, and the social sciences. The journal's first issue appeared in 1939 under the editorship of Dr. Dunbar. Thereafter, research in the field expanded rapidly, but there was no permanent forum other than the journal for the exchange of data and ideas. Accordingly, in December 1942, the advisory board of the journal voted to establish the American Society for Research in Psychosomatic Problems.

Subsequent editors of the Journal were Drs. Carol Binger, Morton F. Reiser, Herbert Weiner, Donald Oken, Joel Dimsdale, and David Sheps.

Society Founders

Gathered together at the organizing meeting were representatives of the several centers where psychosomatic research was under way, including Drs. George Daniels, George Draper, and Helen Dunbar, Columbia-Presbyterian; Drs. Stanley Cobb,

Hallowell Davis, Alexander Forbes, Walter B. Cannon, and Eric Lindeman, Harvard; Dr. Harold G. Wolff and his group at Cornell-New York Hospital; and the group from Temple University in Philadelphia under Dr. Edward Weiss, who, with Dr. O. Spurgeon English, delineated the field in 1943 in their textbook *Psychosomatic Medicine.*

Meetings

The first meeting of the council was held on May 11, 1943, at the Hotel Statler in Detroit under the honorary presidency of Dr. Adolf Meyer. At the meeting, Dr. Tracy Putnam was elected the first president of the Society; Dr. Winfred Overholser, president-elect; and Dr. Edwin G. Zabriski, secretary-treasurer. The first scientific meeting was held jointly with the annual meeting of the American Psychiatric Association in 1943, and a meeting was held in conjunction with the AMA meeting in New York in 1944. That year, the Society was incorporated under the laws of New York State and control of the journal was shifted from the National Research Council to the Society. Beginning in 1946, the annual meetings were held independently of other organizations. In 1948, the Society's name was changed to The American Psychosomatic Society.

Related Entries: American Psychological Association, Society of Behavioral Medicine

AMERICAN PSYCHOSOMATIC SOCIETY

Anderson, Norman B.

Norman B. Anderson, PhD, became the chief executive officer of the American Psychological Association (APA) on January 1, 2003, with the retirement of Raymond D. Fowler. Trained as a practitioner and a scientist, Dr. Anderson has dedicated much of his professional life to studying the relationships between health and behavior and between health and race.

Prior to joining APA, Dr. Anderson was professor of health and social behavior at the Harvard University School of Public Health, where his interests centered on health disparities and mass media approaches to public health. He was the former associate director of the National Institutes of Health (NIH) and the first director of the NIH Office of Behavioral and Social Sciences Research (OBSSR). At NIH, he was charged with facilitating behavioral and social sciences research across all of the then 24 Institutes and Centers of the National Institutes of Health. Under his purview was behavioral and social research in such areas as cancer, heart disease, mental health, diabetes, aging, and oral health.

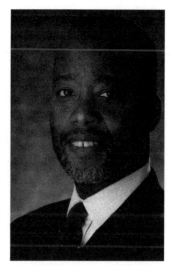

Anderson, Norman B.

Appointed by then NIH Director Dr. Harold Varmus in 1995, Dr. Anderson worked closely with the scientific community nationally to quickly establish the Office's long-term goals and to develop strategies for achieving them, resulting in the first OBSSR Strategic Plan. Under his leadership, the Office organized funding initiatives totaling over $90 million in 5 years.

The success of the Office prompted Congress to triple its budget, enabling it to have greater latitude in developing NIH-wide funding activities. Before leaving NIH, Dr. Anderson initiated several activities to help guide future funding directions in the social and behavioral sciences, including reports on social and cultural dimensions of health and religion and on spirituality and health, and commissioned the National Academy of Science's report on the future of behavioral and social sciences research (*New Horizons in Health Science: An Integrative Approach*).

Prior to going to NIH, Dr. Anderson was associate professor in the Department of Psychiatry and Psychology: Social and Health Sciences at Duke University. There he studied the role of stress in the development of hypertension in African Americans and directed the NIH-funded Exploratory Center for Research on Health Promotion in Older Minorities. He has received several awards for his research, including the 1986 New Investigator Award from the Society of Behavioral Medicine, the 1991 Award for Outstanding Contributions to Health Psychology from the American Psychological Association, and a Research Scientist Development Award from the National Institute of Mental Health.

Dr. Anderson is a Fellow of the American Psychological Association, the American Psychological Society, the Society of Behavioral Medicine, and the Academy of Behavioral Medicine Research and is a past-president of the Society of Behavioral

Medicine. Currently, he is president of the Board of the Directors for Steven Spielberg's STARBRIGHT Foundation of Los Angeles. He is also on the Advisory Committee for Public Issues for the Advertising Council and the Advisory Council for the National Institute on Drug Abuse at NIH and chairs the National Academy of Science Panel on the Future of Research on Race, Ethnicity, and Health in Later Life.

NORMAN B. ANDERSON

Angina Pectoris

Angina pectoris is a medical condition that refers to chest discomfort due to cardiovascular disease. Angina is a symptom of coronary heart disease, where blood flow through the arterial system is inadequate to meet the metabolic demands of the heart. Consequently, the heart muscle receives an insufficient amount of oxygen. Over six million Americans suffer from angina. Risk factors for this condition include cigarette smoking, obesity, high blood cholesterol and hypertension.

Angina feels like a pressing pain, usually in the chest, but it can also occur in the shoulders, arms, neck, and jaw. Stable angina, predictable chest pain occurring from physical exertion or emotional stress, is the most common type. Unstable angina refers to chest pain that can occur both during exertion and at rest. Variant angina is a specific type of unstable angina, perhaps resulting from a coronary artery spasm. Angina may be treatable with lifestyle changes, pharmacological agents, or surgery.

Related Entries: Cardiovascular System, Coronary Heart Disease

BIBLIOGRAPHY

American Heart Association. Available at www.americanheart.org
National Heart, Lung, and Blood Institute. Available at www.nhlbi.nih.gov.
Virmani, R., Atkinson, J. B. & Fenoglio, J. J. (1991). *Cardiovascular pathology.* Philadelphia: Saunders.

ANGELA J. GRIPPO

Anticipatory Nausea and Vomiting

Anticipatory nausea and vomiting (ANV) is the experience of nausea and vomiting (emesis) without the administration of a known emetic agent (i.e., a substance known to provoke such symptoms). This phenomenon most frequently occurs among cancer patients receiving chemotherapy (but also can occur with radiation therapy) and can be explained with a classical conditioning paradigm. Chemotherapy medications (unconditioned stimulus) typically produce nausea and vomiting (unconditioned response). Neutral stimuli such as a cancer clinic and health care providers (conditioned stimuli) are paired with the unconditioned stimulus. After repeated pairing, the conditioned stimulus alone (e.g., oncology nurse) produces a conditioned response of nausea and vomiting.

The majority of chemotherapy patients experience some nausea and approximately 40 percent report one episode of vomiting. ANV develops in 25–30 percent of patients by the fourth chemotherapy treatment cycle and occurs in both adults and children. Several risk factors for ANV have been identified. Women and younger individuals are more likely to experience chemotherapy-related nausea and vomiting and are therefore at a greater risk for developing ANV. Some drugs (e.g., cisplatin) have a higher emetic risk than others. Among patients who do experience posttreatment nausea and vomiting, the risk for developing ANV increases with symptom severity, frequency, and duration. Therefore, as patients complete more chemotherapy cycles, the risk for ANV increases. Other predisposing factors include lengthier infusions, greater sensitivity of the autonomic nervous system, susceptibility to motion sickness, expectations of posttreatment nausea, and emotional distress. Individuals who consume more than five alcoholic beverages a day or have a history of alcohol consumption report less ANV.

ANV can affect patients' compliance with the cancer treatment regimen and may result in the limiting of chemotherapy doses by physicians. Therefore, preventing and treating ANV are critical. Among cancer patients, nausea and vomiting may be the consequence of central nervous system metastases, adhesions, or decreased bowel motility due to medications or inactivity. As nausea and vomiting can result from a wide array of causes, a thorough assessment including history, physical exam, and laboratory tests is necessary. Pharmacologic antiemetic agents are generally not effective in treating ANV and ANV is unlikely to improve spontaneously. Therefore, prophylactic administration of antiemetics to control emesis is advised to reduce the likelihood of developing ANV. This treatment regimen would likely include a 5-HT$_3$ (serotonin) antagonist, a steroid, and a benzodiazepine. Selection of the pharmacologic agents is based on the emetogenic potential of the treatment regimen, potential sideeffects, and patient characteristics.

Should ANV develop, several behavioral strategies including relaxation training, hypnosis, systematic desensitization, and distraction have been shown to reduce symptoms. Progressive muscle relaxation involves systematic tensing and relaxing of muscles. Hypnosis involves learning to induce a state of relaxation incompatible with nausea and vomiting during which time a clinician may introduce suggestions of well-being. Systematic desensitization involves graded exposure to stimuli that elicit nausea and vomiting while simultaneously employing relaxation techniques. In this way, the conditioned stimuli are now associated with the relaxation response. Finally, cognitive distraction techniques, such as playing video games during chemotherapy, focus a patient's attention away from nausea and vomiting and therefore reduce symptoms.

Related Entries: Cancer: Biopsychosocial Aspects, Classical Conditioning

BIBLIOGRAPHY

Abrahm, J. L. (2000). Antiemetic therapy. In R. Hoffman, E. J. Benz, S. J. Shattil, B. Furie, H. J. Cohen, L. E. Silberstein, & P. McGlave (Eds.), *Hematology: Basic principles and practice* (pp. 1529–1531). New York: Churchill Livingstone.

Anthony, L. B. (2003). Nausea and vomiting. In R. E. Rakel & E. T. Bope (Eds.), *Conn's current therapy* (pp. 5–11). Philadelphia: Elsevier.

Burish, T. G., & Carey, M. P. (1986). Conditioned aversive responses in cancer chemotherapy patients: Theoretical and developmental analysis. *Journal of Consulting and Clinical Psychology, 54,* 593–600.

Matteson, S., Roscoe, J., Hickok, J., & Morrow, G. R. (2002). The role of behavioral conditioning in the development of nausea. *American Journal of Obstetrics and Gynecology, 185,* S239–9S243.

Morrow, G. R., Roscoe, J. A., & Hickok, J. T. (1998). Nausea and vomiting. In J. C. Holland (Ed.), *Psycho-oncology* (pp. 476–484). New York: Oxford.

NAN E. ROTHROCK

Arthritis

Arthritis literally means "joint inflammation." The terms arthritis and rheumatic disease are usually used interchangeably. These chronic diseases and conditions, of which there are over 100 different types, involve pain and stiffness in or around the joints. Arthritis symptoms can affect nearly every activity of daily living. Arthritis is a leading cause of disability in the United States and a major public health concern. Costs from arthritis-related medical care and lost wages due to disability amount to billions of dollars each year.

Approximately one of every six Americans has arthritis. This number is expected to increase as the population ages. Although age is a risk factor for some types of arthritis, people of all ages, including young children, can be diagnosed with arthritis. Women are more likely to have arthritis than are men; reasons for this gender difference are not well understood.

The most common type of arthritis among adults is osteoarthritis. It is characterized by degeneration of joint cartilage, often in the knee, hip, back, or fingers. Although osteoarthritis is common among the elderly, it is not an inevitable part of aging. Half of all people in their 70s and 80s have osteoarthritis.

The type of arthritis that has been studied most by health psychologists is rheumatoid arthritis. It is a systemic disease that involves inflammation of the joint lining. The cause is unknown but thought to be autoimmune. Although it most often affects the hands and feet, it may also involve organ systems. Its course is unpredictable, with symptoms that tend to flare and remit. Juvenile rheumatoid arthritis is the most common type of arthritis among children. As with other types of arthritis, juvenile rheumatoid arthritis may be mild or severe. Some of the other types of arthritis are fibromyalgia, systemic lupus erythematosus, gout, ankylosing spondylitis, bursitis, and Lyme disease.

EFFECTS OF ARTHRITIS ON FUNCTIONING

For some people arthritis may be barely noticeable, whereas for others it may erode their quality of life profoundly. Symptoms of arthritis can limit ability to perform basic motions such as bending, walking, grasping, and lifting. Consequently, arthritis may interfere with functioning at work, home, and school; participation in social, leisure, and recreational activities; and personal care activities such as bathing, dressing, and eating. People with arthritis are less likely to be employed than those without arthritis. If they are employed, then on average they earn less.

Disruption in important life activities and roles, reductions in independence, and uncertainly about the future may result in a variety of negative psychological and social consequences. Nonetheless, research also shows that as with other chronic diseases, most people with arthritis report finding positive meaning or benefit in their experience, such as improved relationships, increased empathy, and spiritual growth.

Despite the numerous potential stressors caused by arthritis, most people with arthritis do not experience clinical depression. However, compared to people who do not have a chronic disease, people with arthritis are more likely to experience depression. Depression, which can worsen the pain and disability associated with arthritis, must be recognized and treated. Unfortunately, depression in individuals with arthritis may be difficult to assess. Some types of arthritis manifest symptoms (e.g., fatigue, sleep problems) that may overlap with symptoms of depression, so the diagnosis of one might mask the other. Complicating the clinical picture, medications such as corticosteroids that are used to treat some types of arthritis may induce depressive symptoms.

COPING AND CONTROL

Research on the different ways that individuals cope with arthritis has shown that some coping strategies may be more effective than others. Coping strategies such as actively seeking information and trying to view one's situation in a more positive light have been associated with better psychological functioning. In contrast, wishful thinking and self-blame have been associated with poorer psychological functioning. Experimental research suggests that disclosing emotions through writing or talking also may be an effective coping tool.

The extent to which patients believe that they have control over their symptoms appears to have a significant impact on their adjustment to arthritis. Numerous studies have found that self-efficacy, or patients' confidence in their ability to cope with arthritis, predicts decreased pain, disability, and psychological distress. In contrast, perceived helplessness has been associated with increased pain, disability, and psychological distress. Among people with rheumatoid arthritis, perceived helplessness has also been linked to early mortality.

INTERPERSONAL FACTORS

Family and friends play an important role in patients' adjustment to arthritis. Numerous studies have linked social support to well-being among patients with arthritis. The type and amount of social support that is most helpful may vary during different points in the disease course. Some studies of people with arthritis have also revealed a potential downside of social support. For example, arthritis patients report being negatively affected by critical or well-intended but unwelcome comments from others. Among women with rheumatoid arthritis, interpersonal stress (i.e., conflicts with others) has been shown to affect immune system activity.

Research also has addressed the impact of arthritis on patients' spouses. Partners of individuals with arthritis report feeling distressed and helpless in response to seeing their partner in pain. They also may experience a reduction in pleasurable activities previously shared with their partner, as well as fear and uncertainly regarding the future. Partners may feel reluctant to burden the person with arthritis with their own needs. At the same time, patients may fear burdening their partners. It is important that patients and their partners develop strong support networks to bolster their own mental health as well as the health of their relationship.

BIOMEDICAL INTERVENTIONS

The medications used to treat most types of arthritis control symptoms, and in some cases slow disease progression, but do not cure it. As with other chronic diseases, the effectiveness of treatment is related to the degree to which patients adhere to the prescribed medical regimen. Depending on the type of arthritis, treatment may include nonsteroidal anti-inflammatory drugs, analgesics, biologic response modifiers, corticosteroids, or disease-modifying antirheumatic drugs. Assistive devices such as splints or braces also may be used. Surgical intervention such as joint replacement may benefit some patients. Physical and occupational therapy are also important components of a comprehensive treatment plan.

PSYCHOLOGICAL INTERVENTIONS

In some cases arthritis can be prevented. For example, maintaining a healthy body weight and taking precautions to avoid occupational or sports-related injuries can contribute to the prevention of osteoarthritis, and learning how to reduce the risk of tick bites can contribute to the prevention of arthritis related to Lyme disease. However, these types of primary prevention strategies are not applicable to most cases of arthritis. Therefore health psychologists interested in arthritis have focused their efforts on helping individuals who are living with the disease.

Cognitive–behavioral interventions have been shown to improve physical and psychological functioning among people with arthritis. The cognitive component of these interventions focuses on goals such as understanding pain, gaining an increased sense of control, and developing coping skills. The behavioral component focuses on mastering techniques such as relaxation, goal setting, and activity pacing. Cognitive–behavioral therapy, whether administered in a group or individual setting, also involves home practice.

Randomized, controlled studies of arthritis patients who participate in cognitive–behavioral interventions generally result in positive effects following treatment. Although findings vary across studies, these effects include reductions in pain, disability, psychological distress, and health care utilization. Unfortunately these gains are not always sustained through long-term follow-up assessments. Incorporating strategies for preventing relapse and coping with setbacks into cognitive–behavioral interventions may help patients maintain treatment gains over time.

Cognitive–behavioral techniques are part of the Arthritis Self-Help Course, a widely used educational program sponsored by the Arthritis Foundation. The Arthritis Self-Help Course uses a structured group format and is led by trained volunteers. The course provides disease-related information and teaches self-management skills such as relaxation and problem solving. Research indicates that benefits of the course include increased knowledge, self-care behaviors, and self-efficacy and decreased pain, depression, and number of physician visits.

The Arthritis Foundation also offers an exercise program called People with Arthritis Can Exercise, as well as programs focused specifically on aquatic exercise and walking. In the past arthritis patients were discouraged from exercising, but since the 1970s research findings have consistently shown that moderate-intensity exercise is safe for people with arthritis. Not only does regular exercise improve overall health and fitness, but it also has been shown to relieve symptoms such as joint pain and stiffness. Reported benefits of the People with Arthritis Can Exercise program include increased functional ability and self-care behaviors, decreased pain and depression, and increased self-efficacy.

Arthritis can pose a multitude of daily challenges. The symptoms and stressors associated with arthritis can lead to physical, occupational, social, and psychological impairment. Although most people with arthritis find ways to manage or cope with their disease, depression is not an uncommon response. Arthritis also has an impact on family members, who may play important roles in patients' adaptation to the disease. Interventions such as cognitive–behavioral therapy can positively affect psychological (e.g., self-efficacy, mood) and physical (e.g., pain, disability, health care utilization) outcomes.

Related Entries: Chronic Illness, Pain, Stressful Life Events

BIBLIOGRAPHY

American College of Rheumatology. Available at http://www.rheumatology.org

Arthritis Foundation. Available at http://www.arthritis.org

DeVellis, B. M., Revenson, T. A., & Blalock, S. J. (1997). Rheumatic disease and women's health. In S. J. Gallant, G. P. Keita, & R. Royak-Schaler (Eds.), *Health care for women: Psychological, social, and behavioral influences* (pp. 333–347). Washington, DC: American Psychological Association.

Fries, J. F. (1999). *Arthritis: A take care of yourself health guide for understanding your arthritis* (5th ed.) Cambridge, MA: Perseus.

Keefe, F. J., Smith, S. J., Buffington, A. L. H., Gibson, J., Studts, J. L., & Caldwell, D. S. (2002). Recent advances and future directions in the biopsychosocial assessment and treatment of arthritis. *Journal of Consulting and Clinical Psychology, 70,* 640–655.

Lorig, J. F. (1999). *Arthritis: A take care of yourself health guide for understanding your arthritis* (5th ed.). Cambridge, MA: Perseus.

National Institute of Arthritis and Musculoskeletal and Skin Diseases. Available at http://www.niams.nih.gov

SHARON DANOFF-BURG

Asthma

Asthma is a reversible obstructive respiratory disorder that produces impaired breathing, which may be accompanied by other respiratory symptoms, such as wheezing, coughing, and tightness in the chest. Asthma afflicts many millions of individuals around the world. In the United States, about 17 million people suffer from asthma, and morbidity and mortality rates for the disease are rising. Over 5,000 Americans die of the disorder each year, with mortality rates being higher among the elderly than younger individuals, among Blacks than Whites, and among people from lower than higher social classes; these rates are increasing particularly rapidly among children. Although asthma may emerge at any age, most people who develop asthma have their first episode in early childhood.

The respiratory symptoms in asthma episodes result mainly from temporarily decreased diameters of the airways to the lungs. Asthma is a psychophysiological disorder, and its development and episodes are best understood from a biopsychosocial perspective, involving the interplay of biological, psychological, and social factors in the person's life.

BIOMEDICAL FACTORS IN ASTHMA

During an acute episode of asthma, the airways narrow because they become inflamed, the smooth muscles of the bronchial tubes develop spasms, and the walls of the tubes constrict and produce mucus, which tends to plug the airways. These events result in part from arousal of the autonomic nervous system at the start of and during an episode in reaction to triggers, or precipitating conditions. There are three types of triggers: (1) environmental conditions, such as temperature and allergic substances; (2) physical activities, such as strenuous exercise; and (3) personal factors, such as current infections and emotions or moods. Because emotions arouse the autonomic nervous system, they may produce the initial symptoms in an attack or aggravate existing symptoms as a vicious circle develops.

When an asthma episode is triggered, a chain reaction occurs in the body. For example, when the trigger is an allergen, such as pollen, the immune system reacts with an overproduction of antibodies, which bind to mast cells found throughout the body that break down and release the chemical histamine, a highly reactant form of acetylcholine. In individuals who do not have asthma, histamine has relatively little effect on respiratory function, but in people with asthma, it causes the lining of the bronchial tubes to constrict markedly and secrete excess mucus. Autonomic nervous system activity appears to be mediated by activity in the vagus nerve, which arises from the medulla and connects to and regulates the heart, lungs, and airways by carrying efferent signals via the autonomic nervous system.

Although researchers do not fully understand the etiology of asthma as a disorder, it is known that environmental and genetic factors can play substantial roles in asthma development. An important environmental factor in asthma is respiratory infection. Past respiratory infection has been associated with the development of asthma, and current respiratory infections are major triggers of asthma episodes. There is also considerable evidence that heredity affects the development of asthma. Studies of twins have found much higher concordance rates among identical (monozygotic) than fraternal (dizygotic) twins for the presence of asthma. Family history studies have shown that the relatives of children with asthma have higher asthma prevalence rates than the relatives of children without asthma. Some evidence from research with twins indicates that heredity affects not only the presence of asthma, but also the severity of children's asthma condition and the impact of respiratory infection and physical exertion as triggers of asthma episodes.

Medical treatment for asthma involves advising patients to avoid known triggers and to use medication of two types. First, anti-inflammatory medicines, such as cromolyn and corticosteroids, prevent asthma attacks from starting because they keep the airways open by reducing inflammation. Second, bronchodilators relax airway muscles, thereby stopping asthma episodes once they begin.

PSYCHOSOCIAL FACTORS IN ASTHMA

Research findings and theory have implicated emotional and cognitive processes in the expression of asthma symptoms. Three lines of evidence have linked emotion and asthma. First, survey and interview data indicate that stress and emotion can trigger asthma episodes. Second, studies comparing individuals with and without asthma have found that those with asthma express more emotion when stressed and report greater amounts or degrees of negative emotion in their everyday lives. Because emotions arouse the autonomic nervous system, they may produce the initial symptoms in an asthma episode or aggravate existing symptoms. Despite some inconsistencies in the evidence, most research results support a role of emotions in triggering or exacerbating asthma symptoms.

The role of emotion in asthma suggests that cognitive processes may affect asthma episodes, and these processes have been implicated in both research and theory. Studies have shown, for example, that asthma symptoms can be induced in people who do and do not have asthma via suggestion under placebo conditions, such as inhaling an inactive substance. Thus, individuals with and without asthma who were told that the substance they would inhale would make breathing difficult showed far greater airway resistance while inhaling than people not told the substance would impair breathing. Studies demonstrating that emotion and suggestion can serve as triggers of attacks clearly implicate learning processes in the expression of asthma symptoms. This may occur through respondent (classical) and operant conditioning: respondent conditioning may establish nonallergic conditioned stimuli through association with allergic conditions; operant conditioning enables the reaction to persist via reinforcement processes (e.g., a parents attention when his or her child shows respiratory symptoms).

Another important issue is nonadherence to the medical regimen. Many people with asthma do not avoid triggers or take anti-inflammatory medicines as recommended, making attacks much more likely.

PSYCHOLOGICAL TREATMENTS FOR ASTHMA

Because of the role that conditioning processes appear to play in asthma, efforts to apply psychological approaches have focused on using behavioral methods, which apply principles of operant and respondent conditioning, as adjunctive therapies to medical treatment for the disorder. These methods include relaxation, biofeedback, and systematic desensitization.

Relaxation techniques are muscular and nonmuscular activities that enable people to reduce their levels of emotional and autonomic arousal, which aggravate asthma episodes. The most commonly used muscular relaxation technique is called *progressive muscle relaxation*, which involves having people sit or lie quietly and focus their attention on specific muscle groups while alternately tightening and relaxing these muscles. Nonmuscular relaxation techniques use "mental" or cognitive activities, such as *meditation*, in which individuals spend quiet periods focusing their awareness on a single thing, such as their breathing or a phrase, and *autogenic training*, which involves quietly focusing attention on internal sensations, such as how light or warm parts of the body feel. People generally need much practice to master relaxation techniques. Many studies have examined the value of relaxation methods in treating asthma and found them to be useful, especially if emotions play a strong role in triggering or worsening episodes. The evidence is stronger and clearer for muscular than nonmuscular methods.

Biofeedback is a technique by which individuals can acquire voluntary control over a physiological function by monitoring its status. The feedback the person receives for physiological functioning may be conveyed with high or low numbers on a gauge, pitches or degrees of loudness of tones from an audio speaker, or degrees of brightness of a light. Biofeedback for asthma may be applied in two ways. *Respiratory biofeedback* uses an apparatus to provide feedback regarding airflow to help people learn to control their respiration, particularly by enlarging airway diameters. *Nonrespiratory biofeedback* provides feedback on muscular activity, such as of the forehead, without directly affecting respiration. Studies on the value of respiratory and nonrespiratory biofeedback in treating asthma have produced inconclusive results, with effects being more positive for child than adult asthmatics. This age difference may reflect a generalized ability of children to use biofeedback more effectively than adults.

Systematic desensitization is a respondent conditioning technique for reducing fear or anxiety, replacing it with a calm response by pairing feared objects or situations with pleasant or neutral events, usually with the person employing relaxation techniques. The feared stimuli are presented in a graded series, or stimulus hierarchy. In asthma treatment, for example, the person might imagine or listen to increasingly more fearful descriptions of asthma attacks and various sensations and thoughts. Research has shown that systematic desensitization is a useful technique in treating asthma in children and adults and is more effective than relaxation alone. These studies have usually found large improvements, sometimes even at long-term follow-up, in subsequent symptoms.

In summary, biological, psychological, and social factors affect asthma development and episodes. Respiratory biofeedback, relaxation, and systematic desensitization methods can provide effective adjunctive approaches to medical treatment for asthma, but the utility of nonrespiratory biofeedback is less clear. Respiratory biofeedback is the only behavioral method for treating asthma in which success seems to depend on the patient's age, with children seeming to benefit more than adults. The fact that behavioral methods have not always produced consistent and large (clinically meaningful) group-wide improvements in research may be partly because treatment groups included patients who varied widely in the role of emotions in their condition. Other promising treatment approaches that use psychological methods are hypnosis and asthma education programs, which train people with asthma to understand the disorder, use medications correctly and as scheduled, cope better with stress, and apply breathing and relaxation exercises when attacks begin.

Related Entries: Chronic Illness, Coping

BIBLIOGRAPHY

American Lung Association. *Asthma medications* and *Focus: Asthma*. Retrieved (July 23, 2002) from www.lungusa.org

Asthma and Allergy Foundation of America. *Asthma & allergies*. Retrieved (July 23, 2002) from www.aafa.org

Devine, E. C. (1996). Meta-analysis of the effects of psychoeducational care in adults with asthma. *Research in Nursing and Health, 19,* 367–376.

Lehrer, P., Feldman, J., Giardino, N., Song, H.-S., & Schmaling, K. (2002). Psychological aspects of asthma. *Journal of Consulting and Clinical Psychology, 70,* 691–711.

Lehrer, P. M., Isenberg, S., & Hochron, S. M. (1993). Asthma and emotion: A review. Journal of Asthma, 30, 5–21.

Sarafino, E. P. (1997). *Behavioral treatments for asthma: Biofeedback-, respondent-, and relaxation-based approaches.* Lewiston, NY: Mellen.

Sarafino, E. P., & Goehring, P. (2000). Age comparisons in acquiring biofeedback control and success in reducing headache pain. *Annals of Behavioral Medicine, 22,* 10–16.

Wright, R. J., Rodriguez, M., & Cohen, S. (1998). Review of psychosocial stress and asthma: An integrated biopsychosocial approach. *Thorax, 53,* 1066–1074.

EDWARD P. SARAFINO

Atherosclerosis

PSYCHOSOCIAL ASPECTS OF CARDIOVASCULAR DISEASE

Mental or emotional stress has long been considered among the risk factors for heart attack. To begin to understand why, a brief explanation of what causes a heart attack seems in order.

The underlying cause of cardiovascular disease that most often leads to heart attack is atherosclerosis. Atherosclerosis develops as a response to *endothelial dysfunction*, a malfunction of the inside lining of the arteries supplying the heart muscle with blood. As early as the first decade of life, fatty streaks appear in the large arteries of the body. These fatty streaks are composed of intracellular lipid (fat) accumulation just beneath the inside layer of the artery wall. Beginning in the third decade, the fatty streaks change, developing pools of extracellular fat inside the lining of the artery wall. These pools of fat eventually form a fatty core, which becomes fibrous and, in time, may contain calcium deposits. Under the right conditions, this core in the inside surface of the vessel wall ruptures, and when it does, it bleeds, forming a clot, or *thrombus*. If big enough, the thrombus occludes the flow of blood through the artery, starving the part of the heart muscle it feeds of oxygen, resulting in the death of that portion of the heart muscle. This death of heart muscle is a *myocardial infarction*, the lay term for which is *heart attack*.

What causes the endothelial dysfunction in the first place? Certainly age, gender, and genetics play a roll, but equally important are other risk factors that we now know speed its development. These include mental stress, lack of exercise, high blood pressure (hypertension), high blood cholesterol (specifically high levels of low-density lipoprotein, or LDL), a low level of high-density lipoprotein in the blood (HDL), diabetes, smoking, and, the most recent additions to the list, elevated C-reactive protein (a highly sensitive version of an old test to measure inflammation in the blood vessels) and high levels of homocysteine in the blood. The more risk factors, the more likely it is a person will develop atherosclerosis. Of these, mental stress is probably the most difficult to define, qualify, and quantify, but adds power to the other risk factors.

Mental or emotional stress has been known to trigger various heart problems, but the mechanisms are complicated and somewhat elusive, details of which are beyond the scope of this writing. We know that over time, mental stress can result in hypertension, arterial inflammation, elevated cholesterol, elevated homocysteine levels, elevated glucose, and obesity (one of the hormones that is released during stress, cortisol, is an appetite stimulant). Acutely, mental stress causes the blood vessels to narrow and the blood to clot more readily. When the sympathetic nervous system is stimulated, as it is during mental stress, plasma norepinephrine increases, resulting in rapid, but short-lived (i.e., less than 10 min) vasoconstriction and can precipitate ventricular arrhythmias that, under the right circumstances, can cause sudden death. However, mental stress also causes endothelial dysfunction by preventing the vessel wall from relaxing, resulting in decreased blood flow through the arteries lasting nearly 1 hr. Frequent stressful stimuli thereby result in lengthy states of endothelial dysfunction and vasoconstriction. In addition, cortisol, one of the "stress" hormones produced by the adrenal glands, is elevated in the blood after mental stress, resulting in high blood pressure and high blood glucose, effects that last up to hours.

Other psychosocial stressors include social isolation, anger, and hostility (likely among the toxic components of the Type A behavior pattern) and depression, all of which have been implicated in the development of cardiovascular disease. An abbreviated discussion of each follows.

Social Isolation

Several epidemiologic studies and scientific investigations have demonstrated correlations between social isolation and increased cardiovascular morbidity and mortality. Socially isolated individuals may face a poorer prognosis because of reduced availability of, or reluctance to seek, rapid medical assistance or an adverse response to decreased human contact, or it may be that socially isolated people may be less likely to take actions to prevent cardiovascular disease onset or progression.

Anger and Hostility

An episode of anger more than doubles the risk for acute myocardial infarction for 2 hr. Even recalling the anger associated with a particular situation results in cardiac patients' hearts pumping less blood, an effect not found in normal subjects.

Patients who have high levels of hostility do not do as well as those who do not following procedures to open occluded coronary arteries. Indeed, they are nearly three times more likely to experience a reocclusion of the vessel.

Depression

Several studies have linked depression with cardiovascular morbidity and mortality. In people 65 years of age and older, depressive symptoms independently predict the development of heart disease and total mortality. Depressed patients who have suffered acute myocardial infarction are three to five times more likely to die during the first year than patients who are not depressed. Up to half the time, symptoms of depression precede acute myocardial infarction and are present in those undergoing coronary artery bypass graft surgery. Milani and associates (1996) found that 97 percent of depressed patients who had had a myocardial infarction remained depressed at 6 months if they did not participate in a cardiovascular rehabilitation program, yet only 33 percent of the patients in a cardiovascular rehabilitation program remained depressed at 3 months, suggesting social isolation may also be a factor.

Thus, mental stress, in the form of emotional stress, social isolation, anger and hostility, or depression, is a significant factor in those with or at risk for cardiovascular disease. Comprehensive stress management is an integral element in the management of this population and is necessarily a vital component of cardiovascular rehabilitation programs.

Related Entries: Cardiovascular System, Coronary Heart Disease

BIBLIOGRAPHY

Ariyo, A. A., Haan, M., Tangen, C. M., et al. (2000). Depressive symptoms and risks of coronary heart disease and mortality in elderly Americans. *Circulation, 102,* 1773–1779.

Franklin, B. A. (2001). Psychosocial considerations in heart disease. *J HK Coll. Cardiol. 9*(Supplement), 16–22.

Frasure-Smith, N., Lespérence, F., Gravel, G., et al. (2000). Social support, depression, and mortality during the first year after myocardial infarction. *Circulation, 101,* 1919–1924.

Frasure-Smith, N., Lespérence, F., & Talajic, M. (1993). Depression following myocardial infarction: Impact on 6-month survival. *Journal of the American Medical Association, 250,* 1819–1825.

Goodman, M., Quigley, J., Moran, G., et al. (1996). Hostility predicts restenosis after percutaneous transluminal coronary angioplasty. *Mayo Clinic Proceedings, 71,* 729–734.

Ironson, G., Taylor, C. B., Boltwood, M., et al. (1992). Effects of anger on left ventricular ejection fraction in coronary artery disease. *American Journal of Cardiology, 70,* 281–285.

Milani, R. V., Lavie, C. J., et al. (1996). *American Heart Journal, 132,* 726–736.

Mittleman, M. A., Maclure, M., Sherwood, J. B., et al. (1995). Triggering of acute myocardial infarction onset by episodes of anger. *Circulation, 92,* 1720–1725.

Pirraglia, P. A., Peterson, J. C., Williams-Russo, et al. (1999). Depressive symptomatology in coronary artery bypass graft surgery patients. *Journal of Geriatric Psychiatry, 14,* 668–680.

Pistacella, J. C., & Franklin, B. A. (2003). *Take a load off your heart.* New York: Workman.

Spieker, L. D., Hürlimann, D., Ruschitzka, F., et al. (2002). Mental stress induces prolonged endothelial dysfunction via endothelin-A receptors. *Circulation, 105,* 2817–2820.

Wenger, N. K., Froelicher, E. S., Smith, L. K., et al. (1985). *Cardiac rehabilitation. Clinical practice guideline No. 17* (AHCPR Publication No. 96-0672). Rockville, MD: U.S. Department of Health and Human Services, Public Health Service, Agency for Health Care Policy and Research and the National Heart, Lung, and Blood Institute.

PATRICIA LOUNSBURY

Aversion Therapy

Aversion therapy is a classical conditioning paradigm in which an unwanted behavior is paired with an aversive stimulus or the aversive stimulation is made contingent upon the target behavior, thereby establishing a new link that is successful in eliminating the undesirable response. One such paradigm has been utilized in the treatment of alcoholism. A drug which induces nausea (usually emetine or Antabuse) is paired with the consumption of alcohol, thereby utilizing the same physiological system (gastrointestinal) to classically condition abstinence. Aversive techniques have been applied to a variety of behaviors for decades, including obesity, smoking, homosexuality, and self-mutilation. These attempts have met with varying degrees of success in treatment facilities. A major weakness of aversion therapy, however, is that repeated exposure to the original stimulus without the consequent noxious stimulus (often following patient discharge) tends to weaken the classically conditioned response, usually leading to extinction and eventual relapse in behavior.

Related Entries: Alcoholism, Classical Conditioning, Smoking Cessation

JAMES BUNDE

Bb

Bandura, Albert (1925–)

Albert Bandura is David Starr Jordan Professor of Social Sciences in Psychology at Stanford University. He received his bachelor's degree from the University of British Columbia in 1949 and his PhD degree in 1952 from the University of Iowa. After completing his doctorate, Bandura joined the faculty at Stanford University, where he has remained to pursue his career.

Bandura is a proponent of social cognitive theory. This theory emphasizes the power of social modeling in human self-development of change and the capacity of people to serve as agents of their psychosocial functioning. Bandura regards belief in one's efficacy as the foundation of human motivation and action. Whatever other factors may serve as guides and motivators of human behavior, they are rooted in the core belief that one has the power to achieve personal and social changes by one's actions.

Social cognitive theory provides the health field with a core set of determinants, specifies the mechanisms through which they work, and prescribes guidelines on the optimal ways of implementing them. These core determinants include knowledge of health risks and benefits of different health practices; perceived efficacy that one can exercise control over one's health habits; outcome expectations in the form of expected physical, social, and self-evaluative costs and benefits for different health habits; the health goals people set for themselves and the concrete plans and strategies for realizing them; and the perceived facilitators and social impediments to the changes they seek.

Bandura has applied this theory at different levels for health promotion and disease prevention. At the personal level, the theory has guided development of effective self-management systems combining principles of self-regulation

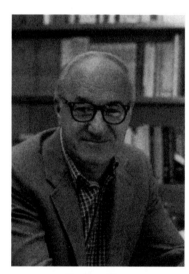

Bandura, Albert

and computer-assisted implementation. This model of self-management is individually tailored to people's needs, and provides continuing personalized guidance and informative feedback that enables participants to exercise control over their own change. It can serve large numbers of people simultaneously under the guidance of a single implementer.

Efforts to get people to adopt healthful practices rely heavily on persuasive communications in health campaigns. Social cognitive theory provides guidelines on how to structure population-based approaches to achieve desired health outcomes. In his approach, Bandura shifts the emphasis in health communications from trying to scare people into health to empowering them with the self-management skills and self-beliefs needed to exercise control over their health habits.

His theory has also promoted global applications to health promotion. This work is founded on three major components.

The theoretical model provides the guiding principles. The translational and implementation model converts theoretical principles into an innovative operational model. The social diffusion model specifies how to promote adoption of psychosocial programs in diverse cultural milieus. This approach promotes personal and social changes in diverse cultural contexts.

Bandura's contributions have earned him election to the American Academy of Arts and Sciences and the Institute of Medicine of the National Academy of Sciences.

BIBLIOGRAPHY

Bandura, A. (1986). *Social foundations of thought and action: A social cognitive theory.* Englewood Cliffs, NJ: Prentice-Hall.
Bandura, A. (1997). *Self-efficacy: The exercise of control.* New York: Freeman.

ALBERT BANDURA

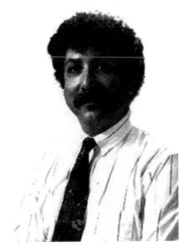

Baum, Andrew

Baum, Andrew (1948–)

Andrew Baum was born on October 3, 1948, in Washington, D.C. He is currently professor of psychiatry and psychology at the University of Pittsburgh and deputy director, University of Pittsburgh Cancer Institute, where he directs the Division of Cancer Control and Population Sciences and the Behavioral Medicine Program. Before coming to the University of Pittsburgh, he was professor of medical psychology, psychiatry, and neuroscience at the Uniformed Services University of the Health Sciences in Bethesda, Maryland, where he also directed the Military Stress Studies Center. He graduated from the University of Pittsburgh (BS) and the State University of New York at Stony Brook (PhD). His early research contributions concerned crowding and the social and psychological effects of architecture. He showed that dormitory designs varying in the nature of shared social spaces affected crowding, stress, and well-being. These studies showed that arrangements of space that affected social experience also affected crowding and marked the beginnings of his interest in chronic stress and its impact on health and well-being. Arguing that the study of severe or extreme stress can provide unique information about how stress operates, he began to study natural and human-caused disasters, naturalistic chronic stressors that could be studied as they unfolded.

Over the next 10 years, he studied a cohort of residents of the Three Mile Island area after the nuclear accident there, documenting a series of physical and psychological sequelae of stress associated with the accident and its aftermath. Persistent distress was more common than is normally observed and a panoply of related effects, including heightened blood pressure and stress hormones, was seen for several years. These studies led to systematic evaluation of the biobehavioral sequelae of chronic stress following more than two dozen natural disasters, toxic hazard exposures, and human-caused accidents, specifying conditions under which stress persisted over long periods of time and leading to conceptual advances that distinguished the effects of natural and human-made disasters. These studies as well as his earlier work identified mechanisms by which stress defeats attempts at adaptation and becomes chronic. This work pioneered the use and integration of biological measures of stress and the naturalistic study of stressors like disasters, motor vehicle accidents, and rescue work following air disasters. Baum also identified and studied the important role of intrusive thoughts in the maintenance of stress and the conditions characterizing vulnerability to posttraumatic stress disorder following stressor exposure.

Since 1990 Dr. Baum's research has focused on psychoneuroimmunology, including studies of stress and natural killer cell activity and biobehavioral aspects of cancer. As a leader in the University of Pittsburgh Cancer Institute, he has been able to achieve unprecedented integration of health psychology research and clinical activity in the Cancer Institute and has conducted or directed studies of successful psychosocial interventions for cancer patients that enhanced life quality and other outcomes and have been integrated into clinical practice. He also studies stress–immune interactions in cancer progression as well as in development and persistence of symptoms such as fatigue, weight loss, and generalized distress.

ANDREW BAUM

Behavioral Medicine

Behavioral medicine is the multidisciplinary field that seeks to integrate knowledge and techniques from both the behavioral and the biomedical sciences. The field is dedicated to the diagnosis, treatment, and prevention of disease and to the promotion and maintenance of physical and mental health. Behavioral medicine emphasizes interdisciplinary integration to a greater degree than some related fields (e.g., health psychology, psychosomatic medicine). Behavioral medicine professionals include both researchers and practitioners from many different professional backgrounds including, for example, medicine, psychology, public health, epidemiology, and nursing. Behavioral medicine research and practice has focused on the prevention and/or treatment of many conditions including cardiovascular disease, diabetes, cancer, HIV/AIDS, renal disease, chronic pain, obesity, and many others. The field of behavioral medicine is rapidly growing and is becoming increasingly seen as critical to an understanding of how to prevent and manage disease and improve health.

Related Entry: Psychosomatic Medicine

ALAN J. CHRISTENSEN

Biofeedback

The term biofeedback has come to be defined as the process of monitoring some biological event with an instrument designed to provide real-time information about that event to the person being monitored. However, clinical biofeedback requires accurate measurement of various physiological processes while providing the client feedback that is sensitive to small changes in his or her physiology. It is also necessary to provide instructions to the client about proper interpretation of the feedback signal and to emphasize why changing the physiology will treat the disorder. Generalization, the ability to transfer what is learned in the clinic to the person's, home, work, and social environments, is also necessary.

Most biofeedback systems are computer interfaced so the feedback signal can be visual and/or auditory. The visual feedback is only limited by the computer graphics, so the signal can be as simple as a line graph where the status of the physiology is depicted by a line that moves across the screen, with the height of the line carrying the information about the level of the physiological event. In some instances, the feedback may be entertaining. This type of feedback is often used with children

and can be, for example, a video game where the game's progress is based on the level of the physiological event. For instance, a maze is presented that must be negotiated, with an object that moves through the maze one step each time the physiological event reaches a predetermined level. In these instances, the feedback is not only informative, but provides an incentive to the client to change his or her physiology in order to "play" such a game.

The physiological parameters used in clinical settings are levels of skeletal muscle activity (tested with electromyograms, EMG), finger skin temperature, sweat gland activity (measured as skin conductance activity, SCA), heart rate, brain wave activity (measured with quantitative electroencephalography, QEEG), and respiration events. Biofeedback of muscle activity is used to reduce sustained muscle activity, which often causes pain; to increase muscle activity after paralysis; and to re-educate specific muscle control after injury to the nervous system such as a stroke. Finger temperature biofeedback is often provided as an indicator of general relaxation because most individuals increase their finger temperature as they go from a stress response to being relaxed. Sweat gland activity is used as a measure of general arousal, especially to emotionally laden cognitive events. Heart rate is also often used as an indication of relaxation because when a person relaxes, the heart rate slows and produces certain rhythms. Brain wave biofeedback is used to treat such disorders as Attention Deficit/Hyperactivity Disorder (ADHD). When brain wave feedback is used it is usually based on findings that indicate the person has a specific brain wave that is related to his or her disorder and the biofeedback system is capable of detecting this activity and letting the person know when it is present. This information allows the person the possibility to either increase or decrease that activity, and thus have less of an unwanted activity and/or more of a wanted activity. Respiration biofeedback is often used as a means to teach correct breathing patterns and as a form of relaxation training.

To present the disorders treated with biofeedback techniques, a table of these disorders was developed (see Table 1). Any listing of disorders should be taken as a guideline as it is always biased by the interpretation and experiences of the author. Some applications appear well established by controlled outcome studies of clinical effectiveness and cost effectiveness, whereas others are based on repeated single-case studies or multiple studies with relatively small sample sizes. Additionally, some applications are based on the clinical literature and the clinical experience of the author. The listing of disorders treated with biofeedback is divided into three categories: A = well established; B = multiple research support; but not enough to firmly substantiate the application; and C = promising but not established at this time.

The following are important when considering the application of clinical biofeedback for an individual: the individual

Table 1. Selected Disorders Treated with Biofeedback Techniques

A	B	C
ADD/ADHD	Dyschezia (anismus)	Dysmenorhea
Anxiety disorders	Esophageal spasm	Hyperfunctional dysphonia
Asthma	Forearm and hand pain from repeated motion syndrome	Mild to moderate depression
Chronic back pain	Hyperhidrosis	Phantom limb pain
Diabetes mellitus	Insomnia	Tinnitus (associated symptoms)
Essential hypertension	Nocturnal enuresis	
Fecal and urinary incontinence	Specific seizure disorders	
Fibromyalgia	TMJ disorder or MFP	
Irritable bowl syndrome	Writers cramps	
Motion sickness		
Muscle rehabilitation		
Raynaud's disease		
Tension and migraine headaches		

Note: ADD/ADHD, Attention Deficit Disorder/Attention Deficit Hyperactivity Disorder; MFP, myogenic facial pain; TMJ, temporomandibular joint.

must be able to tolerate the application of the sensors; be able to understand the instructions regarding the relationship between his or her physiology and the feedback signal; be motivated to change physiology, using the feedback signal to facilitate this process; and, finally, be motivated to practice what has been learned in the clinic in the world outside the clinic. One of the most frequent applications of biofeedback is to use it to facilitate relaxation training. This is referred to as biofeedback-facilitated relaxation training (BFRT).

Example of BFRT Protocol

When using BFRT, it is first necessary to determine whether the client would benefit from such therapy. General relaxation may be helpful in a variety of conditions and it may also be useful as an incompatible response during such procedures as systematic desensitization. BFRT normally takes between 8 and 20 sessions, depending on the acquisition skills and the distress level of the client before and during therapy. After determination of the need for BFRT, the therapist must explain the rationale for biofeedback therapy, outline the basic aspects of the physiological processes that will be trained, and discuss the potential benefits and risks of the training. This author recommends conducting the first BFRT session with frontal EMG feedback while monitoring other modalities such as finger temperature, SCA, and/or heart rate. During the first biofeedback session, facial muscle discrimination training should be demonstrated and the client should be provided time to use his or her relaxation techniques to reduce frontal EMG levels. The therapist should monitor the other modalities during the session

to observe the changes that occur as the client tries to reduce frontal EMG levels. The value of monitoring other modalities is that, for instance, by observing sweat gland activity, it can be determined whether the client is engaging in arousing internal dialogue by noting whether several short duration responses are observed. If so, the therapist could interrupt the session and suggest a change in strategy by the client. During the interruption, the therapist should ask the client what strategy he or she was using and then encourage him or her to select a different strategy, such as diaphragmatic breathing or changes in imagery. The most labile physiological process is usually selected as the target of biofeedback therapy after frontal EMG levels are acceptable.

Another example of an often-used biofeedback procedure is QEEG feedback for treatment of ADHD: First, it is helpful to explain that the QEEG is different than the traditional EEG. The QEEG is the EEG after it has been digitized through the use of an analogue-to-digital converter. This process allows the mathematical determination of the characteristics of specific frequencies. Children with ADHD have been shown to have different patterns of brain waves then non-ADHD children of the same age. The diagnosed children have more electrical activity in the slow frequency range, such as theta (4–8 Hz) and alpha (8–12 Hz), and fewer in the fast frequency range, such as sensorimotor rhythm (SMR; 12–15 Hz) and beta (16–30 Hz). The biofeedback technique trains for a decrease in theta or alpha and an increase in SMR or beta. The treatment protocol requires a QEEG assessment to determine which specific frequencies will need to be trained. Several studies clearly demonstrate that the QEEG patterns change according to the direction of training for some children and that clinical improvements are observed with successful training. The number of sessions necessary is usually 40–60, depending on how quickly the QEEG changes. See Lubar (2003) and Lubar and Lubar (1999) for further information.

SUMMARY

To be effective in the clinical application of biofeedback, one must have the following: a measurable physiological process, feedback about the process provided with enough resolution and speed to allow the individual to obtain volitional control of the physiology, and a change in physiology that alters the physiological processes causing the targeted disorder. In some instances the relationship between the monitored physiological event and the disorder is obvious, such as finger temperature for Raynaud's disease, but for others, such as BFRT for the treatment of asthma and irritable bowel syndrome, the relationship is less obvious. Therefore, the clinician must be aware of the physiology underlying the disorder and the literature that relates to the different biofeedback treatments used to treat it. This information must then be combined with the individual's characteristics such as his or her unique physiological levels and the ability to benefit from the various types of biofeedback techniques available. The clinician must also be skilled in helping the client transfer the control acquired in the clinic to the individual's life situations. Constant advances in computer technology and developments in bioengineering, which provide new sensor technology and signal processing, make the future of clinical biofeedback look very promising.

Related Entries: Nervous System, Operant Conditioning, Pain, Placebo Effect, Psychophysiology, Relaxation Response, Stressful Life Events

BIBLIOGRAPHY

Evans, J. R., & Abarbanel, A. (Eds.). (1999). *Introduction to quantitative EEG and biofeedback*. New York: Academic.

Lubar, J. F. (2003). Neurofeedback for the management of attention-deficit/hyperactivity disorders. In M. S. Schwartz (Ed.), *Biofeedback: A practitioner's guide (3rd ed.).* (pp. 493–522). New York: Guilford.

Lubar, J. F., & Lubar, J. O. (2003). Neurofeedback assessment and treatment for attention deficit/hyperactivity disorders. In J. R. Evans & A. Abarbanel (Eds.), *Introduction to quantitative EEG and neurofeedback* (pp. 103–143). San Diego: Academic.

Kasman, G. S., Cram, J. R., Wolf, S. L., & Barton, L. (1998). *Clinical applications in surface electromyography: Chronic musculosketal pain*. Gaithersberg, MD: Aspen.

Schwartz, M., & Andrasik, F. (Eds.). (2003). *Biofeedback: A practitioners guide*. New York: Guilford.

DOIL D. MONTGOMERY

Biomedical Model

The biomedical model has been the most common model of thinking among medical practitioners for many centuries. The model states that disease is best conceptualized as a malfunction of biological processes. There are three key components to the biomedical model: a reductionistic approach, mind–body dualism, and an emphasis on illness rather than health (Engel, 1977). The reductionistic approach of the biomedical model states that illness is best understood and treated when it can be reduced to the lowest-level somatic process, such as the molecular and cellular levels. It uses a fractional-analytic approach to the human body, deconstructing illness into somatic components (e.g., a virus or a bacterium) and excludes any influence of psychological or social factors. The second component of the biomedical model is mind–body dualism, the belief that the mind and the body operate independently of one another.

The third component of the biomedical model is a focus on illness instead of on health. This results in medical practitioners emphasizing disease and the causes of disease rather than emphasizing the factors that lead to health and the prevention of disease.

Health psychologists and other members of the medical community have identified several concerns with the biomedical model and have proposed an alternative model, the biopsychosocial model, which takes an integrative approach to health and illness. The following four issues have been noted as challenges to the biomedical model and areas in which the biopsychosocial model contributes new insight (Engel, 1977).

First, biochemical deviation has been found to be a necessary but not sufficient cause for disease. To explain AIDS, for example, as simply the result of a viral infection ignores the many psychological and social factors that influence the transmission of the disease. The biopsychosocial model, in contrast, considers the impact of psychosocial variables on disease transmission.

Second, treatment effectiveness often varies among patients. The same HIV treatment regimen, for example, may have different effectiveness among patients. The biomedical model does not have sufficient information to explain these variations to treatment response, which may be influenced by psychosocial factors such as social support, religious beliefs, patient adherence, or others.

Third, practitioner variables have been shown to influence patient outcome. For example, a patient seeking treatment for HIV will be more likely to return to his or her practitioner and continue treatment if he or she does not feel judged or threatened by the practitioner, thereby improving outcome possibilities.

Finally, the biomedical model is unable to account for the lack of a direct relationship between biochemical mechanisms and patient-reported symptoms and treatment-seeking behaviors. For example, a patient's T-cell count may not always correlate with his or her experienced or reported illness symptoms. In addition, the time at which persons with HIV seek treatment for their symptoms is not directly related to any specific cellular measure. Where the biomedical model falls short in explaining disease, the biopsychosocial model is beginning to expand our knowledge of disease and health.

Related Entry: Biopsychosocial Model

BIBLIOGRAPHY

Engel, G. L. (1977). The need for a new medical model: A challenge for biomedicine. *Science, 196*, 129–136.

ELIZABETH MCDADE-MONTEZ

Biopsychosocial Model

George Engel's 1977 article in the prestigious journal *Science* introduced the biopsychosocial model as a replacement for the traditional biomedical explanatory model in medicine. This article both heralded and instigated a paradigm shift in the fields of medicine and the social sciences, and could be said to have functioned as the primary midwife in the birth of the new interdisciplinary fields of behavioral medicine and psychoneuroimmunology.

The biopsychosocial model seeks to identify the behavioral, emotional, genetic, or pathogenic factors that might alter the body's internal milieu and thereby facilitate disease processes. The model encourages the clinician to take into account the patient's attitudes toward illness, life goals, emotional and behavioral reactions, and personality traits and mental disorders, as well as biochemical and structural changes, in understanding the onset and progression of disease. As the model was further articulated, evidence began to amass concerning the role of stress and coping processes in influencing the balance between health and disease. From the other side of the equation, studies demonstrated how an illness alters patients' social and occupational roles and relationships, which in turn affect the duration and intensity of an illness. There was a growing appreciation for the importance of the bidirectional communication between patients and their health care providers as well as the wider psychosocial environment in influencing patients' response to medical care and recovery from illness.

HISTORICAL PATHWAYS

In both research and clinical practice, the biomedical model since the time of Pasteur had focused on discovering discrete, molecular causes of disease. Research conducted according to this largely unchallenged model was often spectacularly successful in uncovering the etiology of acute infectious diseases and developing cures. As these diseases were gradually conquered or controlled and as more chronic disorders such as cancer and heart disease emerged as the predominant causes of death in the second half of the 20th century, both clinicians and researchers began to appreciate the importance of the interaction of multiple factors in the onset, progression of, and recovery from chronic disorders.

Stress

Arguably, the most important of these factors was *stress*, a phenomenon first named by Hans Selye at McGill University. Richard Lazarus, a major theoretician and researcher in this area, defined stressful situations as those novel, unpredictable, and/or uncontrollable situations in which individuals are faced with environmental or other demands that exceed their ability to cope. In the mid-1970s the physician Ray Rosenman and his colleagues reported that the response to stress that they called the Type A behavior pattern was a significant risk factor for coronary heart disease.

Research on the pathogenic components of Type A behavior, particularly hostility, was invigorated and solidified by methodology from the rapidly growing discipline of health psychology, formally recognized in the United States in the late 1970s (and a decade later in Europe), even though psychologists had worked for decades in the areas of health and illness. In the early to mid-1980s the British psychiatrist Steven Greer and the American psychologist Lydia Temoshok led teams investigating the role of emotion management (expression or repression) and coping styles (e.g., the Type C coping style) in the progression of cancer. In the 1990s, The Belgian psychologist Johan Denollet investigated the relationship of Type D personality (high negative affectivity and high social inhibition) to coronary heart disease.

Psychosomatic Medicine

Psychosomatic medicine, a field that grew out of the psychoanalytic approach to medicine, was a parallel and contributory influence on the evolution of the biopsychosocial model. By the 1950s, psychosomaticists had a list of seven ailments thought to have a psychological as well as a physical component to their etiology: peptic ulcers, ulcerative colitis, hypertension, hyperthyroidism, rheumatoid arthritis, neurodermatitis, and asthma. Perhaps the most influential research in this field in terms of foreshadowing the development of the biopsychosocial model was conducted by psychiatrist George F. Solomon and the psychologist Rudolph Moos. Their now-classic 1965 study published in *Psychosomatic Medicine* demonstrated that a psychological variable—integrated and "super healthy" psychological functioning—can prevent the process by which a predisposing biological agent—the rheumatoid factor (an antibody found in the blood of patients with rheumatoid arthritis and considered a genetic marker)—would otherwise lead to overt illness—rheumatoid arthritis, a severe autoimmune disease that affects the connective tissue of the joints.

Immune System Connections

A 1964 theoretical paper by Solomon and Moos on emotions, immunity, and disease was clearly on the threshold of a new paradigm. By 1966, Solomon was using "psychoimmunology" to label his laboratory research with the immunologist Alfred Amkraut, including their remarkable study published in 1972, which showed the importance of individual differences in modulating the effects of stress on tumors in mice. Influenced by pioneering but largely unknown research by Russian scientists, including Elena Korneva on the role of the hypothalamus in immunity, Herbert N. Spector championed the term "neuroimmunomodulation." But it was experimental psychologist Robert Ader, who had worked with the immunologist Nicholas Cohen on the classic experiments showing that rats' immune responses could be behaviorally conditioned, who ended up with the winning term for the field, *psychoneuroimmunology*.

Mind–body Medicine

Research into this uncharted territory received a shot in the arm, so to speak, from the popular press. First published as an article in the *New England Journal of Medicine* in 1976, Norman Cousins' *Anatomy of an Illness,* was an anecdotal account of his personal triumph over severe illness, the healing power of laughter, and the importance of the patient–physician relationship. The book, as well as the cancer surgeon Bernie S. Siegel's 1986 book, *Love, Medicine, and Miracles*, stimulated thousands of articles and books dealing with aspects of mind–body medicine, sometimes referred to as "alternative" or "complementary" medicine. A marker of how far the field has come was the establishment of a National Center for Complementary and Alternative Medicine as part of the National Institutes of Health. Some critics, however, have argued against the "medicalization" of the field of mind–body medicine, in that clinicians in both standard and alternative medicine rely on randomized controlled clinical trials as the only method to document the effectiveness of an intervention, and NIH funding follows. To the extent that such trials seek to control and eliminate multiple factors and interactions, they are antithetical to testing the "real world" application of the biopsychosocial model.

SYSTEMS THEORY

Homeostasis, the ability or tendency of an organism to maintain internal equilibrium and a state of health by regulating its physiological processes, was first described in 1935 by Walter Cannon. This major tenet of systems theory is central to an understanding of health and disease. In 1983, Temoshok adapted elements from stress theories and the systems theories of Tart, Battista, and John concerning consciousness and hierarchically organized mental subsystems to propose a multidimensional theory of emotion, adaptation, and disease. According to this model, the dynamic equilibrium of homeostasis is disrupted when there is too much or too complex information, internal or external, which cannot be integrated into consciousness, causing distress. The process of repression, by which the cognitive content and the affective meaning of the information are split and one or the other relegated to subsystems below the level of consciousness, reduces distress and allows a precarious balance

to be re-established. However, there is a price to pay for this state of uneasy equanimity. To the extent that information salient to mental or physical health is inaccessible to consciousness, this information or cue cannot be acted on nor can the stressful situation be resolved. Temoshok theorized that extreme levels of stress, stress early in life, and/or very inadequate coping resources lead to information accommodation via the process of repression at increasingly more primitive mental subsystems, resulting in maladaptive mental and physical functioning, and, eventually, increasingly severe mental and physical disorders.

Psychologist Gary Schwartz (1990) argued that some attention to levels of distress is needed for feedback mechanisms and homeostasis to function so that the organism maintains health. A repressive style in which the meaning of emotions or bodily sensations is cut off from conscious awareness disturbs these feedback mechanisms such that the normal homeostatic process in which arousal is followed by return to baseline goes awry. Temoshok interpreted her findings on the relationship of the Type C coping style to cancer progression along parallel lines, in that the Type C style has a large repressive component in addition to nonrecognition and nonexpression of emotion. Maladaptive coping patterns such as Type C represent deviations from the inverted U-shaped function that characterizes homeostasis (commensurate arousal in response to stimuli followed by return to baseline) in that they fail to recognize, respond appropriately to, and/or resolve stressors. This coping pattern tends to keep the physiological stress response— and cortisol's immunosuppressive effects—chronically engaged, with implications for vulnerability to immunologically mediated diseases.

These theories implicate as mediating mechanisms the existence of bidirectional pathways between neuroendocrine and immune processes, as established by numerous psychoneuroimmunologic studies. More recent research has demonstrated that, in addition to neurotransmitters and hormones, brain function is modulated by neuropeptides. Receptors for neuropeptides are found throughout the brain, particularly in the limbic system areas that mediate emotion, as well as on various cells in the immune system. Candace B. Pert, now at Georgetown University Medical Center in Washington, D.C., who conducted pioneering research on opiate receptors in the brain, was the first scientist to promulgate the conceptual shift that neuropeptides (or as they are now called more generally, "cytokines" and "chemokines") and their receptors are the communicating link among the mind, the brain, and the endocrine and immune systems (Pert et al., 1985). In 1996, chemokine receptors were discovered to play a key role in HIV's ability to enter cells. The results of studies showing that specific chemokines have been shown to block viral receptors, and thus HIV entry into cells, has opened up new possibilities for biomedical treatments targeted at blocking viral receptors. To the extent that certain psychosocial factors may stimulate chemokine production that inhibits HIV, it is logical that research into how these factors may be

INDEPENDENT VARIABLES   MEDIATING VARIABLES   OUTCOME VARIABLES

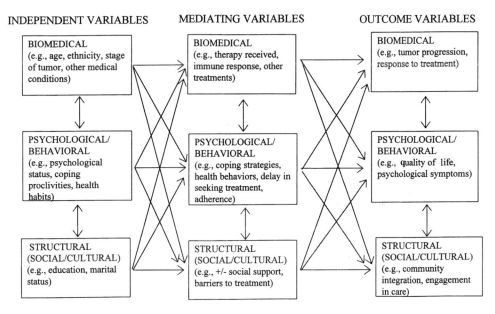

Figure 1.   The biopsychosocial model.

engaged may constitute the basis for a "natural" biopsychosocial anti-HIV intervention.

ELABORATING THE BIOPSYCHOSOCIAL MODEL

A major challenge for researchers in health psychology and behavioral medicine is to understand how stress or other psychosocial factors may mediate the development or exacerbation of an illness. Evidence suggests that there is not just a single route involved (see Figure 1), in that stress may result in negative health outcomes by direct effects on organ systems (e.g., increases in blood pressure, muscle tension, cortisol, gastric motility), by indirect biological effects (e.g., exacerbating or triggering a disease process in an already genetically vulnerable individual), or by increasing risk behaviors (e.g., smoking, alcohol consumption) that contribute to disease processes.

Much research in health psychology has focused on individual beliefs, attitudes, cognitions, and behaviors as well as environmental factors (e.g., social support, the treatment environment, doctor–patient communication) that affect medically salient processes and outcomes (e.g., adherence to medical treatment, risky behaviors). Another vigorous area of research focuses on the psychological concerns and coping of patients with chronic diseases, disabilities, and stressful medical procedures. On the same coin of the realm as behavioral medicine but on the flip side is the field of behavioral health, which encompasses health promotion, education, and prevention (e.g., accident prevention, immunization, nutrition, physical fitness and exercise, occupational safety and health, and changing health-damaging lifestyles.)

Let us consider the phenomenon of HIV/AIDS in the context of the biopsychosocial model and Figure 1, beginning with the premise that HIV not only affects the biomedical sphere of the person with the infection, but also significantly affects the psychological and social realities of any person touched by HIV. A further tenet of the biopsychosocial model is that the health and the sense of well-being of individuals affected by HIV are not dependent solely on the achievements of biomedicine. To the extent that psychosocial and behavioral variables influence susceptibility to HIV infection, quality of life, and possibly progression of HIV disease and longevity, then these variables become critical to consider in HIV prevention and intervention. A problem of this magnitude requires a comprehensive approach to inform medical, psychological, and public health intervention and prevention efforts.

The biopsychosocial model is the logical theoretical underpinning of this comprehensive approach. Elaborating the boxes in Figure 1, understanding the direction and strength of the arrows, as well as which boxes and arrows are highlighted for specific diseases and disorders constitute a worthy challenge for biopsychosocial researchers in the 21st century.

Related Entry: Biomedical Model

BIBLIOGRAPHY

Ader, R. (Ed.). (1981). *Psychoneuroimmunology*. San Diego, CA: Academic.
Cousins, N. (1979). *Anatomy of an Illness*. New York: Norton.
Engel, G. L. (1977). The need for a new medical model: A challenge for biomedicine. *Science, 196*, 129–136.

Pert, C. B., Ruff, M. R., Weber, R. J., & Herkenham, M. (1985). Neuropeptides and their receptors: A psychosomatic network. *Journal of Immunology, 135,* 820–826.

Schwartz, G. E. (1990). Psychobiology of repression and health: A systems approach. In J. L. Singer (Ed.), *Repression and dissociation* (pp. 337–386). Chicago: University of Chicago Press.

Solomon, G. F., Kemeny M. E., and Temoshok, L. (1991). Psychoneuroimmunologic aspects of human immunodeficiency virus infection. In R. Ader, D. L. Felten, & N. Cohen (Eds.), *Psychoneuroimmunology* (2nd ed., pp. 1081–1111). San Diego, CA: Academic.

Solomon, G. F., and Moos, R. H. (1964). Emotions, immunity, and disease: A speculative theoretical integration. *Archives of General Psychiatry, 11,* 657–674.

Temoshok, L. (1983). Emotion, adaptation, and disease: A multidimensional theory. In L. Temoshok, C. Van Dyke, and L. S. Zegans (Eds.), *Emotions in health and illness: Theoretical and research foundations.* (pp. 207–233). New York: Grune & Stratton.

Temoshok, L. (1990). On attempting to articulate the biopsychosocial model: Psychological–psychophysiological homeostasis. In H. Friedman (Ed.), *Personality and disease* (pp. 203–225). New York: Wiley.

Temoshok, L. (2000). Complex coping patterns and their role in adaptation and neuroimmunomodulation: Theory, methodology, and research. *Annals of the New York Academy of Science, 917,* 446–455.

Lydia R. Temoshok

Blood Pressure

Blood pressure is the force resulting from the pumping action of the heart and applied to the interior vessel walls by circulating blood. The consequent stretching of the vessels and their subsequent contraction are crucial for sustaining circulation in the vascular system. The contraction of the heart (systole) produces the highest blood pressure and corresponds to the top number in a blood pressure reading; the relaxation of the heart (diastole) results in the lower figure and is represented by the bottom number in a blood pressure reading. Pressure waves originating in the heart can be detected at points where arteries lie close to the skin; blood pressure is usually measured over the brachial artery (by an instrument called a sphygmomanometer), and both systolic and diastolic pressures are reported. With age and deteriorating artery condition (or in response to physical or emotional strain), blood pressures tend to increase; sustained high pressures can cause blood vessel damage and increased risk of stroke, heart disease, kidney disease, and other heath problems. Treatments for hypertension (persistent high blood pressure) include exercise, weight reduction, and pressure-reducing medications.

Related Entries: Cardiovascular System, Hypertension

James Bunde

Blood–Brain Barrier

The blood–brain barrier (BBB) prevents potentially harmful substances carried in the bloodstream, such as drugs or hormones, from entering the brain. The BBB is formed from thickened capillary walls within the brain, which ensure that only a few selected substances can pass through to the brain.

There are three main ways substances can pass through the BBB. Lipid-soluble substances, such as the gases carbon dioxide and oxygen, can diffuse through the BBB. Certain non-lipid-soluble substances, such as glucose and amino acids, are transported across the BBB by carrier-mediated transport systems, and electrolytes can pass through ion channels.

Not every area of the brain is equally protected by the BBB. Areas such as the posterior pituitary and the circumventricular organs have "leaky" BBBs; however, this is essential for their physiological functions. For example, the posterior pituitary releases hormones into the circulatory system, and the circumventricular organs monitor the levels of various substances within the bloodstream.

Related Entry: Nervous System

BIBLIOGRAPHY

Kandel, E. R., Schwartz, J. H., & Jessel, T. M. (Eds.). (2000). *Principles of neural science* (4th ed.). New York: McGraw-Hill.

Rosenzweig, M. R., Breedlove, S. M., & Leiman, A. L. (2002). *Biological psychology* (3rd ed.). Sunderland, MA: Sinauer.

Adele M. H. Seelke

Body Image

Body image refers to the image we hold in our minds about the size, appearance, and shape of our bodies. Individuals satisfied with their body image are less likely to experience psychological distress than people who are dissatisfied with their body image. For example, obese individuals tend to be more dissatisfied with body image than nonobese individuals. Furthermore, if obese individuals lose weight, their body image clearly improves. At the same time, some normal-weight individuals are extremely dissatisfied with their bodies and such body image concerns seem to be a risk factor for the development of eating disorders such as anorexia nervosa and bulimia nervosa. There is speculation that such body dissatisfaction among normal-weight people is influenced by extreme sociocultural norms for thinness, especially among women.

Related Entries: Eating Disorders; Exercise, Effects and Benefits; Nutrition

BIBLIOGRAPHY

Ricciardelli, L. A., & McCabe, M. P. (2001). Children's body image concerns and eating disturbance: A review of the literature. *Clinical Psychology Review, 21*(3), 325–344.

STEPHEN A. WONDERLICH

Breast Self-Examination

Breast self-examination (BSE) refers to the systematic self-palpation of breast tissue to detect abnormalities that might be indicative of breast cancer. Monthly performance of BSE enables a woman to become familiar with the usual configuration of her breast tissue so that a deviation or lump can be detected. Like clinical breast examination by a health care provider and mammography, BSE is a screening technique used to discover breast cancer early when the treatment prognosis is good. Although most women discover their own malignant tumors, the research evidence is ambiguous regarding the impact of BSE on cancer mortality.

A thorough breast self-examination can be conducted in less than 10 min. The exam is performed while lying down, using the right hand to palpate the left breast and the left hand to palpate the right breast. Using small circular finger movements, the woman presses firmly with the flat part of her fingers into her breast tissue and underarm area to search for a lump. To ensure complete coverage of the area, a systematic coverage pattern, such as concentric circles or vertical strips, is recommended.

Lump identification may be difficult at first because breast tissue is not uniform. For this reason, it is desirable for women to perform their BSE at the same time each month so that they know what their breast tissue normally feels like. Menstruating women are encouraged to practice BSE the day after their periods end when the breasts are less swollen and tender. Nonmenstruating women should select a day each month to conduct their BSE.

If a lump is discovered, it should be reported to a health care provider. Most lumps just require checking by a doctor. Of those requiring removal, about 80 percent are harmless and can be removed in a doctor's office. If the lump is a malignant tumor, early treatment can save one's life.

It is estimated that between 25 and 40 percent of women in the United States perform BSE on a monthly basis. These data are based on self-report and may overestimate performance frequency. Data from numerous studies suggest that women of higher education are more likely to practice monthly BSE. Barriers that hinder monthly performance include lack of confidence in one's ability to conduct a thorough exam and difficulty remembering to do the exam monthly.

Confidence in BSE performance and quality of BSE can be enhanced by instruction that includes modeling proper technique and giving corrective feedback. Women achieve the greatest improvement in lump detection skills through practice with synthetic breast models containing embedded lumps. This practice enables women to discriminate between normal tissue and lumps that warrant scrutiny.

BSE maintenance is increased by prompting strategies that cue monthly exams in a timely manner. Rewards contingent on BSE performance also appear to improve maintenance. However, even with prompts and rewards, long-term adherence to monthly practice is less than optimal, and women least likely to engage in other cancer screening activities (e.g., clinical breast exam and mammography) are least likely to practice monthly BSE.

Related Entry: Testicular Self-Examination

BIBLIOGRAPHY

Mayer, J. A., & Solomon, L. J. (1992). Breast self-examination skill and frequency: A review. *Annals of Behavioral Medicine, 14,* 189–196.

O'Malley, M. S., & Fletcher, S. W. (1987). Screening for breast cancer with breast self-examination: A critical review. *Journal of the American Medical Association, 257,* 2197–2203.

LAURA J. SOLOMON

Brownell, Kelly D. (1951–)

Kelly D. Brownell, PhD, is professor of psychology at Yale University, where he also serves as professor of epidemiology and public health and as director of the Yale Center for Eating and Weight Disorders. He has served as president of several national organizations, including the Society of Behavioral Medicine, the Association for the Advancement of Behavior Therapy, and the Division of Health Psychology of the American Psychological Association. He has received numerous awards and honors for his work, including the James McKeen Cattell Award from the

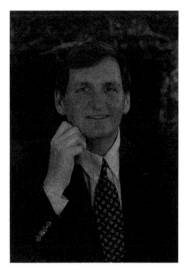

Brownell, Kelly

New York Academy of Sciences, the award for Outstanding Contribution to Health Psychology from the American Psychological Association, and Distinguished Alumni Award from Purdue University. He has published 13 books and more than 200 scientific articles and chapters.

Dr. Brownell is an internationally known expert on obesity, eating disorders, and body weight regulation. His work has been marked by an ability to develop integrative theoretical models of obesity that have provided the framework for other investigators to conduct further research. For example, he was one of the initial investigators to identify that obesity is a chronic condition with high risk for relapse. He coined the term "yo-yo dieting" to describe the phenomenon of weight cycling, or repeated weight loss and regain, among obese individuals. In his paper Understanding and Preventing Relapse published in the *American Psychologist*, he identified common processes associated with relapse across physical and mental health conditions, it is listed as one of the most frequently cited papers in psychology.

Dr. Brownell was one of the first researchers to develop integrated theoretical models for understanding the interaction between eating disorders and obesity. His work particularly focused on the psychological consequences of having a comorbid eating disorder in the obese population. His coedited *Eating Disorders and Obesity: A Comprehensive Handbook* represents a definitive handbook on integrating the two fields, and provides an excellent example for future researchers investigating links between psychopathology and physical health.

Perhaps Dr. Brownell's most important contribution to the field of health psychology has been his work examining the role of social environment in the etiology, prevention, and treatment of obesity. He was the first investigator to examine whether integrating family members into behavioral treatments for obesity could improve outcomes. His cognitive–behavioral treatment for obesity, *LEARN*, still extensively used in both clinical and research settings, represents one of the first weight loss manuals to explicitly discuss the role of interpersonal relationships in weight loss. In addition, he has conducted extensive work identifying the role of stigma in psychological functioning in obesity.

Dr. Brownell's most recent work has involved identifying the role of the "toxic environment," in which energy-rich foods are widely available, inexpensive, and promoted heavily, in combination with energy-saving devices and other changes in lifestyle that increase sedentary behavior in perpetuating the high incidence and prevalence of obesity. In a landmark editorial in the *New York Times*, he outlined the possible role of public policy interventions that may be the key to the management of this public health crisis. His bold proposals of holding food companies accountable for faulty advertising and taxing foods of poor nutritional value has framed the debate over how to handle the obesity epidemic in this country.

MICHAEL A. FRIEDMAN

Cc

Caffeine

Caffeine is the most widely used central nervous system stimulant, regularly consumed by 80 percent of adults throughout the world. It is present in coffee, tea, many soft drinks (including colas, Mountain Dew, and Mello Yello), and chocolate. Recently, it has been added to bottled spring water, such as Verifine Fruit2$_O$ Plus: Citrus Energy. Caffeine is a component of most beverages marketed as energy drinks, including AMP, Venom, and Adrenaline Rush. Caffeine is also an ingredient of some cold medications, diet pills, headache remedies, pain relievers, allergy tablets, antacids, and sleep prevention compounds.

Caffeine has been shown to have a number of physiological effects. Perhaps the most researched is that caffeine consumption causes a small increase in blood pressure. Although the magnitude of the increase is most likely not harmful to healthy individuals, those with hypertension or borderline high blood pressure may be adversely affected. Although there are inconsistencies in the literature, caffeine may also be associated with osteoporosis, or loss of bone density in postmenopausal women. Again, although the literature is inconsistent, research suggests negative effects of use in pregnant women including low birth weight and increased risk of spontaneous abortion. Research has also examined the association between caffeine use and numerous types of cancer. The current pattern of results, although not entirely consistent, demonstrates little evidence of any association between caffeine consumption and the development of cancer.

The physiological effects of caffeine use are not all negative. Research has suggested that caffeine when used in combination with an additional analgesic decreases pain, especially headache pain. Because caffeine is a stimulant, it is reliably associated with decreased fatigue and increased arousal. One area of application of this finding is improvement in tasks requiring sustained attention. Caffeine has also been used to assist individuals with diabetes recognize when they are experiencing hypoglycemia, or low blood sugar. Research also suggests that caffeine use may be associated with a lower risk of developing Parkinson's disease. Although this finding is provocative, other explanations are possible, including a decision by individuals who are in the very early stages of Parkinson's disease not to consume any caffeine.

The debate on whether caffeine is an addictive drug focuses on withdrawal or physical dependence, tolerance, and the reinforcing effects of caffeine. There is a set of recognized withdrawal symptoms, including headache, drowsiness, increased work difficulty, decreased feelings of contentment, decreased sociability, flu-like feelings, and blurred vision. Depression and anxiety may also increase. The severity of withdrawal increases with the dose of caffeine. Although not all caffeine users experience significant symptoms, withdrawal may be of clinical importance in diagnosing and treating ailments such as headache and fatigue. Tolerance also develops to some of the effects of caffeine, although it is generally not complete, and may disappear after overnight abstinence. At low to moderate doses, caffeine has been shown to have reinforcing effects, with a proportion of caffeine users reliably selecting caffeine over placebo in studies where choice is provided.

Related Entries: Addiction, Fight-or-Flight Response, Nervous System

BIBLIOGRAPHY

Cnattingius, S., Signorello, L. B., Anneren, G., Clausson, B., Ekbom, A., Ljunger, E. et al. (2000). Caffeine intake and the risk of first-trimester spontaneous abortion. *New England Journal of Medicine, 343*, 1839–1845.

Debra, K., Sherwin, R. S., Murphy, J., & Kerr, D. (1996). Effect of caffeine on recognition of and physiological responses to hypoglycaemia in insulin-dependent diabetes. *Lancet, 347,* 19–24.

Green, P. J., Kirby, R., & Suls, J. (1996). The effects of caffeine on blood pressure and heart rate: A review. *Annals of Behavioral Medicine, 18,* 201–216.

Griffiths, R. R., & Mumford, G. K. (1995). Caffeine—A drug of abuse? In E. Floyd Bloom & D. J. Kupfer (Eds.), *Psychopharmacology: The fourth generation of progress* (pp. 1699–1713). New York: Raven.

Honig, L. S. (2000). Relationship between caffeine intake and Parkinson disease. *Journal of the American Medical Association, 284,* 1378–1379.

James, J. E. (1997). Understanding caffeine: A biobehavioral analysis. In R. Rick Turner (Series Ed.), *Behavioral medicine and health psychology* (Vol. 2, pp. 00–00). Thousand Oaks, CA: Sage.

PETER J. GREEN

Table 1. 2001 Estimates of Cancer Incidence and Mortality by Site and Gender for the Six Leading Sites

	Male		Female	
	Site	Number (%)	Site	Number (%)
Cancer incidence				
	Prostate	198,100 (31)	Breast	192,200 (31)
	Lung	90,700 (14)	Lung	78,800 (13)
	Colon/rectum	67,300 (10)	Colon/rectum	68,100 (11)
	Bladder	39,200 (6)	Uterine	38,300 (6)
	Lymphoma	31,100 (5)	Lymphoma	25,100 (4)
	All sites	643,000 (100)	All sites	625,000 (100)
Cancer mortality				
	Lung	90,100 (31)	Lung	67,300 (25)
	Prostate	31,500 (11)	Breast	40,200 (15)
	Colon/rectum	27,700 (10)	Colon/rectum	29,000 (11)
	Pancreas	14,100 (5)	Pancreas	14,800 (6)
	Lymphoma	13,800 (5)	Ovary	13,900 (5)
	All sites	286,100 (100)	All sites	267,300 (100)

Source: From *Cancer Facts and Figures 2001.* Copyright 2001 by the American Cancer Society, Inc. Adapted with permission.

Cancer: Biopsychosocial Aspects

Cancer, the uncontrolled abnormal growth of cells, is diagnosed in over one million Americans each year (American Cancer Society). This entry provides an overview of the biomedical, psychological, and socioenvironmental aspects of cancer. By way of introduction, data on cancer incidence, death rates, and gender differences are provided. The overview focuses on important health psychology issues, with research findings organized by the different phases of the cancer experience, from prevention through diagnosis and treatment to long-term survival and terminal illness. Psychological interventions with demonstrated effectiveness for treating cancer patients are highlighted in each section. The conclusion provides a brief summary and discusses research directions for the 21st century.

CANCER INCIDENCE, DEATH RATES, AND GENDER DIFFERENCES

The risk of developing cancer over the course of a lifetime is 1 in 2 for men and 1 in 3 for women. Cancer is the second leading cause of death, with the number of deaths exceeded only by those from heart disease. Eighty percent of all cancer diagnoses are made in people over the age of 55 years. Table 1 displays data from the United States on the incidence and death rates by specific types of cancer diagnoses and gender. These data indicate, for example, that women are most commonly diagnosed with breast cancer and men with prostate cancer, but that lung cancer is the number one cause of cancer-related death for both genders.

BIOMEDICAL, PSYCHOLOGICAL, AND SOCIOENVIRONMENTAL ISSUES IN CANCER: FROM PREVENTION TO DISEASE OUTCOMES

Prevention

Lifestyle behaviors such as tobacco use, poor dietary habits, physical inactivity, and alcohol consumption account for an estimated 68 percent of all cancer deaths in the United States. Therefore, cancer incidence and premature death can be diminished through changes in lifestyle. Prevention efforts focus on reducing the probability of cancer onset by decreasing toxic exposures (e.g., asbestos) and providing information on risk factors (e.g., warning labels on tobacco products). Besides tobacco use, other lifestyle behaviors linked to increased cancer risk, such as dietary habits and amount of sun exposure, are targets of intervention. Diet modification, particularly reductions in fat intake and increases in fiber, are emphasized in the prevention of colorectal cancers, whereas increased avoidance of the sun and use of sun block are important in skin cancer prevention. Other prevention efforts are used to identify cancer in its earliest and often asymptomatic stages (e.g., mammography, prostate and colorectal screening). Lower socioeconomic status, lack of insurance, and rural residence can hinder awareness and access to prevention and screening interventions.

Symptom Appearance

In view of the magnitude of the cancer problem and the potential for life threat, delay in seeking medical treatment for symptoms is a surprisingly common occurrence. Whether the time lag occurs when seeing a physician for symptoms, being diagnosed, or beginning treatment, all individuals, and even some physicians, can be "delayers." Most delay occurs in deciding whether to seek medical attention for physical symptoms (e.g., pain, loss of appetite, bleeding). Unfortunately, the development and appearance of cancer symptoms can occur over months or even years, extending delay, unlike the presentation of other serious medical problems (e.g., heart attack). Although cancer is a life-threatening disease, it is a low probability one for many individuals. Thus, delay may lengthen as people think it unlikely that their symptoms indicate a condition as serious as cancer. Economic factors such as cost of medical care, social factors such as family influence and support, personal health beliefs, and an avoidant coping style can also influence the length of delay. Barbara Andersen and colleagues have developed a model to identify factors related to medical delay (Andersen, 1992, 2002; Andersen et al., 1994, 1995). Prevention/screening efforts and shortening the delay in seeking medical care for symptoms are linked to improved survival rates for many cancers (e.g., cancers of the cervix, breast, colon, and prostate).

Diagnosis

Cancer is one of the most stressful medical diagnoses a person can receive and is accompanied by high levels of emotional distress (Weisman & Worden 1976). Depressive symptoms are the most common emotional symptoms reported by cancer patients, although anxiety symptoms are reported as well. The average rate of depression for cancer patients is 24 percent, a rate consistently higher than rates for patients with other medical diagnoses. It is not uncommon for psychological symptoms in cancer patients to wax and wane over time, with initial adjustment difficulties developing into depressive or anxiety disorders. This situation is of particular importance because psychological symptoms are not only associated with lower quality of life but may lead to other difficulties such as poorer treatment adherence.

Importantly, the emotional problems of diagnostic-related distress are alleviated through psychological interventions (Andersen, 1992). The most effective interventions focus on stress reduction via relaxation training. Other common intervention strategies include a focus on health education, problem-solving skills, and group support. Improvements in mood, specifically stress reduction, and enhanced coping, including the use of active-behavioral strategies, can be achieved with brief, cost-effective interventions (i.e., group meetings occurring over several weeks or months).

Treatment

Some of the emotional distress occurring at diagnosis is due to the anticipation of treatment. Standard cancer therapies include any combination of surgery, radiation, chemotherapy, hormonal therapy (e.g., tamoxifen), and immunotherapy. Most treatments are preceded or followed by physical examinations, body scans (e.g., x-rays), and laboratory tests (e.g., blood tests). Thus, getting cancer treatment often represents multiple stressors for patients. What may distinguish cancer patients undergoing surgery from noncancer surgical patients are higher overall levels of presurgery distress and slower rates of emotional recovery. The scenario for radiation and chemotherapy patients is similar, but because these treatments can be lengthy (weeks or months), heightened anxiety often occurs when treatments end. At this time patients can feel "on their own" and as if they are playing a "waiting game" for cancer recurrence.

Psychological interventions to reduce patients' treatment anxiety are frequently incorporated into routine medical care. Such efforts include procedural information (e.g., how surgery or radiation is done), information on the actual physical sensations that can be produced by treatments, and instruction in relaxation and hypnosis. These interventions produce many benefits including reduced emotional distress, decreased pain medication use and length of hospital stay, and decreased overall recovery time (e.g., amount of time until patients return to work and social activities).

Psychological intervention efforts have focused on alleviating three common treatment-related complications—adherence, fatigue, and appetite and weight changes. Adherence with treatment is important, because the expectation and experience of unpleasant side effects such as fatigue and nausea/vomiting not only diminish patients' quality of life, but can also be so discouraging or annoying that a patient may be reluctant to continue treatment. Nonadherence with treatment has also been related to emotional distress, lower income, and age (e.g., adolescent patients). It is a behavioral problem that can directly affect the effectiveness of cancer therapy. For instance, when patients do not adhere to medical recommendations, treatment dosage may be reduced, which can, in turn, lower the cure rate. Psychological interventions to improve patient adherence focus on a variety of techniques, including appointment and medication reminders, clearly written and specific treatment communications, and home visits. Additionally, preparatory hospital-based interventions such as offering a tour of the oncology clinic, videotape presentations about treatment, discussion/question sessions, and take-home information are especially effective in improving coping with treatment.

Fatigue is the most common symptom reported following treatment, especially by cancer patients receiving radiation or chemotherapy. Importantly, fatigue is distinct from depression. Symptoms of fatigue (e.g., feeling tired, a lack of energy, sleepy, confused) have been related to decreased quality of life, reduced overall daily functioning, and poor treatment adherence. Psychological interventions focus on increasing tolerance to fatigue in a number of ways: (1) providing information on side effects and activity/rest cycle recommendations (e.g., naps in the afternoon), (2) increasing physical activity (e.g., walking, flexibility, or strengthening exercises), (3) enhancing coping efforts (e.g., planning and scheduling activities, decreasing nonessential activities, reliance on others for assistance), and (4) improving nutritional status (e.g., protein intake).

Appetite and weight changes are also significant problems for cancer patients. Malnutrition is associated with increased morbidity and mortality. Food aversions learned in connection with chemotherapy are rapidly acquired (usually after one to three treatments) and although these aversions may not involve appetite or weight loss, patients may unknowingly develop aversions to their favorite foods. These aversions can affect patients' daily routine and perceived quality of life. Since the late 1980s, research has revealed that many cancer patients will develop nausea and/or vomiting in response to chemotherapy treatments (Carey & Burish, 1988). However, anti-nausea/vomiting drug treatments have dramatically reduced the incidence of such problems. Psychological treatments for these problems include hypnosis, progressive muscle relaxation with guided imagery, systematic desensitization, cognitive distraction, and biofeedback. Effective preventive care also reduces the likelihood of conditioned anticipatory reactions (i.e., nausea and vomiting associated with previously neutral events such as going to the hospital and sitting in the waiting room). Weight gain resulting from chemotherapy or hormonal treatments is an important issue for women with cancer and appears to be a risk factor for breast cancer recurrence. Behavioral weight management interventions teach healthy eating habits (e.g., reducing daily fat intake and increasing fiber) and promote exercise to maintain or lose weight.

Recovery and Survivorship

The term "survivor" typically refers to individuals who have survived cancer at least 5 years, as the probability of recurrence declines significantly after that time for most cancers. As the prognoses for many cancer diagnoses have improved, there is increased attention to quality of life, particularly for long-term survivors of cancer. Studies suggest that by 1 year following treatment the severe distress of diagnosis and treatment declines and emotions stabilize. Emotional difficulties, therefore, do not persist for the majority of cancer survivors. In fact, many survivors report positive life changes (e.g., greater empathy and appreciation for life, closer relationships, living life more fully in the present moment). Still, many cancer survivors do report specific problems beyond treatment including premature menopause, sexual disruptions, financial concerns, and fears of recurrence.

Premature or abrupt menopause is a difficult circumstance for many women receiving chemotherapy, and occurs more frequently in older women or women receiving higher doses of chemotherapy. The consequences of chemotherapy-induced menopause include sleep disturbances, hot flashes, mood swings, difficulties with vaginal lubrication, cessation of menses, and infertility. These symptoms may be even more severe than those experienced during naturally occurring menopause. In addition, for young women, fertility concerns can have a major impact on quality of life. Issues related to premature menopause and infertility should be discussed early and often to promote coping and adjustment during survivorship.

Sexuality is also disrupted for many cancer survivors. All patients with solid tumors (85 percent) and many treated for blood-related cancers (e.g., lymphoma and leukemia) are vulnerable to sexual dysfunction (e.g., desire and arousal problems and painful intercourse). Estimates of cancer-related sexual dysfunction range from 10 to 20 percent for breast cancer patients treated with lumpectomy to 100 percent for men having surgical prostate removal. Disease and treatment side effects are the primary cause of sexual problems. Feelings related to perceived attractiveness and body image changes associated with treatment (e.g., facial or genital surgery, loss of hair due to chemotherapy) may also play a role in sexual dysfunction. If sexual problems do develop, they usually do so when intercourse resumes, and, if untreated, are unlikely to resolve. Several psychological interventions facilitate sexual adjustment including (1) consideration of the optimal timing for sexual activity (e.g., when fatigue is at its lowest), (2) use of strategies to facilitate desire (e.g., fantasy and erotic materials), (3) expanding the behavioral repertoire (e.g., sexual activities in lieu of intercourse and alternative intercourse positions), and (4) use of lubricants to counter vaginal dryness. Interventions to enhance couples' sexual communication or rehearse sharing information about cancer with a prospective partner are also beneficial.

Other difficulties experienced by cancer survivors include financial disruption and fears of recurrence. Cancer treatments are expensive and occupationally disruptive. Some cancer survivors report chronic economic stress including increased insurance premiums, loss of insurance, and income reductions due to work absences. In addition, the majority of survivors report ongoing concerns about cancer recurrence that are exacerbated during subsequent medical appointments. Psychological interventions during this phase of the cancer experience include referrals for potential financial and insurance assistance, open discussion of concerns regarding potential recurrence, and relaxation training to reduce stress at follow-up medical appointments.

Recurrence and Metastatic Cancer

Many patients experience a rebound in emotional distress when cancer recurs, with as many as 45 percent reporting symptoms of anxiety or depression at the time of recurrence diagnosis. Persons experiencing a greater number of current stressors, particularly financial difficulties, have an elevated risk of emotional distress during recurrence. Younger patients and patients with greater pain or discomfort and less hopefulness also report greater distress. In addition, partners or spouses may be more distressed by a recurrence diagnosis than the initial cancer diagnosis, and may become more distressed than the cancer patient. The partner or spouse plays an essential role in supporting the patient through this difficult experience. However, many couples are reluctant to discuss the meaning of the recurrence and fears of loss. Psychological interventions designed to improve couple communication can be useful to address these concerns. Supportive–emotionally expressive group interventions and problem-solving approaches also bring about important emotional benefits such as decreased distress, enhanced coping, and improved self-esteem.

Two of the most distressing aspects of metastatic cancer are pain and delirium. Pain is more common and less controllable for individuals with metastatic cancer (i.e., disease that has spread from the original site). Eighty percent of patients with metastatic cancer report moderate to severe pain as compared to 40 percent of earlier-stage patients. The major cause of cancer pain is direct tumor involvement (e.g., metastases to bone and nerve compression), but pain can also be the result of treatment (e.g., surgery and radiation). If pain worsens or is difficult to control, daily functioning can be impaired, social interactions may suffer, and quality of life may deteriorate. Pain is associated with depression and anxiety and inadequately controlled pain has been cited as a primary reason for requests for physician-assisted suicide. In addition to pain-controlling medications, psychological interventions for advanced cancer pain benefit both patients and family members. Interventions include dispelling myths about addiction to pain medication, teaching self-control techniques such as hypnosis and relaxation, and offering education regarding early identification of pain symptoms and assertive communication leading to more effective pain control.

Another frequent complication of metastatic cancer is delirium. Approximately 75 percent of patients with metastatic cancer meet criteria for delirium as compared to 8 percent of patients during other illness phases. Delirium is characterized by problems with awareness, attention, and memory. Individuals with delirium may also be restless and disoriented, which is distressing to family members and caregivers. Delirium in cancer patients is caused by a number of factors including chemotherapy, narcotics used for pain control, and brain metastases. Although delirium is a reversible brain disorder, it is often misunderstood and misdiagnosed, with symptoms often attributed to depression and anxiety. Psychological interventions aimed at the early identification of symptoms and helping patients and caregivers understand the transient nature of delirium can reduce anxiety and create immediate emotional benefits. Organization of the patient's environment to include calendars, clocks, and objects of personal significance also helps to orient the patient to the date, time, and location.

Terminal Cancer

Cancer is considered terminal when the disease is no longer responsive to treatment. At this point, the focus is on palliative care. The World Health Organization (1990) defines palliative care as "the active total care of patients . . . including control of pain, of other symptoms, and of psychological, social, and spiritual problems. The goal of palliative care is achievement of the best possible quality of life for patients and their families." The most common physical symptoms of terminal cancer include pain, difficulty breathing, fever, nausea or vomiting, constipation or diarrhea, loss of appetite, and weight loss. Up to 60 percent of individuals with terminal cancer also experience psychological difficulties including adjustment disorders, depression, anxiety, and delirium. At this phase of illness, patients report distress associated with unmanaged physical symptoms, inability to carry on meaningful activities, and insufficient emotional support, especially for the unmarried or those living alone. During terminal illness many individuals seek emotional support related to their worries or fears. These fears are often existential in nature (e.g., concerning the meaning of life and death), or more pragmatic, related to the families' ability to carry on beyond the death of the patient.

The terminal phase is especially difficult for family members. Many family members experience a period of anticipatory grieving that involves physical or emotional distancing from patient suffering as a means of managing the eventual death of the loved one. Some caregivers have chronic health problems of their own that can be exacerbated by exhaustion or sleep deprivation. Many caregivers also suffer significant reductions of income due to work absenteeism resulting in financial distress. Family members report needs for assistance to assure the patient's comfort, frequent information regarding the patient's condition, needs for the support of other family members, and acceptance and support from health care professionals. Psychological interventions that focus on the quality, not quantity, of survival are important when death is inevitable. These efforts emphasize patient control over the environment, attention to unfinished family business, and continued involvement in feasible, but meaningful activities. Listening to patients' reminiscences, helping them develop meaning, and offering support to struggling family members are important in enhancing quality of life during terminal illness.

SUMMARY AND CONCLUSIONS

Psychological interventions are a valuable addition to medical treatment across all phases of the cancer experience, from efforts to enhance health-promoting behaviors and consequently prevent cancer, to efforts to facilitate meaning in the face of terminal disease. Psychological interventions have an established impact on symptom management (i.e., nausea and vomiting, fatigue, pain control), stress reduction, mood improvement, and overall quality of life. Psychological interventions may also improve treatment adherence and facilitate healthy lifestyle changes (e.g., diet and exercise), although maintenance of these changes is challenging for many patients.

Since the late 1980s, research efforts have also focused on the effect of psychological interventions on immune functioning and survival. A study published by David Spiegel and colleagues at Stanford University in 1989 reported an 18-month survival benefit for women with metastatic breast cancer who participated in a year-long supportive–emotionally expressive therapy group. However, the studies published since Spiegel's original work report inconsistent results. A biobehavioral model of cancer stress and disease course has also been developed to describe the mechanisms by which the stress could influence survival. Thus far, significant progress has been made in understanding the biomedical, psychological, and socioenvironmental aspects of cancer. Psychological interventions are known to improve quality of life from diagnosis to terminal illness, regardless of the duration of the cancer experience.

Related Entries: Anticipatory Nausea and Vomiting, Chronic Illness

BIBLIOGRAPHY

American Cancer Society. (2001). *Cancer facts and figures 2001.* Atlanta, GA: American Cancer Society.

Andersen, B. (1992). Psychological interventions for cancer patients to enhance quality of life. *Journal of Consulting and Clinical Psychology, 60,* 552–568.

Andersen, B. (2002). Biobehavioral outcomes following psychological interventions for cancer patients. *Journal of Consulting and Clinical Psychology, 70,* 590–610.

Andersen, B., Cacioppo, J., & Roberts, D. (1995). Delay in seeking a cancer diagnosis: Delay stages and psychophysiological comparison processes. *British Journal of Social Psychology, 34,* 33–52.

Andersen, B., Kiecolt-Glaser, J., & Glaser, R. (1994). A biobehavioral model of cancer stress and disease course. *American Psychologist, 49,* 389–404.

Auchincloss, S. (1989). Sexual dysfunction in cancer patients: Issues in evaluation and treatment. In J. Holland & J. Rowland, *Handbook of psychooncology: Psychological care of the patient with cancer.* New York: Oxford University Press.

Baider, L., Cooper, C. L., & Kaplan De-Nour, A. (2000). *Cancer and the family.* London: Wiley.

Baum, A., & Andersen, B. (2001). *Psychosocial interventions for cancer.* Washington, DC: American Psychological Association.

Carey, M., & Burish, T. (1988). Etiology and treatment of the psychological side effects associated with cancer chemotherapy: A critical review and discussion. *Psychological Bulletin, 104,* 307–325.

Cherny, N., Coyle, N., & Foley, K. (1994). Suffering in the advanced cancer patient: A definition and taxonomy. *Journal of Palliative Care, 10,* 57–70.

Demark, W., Winer, E. P., & Rimer, B. (1993). Why women gain weight with adjuvant chemotherapy. *Journal of Clinical Oncology, 11,* 1418–1429.

Ganz, P. A., Desmond, K. A., Leedham, B., Rowland, J. H., Meyerowitz, B. E., & Belin, T. P. (2002). Quality of life in long-term, disease-free survivors of breast cancer: A follow-up study. *Journal of the National Cancer Institute, 94,* 39–49.

Given, B., & Given, C. W. (1992). Patient and family caregiver reaction to new and recurrent breast cancer. *Journal of the American Medical Women's Association, 47*(5), 201–206.

Gotay, C. C., & Muraoka, M. (1998). Quality of life in long-term survivors of adult-onset cancers. *Journal of the National Cancer Institute, 90,* 656–667.

Jacobsen, P. B., & Schwartz, M. D. (1993). Food aversions during cancer therapy: Incidence, etiology, and prevention. *Oncology, 7,* 139–143.

Massie, M. J., & Holland, J. C. (1992). The cancer patient with pain: Psychiatric complications and their management. *Journal of Pain and Symptom Management, 7,* 99–109.

Massie, M. J., Holland, J. C., & Glass, E. (1983). Delirium in terminally ill cancer patients. *American Journal of Psychiatry, 140,* 1048–1050.

McDaniel, J. S., Musselman, D., & Nemeroff, C. (1997). Cancer and depression: Theory and treatment. *Psychiatry Annuals, 27,* 360–364.

Mererowitz, B. E., Richardson, J., Husdon, S., & Leedham, B. (1998). Ethnicity and cancer outcomes: Behavioral and psychosocial considerations. *Psychological Bulletin, 123,* 47–70.

Pinto, B., Eakin, E., & Maruyama, N. (2000). Health behavior changes after a cancer diagnosis: What do we know and where do we go from here? *Annals of Behavioral Medicine, 22,* 38–52.

Richardson, J., Marks, G., & Levine, A. (1988). The influence of symptoms of disease and side effects of treatment on compliance with cancer therapy. *Journal of Clinical Oncology, 6,* 1746–1752.

Spiegel, D. (2001). Mind matters—Group therapy and survival in breast cancer. *New England Journal of Medicine, 345,* 1767–1768.

Spiegel, D., Bloom, J. R., Kraemer, H., C., & Gottheil, E. (1989). Effect of psychosocial treatment on survival of patients with metastatic breast cancer. *Lancet, 14,* 888–891.

Wachtel, T., Allen-Masterson, S., Reuben, D., Goldberg, R., & Mor, V. (1988). The end-stage cancer patient: Terminal common pathway. *Hospice Journal, 4,* 43–80.

Weisman, A., & Worden, J. W. (1976). The existential plight in cancer: Significance of the first 100 days. *International Journal of Psychiatry in Medicine, 7,* 1–15.

WHO Expert Committee. (1990). *Cancer pain relief and palliative care* (Technical Report Series, No. 804). Geneva: World Health Organization.

Winningham, M., Nail, L., Burke, M. B., Brophy, L., Cimprich, B., Jones, L., et al. (1994). Fatigue and the cancer experience: The state of knowledge. *Oncology Nursing Forum, 21,* 23–26.

DEANNA M. GOLDEN-KREUTZ
SHARLA WELLS-DI GREGORIO

Cardiac Invalidism

Cardiac invalidism describes prolonged limits in physical abilities suffered by some people who have experienced a heart attack. Patients continue to function at a level below what could be expected based on illness severity alone and the patient's abilities are underestimated. People who experience cardiac invalidism show exaggerated signs of emotional distress, helplessness, and interpersonal dependency as a result of their new perceptions of poor health. Family members often contribute to cardiac invalidism by exaggerating the amount of care heart attack patients need and overprotecting them. Whereas overprotectiveness has been shown to be beneficial during the first month of recovery for heart attack patients, it can be detrimental if it persists. Although it can be disadvantageous to be overprotected, patients who do not receive the necessary support may be even worse off. Instead of engaging in overprotective behavior, encouragement from family members can lead to shorter recovery times and better adherence and adjustment.

Related Entries: Cardiovascular Rehabilitation, Coronary Heart Disease

S. BETH BELLMAN

Cardiovascular Rehabilitation

In the United States, cardiovascular disease is the leading cause of death and disability, accounting for nearly half of all deaths. Coronary artery disease (CAD), the major category in cardiovascular disease, manifests clinically as myocardial infarction ("heart attack"), angina pectoris (discomfort due to insufficient blood supply to the heart muscle from one or more coronary arteries), and sudden cardiac death. Heart failure, another major heart problem and often a result of CAD, is increasing in prevalence as the population ages and more people survive cardiovascular diseases; for many of these patients, heart transplantation and/or mechanical heart pumps (ventricular assist devices, or VADs) have become common treatment. Thus, for the several million survivors of CAD and heart failure each year, cardiovascular rehabilitation is a safe, efficacious, enjoyable, and economical treatment for improving functional capacity and quality and quantity of life.

The goals of cardiovascular rehabilitation include the following:

- Improved exercise tolerance resulting in increased functional capacity, lower body weight, blood pressure, and triglyceride levels, better stress management, and improved sleep.
- Improved symptoms including less discomfort from angina pectoris, claudication (aching in the legs from insufficient blood supply during activity), and shortness of breath, resulting in increased functional capacity and quality of life.
- Achieving and maintaining therapeutic levels of blood lipids, such as cholesterol, triglycerides, and low-density lipoproteins (LDL or "bad" cholesterol) and a higher level of high-density lipoproteins (HDL or "good" cholesterol), resulting in weight loss and improved symptoms.
- Cessation of tobacco use resulting in increased HDL, improved exercise tolerance, and decreased symptoms of angina, claudication, and shortness of breath.
- Stress management resulting in decreased blood pressure, improvement in blood lipids, improved sleep, and improved psychosocial well-being.
- Decreased mortality and cardiovascular morbidity.

It should be apparent that these goals are inextricably interdependent and interrelated, comprising the components of a successful comprehensive cardiovascular rehabilitation program that can be successfully implemented by a team of dedicated multidisciplinary professionals. Cardiovascular rehabilitation programs are long term (thrice weekly for several weeks), individualized, and comprehensive, involving medical evaluation, supervised electrocardiograph-monitored exercise and strength training, CAD risk factor modification (cessation of tobacco use, attaining and maintaining ideal body weight and blood lipid values, stress management, and medical management), education, and counseling. Led by a qualified physician, the health care team usually consists of registered nurses, exercise physiologists, physical therapists, registered dietitians, psychologists, and/or social workers, with occupational or vocational therapists and pharmacists involved as necessary.

It is imperative to recognize the importance of long-term adherence. Without sustained risk factor modification and behavioral change, a course in cardiovascular rehabilitation will not have maximum long-term benefit. Thus, the importance of psychosocial variables cannot be overemphasized. Depression, the hostility component of the Type A behavior pattern, stress management, social isolation, low socioeconomic status, tobacco abuse, some eating habits, and long-term behavioral change require targeted assessment and intervention by qualified clinicians. Without effective management, such psychosocial variables often sabotage even the best-planned cardiovascular rehabilitation program.

Related Entries: Cardiac Invalidism, Coronary Heart Disease

PATRICIA LOUNSBURY

Cardiovascular System

The cardiovascular system circulates blood and certain chemicals continuously throughout the body, providing oxygen, nutrients, and hormones to live body organs and tissues and removing waste products from them. Its remarkably flexible and

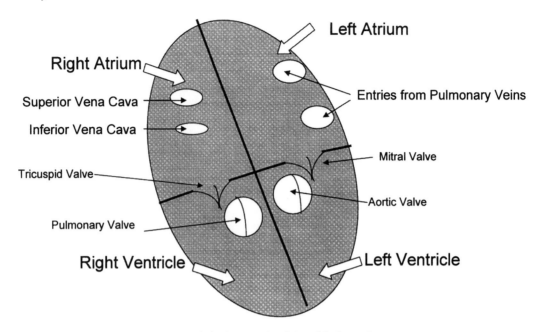

Figure 1.   Stylized cross-sectional view of the human heart.

adaptive nature allows the cardiovascular system to increase and decrease blood flow to specific areas of the body as a function of regional metabolic demands and other factors. During digestion, for example, blood flow to the stomach and intestines increases relative to the large muscle beds in the arms and legs, whereas during intense aerobic exercise, the reverse occurs. Highly evolved physical structures and control systems regulate the operation of the cardiovascular system.

THE HEART

The heart is best described as a sophisticated four-chambered, two-cycle pump that circulates blood throughout the cardiovascular system and hence the body. The size and shape of a clenched fist, the heart consists mostly of specialized striate muscle sometimes labeled cardiac muscle. The major physical anatomical structures of the heart include chambers and valves (see Figure 1). Sophisticated neural and endocrine control systems regulate the operation of the heart.

Anatomical Structures

Chambers

The heart consists of four chambers, two *atria* ("left" and "right") located toward the top of the heart and two *ventricles* ("left" and "right") located toward the bottom of the heart. The atrial pair operates (i.e., contracts) in tandem, as does the ventricular pair. Each atrium is paired with a ventricle (left with left, right with right) and they are connected via a valve.

Blood returning from bodily tissues and organs flows into the atria, the right atrium receiving oxygen-deficient blood from the body, the left receiving oxygenated blood from the lungs. When contracting (the first pumping cycle), the atria operate as "primer pumps," each forcing a bolus of blood into its respective ventricle. Considered the "power pumps" of the heart, the ventricles function primarily to pump blood to the lungs and body. When contracting (the second pumping cycle), the right ventricle pumps the oxygen-deficient blood received from the right atrium to the lungs and the left ventricle pumps oxygenated blood received from the left atrium to the rest of the body.

Valves

The heart contains four valves, which control the direction of blood flow within and from the heart. The valves operate in conjunction with atrial and ventricular contraction. The atrioventricular (AV) valves, tricuspid and mitral, located near the bottom of each atrium, connect the right atrium to the right ventricle, and the left atrium to the left ventricle, respectively. These "one-way" valves control blood flow into the ventricles and normally prevent blood from flowing back into the atria when the ventricles contract. Blood flowing in the reverse direction (e.g., due to deficient valve operation) causes distinctive sounds known as "heart murmurs."

Two semilunar valves, each a "one-way valve," located near the top of each ventricle, regulate the outflow of blood from the heart, thereby controlling blood flow from the ventricles to the arteries, and normally prevent backflow from the arteries. The pulmonary or right semilunar valve opens during systole (ventricular contraction), allowing deoxygenated blood flow to the lungs. The aortic or left semilunar valve also opens during systole, allowing oxygenated blood flow to arteries serving the body.

Control Systems

A sophisticated control system regulates the operation of the heart. It includes autoregulatory, neural, and hormonal components, each capable of dominating regulation, thereby providing redundancy, but normally working in concert.

Autoregulation

Its autoregulatory system can drive the heart independently of neural and endocrine control. Indeed, hearts can beat for relatively lengthy periods of time when removed from the body. Specialized spontaneously firing pacemaker cells comprise this autoregulatory system, causing the heart to beat at approximately 100 beats per minute. The sinoatrial node, located in the right atrial wall near the opening of the superior vena cava, serves as the heart's internal pacemaker. Neural and endocrine control mechanisms modulate the autoregulatory function of the pacemaker cells.

Neural Control

Neural regulation of the heart occurs via the autonomic branch of the peripheral nervous system. Both major branches of the autonomic nervous system synapse with the sinoatrial node, regulating its firing rate; sympathetic innervation increases or accelerates its rate, and parasympathetic (via the vagus) innervation decreases or brakes its rate. Normally, parasympathetic stimulation predominates, causing the sinoatrial node to fire (and the heart to beat) between 60 and 80 times per minute.

When the sinoatrial node fires, depolarization spreads across and down the striate muscle fibers of the atria, causing them to contract. Eventually this depolarization reaches and fires the atrioventricular node located in the wall of the right ventricle near the tricuspid valve. Functionally, the atrioventricular node delays the cardiac signal (i.e., the spread of depolarization to the striate muscles of the ventricles) by approximately 110 msec, thereby allowing the atria to pump their contents via atrial contraction into the ventricles.

Subsequently, the atrioventricular node transmits the cardiac signal to the striate muscle fibers of the ventricles via the atrioventricular bundle also know as the Bundle of His. This bundle consists of Purkinje fibers, which branch slightly below the atrioventicular node following the line of the ventricular septum that separates the left from the right ventricles to the apex of the ventricles located at the "bottom" of the heart. The Purkinje fibers of the bundle then separate and spread branching upward and outward over the ventricular striate muscle. When the atrioventricular node fires, the neural signal travels down the atrioventricular bundle branches and the up the Purkinje fibers, causing the ventricles of contract from the bottom upward and forcing their contents toward the tops of the ventricles, thereby putting pressure on the semilunar valves to open. When sufficient contraction has taken place, the valves open, allowing their contents to flow outward to the lungs (from the right ventricle) and the aorta (from the left ventricle).

Endocrine Control

Hormonal control of the heart occurs via sympathetically regulated adrenal medullary activity and the hypothalamic pituitary adrenal cortical activity. When fired (e.g., during a potentially stressful or threatening situation) sympathetic projections to the adrenal medullae stimulate the release of ephinephrine (adrenaline) into the blood stream. This hormone increases the firing rate of sympathetic nerves synapsing at the heart (i.e., sinoatrial node), causing the heart to beat faster and circulating more blood to the lungs and body. Circulating epinephrine also tends to dilate the arteries and thicken the blood. However, certain effects of sympathetic adrenal medullary release of epinephrine can be moderated by pituitary adrenal cortical activity that inhibits the former's inotropic (cardiac output) and vasodilatory effects.

THE VASCULATURE

Blood pumped from the heart flows to bodily tissues and organs via an elaborate system of vessels that form the vasculature. Arteries and arterioles carry blood away from the heart; venuoles and veins carry blood back to the heart. Arteries eventually branch into the smaller arterioles, which feed even smaller vessels called capillaries (vessels with thin, permeable walls). Exchange of oxygen and nutrients for carbon dioxide and waste products occurs at the level of the capillaries. The deoxygenated blood then flows to venuoles and then into the large veins and eventually returns to the right atrium of the heart via the inferior and superior vena cavae. Arteries and arterioles regulate the regional flow of blood in the body via their vasodilatory and vasoconstrictive capabilities.

BLOOD

As described in the foregoing, blood has a number of important biological functions. First, blood carries the oxygen and nutrients that the cardiovascular system delivers to the body. Second, blood carries carbon dioxide and waste products to specialized organs that help eliminate them from the body (e.g., lungs, liver, kidneys). Third, blood transports hormones (e.g., epinephrine) to target organs. Fourth, blood helps regulate body temperature.

Blood has three major components: cells, platelets, and plasma. Cells fall into two major categories (and several subcategories): red and white. Red blood cells (erythrocytes), which comprise about 45 percent of blood volume, transport oxygen. They are composed largely of hemoglobin, the chemical agent that carries oxygen. White blood cells (leukocytes), which normally comprise 1 percent of blood volume, attack and destroy agents foreign to the body (e.g., viruses, bacteria, parasites, cancer cells). Platelets (thrombocytes) function to form clots at the sites of ruptures to blood vessels. Like white blood cells, platelets normally comprise 1 percent of blood volume. Blood cells and platelets are suspended in plasma, which comprises the remaining blood volume (approximately 53 percent) and is 90 percent water.

CARDIOVASCULAR DYSFUNCTION

Remarkably, given its complicated nature, the cardiovascular system can sustain human life for more than a century despite the repeated loads put on it during both routine and nonroutine daily activities. Nevertheless, various problems can plague the cardiovascular system and reduce its effectiveness or lead to death. Heart problems form the single largest cause of human morbidity and mortality (>50 percent). Notable among these problems are hypertension, ischemic heart disease, valve malfunctions, and leukemias (cancers of the blood). Behavioral processes, especially those involving stress responses, have increasingly been shown to play a major role in many aspects of cardiovascular dysfunction. These problems can be addressed via preventive behavioral (e.g., diet, exercise, stress reduction) and ameliorative biomedical measures (e.g., pharmacological agents, surgery).

Related Entries: Angina Pectoris, Atherosclerosis, Blood Pressure, Coronary Heart Disease, Hypertension

JIM BLASCOVICH

Cholesterol

Cholesterol is one of several lipids or fats that circulate in the body; it can originate from both endogenous and exogenous sources. Other related lipids include trigylcerides, fatty acids, phospholipids, and cholesterol esters. Because lipids are hydrophobic, most of the time they circulate through the blood after combining with particular proteins called apolipoproteins. The resulting particles are called lipoproteins, and include high-density lipoprotein (HDL), low-density lipoprotein (LDL), very low density lipoprotein (VLDL), chylomicrons, as well as others. Thus, lipoproteins transport lipids from one tissue site to another. The lipoproteins are classified according to their chemical composition (i.e., the amount and type of lipid and protein), size, density, and electrophoretic mobility. While the lipoproteins are in the circulation, they undergo rapid and repeated changes in their structure, composition, and function. Once the lipoproteins are internalized into a cell, the various portions of the particles are delivered to specific sites to be ultimately used for energy, cell membrane structure, and/or synthesis of steroid hormones and bile acids.

Most cells in the body are not well equipped to store lipids, and excess lipids therefore can accumulate in the blood and ultimately become deposited in the arterial walls. These fibrous plaques gradually build and ultimately occlude the lumen of the arterial wall. When blood can no longer flow through the vessel adequately, a clinical event such as myocardial infarction (heart attack) or angina (chest pain and shortness of breath) occurs. LDL is the major carrier of cholesterol in the blood, and epidemiologic and clinical investigations have demonstrated that high concentrations of LDL are a risk factor for cardiovascular disease (CVD). Similar types of investigations have shown that high concentrations of HDL appear to be cardioprotective.

Blood concentrations of the lipids are determined by behavioral influences and by genetics. Some lipoproteins (i.e., chylomicrons, triglycerides, and VLDL) are much more strongly influenced by lifestyle factors, whereas others [e.g, Lp(a)] are almost entirely influenced by genetic contributions. Heritability estimates for the major lipoproteins commonly linked with risk of CVD, namely LDL and HDL, are around 0.5.

Various interventions have been aimed at changing the concentrations of lipids and lipoproteins with the overall aim of reducing subsequent risk of CVD. Although most interventions have focused on reducing total cholesterol, LDL-c, and, to a lesser extent, Lp(a), some have also targeted increasing HDL-c. Interventions include reducing dietary fat consumption and body weight, increasing activity level, increasing smoking cessation rates and adherence, and initiating various pharmacologic treatments (see Table 1). In general, lipid lowering is most successful when a combination of these interventions is employed, particularly among individuals with greatly elevated lipid concentrations.

Ironically, although the number of cardiovascular events decreases in those with lowered cholesterol, overall mortality is not significantly reduced. Various multiethnic studies have found that patients with low cholesterol are at an increased risk for non-illness-related deaths including suicide, homicide, and accidents. Personality characteristics, such as hostility,

Table 1. Average Percentage Change in Lipids with Various Cholesterol-Lowering Interventions

Intervention	Change in total cholesterol	Change in LDL-c	Change in HDL-c
Medications			
Statins[a]	▼ 19	▼ 27	▲ 4
Fibrates[b]		▼ 5–20	▲ 10–20
Resins[b]		▼ 10–20	▲ 4–6
Dietary changes			
Low-fat[b,c,d]	▼ 5–13	▼ 3–17	▲ 2
Low-fat vegetarian[e]	▼ 13.2	▼ 16.9	▲ 16.5
Dietary supplements			
Soy[f]	▼ 9.3	▼ 12.9	▲ 2.4
Plant sterol[b]	▼ 9–20	▼ 9–20	▲ 5.5
Combined interventions			
Diet + exercise[c,d]	▼ 4–6	▼ 6	▲ 1–13

[a] MacMahon, S., Sharpe, N., Gamble, G., Hart, H., Scott, J., Simes, J., et al. (1998). Effects of lowering average or below-average cholesterol levels on the progression of carotid atherosclerosis. *Circulation, 97*, 1784–1790.

[b] Mosca, L. J. (2002). Contemporary management of hyperlipidemia in women. *Journal of Women's Health and Gender-Based Medicine, 11*, 423–432.

[c] Lalonde, L., Gray-Donald, K., Lowensteyn, I., Marchand, S., Dorais, M., Michaels, G., et al. (2002). Comparing the benefits of diet and exercise in the treatment of dyslipidemia. *Preventive Medicine, 35*, 16–24.

[d] Wood, P. D., Stefanick, M. I., Williams, P. T., & Haskell, W. L. (1991). The effects on plasma lipoproteins of a prudent weight-reducing diet, with or without exercise, in overweight men and women. *New England Journal of Medicine, 325*, 461–466.

[e] Barnard, N. D., Sciallo, A. R., Bertron, P., Hurlock, D., Edmonds, K., & Talev, L. (2000). Diet in altering serum lipids in healthy premenopausal women. *American Journal of Cardiology, 85*, 969–972.

[f] Anderson, J. W., Johnstone, B. M., & Cook-Newell, M. E. (1995). Meta-analysis of the effects of soy protein intake on serum lipids. *New England Journal of Medicine, 333*, 276–282.

depression, impulsivity, and violent behavior, have been linked with low or lowered cholesterol levels in both the general population and in psychiatric populations. It has been hypothesized that reducing cholesterol, specifically the intake of polyunsaturated fatty acids, may lead to the irregularities in serotonin that are often observed in suicidal individuals.

A more comprehensive understanding of the mechanisms linking personality, behavior, and environment with lipid concentrations will ultimately help to further our understanding of how lipids are regulated.

Related Entries: Coronary Heart Disease, Nutrition

BIBLIOGRAPHY

Bucher, H. C., Griffith, L. E., & Guyatt, G. H. (1999). Systematic review on the risk and benefit of different cholesterol-lowering interventions. *Arteriosclerosis, Thrombosis, and Vascular Biology, 19*, 187–195.

Hillbrand, M., & Spitz, R. T. (Eds.). (1997). *Lipids, Health, and Behavior.* Washington, DC: American Psychological Association.

Stoney, C. M., & Finney, M. (2000). Cholesterol and lipoproteins. In G. Fink (Ed.), *Encyclopedia of Stress* (Vol. 1). New York: Academic.

CATHERINE M. STONEY
KRISTIN KUNTZ

Chronic Fatigue Syndrome

Chronic Fatigue Syndrome (CFS), also known as chronic fatigue and immune dysfunction syndrome (CFIDS) and myalgic encephalomyelitis (ME), is a serious health concern. CFS is a debilitating condition characterized by severe and persisting fatigue, not attributable to ongoing exertion or lack of rest, and worsened by physical or mental activity. There is widespread disruption of central and peripheral nervous system and physiological function, which waxes and wanes over time. Little is known about the etiology and pathophysiology of this condition; in ignorance, people with CFS have been accused of malingering or faking. Historically, case descriptions of CFS date to the late 18th century. The lack of understanding of this syndrome by the medical community has provided tremendous hardship and obstacles for persons with CFS seeking treatment. Recent estimates indicate that about 1.3 million people in the United States have CFS, but 85–90 percent of these persons go undiagnosed and untreated. These individuals are either unaware that they are suffering from CFS or they are fearful of the stigma attached to such a diagnosis. At this time, treatment plans are symptom focused and relatively ineffective in ameliorating the symptomatology. However, there are significant clues that have led to scientific investigation and have provided hope for more rapid progress in establishing the underlying pathological mechanisms.

DEFINITION, SYMPTOMS, AND DIFFERENTIAL DIAGNOSIS

The term "chronic fatigue syndrome" was proposed by the U.S. Centers for Disease Control and Prevention in 1988 and revised in 1994. To exclude other mental and physical causes of their symptoms, persons with CFS must undergo an extensive battery of tests before the CFS diagnosis is considered. The International CFS Working Group's 1994 CFS case definition criteria include 6 months or more of clinically evaluated, unexplained, persistent or relapsing fatigue and four of eight concurrent symptoms that do not predate the fatigue. The fatigue must (1) be of new or definite onset, (2) not be the result of ongoing exertion, (3) not be substantially alleviated by rest, and (4) result in substantial reduction in previous levels of occupational, educational, social, or personal activities. Concurrent symptoms include four or more of the following symptoms: (1) impaired short-term memory or concentration, (2) sore throat, (3) tender lymph nodes, (4) muscle pain, (5) multijoint pain without arthritis, (6) headaches of a new type, pattern, or severity, (7) unrefreshing sleep; and (8) postexertional malaise lasting more than 24 hr.

Fatigue is a prominent symptom in a number of other clinical disorders including fibromyalgia, irritable bowel syndrome, major depression, anxiety, and somatoform disorders. In persons with these disorders there are also several symptoms that overlap with CFS symptomatology including sleep disturbance, neurocognitive impairment, mood changes, and musculoskeletal pain. For example, CFS and fibromyalgia are so similar that an emphasis on musculoskeletal pain symptoms is the main characteristic that distinguishes them. In addition, up to 75 percent of CFS patients report either current or past major depression, whereas lifetime prevalence of depressive disorders in the general population is only 13–25 percent. Such comorbidity is not surprising, as diagnostic criteria for both CFS and major depression includes fatigue, sleep disturbance, and cognitive impairment. Even more challenging is the distinction between CFS and somatoform disorders, as the latter describe persons with unexplainable physical symptoms that are believed to result from underlying psychological processes. Other comorbid conditions include irritable bowel syndrome, multiple chemical sensitivities, temporomandibular disorder, interstitial cystitis, postconcussion syndrome, tension headache, chronic low back pain, chronic pelvic pain (women), and chronic nonbacterial prostatitis (men). Therefore, when making a CFS diagnosis, a careful assessment to exclude alternative diagnoses is essential.

PREVALENCE AND DEMOGRAPHICS

CFS primarily affects individuals between 20 and 50 years of age. Accurate prevalence studies are difficult to conduct in absence of a sensitive laboratory marker. Although fatigue is a relatively frequently reported symptom, affecting up to 74 percent of all people visiting general practitioners, CFS prevalence following the exclusion of comorbid conditions is considerably lower, with 200–1000 cases occurring per 100,000 adults, or 0.2–1 percent. A recent epidemiologic study estimates the CFS prevalence at approximately 422 per 100,000 adults in the United States. Thus, as many as 1.3 million people nationwide may suffer from the condition. To put CFS prevalence into perspective, systemic lupus affects 50 per 100,000, multiple sclerosis affects 104 per 100,000, and rheumatoid arthritis affects 1,022 per 100,000 adults. In addition, CFS has been identified in children and adolescents, albeit with diminished prevalence; an Australian study reported 5 cases per 100,000 children up to age 9 years and 48 pediatric cases per 100,000 for ages 10 to 19 years.

Of those diagnosed with CFS, about 70 percent are women. This sex specificity may be because women seek medical care more frequently than men do. However, studies indicate that fatigue symptoms appear to be more prevalent in people from more socially disadvantaged groups, who have poorer access to medical care. There is now evidence that CFS affects all racial and ethnic groups. Another study has indicated that a high rate of CFS occurs in nurses, suggesting that specific environmental influences may pose additional risk.

ETIOLOGICAL CLUES

Although twin studies suggest a genetic vulnerability to the disorder, there is growing evidence that CFS is heterogeneous, and it is likely that it will have no single cause. There is no evidence that CFS is caused by a neuromuscular pathology. Several other possible etiologies have been proposed, including central nervous system (CNS), neuroendocrine and autonomic nervous system functional dysregulation, infections, and immunological factors.

CNS, Neuroendocrine, and Autonomic Nervous System

Among psychological factors, no link has been found between psychological events (e.g., childhood abuse) and CFS. However, CFS patients were more likely to have experienced critical life events prior to disease onset. Although several other lines of investigation suggest altered CNS function in CFS, including high rates of major depression, the pattern of psychological changes observed in CFS patients is different from that seen in people with depression; hence, different pathophysiologic processes are indicated. No conclusive evidence of a link to CFS from other premorbid psychiatric disorders has been documented.

CFS patients frequently suffer from sleep disturbances; research on increased sensitivity to serotonin and on changes in brain structure and function has yielded no definitive findings. Impairments in neuroendocrine function, namely in hypothalamic–pituitary–adrenal axis (HPA) activation, have also been reported in CFS patients. Physical, emotional, and mental challenges induce fatigue and other CFS symptoms that may last about 2–4 days. Such stressful challenges induce HPA axis activation and result in cortisol and corticotrophin-releasing hormone (CRH) secretion. These substances influence immune function by suppressing inflammation and cellular immunoactivation and also affect other systemic function. Some studies have shown a reduction in cortisol levels and HPA axis/CRH functionality in CFS patients. Therefore, depressed HPA axis function may affect CFS patients by its influence on systemic function.

There is accumulating data that most CFS patients have difficulty sustaining an upright posture. Significant hypotension, racing heart rate, and light-headedness are common observations during postural challenges. These confluent signs are consistent with autonomic dysregulation of circulation, manifesting as orthostatic intolerance in which postural tachycardia syndrome and/or hypotensive syncope, dizziness, and a transient loss of consciousness and postural tone may be observed. Moreover, there is evidence that many CFS patients have diminished red blood cell volume. Because the red blood cell transports oxygen and blood sugar to the cells, the impairment of this function could account for persistent fatigue and circulatory dysfunction in CFS.

Infection

In addition to fatigue, CFS is associated with chronic or recurrent flulike symptoms, including sore throat, lymph node pain and tenderness, headache, and muscle and joint pain, suggesting an infectious etiology. A majority of patients self-report an infectious onset to their illness. Epstein–Barr virus, triggering infectious mononucleosis, has been shown to precede CFS onset. However, Epstein–Barr viral reactivation is not more prevalent in CFS. There is a strong support against a role in CFS of retroviruses, viruses such as human immunodeficiency virus, spumavirus, and leukemia virus that use the DNA machinery of the cell to reproduce. However, evidence is conflicting for a role of enteroviruses, such as human herpesvirus-6 and borna disease virus, which are small viruses that multiply in the gut lining and are transmitted from person to person by the fecal-oral route. Among the nonviral infections, Lyme disease and Q fever have been implicated. The consensus is that CFS is not contagious and cannot be caused exclusively by any single recognized infectious agent.

Immunological Factors

CFS patients demonstrate altered immunological profiles including increased numbers of neutrophils and activated lymphocytes but depressed amounts of some kinds of antibody and decreased numbers and function of other immune cells, suggesting that chronic and perhaps multiple infectious and/or allergic sources are exerting an etiological role. Still, some cells are working too hard, making chemical messengers called cytokines that cause inflammation, which are associated with that "flulike" feeling. The fine tuning of the immune system does not seem to turn off this inflammatory process. Among proinflammatory conditions associated with CFS, serum elevations of immune cytokines (e.g., IL-6) have been reported. Proinflammatory mediators produced, for example, in response to infectious or allergic sources have been shown to induce fatigue, sleep–wake cycle disruption, mental confusion, and diminished red blood cell production. In addition, studies of CFS patients have reported reduced numbers of natural killer (NK) cells along with a reduction in their function. The NK cell is an immune cell that provides first-line defense against infection and also releases perforin, a chemical messenger that turns off proinflammatory

activity. The lack of perforin may to lead to prolonged persistence of inflammatory conditions. In sum, there are a number of findings that suggest an immune-mediated CFS etiology exists that has system-wide biobehavioral impact.

TREATMENT

The several clinical treatment approaches available are symptom focused. No specific diagnostic test for CFS has been identified. Laboratory blood tests are conducted primarily to rule out underlying medical conditions. Initially, control of key symptoms such as pain, sleep disturbance, and depressed mood with standard pharmacologic treatments is explored. Once these methods prove helpful for the patient, treatment may be coordinated with nonpharmacologic forms of care.

Pharmacologic Treatments

Drug treatment clinical trials based on immune/allergy approaches have demonstrated only marginal improvements in some studies. Antidepressants have also been assessed, but limited improvements in fatigue have been observed. Although serotonin reuptake inhibitor agents are popular for treating depression and mood instability, there has been little evidence of their usefulness in alleviating CFS symptoms. Corticosteroid trials demonstrated some reduction in fatigue, but the observed effect was due to a significant depression of adrenal function; long-term use of corticosteroids is associated with serious morbidity and cannot be recommended.

Nonpharmacologic Approaches

Due to some reports of nutritional deficiencies in CFS patients, studies were undertaken to provide nutrient supplements, such as folic acid, vitamins B12 and C, magnesium, zinc, and omega 3 fatty acids. Results from these studies are inconclusive. Trials evaluating graded exercise therapy reported overall but limited improvements in fatigue, functional work capacity, and fitness of CFS patients. Cognitive–behavioral therapy also has produced positive outcomes for a majority of CFS patients, for whom decreased frequency of primary care visits, improvements in fatigue severity, physical functioning, and increased self-confidence were observed. In addition to skill-training methods for coping with stressful challenges, the cognitive component of this therapy is aimed at identifying beliefs and behaviors that may impair recovery. In contrast with earlier treatment beliefs, which advocated prolonged rest and social withdrawal, current evidence suggests that behavioral approaches may be an essential component of managing CFS. Alternative treatments, including herbal supplements, physical rehabilitation, acupuncture, homeopathy, chiropractic, guided imagery, self-hypnosis, massage therapy, energy healing, religious healing, oxygen therapy, and dietary restrictions, have been proposed, but scientific evidence for these approaches is lacking.

CONCLUSION

The historical record indicates that CFS is an old clinical problem derailed by ignorance and biases. Scientific examination of this syndrome is in its infancy. From what is known about CFS, it can be characterized as an illness that has widespread and complex physiological and psychological impact. Together, the difficulty in diagnosing CFS, the broad range of prevailing symptomatology, and the evidence of multisystem (i.e., CNS, immune, neuroendocrine, and circulatory) abnormalities suggest that multifactorial interactive biobehavioral processes are likely underlying its etiology. Hence a formidable scientific challenge exists that perhaps requires a more multidisciplinary biobehavioral approach to ascertain an understanding of the pathophysiologic basis of CFS.

Related Entry: Depression

BIBLIOGRAPHY

Center for Disease Control and Prevention, National Center for Infectious Diseases. (2002). *Chronic Fatigue Syndrome.* Available at www.cdc.gov/ncidod/diseases/cfs/info.htm

Demitrack, M. A., & Crofford, L. J. (1998). Evidence for and pathophysiologic implications of hypothalamic–pituitary–adrenal axis dysregulation in fibromyalgia and chronic fatigue syndrome. *Annals of the New York Academy of Science, 840,* 684–697.

Evengard, B., Schacterle, R. S., & Komaroff, A. L. (1999). Chronic fatigue syndrome: New insights and old ignorance. *Journal of Internal Medicine, 246*(5), 455–469.

Freeman, R., & Komaroff, A. L. (1997). Does the chronic fatigue syndrome involve the autonomic nervous system? *American Journal of Medicine, 102*(4), 357–364.

Fukuda, K., Straus, S. E., Hickie, I., Sharpe, M. C., Dobbins, J. G., & Komaroff, A. L. (1994). The chronic fatigue syndrome: A comprehensive approach to its definition and study. International Chronic Fatigue Syndrome Study Group. *Annals of Internal Medicine, 121,* 953–959.

Glaser, R., & Kiecolt-Glaser, J. K. (1998). Stress-associated immune modulation: Relevance of viral infections and chronic fatigue syndrome. *American Journal of Medicine, 105*(3A), 35S–42S.

Hurwitz, B. E., Brownley, K. A., Fletcher, M. A., & Klimas, N. G. (2000). Chronic fatigue syndrome: Evidence supporting the hypothesis of a behaviorally-activated neuromodulator of fatigue. *Journal of Chronic Fatigue Syndrome, 6*(2), 45–63.

Jason, L. A., Richman, J. A., Rademaker, A. W., Jordan, K. M., Plioplys, A. V., Taylor, R. R., et al. (1999). A community-based study of chronic fatigue syndrome. *Archives of Internal Medicine, 159*(18), 2129–2137.

Patarca, R. (2001). Cytokines and chronic fatigue syndrome. *Annals of the New York Academy of Science, 933,* 185–200.

Strauss, S. E. (1991). History of chronic fatigue syndrome. *Review of Infectious Diseases, 13*(Supplement 1), S2–S7.

Whiting, P., Bagnall, A.-M., Sowden, A. J., Cornell, J. E., Mulrow, C. D., & Ramirez, G. (2001). Interventions for the treatment and management of chronic fatigue syndrome. *Journal of American Medical Association, 286,* 1360–1368.

Barry E. Hurwitz

Chronic Illness

A chronic illness is defined as an illness that is enduring. The course of the disease may be progressive or characterized by symptom flare-ups and remissions. The unique feature of a chronic illness is that it is not reversible. It is long lasting, which distinguishes it from an acute illness, such as a cold or a flu or even appendicitis.

Two of the most common chronic illnesses in our culture, heart disease and cancer, are also the first and second leading causes of death. Heart disease is not considered curable or reversible, but is treatable. People who have coronary artery disease (blockages in the arteries that provide blood to the heart) are often treated with medication, coronary angioplasty, or bypass surgery. It is difficult to discuss cancer as a broad category of chronic illness because there are over 150 kinds of cancer. The most prevalent kind of cancer in men is prostate cancer and the most prevalent kind of cancer in women is breast cancer. Both are highly treatable because the majority are diagnosed at an early stage. The leading cause of cancer death in both men and women is lung cancer because it is typically diagnosed at a more advanced stage of disease and is less treatable. Common cancer treatments include surgery, chemotherapy, and hormonal therapy.

A large class of chronic illnesses are those in which the immune system attacks and destroys healthy tissue. In other words, the immune system cannot discriminate between tissue that belongs to the self and tissue that is foreign. These are known as autoimmune disorders. One autoimmune disease that has increased dramatically in our country since the 1980s is acquired immunodeficiency syndrome (AIDS), which caused by the human immunodeficiency virus (HIV), which destroys the white blood cells of the immune system. Early symptoms of HIV infection include a low-grade fever, fatigue, diarrhea, and rashes. When the virus has spread to the point of severe damage to multiple parts of the body, the person is said to have AIDS. AIDS is the end stage of HIV infection. HIV is thought to be terminal, meaning that there is no cure. However, treatments for HIV can prolong life, sometimes by more than 10 years.

Other common autoimmune disorders include lupus, arthritis, and multiple sclerosis. Systemic lupus erythematosus, or lupus, is a chronic inflammatory disease of the connective tissue (muscles, tendons) and is incurable. It affects multiple systems of the body and is accompanied by symptom flare-ups (e.g., achiness, fatigue, fever) but is generally not fatal. Arthritis affects one in seven Americans and there are more than 100 kinds of arthritis. Osteoarthritis is the most common form and involves the breakdown of cartilage and bones. It is a disease that increases in prevalence with age. Rheumatoid arthritis is the most severe form of arthritis and is manifested by an inflammation of peripheral joints (e.g., knees), pain, swelling, and stiffness. As it progresses, it may affect the heart and lungs. Multiple sclerosis (MS) is a progressive disorder of the central nervous system and results from the loss of the myelin sheath that surrounds neurons and facilitates neural transmission. People with MS vary in the severity of impairment from mild disabilities to a disabling form of the disease that requires use of a wheelchair. The cause of these autoimmune disorders is largely unknown.

Diabetes is an autoimmune disease that occurs when the immune system attacks the beta cells in the islets of Langerhans on the pancreas. Beta cells produce insulin, a hormone necessary for glucose metabolism. Someone with Type 1 diabetes must administer insulin on a daily basis because the body no longer produces any insulin. Someone with Type 2 diabetes may be able to control blood sugar levels through diet or medication because insulin production is impaired but not absent. There are long-term consequences of diabetes, including blindness, kidney disease, nerve disease (which may result in amputations), heart disease, and stroke. The management of diabetes by diet, testing, exercise, and medication influences whether these complications occur.

Chronic illnesses differ in controllability, predictability, severity, and progression. For example, the long-term complications from diabetes are amenable to personal control. The behaviors required to exert this control, however, are extensive (i.e., medication, exercise, diet). The disease course of breast cancer, by contrast, is much less amenable to personal control. Treatments may prolong life but there are not a set of behaviors that one can advise a patient to perform to keep the breast cancer from progressing. Chronic illnesses also vary in predictability. Many people with heart disease have symptoms of the disease, such as chest pain and shortness of breath, that would lead them to seek medical attention or signify disease progression. People diagnosed with breast or prostate cancer, by contrast, often feel healthy just prior to diagnosis and have few if any warning signs of the disease. Many illnesses naturally progress in severity over time, such as heart disease with age, but other illnesses, such as asthma, may remain stable over a long time.

These dimensions of chronic illness may influence how one adjusts to the disease psychologically as well as physically. A less controllable, less predictable, and more severe disease will be associated with greater emotional distress and more disruption to daily life. There are also characteristics of the person and the environment that influence psychological and physical adjustment to disease.

PERSONALITY

Personality characteristics can be grouped into vulnerability factors and resistance factors. One of the first vulnerability factors identified in the history of behavioral medicine was the Type A behavior pattern. People characterized as Type A are hard driving, impatient, and hostile. In large epidemiologic studies of healthy people, this behavior pattern prospectively predicted the onset of heart disease. In more recent years, researchers have learned that the toxic component of Type A is hostility (Williams, 1989). Depression is another vulnerability factor to disease. Depression has been most strongly linked to heart disease. A vulnerability factor, which has been associated with depression and also mortality, is the pessimistic attributional style. People who tend to attribute negative outcomes to internal, stable, and global causes while attributing positive outcomes to external, unstable, and specific causes are characterized by a pessimistic attributional style. This style has been examined from records of Harvard student interviews and newspaper quotes from baseball Hall of Famers and shown to predict poor health (Seligman, 1990).

One of the first resistance factors to disease identified was hardiness. Hardy people were characterized by the three c's: a sense of commitment, control, and challenge (i.e., they view obstacles as challenges). Early research showed that hardy people were less vulnerable to illness during times of stress. More recent research has examined the separate components of hardiness. The construct of control has received a large amount of attention. People with a sense of personal control typically adjust better to chronic illness.

One theory about how people would adjust better to traumatic events, including chronic illness, is cognitive adaptation theory. According to cognitive adaptation theory (Taylor, 1989), people who have a high regard for themselves (positive self-esteem), an optimistic view of the future, a sense of personal control, and the ability to derive meaning from a negative experience adjust better to disease. This theory has been supported among women with breast cancer, people with heart disease, and men with HIV. Optimism is one component of the theory that has generated a research area of its own. Optimism has predicted quicker recovery from bypass surgery, fewer heart attacks during bypass surgery, and reduced mortality among people with cancer (Carver & Scheier, 1998).

SOCIAL ENVIRONMENT

The impact of the social environment on the onset of disease and adjustment to disease has been examined from three perspectives. First, measures of social networks have been calculated. This is a quantitative indicator of the number of social contacts and/or the amount of social contact one has. In epidemiologic studies, social network variables have predicted mortality (House, Landis, & Umberson, 1988). Second, the quality of people's relationships has been studied and measures of their supportiveness examined. Typologies of social support include three core components: emotional, informational, and instrumental. Among these, emotional support has the strongest links to psychological and physical adjustment to disease. More recently, researchers have realized that not all relationships are supportive, and unsupportive interactions have been identified. When both positive and negative features of relationships are measured, the negative aspects are often stronger predictors of disease adjustment.

A third way that the impact of the social environment has been studied is from studies of support interventions. Peer support groups exist in communities for a wide array of chronic illnesses (e.g., cancer) or chronic strains (e.g., caregivers of Alzheimer patients). A review of group support interventions for people with cancer concluded that peer support groups with an education focus (i.e., informational support) were more effective than peer support groups with a focus on emotional support (Helgeson & Gottlieb, 2000).

The impact of personality factors and the social environment on disease depends on a host of factors, such as age, severity, and controllability of the situation. For example, some studies have found that personality variables are more strongly related to health among younger people (Scheier & Bridges, 1995). The stress-buffering hypothesis says that social support is only related to good health among people who are under high levels of stress (Cohen & Wills, 1985). There is some evidence that perceptions of personal control are more strongly related to positive health outcomes when situations are amenable to control. Thus, the etiology of chronic illness as well as the disease course and adjustment process are determined by multiple factors that cut across the mind, the body, and the environment.

BIBLIOGRAPHY

Carver, C. S., & Scheier, M. F. (1998). *On the self-regulation of behavior.* New York: Cambridge University Press.

Cohen, S., & Wills, T. A. (1985). Stress, social support and buffering. *Psychological Bulletin, 98,* 310–357.

Helgeson, V. S., & Gottlieb, B. H. (2000). Support groups. In S. Cohen, L. G. Underwood, & B. H. Gottlieb (Eds.), *Social support measurement and intervention: A guide for health and social scientists.* (pp. 00–00). New York: Oxford University Press.

House, J. S., Landis, K. R., & Umberson, D. (1988). Social relationships and health. *Science, 241,* 540–545.

Scheier, M. F., & Bridges, M. W. (1995). Person variables and health: Personality predispositions and acute psychological states as shared determinants for disease. *Psychosomatic Medicine, 57,* 255–268.

Seligman, M. E. P. (1990). *Learned optimism.* New York: Springer-Verlag.

Taylor, S. E. (1989). *Positive illusions: Creative self-deception and the healthy mind.* New York: Basic Books.

Williams, R. (1989). *The trusting heart.* New York: Times.

VICKI S. HELGESON

Chronic Obstructive Pulmonary Disease

Chronic obstructive pulmonary disease (COPD) is a progressive disease that cannot be reversed. Obstructed breathing is due to swelling of the airway walls, excess mucus clogging the airways, and constriction of the muscles around the airways. In addition, air sacs within the lungs lose their supporting structure and elasticity, making it harder to push the air out. When this happens, air can be trapped inside the lungs, causing shortness of breath, increased work of breathing, decreased ventilation, and, eventually, depletion of oxygen to the body.

COPD is the fourth leading cause of death in the United States and is the only one of the top 10 causes that is continuing to rise. In the year 2000, estimates from the Centers for Disease Control and Prevention ranged from 10 adults with doctor-diagnosed COPD to 24 million with self-reported lung function impairment, suggesting many people with undiagnosed COPD. COPD is more prevalent among older adults, ranging between 20 and 50 percent in the 65- to 75-year-old age group, depending on race and smoking history.

Cigarette smoking is the primary risk factor for COPD. However, because not all smokers develop significant COPD, it is generally felt that COPD is caused by an interaction between personal factors and environmental exposures. Personal factors may include genetics, gender, lung size, and allergies and asthma.

Cigarette smoking is the primary environmental cause of COPD, due to prolonged irritation of the lungs by tobacco smoke. Smokers have the fastest disease progression and the highest death rates due to COPD. Even exposure to second-hand smoke may increase the risk of COPD. People who work around dusts and chemicals are at greater risk for developing COPD whether or not they smoke cigarettes. Both indoor and outdoor air pollution may also be related to developing COPD, but the risk is much lower compared to that for cigarette smoke.

The goal of COPD treatment is to relieve symptoms and improve the person's ability to function normally day to day. People with COPD are advised to stop smoking. A person who is diagnosed early with COPD and stops smoking can dramatically slow progression of the disease. Research sponsored by the National Heart, Lung and Blood Institute has demonstrated that smoking cessation can significantly slow the decline in lung function, with quitters' lung function declining at half the rate of continuing smokers' over 5 years.

Treatment of COPD includes several self-management activities such as a medication regimen, which can be complex. In addition to taking daily medicines, patients must recognize when to take additional medicine and when to call the doctor. Those with severe disease have more restricted activities due to the need to conserve energy, avoid exposure to airborne irritants, and keep up with medication and oxygen requirements. Over time, patients become deconditioned and can benefit from medically supervised exercise therapy.

Persons who have chronic disease such as COPD are not necessarily motivated to carry out self-management activities. Understanding the factors that influence whether or not a person stops smoking, takes medicine, and makes other lifestyle changes is a concern in health psychology research. Factors such as people's confidence in their ability to take these steps and their beliefs that taking the steps will have personal benefits are among those under study.

Related Entries: Asthma, Respiratory System

BIBLIOGRAPHY

Anthonisen, N. R., Connett, J. E., Kiley, J. P., Altose, M. D., Bailey, W. C., Buist, A. S., et al. (1994). Effects of smoking intervention and the use of an inhaled anticholinergic bronchodilator on the rate of decline of FEV1. The Lung Health Study. *Journal of the American Medical Association, 272*(19), 1497–1505.

Maninno, D. M., Gagnon R. C., Petty T. L., & Lydick E. (2000). Obstructive lung disease and low lung function in adults in the United States: Data from the National Health and Nutrition Examination Survey, 1988–1994. *Archives of Internal Medicine, 160*(11), 1683–1689.

Mannino, D. M., Homa, D. M., Akinbami, L. J., Ford, E. S., & Redd, S. C. (2002). Chronic obstructive pulmonary disease surveillance—United States, 1971–2000. *Respiratory Care, 47*, 1184–1199.

Scanlon, P. D., Connet, J. E., Waller, L. A., Altose, M. D., Bailey, W. C., & Buist, A. S. (2000). Smoking cessation and lung function in mild-to-moderate chronic obstructive pulmonary disease. The Lung Health Study. *American Journal of Respiratory and Critical Care Medicine, 161*(2 Part 1), 381–390.

U.S. Department of Health and Human Services. (2002). *Global strategy for the diagnosis, management, and prevention of COPD: NHLBI/WHO workshop report. Executive summary* (NIH Publication No. 02-2701). Washington, DC: Author.

U.S. Department of Health and Human Services. (2002). *What you can do about a lung disease called COPD. An information booklet for patients and their families.* Washington, DC: Author. Available from http://www.goldcopd.com

CONNIE L. KOHLER
WILLIAM C. BAILEY

Classical Conditioning

Classical conditioning, also called respondent conditioning, is a form of associative learning that involves repeatedly pairing two stimuli to elicit a reflexive response. This training results in the elicitation of a reflexive response by an environmental stimulus that would otherwise not elicit such a response. For example, when a puff of air is introduced to the eye, an organism blinks. This type of behavior can be called a reflex; an organism has no control over the blink when the puff of air is delivered to the eye. If the puff of air is repeatedly presented after a tone, then blinking will be elicited when the tone is subsequently presented alone. In this example, the puff of air is an unconditioned stimulus (UCS) that naturally elicits an eye blink, the unconditioned response (UCR). After the tone is repeatedly paired with the puff of air, it is called a conditioned stimulus (CS) because presentations of the tone by itself will elicit an eye blink, now called the conditioned response (CR).

Ivan Petrovitch Pavlov (1849–1936), a Russian physiologist, discovered classical conditioning during his study of digestion in dogs. When Pavlov presented a dog with food (UCS), the dog salivated (UCR). Pavlov noticed, however, that a bell (CS) that always rang before the food was delivered also began to elicit salivation (CR). After his initial discovery, Pavlov went on to study classical conditioning in humans and several different species of animals. His experimentation with different temporal arrangements of the stimuli showed that this type of associative learning is a general form of learning that can become increasingly complex.

Classical conditioning has been used to explain certain health phenomena in the field of health psychology. It has been found that immune system responses can be suppressed or enhanced through classical conditioning. Immunosuppression can be classically conditioned in rats by pairing certain dugs (e.g., cyclophosphamide) that cause immune system suppression with a saccharin solution. Later presentations of the saccharin solution alone elicit a decreased immune response. Conditioned immunoenhancement can be explained in the same way as drug tolerance. Drug tolerance is a conditioned anticipatory response to a drug. After several pairings, drug paraphernalia may elicit a metabolic response by the body in anticipation of the drug and the drug will not have the same psychological effects with the same dosage.

Classical conditioning has also been used to treat alcohol addiction and cigarette smoking through the use of aversion therapy. To treat alcohol addiction, for example, a person is given Antabuse (disulfiram), a drug that prevents the metabolism of alcohol. Several unpleasant side effects (e.g., nausea, vomiting) occur when alcohol is consumed after taking Antabuse. The association of these unpleasant side effects with alcohol typically results in a conditioned aversion to alcohol, which discourages subsequent alcohol consumption. Classical conditioning has also been used to treat both physical and mental health concerns, such as severe anxiety, by using more complicated methods from the classical conditioning paradigm. Classical conditioning methods continue to be a useful tool in the field of health psychology.

Related Entry: Operant Conditioning

BIBLIOGRAPHY

Ader, R., & Cohen, N. (1975). Behaviorally conditioned immunosuppression. *Psychosomatic Medicine, 37,* 33–340.

Bakal, D. A. (1992). *Psychology and health* (2nd ed.). New York: Springer.

Barker, L. M. (1994). *Learning and behavior: A psychobiological perspective.* New York: Macmillan.

Bernard, L. C., & Krupat, E. (1993). *Health psychology: Biopsychosocial factors in health and illness.* Orlando, FL: Holt, Rinehart and Winston.

Krank, M. D., & MacQueen, G. M. (1988). Conditioned compensatory responses elicited by environmental signals for cyclophosphamide-induced suppression of antibody production in mice. *Psychobiology, 16,* 229–235.

Martin, G., & Pear, J. (1992). *Behavior modification: What it is and how to do it* (4th ed.). Englewood Cliffs, NJ: Prentice-Hall.

Pavlov, I. P. (1967). *Lectures on conditioned reflexes* (W. H. Gantt, Trans.). New York: International. [Original work published 1928].

Pavlov: The conditioned reflex (1993). Princeton, NJ: Films for Humanities.

Schwarz, B., Wasserman, E. A., & Robbins, S. J. (2002). *Psychology of learning and behavior* (5th ed.). New York: Norton.

ANDREA J. FRANK

Clinical Psychology

As a subfield of psychology, clinical psychology involves the study of behavior and mental processes. However, several aspects of clinical psychology differentiate it from its parent discipline. First, clinical psychologists are mainly concerned with human, rather than animal, behavior. Second, clinical psychologists apply what they know about human behavior to help people who are psychologically distressed. These activities involve assessment of the abilities, characteristics, and behavior of individual human beings as well as interventions such as psychotherapy, crisis intervention, behavior modification, and prevention strategies. Perhaps the most unique feature of clinical psychology is what has been termed the *clinical attitude,* which refers to the combining of general knowledge gained from research on human behavior with deliberate efforts to understand (through formal assessment) and help (through professional interventions) a particular person.

Several definitions of clinical psychology have been offered during the field's approximately 100-year history. One recent definition, which captures the breadth of the field, comes from the Society of Clinical Psychology, a division of the American Psychological Association (APA):

> Clinical Psychology integrates science, theory, and practice to understand, predict, and alleviate maladjustment, disability, and discomfort as well as to promote human adaptation, adjustment, and personal development. [It] focuses on the intellectual, emotional, biological, psychological, social, and behavioral aspects of human functioning across the life span, in varying cultures, and at all socioeconomic levels.

HISTORY OF CLINICAL PSYCHOLOGY

The roots of clinical psychology grew from three historical factors, each of which is prominent in the work of current clinicians.

First, clinical psychology is grounded in the research tradition of psychology and its 19th-century predecessors and pioneers such as the psychophysicist Gustav Fechner, the physiologist Hermann Helmholtz , and the first "official" psychologist, Wilhem Wundt. From its inception, psychology sought to establish itself as a science that discovered knowledge through empirical research. Although psychology had roots in philosophy, its early history embraced the conviction that the best way to study human behavior was through the tools of science—observation, theory development, and experimentation. This scientific orientation forms the basis for clinical psychologists' contemporary reputation for research expertise.

The second defining force behind clinical psychology was an interest in measuring individual differences in behavior and psychological functioning. Among the most important contributors to this tradition was Alfred Binet, a French lawyer and scientist, who developed tests of children's mental abilities such as attention, comprehension, and memory; these measures were the forerunners of formal intelligence or IQ tests. In the latter half of the 19th century, Sir Francis Galton, a cousin of Charles Darwin, designed several questionnaires (the word association test is one still-popular example) to assess mental abilities such as imagery and the ability to make sensory discriminations. The individual most credited with merging the measurement of individual differences with the scientific method of psychology was James McKeen Cattell, an American who trained with Wundt. Cattell developed a battery of mental tests, and was one of the first to appreciate their practical utility in diagnosing disorders and selecting people for certain tasks. This emphasis on measuring individual differences gave clinical psychology its first specific identity—a profession specializing in psychological assessment.

The final historical influence was the gradually evolving idea that mental disorders might be caused by psychological and social factors instead of, or in addition to, organic problems. Among many individuals advancing this notion, none was as influential as the Viennese neurologist Sigmund Freud. At the beginning of the 20th century, Freud was still refining the principles of psychoanalysis. This theory proposed that many mental disorders were due to a dynamic struggle between psychological forces that were activated in early childhood and that persisted, albeit in a mostly unconscious murkiness, throughout adult life. Although the psychoanalytic perspective is no longer dominant among clinical psychologists, its emphasis on psychological causes of disorders and on psychotherapy as an intervention was crucial to clinical psychology becoming a full-fledged mental health profession.

Clinical psychology began formally in 1896, when Lightner Witmer established the first psychological clinic at the University of Pennsylvania. The clinic specialized in the assessment of children with learning problems; Witmer did not practice psychotherapy, did not see adults in his practice, and did not espouse the Freudian approach to mental disorders. However, a different nature for the field emerged following World War I. Large numbers of military recruits had to be assessed in terms of their intellectual ability and psychological stability. Slowly, clinical psychologists began to add psychotherapy to their assessment activities. They began to practice more often in hospitals and other institutions and they worked more frequently with adults. By the mid-1930s, at least 50 psychological clinics and more than a dozen child guidance clinics had been created.

Clinical psychology became a fully recognized professional field following World War II. As a result of the war, many more clinicians were needed to assess and treat veterans of combat, and new job opportunities were created in the civilian sector as well. With the impetus of funding from the Veterans Administration, clinical psychology training programs were created at major universities across the United States. By 1948, 22 accredited clinical training programs had been established; that number grew to 83 by 1973 and to approximately 190 by 2003.

TRAINING OF CLINICAL PSYCHOLOGISTS

To be licensed as a clinical psychologist, a person must have earned a doctoral degree (including a year-long internship) and completed an additional year or more of supervised professional experience. Licensure is necessary for a clinician to practice psychology and to claim the title "clinical psychologist."

Most clinicians have earned either a PhD or a PsyD. The PhD is the degree of choice for individuals who want to be educated as *scientist-practitioners*; it emphasizes research training and empirical science as the foundation upon which clinical practice should rest. The PsyD is primarily a practitioner degree, emphasizing training in assessment and treatment over research. Most PhD programs are located in university-based departments of psychology, whereas PsyD programs are usually housed in free-standing professional schools of psychology. The APA establishes standards for these programs, which, when satisfied, results in a program being APA accredited.

PROFESSIONAL ROLES AND SPECIALIZATION

Clinical psychologists spend their professional time in some combination of six activities:

1. Assessment. Clinicians use tests, interviews, and observational methods to diagnose mental disorders, select job candidates, assess personality characteristics, measure treatment progress, and offer guidance concerning career and educational planning.
2. Treatment. Clinicians help people better understand and solve psychological problems through interventions such as psychotherapy, group therapy, and crisis intervention. These treatments are delivered on both an inpatient and outpatient basis and vary greatly in techniques, depending on the theoretical orientation of the clinician.
3. Research. Clinical research is conducted in the confines of a formal laboratory or in natural settings such as schools, hospitals, prisons, and clinics. The importance of research is that it is the basis on which clinicians evaluate the effectiveness of their treatments and the trustworthiness of their assessments.
4. Teaching. A considerable portion of many clinicians' time is spent in educational activities, including formal classroom teaching, supervision of students in training, or in-service training of other professionals.
5. Consultation. Combining aspects of research, assessment, and teaching, clinical psychologists offer advice and guidance to organizations about a variety of problems and decisions that they face
6. Administration. Many clinicians manage on a day-to-day basis organizations such as mental health clinics, counseling centers, academic departments or institutions, government agencies, hospitals, and social service agencies.

In the past, the standard training for clinical psychologists involved a core curriculum covering knowledge about the fundamentals of behavior, training in research methods, and courses in, and experience with, psychopathology, assessment, intervention, and ethics. This core curriculum model has come under challenge, especially in the past 10–15 years, mainly because clinical psychologists are increasingly working in new specialized areas that demand advanced training not typically covered in traditional graduate programs. Usually, this specialized training is provided through postdoctoral traineeships lasting 1–2 years.

Some specializations reflect the increasing biological orientation of clinical psychology. Examples are health psychology or behavioral medicine (the application of psychological knowledge and techniques to how people stay healthy, why they become ill, and how they respond to illness) and neuropsychology (the study of the relationship among brain processes, human behavior, and psychological functioning). Other popular specializations are forensic psychology (the application of psychological knowledge and techniques to legal questions and problems) and community psychology (the application of psychological principles to understanding social as well as individual problems and to preventing these problems through community-level and individually oriented interventions). Clinical psychology is also now subgrouped according to developmental periods; increasing numbers of clinicians consider themselves to be specialists in clinical child psychology, pediatric psychology (clinical child psychology with an emphasis on health care), adolescent psychology, and geropsychology. In summary, growing from a number of 18th-century ideas and traditions, clinical psychology formally emerged as a subfield of psychology in 1896. Clinicians apply empirically based knowledge to the assessment and treatment of psychological problems and to attempts to prevent these problems; their roles include assessment, treatment, research, teaching, consultation, and administration. As the field has grown, it has broadened its scope of services, diversified its approaches to training, and increased its area of specializations in response to growing social needs for psychological services.

Related Entry: Social Psychology

MICHAEL T. NIETZEL

Cognitive Appraisal

Cognitive appraisal is the process of applying previous experience and knowledge to develop an interpretation of incoming information. Cognitive appraisal is a central aspect of the manner in which we engage in health protective behavior, how we manage our health, and our adjustment to minor and major illnesses. These connections between cognitive appraisal and health are considered in turn.

Cognitive appraisal is a pivotal part of how we evaluate health risk information. For example, when presented with information on the risks of smoking in the development of lung cancer, an individual will make a series of judgments about this information, including the seriousness of lung cancer and whether they perceive themselves to be susceptible to it. This appraisal process will, in turn, affect the likelihood of an individual attempting to quit smoking. Research on the cognitive appraisal process and health risk has been applied to a variety of health behaviors including exercise, smoking, alcohol use, screening behaviors (e.g., HIV, cholesterol, blood pressure), and safer sex practices. Additionally, cognitive appraisal is central to understanding when and why individuals relapse after making health behavior changes. Of particular importance is the manner in which individuals appraise their own coping abilities in situations that represent a high risk for relapse.

When physical changes occur in our bodies, we engage in cognitive appraisal to determine their meaning. For example, we must evaluate whether physical changes are a symptom of an illness or are normal fluctuations in our physical state, and label the problem. Subsequently, there may be cognitive appraisal of the timeline and course of the identified health threat and the cause, the controllability, the appropriate treatment, and the consequences of a particular illness.

Research has demonstrated that cognitive appraisal is also central to our response to receiving medical diagnoses and other health-related information from health care providers. We evaluate medical diagnoses on a variety of dimensions, such as seriousness, which in turn influences how we attend to subsequent medical information and how strictly we adhere to medical advice on the management of the diagnosis. A related and important recent focus of cognitive appraisal research has been in investigating how individuals respond to genetic testing for serious health conditions, such as breast cancer and Huntington's disease.

Cognitive appraisal processes have also been shown to influence adjustment to chronic health conditions, such as chronic pain and coronary heart disease. One specific focus has been the application of cognitive theories of depression to both physical and mental health outcomes in chronically ill populations. Cognitive models of depression posit that when individuals make cognitive errors in appraising life events they are at risk for the development of depression. Cognitive errors involve interpreting everyday events in negative ways, such as viewing a small setback as a catastrophe. Research has demonstrated that when chronically ill individuals make these kinds of errors, particularly when evaluating their health, they are more likely to be depressed, are more disabled by their condition, and may respond more poorly to rehabilitation.

Related Entries: Cognitive Representations of Illness, Depression, Stress Appraisal

BIBLIOGRAPHY

Christensen, A. J., Edwards, D. L., Moran, P. J., Burke, R., Lounsbury, P., & Gordon, E. E. I. (1999). Cognitive distortion and functional impairment in patients undergoing cardiac rehabilitation. *Cognitive Therapy and Research, 23*, 159–168.

Leventhal, H., Leventhal, E. A., & Cameron, L. (2001). Representations, procedures, and affect in illness self-regulation: A perceptual–cognitive model. In A. Baum, T. A. Revenson, & J. E. Singer (Eds.), *Handbook of health psychology* (pp. 00–00). Mahwah, NJ: Erlbaum.

Weinstein, N. D. (2000). Perceived probability, perceived severity, and health-protective behavior. *Health Psychology, 19*, 65–74.

PAULA G. WILLIAMS

Cognitive–behavioral therapy

In the 1930s to the 1960s, the field of psychosomatic medicine dominated the application of psychological theory and intervention to health-related problems. Psychosomatic medicine practitioners, guided by psychoanalytic or psychodynamic theory, conceptualized and treated patients with various stress-related diseases or whose behavior contributed to their illnesses. At the same time, basic research on learning principles flourished in psychology laboratories, which led to behavior change strategies that were applied to humans. In addition, psychodynamic theory and therapy evolved by increasingly emphasizing the rational, conscious aspects of people (the "ego"). Furthermore, by the 1970s, health practitioners realized the limitations of the biomedical model for people with chronic pain and other chronic conditions, people whose lifestyle caused their illness, or people with physical symptoms related to stress. Both patients and providers sought interventions for these problems that were briefer, more effective, and more acceptable to a wide variety of people than were currently available. Thus, by the late 1970s, behavior therapy, and subsequently cognitive–behavioral therapy (CBT), replaced psychosomatic medicine as the dominant model of theory and intervention among health psychologists, many of whom aligned with the new field of behavioral medicine.

THEORETICAL FOUNDATIONS OF CBT

Cognitive–behavioral therapy has its theoretical foundations in classical conditioning, operant conditioning, social learning, and research on cognitive processes. Generally, classical and operant conditioning view behavior as a response to environmental stimuli and consequences. At its simplest, classical conditioning occurs when a neutral environmental stimulus is repeatedly paired with a biologically relevant stimulus that automatically elicits an unlearned, biological response, resulting in the neutral stimulus acquiring the ability to elicit the biological response. Operant conditioning occurs when environmental consequences increase or decrease the frequency of previous behavior and when antecedent stimuli signal the likelihood of those consequences. These two types of learning were studied initially in animals, and the application of their principles to improve human functioning—behavior therapy—emphasized that behavior change follows from changes in the environment. Thus, a primary focus of behavior therapy is a systematic examination and modification of the environment to alter a person's behavior in a desired direction.

The rise of social learning theory in the 1960s, which emphasized modeling or observation and verbal instruction, shifted the research focus from animals to humans and introduced cognition into learning theory. Various cognitive models of human behavior subsequently flourished, and cognitive research established the value of beliefs, appraisals, and attributions as intervening variables between environmental stimuli and behavioral responses. CBT strategies derived, in part, from these cognitive models and from other influences (e.g., covert conditioning, ego psychology). Cognitive strategies emphasize that changes in behavior, symptoms, and moods follow cognitive change.

BASIC PRINCIPLES OF CBT

Several principles distinguish CBT from other forms of psychotherapy. First, CBT views problematic behavior as fundamentally learned via interaction with the environment; therefore, undesired behavior can be unlearned, and desired behavior, such as new skills, can be learned. Although factors other than a person's learning history are acknowledged (e.g., genetics or socioeconomic forces), CBT maintains the rather optimistic attitude that behavior is generally malleable by creating changes in learning experiences. Second, CBT is guided by the principle of parsimony to prioritize its explanations of problems, its clinical targets, and its interventions. According to this principle, the most straightforward and least inferential explanations, problems, and treatments are considered first, whereas more complex or inferential explanations and treatments are considered only if initial approaches prove insufficient. Thus, CBT typically avoids explanations that are difficult to verify (e.g., involving unconscious psychodynamic processes), targets of change that are broad or pervasive (e.g., personality), and interventions that are indirect or overly general (e.g., interpretations). Third, CBT bases it approach on the cumulative body of scientific psychological knowledge as opposed to other sources of knowledge such as personal intuition, clinical experience, persuasive leaders, or tradition. This scientific attitude also is manifest in clinical work with individual cases. In administering CBT, one first generates hypotheses about the factors influencing the problem behavior and then tests these hypotheses by using targeted interventions, followed by an assessment of change. In this way, hypotheses about behavior can be supported if change occurs as expected or refuted if change does not occur, which leads to alternative hypotheses and interventions.

SPECIFIC THERAPEUTIC STRATEGIES

There is a plethora of CBT approaches for health-related problems, and many of these strategies have direct links to the various theories noted previously. Classical conditioning has given rise to procedures designed to alter the responses of the body. For example, exposure-based strategies (e.g., systematic desensitization, flooding, and response prevention) present clients with stimuli that elicit negative emotions or bodily reactions in order to extinguish or habituate these reactions. Operant theory has given rise to stimulus control, in which the eliciting stimuli for behavior are changed, and to contingency management, in which environmental consequences are altered. Other popular CBT strategies are various arousal reduction techniques, particularly relaxation training and related approaches (biofeedback, meditation, breathing retraining). Social learning theory has encouraged interventions in which clients learn complex behaviors, particularly interpersonal behavior, including assertiveness training, which incorporates modeling, role playing, practice, and feedback. Cognitive therapy approaches take advantage of the powerful capacity of cognitive processes. Thus, education and information provision are used to increase predictability and control in stressful situations. Mental control techniques such as thought stopping, distraction, or imagery are also used to control emotions. More importantly, however, cognitive therapy generally views most dysfunctional behavior, moods, and symptoms as resulting from beliefs or thinking patterns that are inflexible, erroneous, overly narrow, or otherwise distorted. Cognitive restructuring identifies the underlying beliefs that support the dysfunctional behavior and attempts to change those beliefs by using logical analysis, rational persuasion, and clinical experimentation.

In CBT practice, therapist and client collaborate to change the client's environment, help the client learn new skills, and modify the client's thinking patterns. Sessions tend to be structured and didactic, various techniques are taught and practiced, homework between sessions is routinely prescribed, and changes in the target problem are tracked over time. There is an emphasis on self-management or self-control procedures, in which clients are encouraged to make changes and apply the skills in their daily lives. This focused and direct intervention approach typically is shorter in duration than most other psychotherapeutic approaches, and much research has demonstrated its efficacy with many health-related problems.

APPLICATIONS TO HEALTH PSYCHOLOGY PROBLEMS

Numerous problems encountered by health psychologists have been conceptualized in cognitive–behavioral terms and effectively treated using CBT strategies. For some clinical problems, a single strategy is useful. For example, by changing environmental contingencies, some unhealthy behaviors (medication non-adherence, excessive sun exposure) can be reduced, and some adaptive behaviors (e.g., exercise, nutritious eating) can be increased. Problems that have strong negative emotional components (e.g., panic disorder and its medically relevant variants, blood and needle phobia, conditioned nausea and vomiting, and posttraumatic stress) can be redressed with conditioning or exposure-based interventions. Relaxation strategies are efficacious for many psychophysiologic or stress-related health problems such as hypertension, irritable bowel syndrome, and headaches. Education or information provision helps to prepare children for stressful medical procedures such as anesthesia induction.

Yet, most health psychology problems are multifaceted and require several CBT intervention strategies and a greater focus on cognitive change. For example, addictive behaviors, including smoking, alcohol abuse or dependence, and obesity-related behaviors (diet and exercise) are complex, and CBT treatment protocols usually incorporate several strategies, including stimulus control and contingency management, cognitive restructuring, problem solving, and relapse prevention. An empirically supported approach to chronic pain is coping skills training, which includes education in pain mechanisms, relaxation training, self-reinforcement via pleasant activity scheduling, substituting positive self-statements for negative thoughts, and problem solving. Depression, which is relatively common in medical patients, is often treated not only with cognitive therapy, but also by behavioral activation, increasing pleasant activities, and even modeling and assertiveness training. A leading CBT approach to decreasing hostility in people at risk for coronary events prescribes 17 strategies including rational analysis, relaxation, distraction, thought stopping, assertiveness, intimacy development, humor, and forgiveness exercises. Although all of these clinical problems could be conceptualized in a more complex fashion (e.g., in psychodynamic terms), CBT focuses on relearning in the most direct and efficient manner possible. This "skills" approach is particularly attractive to many medical patients, who may avoid more traditional psychological explanations and approaches.

THE FUTURE OF CBT

CBT is not static, but continues to evolve, both conceptually and pragmatically. For example, there is increasing agreement that a limited number of common mechanisms or change factors likely underlie the myriad of CBT technical procedures. Leading candidates include exposure to avoided stimuli, increases in self-efficacy, and coping skills. Further, as limitations of CBT are recognized and alternative approaches are validated, the repertoire of acceptable interventions broadens.

For example, biological factors are increasingly recognized as vital to addictive behaviors, and pharmacologic treatments are being integrated into CBT models to yield "biobehavioral" interventions. Practitioners of CBT are increasingly viewing emotional factors as potentially useful and adaptive components of behavior change, and techniques such as emotional disclosure and emotional processing are making inroads into CBT. It is expected that CBT will continue to evolve into an integrated, empirically supported set of interventions that, ideally, are matched to particular clients and specific problems.

Related Entries: Cognitive Appraisal, Cognitive Representations of Illness, Operant Conditioning, Psychotherapy, Shaping

BIBLIOGRAPHY

Brewin, C. R. (1996). Theoretical foundations of cognitive behavior therapy for anxiety and depression. *Annual Review of Psychology, 47,* 33–57.

Hollon, S., & Beck, A. (1994). Cognitive and cognitive–behavioral therapies. In A. Bergin & S. Garfield (Eds.), *Handbook of psychotherapy and behavior change* (4th ed., pp. 428–466). New York: Wiley.

Keefe, F., & Caldwell, D. (1997). Cognitive behavioral control of arthritis pain. *Medical Clinics of North America , 81,* 277–290.

McGinn, L., & Sanderson, W. (2001). What allows cognitive behavioral therapy to be brief: Overview, efficacy, and crucial factors facilitating brief treatment. *Clinical Psychology: Science and Practice, 8,* 23–37.

Meichenbaum, D. (1995). Cognitive–behavioral therapy in historical perspective. In B. Bongar & L. Beutler (Eds.), *Comprehensive textbook of psychotherapy: Theory and practice* (pp. 140–158). New York: Oxford University Press.

Samoilov, A., & Goldfried, M. (2000). Role of emotion in cognitive–behavior therapy. *Clinical Psychology: Science and Practice, 7,* 373–385.

Smith, T., Kendall, P., & Keefe, F. (Eds.). (2002). Behavioral medicine and clinical health psychology [Special issue]. *Journal of Consulting and Clinical Psychology, 70*(3).

Tunks, E., & Bellissimo, A. (1991). *Behavioral medicine: Concepts and Procedures.* New York: Pergamon.

Turk, D., Meichenbaum, D., & Genest, M. (1983). *Pain and behavioral medicine: A cognitive–behavioral perspective.* New York: Guilford.

Williams, R., & Williams, V. (1993). *Anger kills. Seventeen strategies for controlling the hostility that can harm your health.* New York: HarperCollins.

MARK A. LUMLEY
MAZY E. GILLIS

Cognitive Representations of Illness

How do people understand and think about ("mentally represent") health and illness? What rules govern the way people create, maintain, and modify conceptions of their own and others' health status? How do the cognitive processes and structures of illness representations affect individuals' emotional and behavioral responses to health threats? Such questions form the core of health psychologists' study of illness representations.

Western middle-class people use "illness" to refer to a biological condition of the body. However, medical anthropologists and sociologists have sensitized health psychologists to the cultural and role-related meanings packed into concepts of illness. Learning that one has arthritis, diabetes, or hypertension has effects that go beyond merely registering an item of information about one's biological condition. In part, these effects arise because medical and everyday language are not equivalent. The quasi-medical field of patient education fulfills a need to translate between these "dialects," but it assumes that the language of medical professionals is the standard by which to judge patients' understanding. Psychologists who study illness representations, on the other hand, believe that studying the lay person's understanding of illness is worthwhile in its own right because that understanding (no matter how medically accurate) motivates people's health-related activities.

COMPONENTS OF ILLNESS REPRESENTATIONS

Research beginning in the mid-1980s verified that people's mental representations of illness include the following elements:

- *Identity,* a set of one or more bodily symptoms (e.g., fever and diarrhea) and an identifying label (e.g., flu) that names the illness.
- *Timeline,* beliefs about the temporal course of the illness. Is it an acute problem that will be resolved by treatment or by the passage of a few days? Or is it a long-term, chronic illness that will worsen over time? Is it a condition that will wax and wane periodically, going through cycles?
- *Cause,* beliefs about why the illness has occurred. Is it because of contact with an infected family member or environmental toxins? Has it been brought on by overwork or other strains, which have undermined one's resistance to pathogens? Is it the result of bad genes?
- *Controllability,* beliefs about the curability or at least the manageability of the illness. For infectious diseases with which Western middle-class people are most familiar, curability beliefs are strong. For many chronic conditions, the major issue is how to manage the illness—to retard its progress, to make lifestyle adjustments, and so on.
- *Consequences,* people's answers to such questions as, What will be the effect on me of this illness? Will it prevent me from completing a work assignment or joining the family vacation? Will it require mutilating surgery? Will it force me to retire earlier than I planned? Some

consequences may be immediate; others may be anticipated over the long run.

Changing any component of the representational system will influence other components. A cough that was initially identified as a bronchitis episode is transformed as it persists for several weeks. Because the timeline has changed, causal explanations and potential cures that applied to an acute episode are no longer plausible. The person wonders and worries about what the cough signifies—both its identity and its consequences.

CONSEQUENCES OF ILLNESS REPRESENTATIONS

Health psychologists are interested in illness representations because they assume that these motivate and direct coping with health problems. This assumption has been vindicated by research connecting patients' mental representations of chronic diseases, such as hypertension, diabetes, and arthritis, with adherence to treatment. For example, persons who are newly diagnosed with high blood pressure tend to drop out of treatment if they think they have an acute disease. Because hypertension has no reliable symptoms, such patients cannot use symptom remission to judge whether treatment was successful. Instead, they believe they have been cured by temporary changes in diet and a course of medication. Individuals who stick with treatment overwhelmingly believe it has had beneficial effects on such felt symptoms as headaches. These patients readily acknowledge that "most people" cannot detect variations in blood pressure, thereby conforming to the accepted medical view; however, they regard themselves as exceptions to this general rule. Moreover, they report varying self-treatment according to whether they are experiencing symptoms. Such findings highlight the centrality of the "identity" component in illness representations and indicate that illness representations are grounded in people's somatic experience. They also illustrate the *symmetry rule*: People expect symptoms to denote an illness entity, and they expect illnesses to be accompanied by symptoms. In contrast to hypertension, symptoms of unregulated diabetes are readily evident. As a result, "controllability" beliefs play a very important role for persons with diabetes. Individuals who believe treatment is effective in controlling symptoms are more likely to maintain their regimen than those who regard treatment as ineffective.

Besides the symmetry rule, people apply other commonsense heuristics to understanding symptoms and illness. For example, they are less likely to seek treatment for ambiguous symptoms occurring in conjunction with short-term life stresses than when stress is prolonged or symptoms are obviously medical. The *stress–illness rule* shows that "stress" may serve as an alternative explanation for symptoms. However, this rule may be applied in conjunction with stereoypes about what kind of person is most likely to exhibit symptoms. For example, people are less likely to recommend treatment for women who report chest pains and concurrent life stress than for men who report identical conditions. Given the growing incidence of heart disease among women, misapplication of a gender stereotype in informal diagnosis could have catastrophic effects.

Similar to the tendency to discount illness explanations for symptoms associated with short-term life stress, the *aging–illness rule* leads to delays in seeking treatment for symptoms that are attributed to normal aging processes. As individuals age, their sense of vulnerability to disease grows, but they also feel less confident that illness is controllable. One result is a reduced likelihood of seeking treatment unless symptoms are very severe.

THE FUTURE

How universal is the five-component model of illness representations? Examinations of illness descriptions written during the 17th and 18th centuries suggest that it has some historical generality, at least in Western Europe. As to its applicability to non-Western and/or non-middle-class persons, we do not know. Most researchers have concentrated on extending the five-component model to disease entities that, by definition, presuppose a Western medical framework. One criticism of research on the five-component model is that persons whose beliefs about illness causation include the supernatural or retribution may be reluctant to voice views that deviate from the biologically oriented norm. Further validation of the model can address such shortcomings. Only a few psychologists are actively studying illness representation in Africa or Asia, and even these tend to be in urban and Western-influenced settings. It is difficult to see how this latter problem will be overcome in the foreseeable future.

BIBLIOGRAPHY

Baumann, L. J., Cameron, L. D., Zimmerman, R. S., & Leventhal, H. (1989). Illness representations and matching labels with symptoms. *Health Psychology, 8*(4), 449–469.

Bishop, G. D. (1998). East meets West: Illness cognition and behaviour in Singapore. *Applied Psychology: An International Review, 47*(4), 519–534.

Cameron, L., Leventhal, E. A., & Leventhal, H. (1995). Seeking medical care in response to symptoms and life stress. *Psychosomatic Medicine, 57*(1), 37–47.

Hampson, S. E. (1997). Personal models and the management of chronic illness: A comparison of diabetes and osteoarthritis. *European Journal of Personality, 11*(5), 401–414.

Keller, M. L., Leventhal, H., Prohaska, T. R., & Leventhal, E. A. (1989). Beliefs about aging and illness in a community sample. *Research in Nursing and Health, 12*(4), 247–255.

Landrine, H., & Klonoff, E. A. (1992). Culture and health-related schemas: A review and proposal for interdisciplinary integration. *Health Psychology*, *11*(4), 267–276.

Martin, R., & Lemos, K. (2002). From heart attacks to melanoma: Do common sense models of somatization influence symptom interpretation for female victims? *Health Psychology*, *21*(1), 25–32.

Meyer, D., Leventhal, H., & Gutmann, M. (1985). Common-sense models of illness: The example of hypertension. *Health Psychology*, *4*(2), 115–135.

Prohaska, T. R., Keller, M. L., Leventhal, E. A., & Leventhal, H. (1987). Impact of symptoms and aging attribution on emotions and coping. *Health Psychology*, *6*(6), 495–514.

J. A. SKELTON

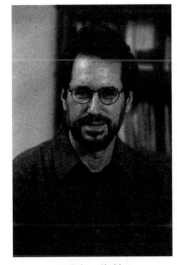

Cohen, Sheldon

Cohen, Sheldon (1947–)

Sheldon Cohen was born on October 11, 1947. He was assistant to associate professor of psychology at the University of Oregon from 1973 through 1982, and has been a professor of psychology at Carnegie Mellon University since 1982. Since 1990 he has also been an adjunct professor of pathology and psychiatry at the University of Pittsburgh Medical School as well as a member of the Pittsburgh Cancer Institute. In 1992, he served as the interim director of Pittsburgh Cancer Institute's Behavioral Medicine Program and has been the codirector of Pittsburgh's Brain Behavior and Immunity Center since its inception in 1990. He is also a member of the core groups of the John D. and Catherine T. MacArthur Foundation Research Network on Socioeconomic Status and Health and the Fetzer Institute's Research Network on Psychosocial Factors in Asthma. Dr. Cohen is the recipient of the American Psychological Association's Award for Outstanding Contributions to Health Psychology and the National Institute of Mental Health's Research Scientist Development and Senior Scientist Awards. He has also been an APA Distinguished Scientist Lecturer and British Psychological Society Senior Fellow.

Dr. Cohen's work focuses on the roles of stress, affect, and social support systems in health and well-being. He has published pioneering theoretical and empirical work on the effects of aircraft noise on health and development of school children and on the roles of stress and social networks in physical and mental health. Over the last 17 years he has studied the effects of psychological stress and social support on immunity and susceptibility to infectious disease. This work attempts to identify the neuroendocrine, immune, and behavioral pathways that link stress, personality, and social networks to disease susceptibility. His research on the role of psychosocial factors in susceptibility to the common cold has been published in the *New England Journal of Medicine* and the *Journal of the American Medical Association*. He is also involved in studies of the effects of psychosocial factors on the onset and progression of asthma and on the effectiveness of social support interventions in facilitating psychological adjustment and disease progression in women with breast cancer. His current work focuses on how interpersonal relationships and positive affect influence immunity and host resistance to infectious disease. This work focuses on the role of endocrine and immune function in linking positive psychological states and susceptibility to infectious disease.

JAMIE A. CVENGROS

Community Interventions

There is a long history of community intervention in the field of public health. Mitler's review of contemporary approaches to community health promotion traces them to the late 1800s. The goals of community interventions are diverse, ranging from decreasing morbidity or mortality, to increasing the practice of a healthy behavior or healthy organizational practices, to securing passage of public healthy policy. Policies can be oriented to active prevention (i.e., policies that require individuals to take action in order to be protected) or passive prevention (i.e., policies that protect individuals without the individual engaging in a health-protective behavior).

Community interventions typically employ an array of programmatic approaches including those that focus on changing individual behavior and those that target contextual influences that facilitate or impede individual behavior. Thus, a predominant theme in community intervention is the need for comprehensive intervention at multiple levels including individual, organizational, and community levels.

CHARACTERISTICS OF SUCCESSFUL INTERVENTIONS

Several characteristics of intervention strategies have been found to be successful. Interventions that utilize data-based planning and feedback systems (epidemiologic, public opinion, strategic) are effective in the development and refinement of interventions. Successful interventions also involve the target population in some aspects of the effort. Success is also related to developing clearly articulated, highly focused, agreed-upon goals and objectives, maintaining flexibility at the tactical (programmatic) level, and emphasizing passive prevention approaches whenever possible so that people are protected automatically rather than having to engage in an active behavior. Furthermore, effective interventions often change the social norms around which individual behavior occurs and target the root causes of problems, especially those in the sociocultural environment. Finally, community intervention strategies that take into account the resources available (i.e., ends being adjusted to the means) and consider the timing and location of intervention in design and implementation are typically more successful.

Although in practice, health promotion is implemented through multiple levels (from the individual through policy), the community level is key to building a comprehensive strategy to promote health and prevent disease among the population at large. The importance of community intervention is often based on the assumption that greater improvement in health can be obtained by small changes in the behaviors (or environments) of large numbers of people than by large changes among a small number of people at high risk. That is, the goal of many community interventions is to affect small shifts in the distribution of risk and protective factors.

THEORY

Ecological Perspective

From an ecological perspective, the potential to change individual risk behavior is best considered within the social and cultural context in which behavior occurs. Interventions that are informed by a social–ecological perspective attend to extraindividual level factors such as community norms and the structure of community services including their comprehensiveness, coordination, and linkages, in addition to individual motivations and attitudes. Thus, individual change is understood within the social and cultural context in which it is to occur.

Social Cognitive Theory

Social cognitive theory has been a key theory guiding the development of community health promotion interventions. Bandura noted that self-efficacy, outcome expectancies, and perceived incentive value are key aspects of social cognitive theory. Self-efficacy refers to a person's belief about how capable he or she is to perform a specific behavior and relates to a person's willingness to participate in community change. Outcome expectancy refers to a person's belief that a behavior will result in a specific outcome. A person will be more willing to spend time and effort to bring about a change to the extent he or she perceives the change will have the intended effect. Perceived incentive value refers to the relative importance one places on a possible outcome. In general, a person is more likely to engage in a behavior if he or she considers the behavior to be important (i.e., valuable).

Social Marketing Approach

Social marketing has also influenced the design of community interventions. Social marketing is the extension of marketing principles to social and health issues, and focuses on the marketing context structure, made up of product, price, promotion, position, and place. The social marketing approach emphasizes the context (marketplace) and the needs of the target population (consumer) so that tailored interventions are designed and delivered. Social marketing is based on two general assumptions: (1) programs/messages should be designed on the basis of the perceived needs and expectation of consumers and (2) successful programs are those that achieve a successful exchange between message sender and receiver.

Community Development Approach

Community development (or community organization) is the study of or intervention around the natural organization of persons and institutions in community systems. A key to this approach involves comprehensive planning and community diagnosis/analysis. There are three critical dimensions at the core of successful community development: (1) multisectoral inclusion, (2) organizational linkages, and (3) enabling and support. Multisectoral inclusion refers to the involvement and subsequent active participation of diverse community members and organizational constituencies in planning, implementing, and evaluating community health programs. Organizational linkages can be described as the communication, coordination, and collaboration among multiple community sectors toward joint goals and objectives. Enabling and support refers to a community's ability to determine its own "health." An enabling approach will change the typical hierarchical relationship between researchers (giving direction) and community groups (taking direction).

Mass Media Approach

The mass media are often used in community interventions. Mass media can influence awareness, interest (or motivation), trial attempts (or experimentation), and adoption of behavior. The media are important in setting the public agenda about health issues (i.e., what people think about and how issues are framed). Thus, the media can create and reinforce public awareness about an issue, contribute to its salience, serve as a cue to action, and reinforce action is that taken.

EMPOWERMENT

Empowerment, defined as efforts at individual, organizational, and community levels of analysis to exert control and gain mastery over salient issues, has also influenced community intervention. Wallerstein (1992) and Zimmerman (1990) defined empowerment by the absence or low levels of normlessness, powerlessness, social isolation, and helplessness. Critical components of empowerment include participation, control, and critical awareness. Community coalition and other strategic alliances such as networks, consortia, leadership councils, and citizen panels exemplify the "empowering" process. Members pool their individual resources to develop a critical mass in leveraging community change. Important benefits result from participating if the group climate is supportive of members, the group is highly committed to the work, and the group has a strong identification with its community.

EVALUATION OF COMMUNITY INTERVENTIONS

Evaluation of the success of community interventions has resulted in mixed findings. Multiple factors may account for the inconsistency in success of community interventions, including methodological or implementation concerns and measurement issues. Difficulties in detecting outcomes often stem from issues such as random assignment, appropriate control sites, and measuring intermediate and long-term outcomes. Difficulties in producing effective outcomes may also result from a lack of use of "best practices" and difficulty implementing intervention strategies.

CONCLUSIONS

Community interventions are popular because they have the potential to improve health above and beyond what can be achieved by individual approaches alone. Indeed, part of the rationale underlying the efficacy of community intervention is the belief that changing the community at large is a more cost-effective means of achieving societal health goals then reaching individuals one person at a time. Also, community interventions have the potential advantage of delivering beneficial programs both to those who explicitly desire assistance as well as those who could benefit from intervention but who do not know they could benefit or who do not have access through more traditional service delivery mechanisms.

BIBLIOGRAPHY

Bandura, A. (1997). *Self-efficacy: The exercise of control.* New York: Freeman.

Farquhar, J. W., Fortmann, S. P., Flora, J. A., Taylor, C. B., Haskell, W. L., Williams, P. T., et al. (1990). Effects of communitywide education on cardiovascular disease risk factors: The Stanford Five-City Project. *Journal of the American Medical Association, 264,* 359–365.

Minkler, M. (1990). Improving health through community organization. In K. Glanz, F. M. Lewis, & B. K. Rimer (Eds.), *Health behavior and health education: Theory, research, and practice* (pp. 00–00). San Francisco: Jossey-Bass.

Wallerstein, N. (1992). Powerlessness, empowerment, and health: Implications for health promotion programs. *American Journal of Health Promotion, 6,* 197–205.

Zimmerman, M. A. (1990). Toward a theory of learned helplessness: A structural analysis of participation and empowerment. *Journal of Research in Personality, 24,* 71–86.

HEATHER CHAMPION
DAVID G. ALTMAN

Conscientiousness

Conscientiousness is one of five personality traits, or characteristics, that made up the five-factor model of personality. This model, based primarily on the extensive analysis of lexical and personality test data, describes the major dimensions of normal personality in somewhat broad terms, with additional detail being included in subcategories (or "facets") of each trait. The domain of conscientiousness includes many qualities, with highly conscientious people being responsible, dependable, well organized, dutiful, disciplined, and persevering. People low on conscientiousness tend to be impulsive, irresponsible, undependable, disorganized, and careless.

Conscientiousness has been empirically linked to better health and even to longevity, and these associations seem to be at least partly due to the better health behaviors that conscientious individuals share. Conscientious individuals are more likely to engage in a variety of health-promoting behaviors, including avoidance of risks (such as smoking) and adhering to treatment regimens. However, engagement in good health practices is not enough to explain the association between conscientiousness and health. In one seven-decade-long prospective longitudinal study, H. S. Friedman and his colleagues (Friedman, 2000; Friedman et al., 1993, 1995) found that even when behavioral factors such as smoking and drinking were statistically controlled, conscientiousness remained a significant predictor of mortality risk. This suggests that psychosocial processes may be meaningfully related to levels of conscientiousness and may thereby play an important role in the maintenance of physical health, perhaps in combination with health behaviors. These processes might include things like social support (those who are dependable might attract more friends) or proactive coping (those who are responsible and well organized might anticipate challenges and meet them more effectively).

Through the early 1990s, the personality characteristic of conscientiousness was largely neglected in health psychology studies, with more attention being focused on the traits of neuroticism, extraversion, and agreeableness. Researchers are now recognizing that conscientiousness plays a crucial role in understanding the complex pathways that connect personality to physical health.

Related Entries: Five-Factor Model of Personality, Neuroticism

BIBLIOGRAPHY

Booth-Kewley, S., & Vickers, R. R., Jr. (1994). Associations between major domains of personality and health behavior. *Journal of Personality, 62,* 281–298.

Friedman, H. S. (2000). Long-term relationships of personality and health: Dynamisms, mechanisms, tropisms. *Journal of Personality, 68,* 1089–1107.

Friedman, H. S., Tucker, J. S., Schwartz, J. E., Martin, L. R., Tomlinson-Keasey, C., Wingard, D. L., et al. (1995). Childhood conscientiousness and longevity: Health behaviors and cause of death. *Journal of Personality and Social Psychology, 68,* 696–703.

Friedman, H. S., Tucker, J. S., Tomlinson-Keasey, C., Schwartz, J. E., Wingard, D. L., & Criqui, M. H. (1993). Does childhood personality predict longevity? *Journal of Personality and Social Psychology, 65,* 176–185.

Goldberg, L. R. (1990). An alternative "description of personality:" The big-five factor structure. *Journal of Personality and Social Psychology, 59,* 1216–1229.

Hampson, S. E., Andrews, J. A., Barckley, M., Lichtenstein, E., & Lee, M. E. (2000). Conscientiousness, perceived risk, and risk-reduction behaviors: A preliminary study. *Health Psychology, 19,* 496–500.

Marshall, G. N., Wortman, C. B., Vickers, R. R., Jr., Kusulas, J. W., & Hervig, L. K. (1994). The five-factor model of personality as a framework for personality–health research. *Journal of Personality and Social Psychology, 67,* 278–286.

Skinner, T. C., Hampson, S. E., & Fife-Schaw, C. (2002). Personality, personal model beliefs, and self-care in adolescents and young adults with Type I diabetes. *Health Psychology, 21,* 61–70.

LESLIE R. MARTIN

Contingency Management

Contingency management is used as treatment component aimed at increasing adaptive behavior and decreasing nonadaptive behavior. Learning principles are utilized in this strategy, including positive reinforcement, negative reinforcement, punishment, extinction, and shaping procedures, to reach a designated goal. An example of positive reinforcement is rewarding children with prizes for adhering to strict dietary regimens and fluid intake restrictions while on hemodialysis. Contingency management has also been utilized as a central component of comprehensive pain rehabilitation programs, illustrating the use of extinction. Central goals within this forum often include the elimination of behavior designed to elicit attention (e.g., facial expressions) or diminishing complaining or sick-role behavior. For example, contingency management may include the elimination of positive reinforcements (e.g., attention paid to patient) previously elicited by, and reinforcing, complaining or attention-seeking behavior. Alternatively, positive reinforcement, such as attention, may be utilized in order to increase well behavior.

Related Entry: Operant Conditioning

KATHERINE RAICHLE

Contraception

Contraception refers to preventing conception, the process by which a sperm from a fertile male joins with an ovum (egg) of a fertile female during vaginal sexual intercourse. Any fertile female who has vaginal intercourse without contraception with a fertile male may become pregnant. If a couple prefers not to conceive a child, then the use of contraception or "birth control" is advised.

CONTRACEPTIVE METHODS

There are many forms of contraception: (1) "natural" methods, to avoid vaginal intercourse or to time intercourse so that it does not occur during the days in each menstrual cycle when a woman is most fertile; (2) chemical methods, to inactivate sperm; (3) barrier methods, to prevent the male sperm from reaching the female egg; (4) hormonal methods, to alter the process of ovulation (release of the female egg) or other biological conditions necessary for conception; (5) use of intrauterine devices, to influence the condition of the uterine lining; and (6) surgical methods, to prevent the release or availability of sperm or eggs. Each contraceptive method has its own advantages and disadvantages.

Natural Methods

Abstinence and other nonpenetrative sexual behaviors are 100 percent effective ways to avoid unintended conception. *Abstinence* involves no sexual contact, whereas *nonpenetrative sexual behavior* refers to activities such as mutual masturbation (sexual touching that can lead to orgasm). Oral and anal sex also avoid conception but these penetrative activities may lead to sexually transmitted infections (STIs) such as HIV, chlamydia, and gonorrhea.

Natural methods can also be used in conjunction with vaginal intercourse. The *withdrawal* method, also known as *coitus interruptus*, requires that the man withdraw his penis from his partner's vagina prior to ejaculation (the release of semen during orgasm). Although commonly practiced, especially among adolescents, withdrawal has a relatively high (24 percent) failure rate because it can be difficult for a man to withdraw in time and because there are fluids that escape the penis prior to ejaculation that may contain viable sperm.

Natural family planning methods are based on the idea that fertilization is most likely to occur around the time of ovulation, and that by avoiding intercourse during those times, conception is less likely to occur. These are several ways to determine the time of ovulation, including the *basal body temperature approach* (use of a woman's daily morning temperature), the *cervical mucus method* (careful monitoring of vaginal wetness), and the *calendar method* (tracking menstrual cycles carefully). Overall, failure rates tend to be relatively high (21 percent) for these methods because they require very careful and accurate monitoring as well as discipline to avoid intercourse during ovulation. However, they have no side effects, are inexpensive, and enjoy greater acceptability among some religious traditions.

The *lactational amenorrhea method* is available only to women who are nursing, and involves the use of breastfeeding to suppress ovulation. This method is effective only when (1) the infant is less than 6 months old, (2) the mother's menses has not returned, and (3) a nursing mother breastfeeds for almost all feedings.

Chemical Methods

Spermacides such as nonoxynol-9 and octoxynol-9 are chemicals placed in the vagina just prior to intercourse to inactivate sperm. They are available without a prescription, and can be used easily by a woman without her partner's knowledge; they are available in the form of cream, foam, gels, suppositories, and film. When spermacides are used by themselves (without a

barrier), they have a failure rate of 26 percent. However, recent research suggests that use of spermacides may irritate the lining of the vagina and increase the likelihood of HIV transmission if a woman's partner is infected.

Barrier Methods

Male condoms or "rubbers" refer to a sheath (covering) that is worn over the penis during intercourse. Condoms are made from latex (rubber), polyurethane (plastic), or lamb intestines ("lambskin"). To be effective, condoms must be applied correctly prior to intromission (insertion of the penis into the vagina) and not removed until the man has withdrawn his penis from his partner's vagina. The estimated failure rate for condoms is 14 percent. A major advantage of the male latex (and polyurethane) condom is that it also protects against HIV and many other STIs.

The *diaphragm* is a flexible rubber disk with a rigid rim that is used with a spermacide; it is inserted into the vagina by a woman prior to intercourse and must be left in place for a minimum of 6 hr after intercourse. The *cervical cap* is a dome-shaped rubber cap that is inserted into the vagina by a woman prior to intercourse; it can be left in place for up to 48 hr. Both the diaphragm and the cervical cap must be fitted by a health professional, are used with a spermacide, and have a failure rate of 12 percent.

The *contraceptive sponge* is made of polyurethane, used with a spermacide, and inserted into the vagina prior to intercourse. It is available without a prescription, is easy to use, and can be left in place for up to 24 hr; however, it has a failure rate of 18–28 percent.

The most recent female barrier method to be developed is the *female condom*, which consists of a lubricated polyurethane sheath with a flexible ring on each end; one end is inserted into the vagina and the other remains outside; thus, the female condom is visible to the partner. The failure rate is estimated at 21–26 percent; like the male latex condom, the female condom protects against HIV and other STIs.

Hormonal Methods

The use of progestin only or estrogen and progestin together is common. These hormones are taken well in advance of vaginal intercourse and may be administered by mouth (i.e., the *pill*), by an *injection* (e.g., Depo-Provera), or *implanted* under the skin (e.g., Norplant). The implants and injectables have the lowest failure rates (2–3 percent), followed by the pill (8 percent). For some women, use of the estrogen and progestin combination also provides additional health benefits including protection against some cancers and pelvic inflammatory disease (PID). For other women, especially those who smoke or who have a history of cardiovascular difficulties, the use of such hormones can have serious side effects. Although very effective, the use of steroids requires careful medical supervision.

Intrauterine Devices

Intrauterine devices (IUDs) are small, plastic, and flexible devices that are inserted into the uterus though the cervix by a trained health professional well in advance of intercourse. IUDs alter uterine and tubal fluids and inhibit the movement of sperm through the cervical mucus and uterus. IUDs have a 4–5 percent failure rate and carry a small risk of PID among some women.

Surgical Methods

Vasectomy is an operation to cut or tie off the tube (the vas deferens) that sperm use to travel from the testicles to the penis. *Tubal ligation* involves surgery to close the fallopian tubes, making it impossible for sperm and egg to unite. Both surgical procedures have an extremely low failure rate (<1 percent) but they are usually irreversible; thus, these procedures tend to be used by adults who have already had, or do not wish to have, children. Also, tubal ligation is a complex medical procedure that leads to complications in 2 percent of cases.

COMBINING CONTRACEPTION AND DISEASE PREVENTION

Most contraceptive methods do *not* protect against HIV and other STIs. Of the methods discussed, only abstinence, nonpenetrative sexual behaviors, and latex and polyurethane male and female condoms prevent both conception and STI transmission. Sexually active couples are advised to seek testing (provided by most health departments) prior to sexual activity to be sure that neither partner is infected with a STI. Testing for STIs is important because a person can have an STI without any symptoms. After test results confirm that both partners are "negative" (i.e., not infected), then the contraceptive methods described can be used within the context of a mutually monogamous relationship (both partners agree to have no other relationships or sexual partners) without fear of acquiring an STI. If there is any doubt about the commitment of either partner, then continued use of a male or female condom is advised.

FACTORS THAT PREDICT CONTRACEPTIVE USE

Unintended pregnancies occur commonly in the United States due to nonuse or incorrect use of contraceptive methods. In the United States, approximately 60 percent of all pregnancies

(86 percent of all pregnancies among unmarried adolescents) are unintended.

Contraceptive use is associated with a wide range of psychosocial and economic factors, including knowledge about contraception and reproductive health, skill in using contraceptives properly, the quality of a couple's relationship, access to reproductive health services and contraceptives, personal and cultural comfort with sexuality, religious and political preferences, and media influences. Ongoing research seeks to increase current understanding of the causes of contraceptive use and nonuse and to identify educational, psychological, medical, and public health programs that can promote contraceptive use among persons who choose to be sexually active.

Related Entries: Human Sexuality, STD Prevention

BIBLIOGRAPHY

Brown, S. S., & Eisenberg, L. (Eds.). (1995). *The best intentions: Unintended pregnancy and the well-being of children and families.* Washington, DC: Institute of Medicine.

DiCenso, A., Guyatt, G., Willan, A., & Griffith, L. (2002). Interventions to reduce unintended pregnancies among adolescents: Systematic review of randomised controlled trials. *British Medical Journal, 324,* 1426–1434.

Fu, H., Darroch, J. E., Haas, T., & Ranjit, N. (1999). Contraceptive failure rates: New estimates from the 1995 National Survey of Family Growth. *Family Planning Perspectives, 31,* 56–63.

Michael P. Carey

Conversion Hysteria

Patients with conversion hysteria complain of numerous puzzling symptoms such as weakness, paralysis, or sensory impairments. They are often referred to neurologists or psychiatrists, who detect no anatomical or physiological basis for the symptoms.

Hysteria was relatively common in late 19th century when Josef Breuer and Sigmund Freud's experiences with hysterical patients yielded the classic psychoanalytic premise, namely, that repressed intrapsychic conflict can be transformed into physical disease.

The similarity of hysteria and hypnotic states has long been recognized, and empirical data support this view. Brain areas activated in hypnotic paralysis are similar to those activated in hysteria. Conversion patients are more responsive to hypnotic suggestions and may be more suggestible (easily influenced) in general.

An accurate diagnosis of hysteria is difficult to make. The development and testing of adequate treatments has thus been severely compromised. Although there are no controlled treatment studies, cognitive–behavioral treatments may be effective.

Related Entries: Psychosomatic Medicine, Somatization

PAUL R. DUBERSTEIN

The Cook–Medley Hostility Scale

PSYCHOMETRICS AND APPLICATIONS IN THE STUDY OF HEALTH AND DISEASE

The Cook–Medley Hostility (Ho) Scale is the most widely researched self-report measure of trait hostility in health psychology. This popularity stems from the measure's origins in basic personality assessment and its association with a wide variety of health outcomes including coronary heart disease (CHD), hypertension, heart attacks or myocardial infarctions (MI), chest pain (angina), carotid artery disease, stroke, atherosclerosis, and premature death. The measure consists of 50 True/False items taken from the original Minnesota Multiphasic Personality Inventory. Several studies have shown that the scale demonstrates both convergent and discriminant validity, properties important for its use as a valid instrument for the measurement of hostility. Originally designed to predict teacher rapport with students, the scale is associated with experiential aspects of hostility including anger-proneness ("I have at times had to be rough with people who were rude or annoying"), resentment ("There are certain people whom I dislike so much that I am inwardly pleased when they are catching it for something they have done"), and mistrust ("it is safer to trust nobody"). Consistent with this characterization, people who score higher on the Ho measure experience more frequent interpersonal and relationship problems, lower satisfaction in their marriages, and lower social support and are less satisfied in their jobs.

Evidence also supports the Cook–Medley Hostility Scale as an important predictor of physical health. In particular, hostility as assessed by the scale has been investigated as a risk factor for the development and progression of CHD and essential hypertension. For example, a recent meta-analysis of six prospective studies of initially healthy people found that Ho scores were predictive of CHD development. Evidence also supports the scale as a predictor of future acute clinical events such as MI. For example, J. C. Barefoot and colleagues found that Ho scores obtained in a sample of 730 men and women in the 1960s were predictive of MI and all-cause mortality over a 30-year follow-up after controlling for traditional medical factors.

Cardiovascular reactivity is one hypothesized mechanism linking psychosocial risk factors to cardiovascular disease and acute events. A growing literature shows that risk factors such as that measured by the Cook–Medley Hostility Scale are associated with larger and longer increases in heart rate and blood pressure in response to psychological stress. For example, Christensen and Smith (1993) found that individuals who scored high on the Cook–Medley Hostility Scale and were assigned to give a self-disclosing speech to a stranger displayed significantly greater blood pressure reactivity than low-Ho individuals. Similar findings have been shown in response to a variety of social and nonsocial mental stress tasks. Hence, Ho as measured by the Cook–Medley Hostility Scale is well-supported risk factor for psychosocial well-being and physical health.

Related Entry: Hostility and Health

BIBLIOGRAPHY

Barefoot, J. C., Larsen, S., von der Lieth, L., & Schroll, M. (1995). Hostility, incidence of acute myocardial infarction, and mortality in a sample of older Danish men and women. *American Journal of Epidemiology, 142,* 477–484.

Barefoot, J. C., & Lipkus, I. M. (1994). The assessment of anger and hostility. In A. W. Siegman & T. W. Smith (Eds.), *Anger, hostility, and the heart* (pp. 43–66). Hillsdale, NJ: Erlbaum.

Blascovich, J., & Katkin, E. S. (1993). *Cardiovascular reactivity to psychological stress and disease.* Washington, DC: American Psychological Association.

Christensen, A. J., & Smith, T. W. (1993). Cynical hostility and cardiovascular reactivity during self-disclosure. *Psychosomatic Medicine, 55,* 193–202.

Cook, W. W., & Medley, D. M. (1954). Proposed hostility and pharisaic–virtue scales for the MMPI. *Journal of Applied Psychology, 38,* 414–418.

Hathaway, S. R., & McKinley, J. C. (1943). *The Minnesota Multiphasic Personality Inventory manual.* New York: Psychological Corporation.

Miller, T. Q., Smith, T. W., Turner, C. W., Guijarro, M. L., & Hallet, A. J. (1996). A meta-analytic review of research on hostility and physical health. *Psychological Bulletin, 119,* 322–348.

Pope, M. K., Smith, T. W., & Rhodewalt, F. (1990). Cognitive, behavioral, and affective correlates of the Cook and Medley Hostility Scale. *Journal of Personality Assessment, 54,* 501–514.

Rozanski, A. (1998). Laboratory techniques for assessing the presence and magnitude of mental stress-induced myocardial ischemia in patients with coronary artery disease. In D. S. Krantz & A. Baum (Eds.), *Technology and methods in behavioral medicine* (pp. 47–68). Mahwah, NJ: Erlbaum.

Ruiz, J. M., Smith, T. W., & Rhodewalt, F. (2001). Distinguishing narcissism and hostility: Similarities and differences in interpersonal circumplex and five-factor correlates. *Journal of Personality Assessment, 76,* 537–555.

Smith, T. W. (1992). Hostility and health: Current status of a psychosomatic hypothesis. *Health Psychology, 11,* 139–150.

Smith, T. W., & Frohm, K. D. (1985). What's so unhealthy about hostility: Construct validity and psychosocial correlates of the Cook and Medley Ho scale. *Health Psychology, 4,* 503–520.

Smith, T. W., Sanders, J. D., & Alexander, J. F. (1990). What does the Cook and Medley Hostility Scale measure? Affect, behavior, and attributes in the marital context. *Journal of Personality and Social Psychology, 58,* 699–708.

JOHN M. RUIZ

Coping

When a person experiences a stressful event, he or she has to handle the problem in some way. Some persons, for example, may take direct action to resolve the problem or may ask others for advice. Other persons might go to a movie to distract themselves from the problem or might ignore the problem and hope that it goes away. These are a small sampling of the numerous ways that people can respond to stress. *Coping efforts* or *coping behaviors* are therefore defined as those thoughts and behaviors that a person uses to manage a stressor.

One useful model for understanding coping behavior is the *transactional model*, developed in 1984 by Richard Lazarus and Susan Folkman. When an event occurs, a person evaluates the event to determine whether it is stressful (called *primary appraisal*). Events that pose a threat (e.g., taking an exam that one is not prepared for) or that involve loss (e.g., being fired from a job) are appraised as stressful. Following this primary appraisal, the person reviews options of how to manage the problem (called *secondary appraisal*) and engages in one or more of those options. The result of those coping efforts is to produce either a positive mood state if the stressor is resolved or a negative mood state if the problem remains ongoing. Negative mood states produce physiological reactions that are detrimental to health, and positive moods produce physiological responses that relax the body and are more health protective. The final, crucial piece of the model is that it is a process. A person can continually reappraise the situation and adjust his or her coping efforts as needed. The remainder of this entry discusses the different types of coping, how often they are used and by whom, and their effectiveness at reducing the health-related consequences of stress.

TYPES OF COPING

There is no single way to view or to categorize coping efforts. Several ways of categorizing coping have been offered, and three commonly used models are described here.

One distinction is between *active* and *passive* coping. Active coping efforts include those intended to resolve a problem. Passive coping efforts are avoidant in nature and include such efforts as distraction (focusing one's attention on something other than the stressor) and denial (acting as if the stressor never occurred). Other categorizations view coping efforts as being *problem focused, emotion focused,* or *avoidant* in nature. Problem-focused strategies include those actions taken to resolve a stressor. Emotion-focused strategies include those efforts that make a person feel better about the situation. Avoidant strategies include those that essentially ignore the problem, such as denial.

A student who is struggling in a class, for example, may engage in problem-focused coping such as scheduling extra study time or hiring a tutor. An example of an emotion-focused strategy for the same situation is when the student talks to friends to relieve anxiety while waiting to hear about test results. Denial is an example of an avoidant strategy in which a person insists that things are fine even though she or he is in danger of failing the class.

Although these distinctions are useful, they obscure the variety of ways that people can cope, and efforts turned to identifying specific coping factors. These factors are often labeled differently across studies, but they have common underlying features such as planful problem solving, seeking social support, waiting for the right time to do something, denial or distancing oneself from the problem, reappraising the situation to view it more positively (e.g., "looking for the silver lining"), accepting responsibility, and escape/avoidance (e.g., drinking alcohol to forget a problem), among others. How a particular effort is categorized depends on the nature of the problem and the intent and result of the effort. For example, talking to a friend may be a problem-solving strategy if it results in a plan of action or it may be an attempt to seek social support if the goal is to help the person feel better. Thus, it is more the intent and outcome of the action that determines the type of coping rather than the action itself.

Thus far, coping efforts have been described as specific behaviors. Another way to conceptualize coping efforts is in terms of *coping flexibility*. When first developed, this concept generally referred to one's variability in the use of coping efforts. In 2001, Cecilia Cheng provided a theoretical model of coping flexibility and tested her model in laboratory and real-life settings. Cheng identified five broad categorizations of flexibility: *flexible* (people who could perceive variability in their degree of control over a situation), *active–inflexible* (maintaining an appraisal of control across all situations), *passive–inflexible* (viewing all events as outside of their control such as in a learned-helplessness attitude), *active–inconsistent* (relying somewhat exclusively on active coping efforts even in situations that were outside of personal control), and *passive–inconsistent* (relying somewhat exclusively on emotion-focused coping efforts, even in instances when personal control existed). Compared to the other groups, the flexible group indeed reported greater variability in their perceptions of stress, selection of coping behaviors, and greater coping effectiveness. Consequently, the concept of coping flexibility is important to the understanding of the coping process.

STRATEGIES AND USAGE

When people have personal control over a stressor, they tend to utilize problem-focused coping strategies. When a stressor is outside a person's control, he or she tends to rely more on emotion-focused or avoidant coping strategies. Otherwise, the usage of the different strategies depends on such factors as the person's gender, personality, and cultural background.

Gender Differences in Coping

Many studies throughout the 1970s and 1980s found that men engaged in more problem-focused coping efforts and that women engaged in more emotion-focused coping efforts when managing a stressor. This information, combined with findings that women reported more psychological problems such as anxiety and depression and utilized the health care system more frequently, led people to believe that women were ineffective copers compared to men.

Research in the 1990s and early 2000s painted a more complex picture of the gender differences in coping. Shelley Taylor and her colleagues proposed that women have a greater tendency to "tend-and-befriend" others when stressed, rooted in women's evolutionary investment in producing and protecting offspring (Taylor et al., 2000). According to Taylor, women are more likely to nurture and protect individual people and the larger social network when faced with stress. Taylor also posited that this response is related to an attachment–caregiving biological system that differs from the "fight-or-flight" system used to fight or run away from an adversary. Although some disagreed with Taylor's assertions, the model suggested that gender differences in coping may, in part, be biologically rooted in different evolutionary needs of men and women.

Other research found that men and women tended to select and report on different stressors. When allowed to select a stressor, men tended to select more task-oriented stressors and women tended to select more interpersonal stressors. Consequently, prior gender differences in coping may have been more an outcome of these different stressors than an indication of ineffective coping.

A meta-analysis compared findings across studies published from 1990 to 2000 and found that women were more likely than men to seek emotional support, constantly think about the problem (called rumination), and engage in positive self-talk designed to encourage or reassure oneself. However, gender differences in coping were more apparent when women appraised the stressor as being more stressful. When men and women appraised the stress equally, gender differences disappeared, with one exception: men were more likely to seek nonspecific social support. Furthermore, women reported using more coping strategies overall, including problem-solving strategies, than men did. These findings suggest that, if gender differences in coping exist, women may take a more flexible approach to their coping rather than have a preference for a given strategy.

Cultural Differences in Coping

When comparing coping efforts of people from Western versus Eastern cultures, research suggests that the more collectivist nature of Asian cultures results in a lesser valuation of personal control and a tendency to report less personal control over stressful events. Because appraisals of low control result in using fewer active behavioral coping strategies, one would predict—and research findings support the notion—that people from Western cultures use more active behavioral coping and that people from Asian culture used more emotional or cognitive coping strategies.

In the United States, similar differences in the use of coping efforts have been found between people from European-American versus other cultural backgrounds. In general, people from African-American and Latino backgrounds tend to report less usage of problem-focused strategies and rely more on emotional and spiritual-based coping as compared to Americans of European descent. Like Asian cultures, African-American and Latino cultures also tend to rely on and value community over individuality more so than do people of European descent. Consequently, the lesser reliance on individual action may be a direct result of this value. One should note, however, that members of African-American and Latino ethnic groups are disproportionately represented in the lower socioeconomic strata; therefore, it is unclear whether these differences are due to cultural preferences per se or to the relatively uncontrollable life circumstances that accompany lower socioeconomic status (e.g., crowding, poverty).

Personality Differences in Coping

Yet another way to conceptualize coping efforts is through a person's general *coping style*, also known as *trait coping*. This approach assumes that different personalities interact with the world differently and have preferences for using certain strategies more than others. One example of a coping style is the characteristic of *optimism*, a general outlook on life that maintains the belief that positive things will happen. Optimists use more problem-focused coping, positive reappraisal, and seeking social support. Pessimists report using more denial, distancing, and disengagement in their coping efforts. A second example of a trait coping style is the monitoring versus blunting coping style, which is particularly relevant for people coping with medical problems. Whereas people with a *monitoring coping style* desire and seek out information about their medical conditions, people with a *blunting coping style* avoid and distract themselves from such information. A third example of personality-influenced coping style is the construct of *hardiness*. People who are considered "hardy" exhibit a composite of three characteristics: high commitment (being fully engaged in what one encounters), high control (believing that one can influence the environment and the events in one's life), and high challenge (being open to change and viewing events as opportunities for growth). People who are high in hardiness tend to use more problem-focused and less avoidant coping strategies than people low in hardiness.

EVALUATION OF COPING EFFICACY

The term *coping efficacy* refers to the extent to which coping efforts are effective at helping a person to resolve a problem or feel better about a situation. A large body of research has accumulated on coping efficacy; in fact, it is perhaps the most prolific in psychology research. Several different methods exist for studying coping efficacy. One model asks them how they typically handle stressors and reflects the more trait-oriented type of coping style. A second model provides people with hypothetical examples of stressors and asks them how they would cope with it if they experienced it. A third model asks people to identify a stressor that they have experienced and how they coped with it. People may be asked to retrospectively recall a stressor that occurred in the past week or month. Diaries recorded at the end of a day are used to study coping efforts close in time to when they happened. In the 1990s the development of hand-held computerized diaries allowed researchers to study coping efforts as they occurred throughout a day. The end-of-day and momentary diaries provide the most promise for understanding the process component of coping.

For as many stressors as one can name—job stress, academic difficulties, illness and injury, marital difficulties, and so on—a separate literature has developed to understand how to cope effectively with these problems. Overall, these studies indicate that problem-focused strategies are more effective when the person has personal control over the situation but that avoidant strategies are most effective when personal control is lacking. A 1985 review by Jerry Suls and Barbara Fletcher found that avoidant strategies were more effective in the short term and strategies that focused one's attention on a stressor were more effective in the long term. Thus, distracting oneself may be effective while waiting to hear the results of a medical test, but such avoidance behaviors are not effective for health matters in the long term.

In the late 1990s, interest developed in previously overlooked ways of coping, including spiritual-based coping and expressive writing (i.e., writing about stressful events in a journal). These strategies were found to be effective at helping people to accept stressful experiences in a positive way. Expressive writing in particular was found to help people to process emotional experiences, release emotions in an adaptive way, and improve health-related physical functioning. The effect of spiritual coping efforts on health remains controversial.

HEALTH BENEFITS OF SUCCESSFUL COPING

When considering the health-related benefits of coping, it is important to consider the impact of coping efforts on both physical and mental health outcomes. Also, one can consider how coping efforts help to prevent illness from occurring and how coping efforts help people with medical problems during and after the diagnostic process.

Overall, there are two main ways by which coping efforts can help keep people healthy. The first is through health-related behaviors. When people cope effectively with stress, they are more likely to take care of themselves by eating regular and healthy meals and by getting adequate sleep. People who cope ineffectively with stress are more likely to turn to unhealthy habits such as smoking and eating poorly. Consequently, one path by which coping efforts influence health is by altering the person's health behaviors.

The second way in which coping efforts contribute to health has been more difficult to establish in research findings. This route pertains to how coping efforts ameliorate the physiological effects of stress. When a stressor occurs, the human body engages in a *fight-or-flight response*, which prepares the body to either fight the threat or run away from it. This response includes, for example, increased heart rate and blood pressure to provide more oxygen to those parts of the body needed to respond to the threat. Although these physiological responses are adaptive for handling acute, time-limited stressors (e.g., escaping a predator), they are less adaptive when dealing with the longer term, chronic stressors encountered in our modern lives (e.g., the constant stress that accompanies attending college over several years). Although our stressors have evolved over time, the body's response to those stressors have not and it is believed that our bodies remain in a heightened state of arousal as we go about our daily activities.

The body's physiological responses are set off by such emotional reactions as fear and anger that accompany threatening situations. Coping theory posits that effective coping reduces the emotional reaction and short-circuits the physiological response. Although some research supports this notion, it has by no means been resolved in the literature and problems in these studies exist. Namely, early research relied on retrospective reports of coping with events that had already passed, the memory of which could have been influenced by the passage of time. In the 1990s, the development of computerized diaries allowed researchers to study coping efforts as they occurred during the day. One study found that coping efforts measured on this momentary basis were unrelated to mood measured at the same time. Although contrary to prior findings, the authors suggested that people might view the coping process differently at the momentary level compared to when they retrospectively recall a stressor. Consequently, many researchers in the early

21st century called for a more process-oriented approach to understand the dynamics of coping.

A 2002 paper by Julie Penley and her colleagues reviewed research on the relationship between coping and health. Although the review included a limited number of studies, it nevertheless produced some interesting summations of this relationship. Overall, the use of self-control and problem-focused coping strategies was associated with some improved physical health outcomes, whereas the use of distancing and seeking social support was associated with poorer physical health outcomes. The use of problem-focused coping was associated with improved psychological health and the use of confrontive coping, distancing, self-control, accepting responsibility, escape–avoidance coping, and wishful thinking were associated with poorer psychological health. Planful problem solving and positive reappraisal were unrelated to either physical or mental health outcomes. Although some of these findings are contrary to prior research, the results may be biased by the selection of only a small sample of studies that may not be representative of the larger body of research on coping and health. Furthermore, a cautionary note about the causal nature of these findings needs to be made. Because most of the articles in the meta-analysis focused on how people coped with medical stressors, it is unclear whether the use of certain coping strategies "caused" certain health outcomes or the experience of chronic health problems "caused" people to rely less on problem-focused and more on emotion-focused coping strategies.

EFFECTIVENESS OF COPING SKILLS INTERVENTION

Given that some people cope more effectively with stress than others, it seems reasonable to presume that ineffective copers may be trained to improve their coping skills. Research in this area typically has selected a problem (e.g., substance abuse) and trained people in techniques that helped them to adapt more successfully to the situation. Examples of skills taught in these interventions are problem-solving skills, time management skills, communication skills, managing emotions, and cognitive restructuring in which negative thought patterns (e.g., "This pain I'm in is absolutely unbearable!") are replaced with positive ones (e.g., "This hurts, but I can ride it out and will be okay"), among others.

Although a wealth of research on this topic exists, James Coyne and Melissa Racioppo (2000) criticized it for not identifying the "crucial ingredients" that make such interventions successful and for not understanding how changes in behavior occurred. Furthermore, changes in behavior are difficult to maintain, and Coyne and Racioppo indicated a need to understand how such behavioral changes are maintained. They

recommended that future research work to further our understanding of these issues.

SUMMARY

Coping efforts refer to those thoughts and behaviors used to manage a stressor. Different ways of categorizing coping efforts have been suggested, and individual differences in the use of coping efforts exist based on gender, culture, and personality. Whether a particular strategy is effective depends on the nature of the stressor. In general, those stressors that are under a person's immediate control tend to be coped with more effectively using problem-focused strategies and those stressors that are outside a person's immediate control tend to be coped with more effectively using emotion-focused strategies. Effectively coping with stress can have health-protective effects by helping a person to maintain healthy lifestyles and reducing deleterious physiological responses to stress, although people can learn more effective coping responses via stress management or coping skills training. Finally, research on coping efforts would benefit greatly from a focus on the process of coping and how it can change over time rather than a focus on individual strategies at a single point in time.

Related Entries: Denial, Hardiness, Optimism and Health, Stress Appraisal, Stress Management, Stressful Life Events

BIBLIOGRAPHY

Brantley, P. J., O'Hea, E. L., Jones, G., & Mehan, D. J. (2002). The influence of income level and ethnicity on coping strategies. *Journal of Psychopathology and Behavioral Assessment, 24,* 39–45.

Cheng, C. (2001). Assessing coping flexibility in real-life and laboratory settings: A multimethod approach. *Journal of Personality and Social Psychology, 80,* 814–833.

Coyne, J. C., & Racioppo, M. W. (2000). Never the twain shall meet? Closing the gap between coping research and clinical intervention research. *American Psychologist, 55,* 655–673.

Hwang, C.-E., Scherer, R. F., Wu, Y., Hwang, C.-H., and Li, J. (2002). A comparison of coping factors in Western and non-Western cultures. *Psychological Reports, 90,* 466–476.

Lazarus, R., & Folkman, S. (1984). *Stress, appraisal, and coping.* New York: Springer.

Marco, C. A., Schwartz, J. E., Neale, J. M., Shiffman, S., & Stone, A. A. (1999). Coping with daily events and short-term mood changes: An unexpected failure to find effects of coping. *Journal of Consulting and Clinical Psychology, 67,* 755–764.

Monat, A., & Lazarus, R. (Eds.). *Stress and coping: An anthology* (3rd ed.). New York: Columbia University Press.

O'Connor, D. B., & Shimizu, M. (2002). Sense of personal control, stress, and coping style: A cross-cultural study. *Stress and Health, 18,* 173–183.

Penley, J. A., Tomaka, J., & Wiebe, J. S. (2002). The association of coping to physical and psychological health outcomes: A meta-analytic review. *Journal of Behavioral Medicine, 25*, 551–603.

Snyder, C. R. (1999). *Coping: The psychology of what works.* New York: Oxford University Press.

Somerfield, M. R., & McCrae, R. R. (2000). Stress and coping research: Methodological challenges, theoretical advances, and clinical applications. *American Psychologist, 55*, 620–625.

Suls, J., & Fletcher, B. (1985). The relative efficacy of avoidant and non-avoidant coping strategies: A meta-analysis. *Health Psychology, 4*, 249–288.

Tamres, L. K., Janicki, D., & Helgeson, V. S. (2002). Sex differences in coping behavior: A meta-analytic review. *Personality and Social Psychology Review, 6*, 2–30.

Taylor, S. E., Klein, L. C., Lewis, B. P., Greunewald, T. L., Gurung, R. A. R., & Updegraff, J. A. (2000). Biobehavioral responses to stress in females: Tend-and-befriend, not fight-or-flight. *Psychological Review, 107*, 411–429.

CHRISTINE A. MARCO

Coronary Heart Disease

RISK FACTORS AND BIOBEHAVIORAL MECHANISMS

Coronary heart disease is the leading cause of death in industrialized countries. Several biological, behavioral, and psychological factors are associated with elevated risk for coronary artery disease (CAD) and its clinical manifestations. In the following sections, a brief review is provided of (1) the epidemiology and pathophysiology of CAD, (2) traditional risk factors for first and recurrent cardiac events (e.g., hypertension, elevated cholesterol), (3) common diagnostic procedures and treatments for patients with CAD, (4) biopsychosocial perspective, including the description of the three main categories of psychological risk factors for coronary syndromes (chronic, episodic, and acute psychological risk factors) based on the pathophysiology of coronary artery disease; and (5) potential implications for psychological interventions.

EPIDEMIOLOGY AND PATHOPHYSIOLOGY OF CORONARY HEART DISEASE

Coronary heart disease (CHD) refers to a broad range of disorders of the heart muscle. A total of 13 million individuals in the United States have CHD. Coronary heart disease is the most common cause of mortality in industrialized countries, accounting for one of five deaths—in the United States, 515,204 deaths in 2000. In this section, common cardiologic terminology is discussed because such information is pertinent to interdisciplinary communication with other professionals in cardiovascular medicine.

The pathophysiology of CHD is determined by multifactorial processes. The heart muscle (myocardium) pumps oxygenated blood through the body and, as is the case for all muscles, this requires adequate myocardial blood supply through the coronary arteries. Myocardial ischemia occurs when cardiac demand for oxygenated blood is not met by the supply of oxygenated blood through the coronary arteries, resulting in insufficient blood perfusion of the heart. Disease of the heart valves and weakening of the heart muscle (cardiomyopathy) are sometimes also categorized under CHD, but is not discussed here. Coronary artery disease is caused by gradual plaque formation (atherosclerosis) of the coronary blood vessels. Serious complications (heart attacks and sudden cardiac death) can occur when the coronary blood supply is abruptly blocked as a result of plaque rupture and/or blood clot (thrombus) formation. These "acute coronary syndromes" are commonly caused by myocardial ischemia and include severe chest pain or pressure (unstable angina pectoris), permanent damage to the heart (myocardial infarction), and malignant heart rhythm disturbances (cardiac arrhythmias).

Coronary atherosclerosis is not a linear process and progresses in phases. Early stages of coronary atherosclerosis are characterized by gradual deposition of lipids (e.g., cholesterol) and other blood particles in the vessel wall. At later stages of CAD, immune system-related molecules (cytokines) play a role in formation of lipid-laden cells in the vessel wall, resulting in impairment of coronary function. When severe CAD has developed, several factors may promote instability of the atherosclerotic plaque and thinning of the cap covering the plaque, both increasing the chance of plaque rupture. Plaque rupture causes partial or complete closure of the coronary artery. The sudden transient coronary obstruction that thus results can cause severe cardiac ischemia and chest pain, whereas complete sustained occlusion leads to myocardial infarction. Although plaque ruptures occur at progressed CAD stages, the actual atherosclerotic narrowing of coronary arteries is generally mild to moderate (20–70 percent) rather than severe. Biological and psychological risk factors differentially affect these increasing stages of coronary pathophysiology. The stage of underlying coronary disease is therefore a major determinant of pathophysiologic mechanisms by which psychological risk factors promote the onset of acute coronary syndromes.

In summary, early stages of atherosclerosis are generally asymptomatic because blood supply to the heart is still well preserved. Narrowing of the coronary arteries (i.e., a stenosis >50 percent of the vessel diameter) may lead to decreased coronary blood supply and cause ischemia when cardiac demand exceeds coronary supply (e.g., in response to exercise or acute mental stress). Myocardial infarction may occur as a result of sudden plaque rupture and blood clot formation, causing prolonged and severe myocardial ischemia. Psychological and biological risk factors for clinical manifestations of CAD thus differ with the stage of underlying disease.

RISK FACTORS FOR CORONARY ARTERY DISEASE

The major risk factors for CAD are age, male gender, diabetes mellitus, high blood pressure, adverse lipid profile, positive family history/genetic factors, overweight, physical inactivity, and tobacco smoking. The exact risk for each of these factors ranges from 50 percent to fivefold, depending on the nature of the risk factor, the population under study, the time between risk factor assessment and cardiac endpoint, and the cutoff used for presence versus absence of these risk factors. The odds ratio (OR) reflects the ratio of disease incidence among individuals exposed to a risk factor, divided by disease incidence of individuals without the risk factor. If the OR is significantly greater than one, then the risk factor is more likely to promote a particular disease. If, for example, the OR is equal to 3, than a person with the risk factor is three times more likely to have the disease than a person who does not have the risk factor. The 95 percent confidence interval is a measure of the accuracy of the estimate and ORs are statistically significant at $p < 0.05$ if the interval does not include the value 1.0. Ranges of estimated risks are as follows: positive family history, 1.5–2.0; diabetes mellitus, 2.4–2.8; hypertension, 1.8–2.0; elevated total cholesterol, 1.7–3.4; obesity, 1.2–1.7; and physical inactivity, 1.5–2.4. Risk factors often cluster and are frequently overrepresented in ethnic and racial minority groups. Socioeconomic status plays an important role in these associations, but cannot account for all the observed differences. A detailed review of the interaction of the multiple cardiovascular risk factors for CAD is beyond the scope of this entry. It is important to differentiate between modifiable (e.g., overweight, physical inactivity, and tobacco smoking) and nonmodifiable risk factors (e.g., age, sex, family history).

DIAGNOSTIC PROCEDURES AND INTERVENTIONS

Several diagnostic procedures exist for determining presence or absence of CAD. The most common sequence of events is that patients experience typical or atypical anginal symptoms (chest pain or pressure, shortness of breath, palpitation, or extreme fatigue). These symptoms may lead to referral for cardiac diagnostic testing. Electrocardiographic assessments are made during exercise to determine inducibility of myocardial ischemia by increasing exercise-induced cardiac demand. These assessments are often combined with noninvasive outpatient procedures involving (1) imaging of cardiac blood perfusion by radioisotope labeling of myocardial tissue using thallium or technetium or (2) determination of cardiac function by echocardiography or radionuclide ventriculography. New developments in cardiac electron beam computed tomography scanning allow for detection of subclinical coronary calcification with high sensitivity for detecting CAD. If inducible ischemia is detected, when patients have typical anginal symptoms, in case of severe coronary calcification, or when patients have a very unfavorable risk profile, coronary angiography is performed to visualize the coronary arteries by intracoronary injection of a radioactive dye. This diagnostic procedure takes approximately 1 hr and patients are generally discharged the same day.

Interventions for CAD have three generally overlapping targets: risk reduction of myocardial infarction and other cardiovascular complications, improvement of cardiac function, and alleviation of symptoms plus optimizing quality of life. Risk reduction of CAD and its clinical manifestations involves pharmacological and behavioral modification of risk factors and intervention targeted at improving coronary supply in patients with documented CAD.

When angiography indicates that CAD has progressed to coronary narrowing of >50 percent, various procedures exist that restore coronary blood supply. Percutaneous transluminal coronary angioplasty (PTCA) involves placement of a balloon-tipped catheter at the site of the stenosis, where it is inflated to reopen the blood vessel. Small metal tubes (stents) are commonly placed at the site of angioplasty to prevent recoil of the artery. Recent developments use coated stents with biological agents that can help prevent renarrowing of the opened arteries. Patients generally stay overnight postangioplasty for monitoring purposes. When angioplasty is not possible, coronary artery bypass graft (CABG) surgery is a common treatment option. During CABG, healthy vessels from the leg or near the chest are taken and placed on the coronary arteries to bypass the blockage. CABG is major surgery and requires long-term (1 week) hospitalization and recovery. In addition to these two methods of improving coronary supply (PTCA and bypass surgery), patients with high vulnerability for life-threatening rhythm disturbances can be provided with an implantable cardioverter defibrillator, which delivers a shock when a malignant arrhythmia is detected. Medications are generally used to improve cardiac function, reduce biological risk factors such as high blood pressure (hypertension) and adverse lipid profile, and decrease symptoms. Most medications have side effects that interfere with patients' quality of life, including fatigue, headache, and reduced sexual function or interest. Behavioral and psychological interventions are used to reduce the risks associated with adverse health behaviors (e.g., overweight and smoking) and psychological factors (e.g., depression). In addition, these interventions may also improve quality of life (as discussed later).

BIOPSYCHOSOCIAL PERSPECTIVE

Psychological risk factors for CAD can be classified into three categories, based on their duration and temporal proximity to coronary syndromes: (1) chronic factors, among which are negative personality traits (e.g., hostility) and low socioeconomic status; (2) episodic factors, which are transient, with a duration of several weeks up to 2 years and recurring throughout the life span (e.g., depression and exhaustion); and (3) acute triggers, including mental stress and outbursts of anger. These three types of psychological risk factors are associated with pathophysiologic mechanisms relevant to CAD progression and their effects as risk factors change with progressive stages of coronary disease.

1. Chronic psychological risk factors involve stable characteristics, which are associated with elevated long-term risk of first myocardial infarction. The predictive value for *recurrent* events is less consistent for chronic psychological risk factors. The most common chronic factors are hostile personality (Type A behavior pattern), social isolation, and low socioeconomic status. Recent reports also document the role of Type D personality (a combination of high negative affectivity and high social inhibition) and mixed results have been reported regarding trait anxiety (RR = 1.9; confidence interval [CI] = 0.5–8.6). There has been substantial controversy about the predictive validity of the Type A behavior pattern. Evidence over the past 15 years suggests that hostility is the toxic component of Type A behavior. Meta-analysis indicates that the elevated risk of hostility is often significant, but results are variable (RR = 1.6; CI = 0.7–3.3).

Low socioeconomic status predicts first cardiac events (estimated risk = 2.7), and the increased risk is not limited to the lowest strata only. Among the factors determining socioeconomic status are education level, income, occupation, economic resources, and social standing. Social isolation and elevated psychological distress are more prevalent among individuals of low socioeconomic status. Aspects of low social support can be construed as a chronic psychological risk factor as well. Social support is defined by the availability of social contacts to promote personal goals or needs. Low social support is associated with increased risk of cardiac events (RR = 1.9; CI = 0.3–13.9). Structural social support refers to the number of available individuals (e.g., marital status, number of friends). Functional social support refers to the utility of social support, including instrumental (i.e., actual help in accomplishing tasks), informational, and emotional support. Both domains of social support have been associated with increased risk of CAD. More research is needed to further disentangle the cardiovascular consequences related to socioeconomic status, chronic social stresses related to racism or adverse stigmata among disadvantaged individuals, social isolation, and sustained low perceived social support.

2. Episodic risk factors for CAD include major depressive disorder and (vital) exhaustion.* These factors are transient (with a duration ranging from several weeks to 2 years) and are recurring over the life span. Episodic risk factors predict first as well as recurrent cardiac events. The risk of depression for first myocardial infarction is greater than 50 percent above normal (OR = 1.6, CI = 1.3–2.1), and recurrent events are significantly predicted by depression with risk ratios ranging from 3.0 to 7.8. Depression in patients with coronary disease (and other medical conditions) is often atypical, and not primarily characterized by depressed mood and/or loss of interest. Exhaustion (extreme fatigue, increased irritability, and feelings of demoralization) is a significant risk factor for incident and recurrent cardiac events. Risk associated with episodic risk factors is of similar magnitude to traditional CAD risk factors (see earlier discussion).

Major life events (e.g., loss of a spouse, unemployment and financial crisis) often precede the onset of episodic risk factors. The risk of CAD associated with episodic risk factors is primarily observed within the first 2 years following assessment. The long-term (>2 years) predictive value of depression and other episodic risk factors for adverse cardiac health outcomes is probably explained by the recurring nature of these types of risk factors.

Job-related stress can be episodic or chronic, depending on the nature of the profession. An imbalance between effort and reward, a combination of low control or autonomy and high job demand, and low job satisfaction have been associated with increased CAD risk factors and myocardial infarction. Job strain should be considered in the context of family demands as well. For example, working women with children may be at elevated risk of myocardial infarction, whereas working outside the home by itself is not associated with elevated risk of cardiac events.

3. Acute psychological risk factors (states) can act as triggers of myocardial infarction. Disasters such as earthquakes and missile attacks increase the risk of cardiac events. Acute outbursts of anger are associated with a greater than twofold risk of myocardial infarction. However, these incidents of anger-induced myocardial infarction are very rare, and researchers

---

* The prefix "vital" will not be used in the remainder of this entry. In the original conceptualization of the exhaustion construct, the term "vital" was included to reflect the far-reaching consequences of this condition on daily life function (similar to vital depression).

and clinicians have therefore also focused on acute psychological states of milder intensity (e.g., frustration, tension, annoyance). These acute psychological factors can trigger more common but less severe cardiac events, such as transient myocardial ischemia. Acute mental stress in standardized laboratory conditions causes myocardial ischemia in 30–60 percent of patients with CAD. Mental stress-induced ischemia is generally asymptomatic (silent), in contrast to exercise-induced ischemia, during which chest pain is common.

Mechanisms accounting for chronic psychological risk factors include sympathetic nervous system-mediated proatherogenic processes, including increased lipid deposition and inflammatory processes. These factors play a crucial role in early stages of CAD. In addition to the direct pathophysiologic pathways, chronic psychological factors also promote development of episodic psychological risk factors (e.g., elevated distress levels and depression in low-socioeconomic status groups), and are associated with increased reactivity to acute stressors. Consequently, the predictive value of chronic psychological risk factors for CAD progression is mediated in part by their association with other (episodic and acute) psychological risk factors for CAD. Mechanisms related to episodic risk factors differ from chronic factors because of their transient (i.e., nonchronic) nature. Most studies have not found significant correlations between episodic factors and CAD severity. Therefore, processes involved in the transition from stable to unstable atherosclerotic plaques are probable candidates accounting for the marked predictive value of depression and other episodic factors for acute coronary syndromes. These include autonomic nervous system- and neurohormonally mediated changes in the likelihood of thrombus formation, immune system alterations, and cardiac arrhythmias. Mechanisms related to acute psychological risk factors include sympathetic nervous system-mediated increases in catecholamines, cardiac demand (heart rate and blood pressure), and stress-induced decreases in plasma volume and transient narrowing of the coronary arteries [for a detailed discussion see Krantz et al. (1996) and Kop (1999)]. These stress-induced responses can result in myocardial ischemia and plaque rupture in advanced stages of CAD

In summary, there are three types of psychological risk factors for coronary artery disease: chronic, episodic, and acute. Chronic psychosocial risk factors are involved in the early stages of CAD and play a role at advanced disease stages primarily because of their association with increased presence of co-occurring episodic and acute psychological risk factors. Episodic risk factors play a role in the transition from stable coronary disease to clinical manifestations such as myocardial infarction. Acute risk factors are primarily important at progressed CAD stages because these factors may cause myocardial ischemia and in rare cases plaque rupture or life-threatening arrhythmias.

PSYCHOLOGICAL INTERVENTIONS

The majority of cardiovascular behavioral medicine intervention studies have targeted patients with established coronary disease or those with elevated cardiovascular risk factors. Psychological intervention studies reported in the 1970s and 1980s generally demonstrated beneficial effects on reducing psychological risk factors as well as preventing recurrent cardiac events. In contrast, more recent studies have failed to support the earlier positive results regarding improved cardiovascular health outcomes. A few excellent reviews and meta-analyses have been published on the efficacy of psychological interventions in reducing (recurrent) cardiac events (see Bibliography). On average, psychological and educational interventions reduce cardiac mortality by 34 percent and recurrent myocardial infarction by 29 percent. These effects are similar to traditional medical interventions. In addition, improving the psychological aspects of quality of life is a valid goal irrespective of its impact on CAD. There is also a strong relationship between psychological measures and perceived symptoms such as shortness of breath and chest pain.

Psychological interventions are most effective in reducing recurrent cardiac events if they have initial beneficial effects on proximal medical (e.g., blood pressure, exercise tolerance) and psychological (e.g., depression) measures that are risk factors for these cardiac events. Interventions targeting chronic psychological risk factors often include various forms of stress management. Episodic risk factor interventions typically use common cognitive–behavioral techniques in combination with stress management and group support sessions. In patients with medical disorders, these interventions do generally not fully eradicate episodic risk factors, which in turn interferes with the ability of such interventions to prevent recurrent cardiac events. Psychological interventions can play a key role in reduction of adverse health behaviors such as smoking, physical inactivity, and poor diet. It is likely that a combination of patient-tailored psychological and pharmacological intervention is needed to sufficiently reduce and maintain psychological risk factors in patients at high risk of recurrent cardiac events.

Related Entries: Atherosclerosis, Cardiovascular System

BIBLIOGRAPHY

Kop, W. J. (1999). Chronic and acute psychological risk factors for clinical manifestations of coronary artery disease. *Psychosomatic Medicine, 61*(4), 476–487.

Krantz, D. S., Kop, W. J., Santiago, H. T., and Gottdiener, J. S. (1996). Mental stress as a trigger of myocardial ischemia and infarction. *Cardiology Clinics, 14*(2), 271–287.

Linden, W. (2000). Psychological treatments in cardiac rehabilitation: Review of rationales and outcomes. *Journal of Psychosomatic Research, 48*(4–5), 443–454.

Rozanski, A., Blumenthal, J. A., and Kaplan, J. (1999). Impact of psychological factors on the pathogenesis of cardiovascular disease and implications for therapy. *Circulation, 99*(16), 2192–2217.

Sebregts, E. H., Falger, P. R., and Bar, F. W. (2000). Risk factor modification through nonpharmacological interventions in patients with coronary heart disease. *Journal of Psychosomatic Research, 48*(4–5), 425–441.

WILLEM J. KOP
ALI A. BERLIN
MICAH STRETCH

Correlation Coefficient

The correlation coefficient (r) is a numerical value that indicates the strength of linear association between two variables. Correlation coefficients can have any value between -1.00 and $+1.00$. The absolute value of the coefficient indicates the magnitude of the association, in that the closer this value is to zero, the weaker is the relationship. A value of zero indicates the absence of any linear relationship, although other types of relationships (e.g., curvilinear) could exist. The sign of the coefficient indicates the direction of the association, which is either positive (increase in one variable accompanies an increase in the other) or negative (increase in one variable accompanies a decrease in the other). Researchers use this coefficient to predict values of one variable based on values of another or to explain relationships between variables. For example, one study reported a correlation of $-.62$ between strength of efficacy beliefs to resist temptation to smoke and number of cigarettes smoked, indicating a strong negative relationship (Godding & Glasgow, 1985).

BIBLIOGRAPHY

Godding, P. R., & Glasgow, R. E. (1985). Self-efficacy and outcome expectations as predictors of controlled smoking status. *Cognitive Therapy and Research, 9*, 583–590.

ZLATAN KRIZAN

Cortisol

Cortisol, or hydrocortisone, is a glucocorticoid hormone secreted by the adrenal cortex as part of the hypothalamic–pituitary–adrenal axis response to physical and psychological stress. Cortisol mobilizes the body to respond to stress by promoting the release of energy through stimulating the breakdown of protein and fat and the production of glucose. Cortisol also increases blood pressure through vasoconstriction and aids muscles in sustaining contractions. In addition, cortisol reduces inflammation by decreasing capillary permeability to leakage of plasma and blood cells. It suppresses cellular immune responses including antibody production, lymphocyte proliferation, proinflammatory cytokine production, and natural killer cell activity. Such anti-inflammatory and immunosuppressive effects may impair wound healing and increase susceptibility to infection. Cortisol is used as an index of stress and can be quantified by immunoassay in saliva, plasma, and urine. It has been found to be elevated following stressful laboratory tasks, cognitive challenges such as examinations, surgical procedures, and physical exercise and is chronically elevated in depressed individuals and disaster victims.

Related Entries: Endocrine System, Fight-or-Flight Response, Stressful Life Events

ERIN S. COSTANZO

Dd

Dementia

Dementia is an acquired clinical condition characterized by persistent and often progressive impairment in multiple intellectual domains, such as memory and the ability to think, reason, and use language. Dementia is most common in the elderly. The prevalence of dementia increases with age, from about 1 percent of individuals aged 65 years to approximately 30–50 percent of individuals 85 years suffering from some form of dementia. Because in the United States the number of people over the age of 65 years is expected to double by the year 2030 to approximately 70 million, the diagnosis and treatment of dementia represents a public health concern of vital and increasing importance. There are multiple causes (etiologies) of dementia, but Alzheimer's disease (AD), vascular disease (VaD), and diffuse Lewy body dementia (DLBD) are responsible for the majority of dementia cases.

ALZHEIMER'S DISEASE

In 1906, a German neuropathologist named Alois Alzheimer described a case of a 51-year-old woman with cognitive impairment, delusions, and confusion. After her death, he conducted an autopsy and reported dense material outside the nerve cells and twisted bands of fibers inside the cells. This condition was named "Alzheimer's disease" and is the most common type of dementia, accounting for about 50 percent of all cases. Although estimates vary across studies, AD afflicts about 3 percent of persons between the ages of 65 and 74 years, 20 percent of persons between 75 and 84 years, and up to 47 percent of individuals over the age of 85 years. The incidence of AD increases sharply with age, from approximately 1.2 percent

at age 65 years to about 6.4 percent at age 90 years. Approximately 4.6 million individuals suffer from AD, but projections indicate that by the year 2050 this number could more than triple to 16 million. The estimated annual cost in the United States of AD is between $80 and 100 billion in lost productivity and medical care. The average cost of caring for a patient with AD from the time of their diagnosis to the time of their death (an average of 8 years) is approximately $174,000, making AD one of the most costly illnesses.

The neuropathology of AD begins in the entorhinal cortex in the hippocampus, which is a structure in the brain important for normal memory function. Tiny, insoluble lumps of protein called amyloid begin to accumulate around nerve cells in the brain (neurons), forming insoluble plaques. Although these amyloid plaques are a hallmark of AD, it is not known whether they are a cause or consequence of the disease. A second type of neuropathology in AD is neurofibrillary tangles, which are abnormal twisted fibers that develop inside nerve cell bodies in brains with AD. These tangles are the remains of microtubules, which are a major support structure in healthy neurons. The breakdown of microtubules into neurofibrillary tangles may impair the ability of neurons to communicate with each other and result in cell death. Plaques and tangles develop first in the hippocampus, which coincides with memory impairment, but spread to other areas of the brain as more widespread cognitive impairment (e.g., agnosia, aphasia, impaired judgment and reasoning) occurs.

The hallmark symptom of AD is amnesia, which first manifests as the loss of memory for recent events and newly learned information, but eventually progresses to the loss of remote events and well-learned information. Other cognitive symptoms include agnosia (the inability to recognize familiar words and people), aphasia (difficulties in naming familiar objects), and impaired judgment and reasoning. Ultimately these symptoms progress to a stage that causes problems in common activities of daily living, such as forgetting the route to familiar locations and becoming unable to perform tasks that were once easy (e.g., balancing a checkbook, preparing meals). At later stages of the disease, changes in personality may occur, with afflicted individuals exhibiting high levels of restlessness, becoming prone to wandering and displaying unpredictable anger.

Several genes have been implicated in the development of AD. Familial AD occurs in young individuals, often before the age of 60 years, and is associated with genetic mutations on chromosomes 1, 14, and 21. This type of AD is quite rare, accounting for fewer than 5 percent of all diagnosed cases of AD. Another gene located on chromosome 19, that for apolipoprotein E (APOE), has been linked to the occurrence of AD. In particular, having the E4 allele of this gene is associated with increased risk for AD; however, only 40 percent of AD cases have the E4 allele, indicating that other factors play a role in development of this disease.

VASCULAR DEMENTIA

Vascular dementia (VaD) refers to cognitive impairment that results from problems in the circulation of blood to the brain (cerebrovascular disease). Alone, VaD accounts for approximately 10–15 percent of all dementia cases, and for about another 20 percent in combination with AD. Since criteria for its diagnosis were established in 1993, there has been disagreement regarding how best to diagnose VaD. Lack of a consensus for diagnosing VaD has made estimating its prevalence problematic, but reasonable estimates place the prevalence rate at 0.3 percent at age 65 years, with an increase to 5.2 percent by age 90 years in Western countries. The prevalence of VaD is much higher in some Asian countries.

Vascular dementia can result from a number of causes. Most commonly, it results from the blockage of small blood vessels, or arteries, within the brain, causing death in the cortex, the area of the brain involved in higher order cognitive abilities, such as learning, memory, and language use. This is called a stroke. Sometimes these strokes affect a very small area of the cortex and may go unnoticed for years. After a number of such "ministrokes" have occurred, damage to the brain accumulates and afflicted persons begin to display the behavioral symptoms of dementia. Another common cause of VaD is Binswanger's disease, which affects white matter deep within the brain. Individuals with Binswanger's disease display slowness, impairments in gait, and fluctuations in emotion.

The presentation of symptoms in VaD differs from that of AD. Whereas AD is characterized as a slow, progressive disease with insidious onset, VaD commonly manifests as stepwise deterioration spanning a period of several years. Comparisons of patients with AD and VaD show that the latter group typically exhibits less severe long-term memory impairment. Individual diagnosed with VaD do show more severe impairment on cognitive tests that measure executive function. Tests of executive function measure the ability to develop strategies (e.g., completing a visual maze puzzle) and to coordinate complex behaviors. Individuals with VaD also present with focal neurological symptoms, such gait abnormalities, weakness of an extremity, and impaired reflexes.

DIFFUSE LEWY BODY DEMENTIA

Diffuse Lewy body dementia (DLBD) is perhaps the second most common form of degenerative dementia, accounting for approximately 15 percent of all dementia cases in people over the age of 65 years. Lewy bodies are tiny spherical structures that develop in nerve cells and may contribute to premature neuronal death. Because the neuropathology and symptomology of DLBD are associated with AD and Parkinson's disease, scientists do not yet know whether DLBD is a variant of these two illnesses or is a distinct illness. A hallmark symptom of DLBD is fluctuating cognition, such that on some days individuals exhibit significant impairments in thinking and memory and appear unimpaired on other days. Other core features of DLBD include highly detailed and recurrent visual hallucinations and symptoms consistent with Parkinson's disease, such as falls, slowness, and tremors.

SECONDARY PROBLEMS

There are a number of noncognitive behavioral disturbances in dementia. The most common of these disturbances (and their approximate prevalence in patients with dementia) include agitation (80 percent), incontinence (50 percent), wandering (25 percent), aggression (20 percent), and sexual disinhibition (10 percent). Estimates of the frequency of these noncognitive behavioral disturbances are highly variable because they are very difficult to measure and quantify. Moreover, the frequency and severity of behavioral disturbances increase as the severity of dementia progresses. These disturbances are particularly important because they place increased burden and stress on caregivers and represent symptoms that can be effectively targeted for behavioral and pharmacologic therapeutic interventions.

TREATMENT

There is no cure for AD or the other dementias described here, but there are a number of therapies that can slow disease progression and reduced symptom severity. The neuropathology of AD leads to a loss of the neurotransmitter acetylcholine from the brain. Most of the pharmacologic therapies for AD involve a class of drugs known as cholinesterase inhibitors, which inhibit the breakdown of acetylcholine in the brain. Approved cholinesterase inhibitors include tacrine, donepezil, and rivastigmine. Clinical trials have shown that these drugs slow the progression of symptoms and can even improve activities of daily living and common behavioral disturbances. However, as the disease progresses and the number of viable neurons in the brain decreases, these therapies become ineffective. There are no approved pharmacologic treatments for VaD or DLBD.

Related Entries: Aging, Neuropsychology

BIBLIOGRAPHY

Buckles, V., Coats, M., & Morris, J. (2000). *Dementia.* Available at Best Practice of Medicine—Neurology, http://merck.micromedex.com/bpm/ne/dementia

Jorm, A. F., & Jolley, D. (1998). The incidence of dementia: A meta-analysis. *Neurology, 51,* 728–733.

National Institute on Aging. (2002). *Alzheimer's disease: Unraveling the mystery.* Available at http://www.alzheimers.org/unraveling/

Terry, R. D., Katzman, R., & Bick, K. L. (Eds.). (1994). *Alzheimer disease.* New York: Raven.

MARTIN SLIWINSKI

Denial

Denial refers to both the complete lack of awareness of a distressing thought, emotion, or memory and avoidant processes aimed at reducing awareness of threatening content. Denial processes may occur consciously, as in the case of intentional suppression, or nonconsciously and automatically, as in the case of emotional dissociation or repression. Contemporary views have emphasized variations in the timing and the focus and scope of attention (e.g., a fleeting experience of threat followed by an attentional shift to more benign contents).

Traditional conceptualizations of repression assume only maladaptive health consequences. This view assumes that repressed thoughts and memories push for indirect symbolic representation in the form of somatic symptoms, and that only conscious awareness of the repressed contents can alleviate these symptoms.

More recent conceptualizations have emphasized the costs and benefits of denial-like processes as well as their variability across time, situation, and ethnicity. Much of this work has centered on individual differences. One group of individuals, identified by either questionnaire or behavioral measures

as repressive copers, exhibits an unusual ability to avoid or reduce conscious awareness of threatening content. Repressors also exhibit impoverished recall for negative emotional events.

In threatening laboratory situations, repressors show elevated stress responding in autonomic and hormonal indicators. However, repressors appear to cope unusually well with acute real-life stressors (e.g., the death of a spouse or sexual abuse). During bereavement, repressors evidenced a short-term somatic cost (initial elevations in arousal and somatic complaints) but also a long-term advantage (reduced grief and return to normal levels of somatic symptoms).

A related personality dimension known as self-enhancement is characterized by self-deception and an overly positive or self-serving bias. Self-enhancement is associated with increased self-esteem but also social liabilities, such as narcissism. Self-enhancers are viewed favorably in initial social contacts but less favorably over time. However, self-enhancers are also rated favorably by long-term close friends and report broader social networks. Like repressors, self-enhancers have also been found to cope extremely well with acute stressors.

The relatively automatic and nonconscious nature of repressive coping and self-enhancement are contrasted by more deliberate, conscious denial processes, such as suppression. Laboratory studies have emphasized the maladaptive nature of deliberate suppression. The suppression of specified thoughts has been shown to increase cognitive processing of those thoughts and to lead to form of rumination. Similarly, deliberate emotional suppression in the context of threatening stimuli has been shown to increase autonomic responding. Complimentarily, a large number of studies have demonstrated health benefits, such as decreased medical visits and improved immunocompetence, following the anonymous written expression of traumatic or emotionally distressing events.

It is important to note, however, that disclosure and suppression are not necessarily ends of the same continuum. Recent studies have again pointed to important variability across situations as well as age and ethnicity. For instance, expressing emotion predicts a worse outcome to bereavement, and among older immigrant adults, emotional inhibition appeared to have salutary health consequences for Eastern European ethnic groups.

Related Entries: Coping, Stressful Life Events

BIBLIOGRAPHY

Bonanno, G. A., Keltner, D., Holen, A., & Horowitz, M. J. (1995) . When avoiding unpleasant emotion might not be such a bad thing: Verbal–autonomic response dissociation and midlife conjugal bereavement. *Journal of Personality and Social Psychology, 46,* 975–989.

Consedine, N., Magai, C., & Bonanno, G. A. (2002). Moderators of the emotion inhibition–health relationship: A review and research agenda. *Review of General Psychology, 6,* 204–238.

Lazarus, R. S. (1985). The costs and benefits of denial. In A. Monat & R. S. Lazarus (Eds.), *Stress and coping* (2nd ed., pp. 154–173). New York: Columbia University Press.

Weinberger, D. A., Schwartz, G. E., & Davidson, R. J. (1979). Low-anxious and repressive coping styles: Psychometric patterns of behavioral and physiological responses to stress. *Journal of Abnormal Psychology, 88,* 369–380.

GEORGE A. BONANNO
KARIN COIFMAN

Dentistry and Health Psychology

For more than a quarter-century, health psychology approaches to dentistry and oral health have been active and productive areas of research. Among the topics that researchers have investigated are bruxism (night-time clenching or grinding of the teeth) and other oral habits (e.g., thumb sucking), taste disorders, the impact of craniofacial anomalies, oral health needs of special populations (e.g., the medically compromised and the seriously mentally ill), and a esthetics (orthodontic treatment and tooth whitening). This entry focuses on temporomandibular disorders, dental fears, and adherence to oral health care regimens. These topics address themes important to health psychology, including the impact of chronic conditions on behavior and emotional functioning, the role of behavior in the etiology of disease, and strategies for attaining and maintaining optimal health.

TEMPOROMANDIBULAR DISORDERS

Temporomandibular disorders (TMD) form a heterogeneous collection characterized by orofacial pain and/or masticatory dysfunction. They are frequently organized into three broad diagnostic classes involving masticatory disorders ("chewing") and disorders involving the hard and soft tissues of the temporomandibular joint (TMJ). These diagnostic classes are not mutually exclusive, and patients may be diagnosed with several disorders simultaneously.

Unlike many chronic pain conditions, which are increasingly frequent with age, TMD is more prevalent in those under age 45 years. In population studies, approximately twice as many women are diagnosed with TMD than men, and in clinical samples, women can outnumber men by a ratio of 8:1. Approximately 4.5 percent of the adult population reports pain and dysfunction sufficiently severe to prompt help seeking.

The pain reported by TMD patients is typically located in the muscles of mastication, in the area just in front of the ears, or in the TMJ. TMD patients may also report headache, other facial pains, earache, dizziness, ringing in the ears, and neck/shoulder/upper and lower back pain. TMD patients may report a variety of TMJ problems other than pain, including locking in the open or closed position and clicking, popping, and grating sounds. Patients may report difficulty opening their jaws wide as well as a sense that their occlusion ("bite") feels "off." The spectrum of symptoms leads patients to seek care from dentists, physicians, and other health professionals. Parafunctional tooth contact may be an important mechanism by which individuals develop the muscle pain of TMD. Like other joints, the TMJ is subject to degenerative changes typical of arthritis.

The best-validated measure for assessing TMD, the Research Diagnostic Criteria (RDC) (Dworkin & LeResche, 1992), is unique among chronic pain (and many medical) conditions in requiring comprehensive assessment of both physical and psychological status. This two-axis system codes physical findings under Axis I of the RDC and psychological findings under Axis II.

Like many chronic pain conditions, patients with chronic TMD may experience depression. TMD patients who report chronic muscle pain are more likely to experience psychological distress than those who only report simple clicking or popping noises. Many activities of daily living (e.g., eating, talking, social and recreational activities) are affected by TMD pain.

When rendered by a dentist, treatment of TMD often involves the fabrication of an interocclusal appliance ("splint") that covers the upper or lower teeth and recommendations for use of a nonsteroidal anti-inflammatory drug. Psychological treatments, including biofeedback, relaxation training, habit reversal training, and cognitive–behavioral management of pain, have all been used successfully to treat TMD (e.g., Crider & Glaros, 1999). Evidence shows that psychological treatments are a competitive alternative to dental approaches and may produce better long-term outcomes.

DENTAL FEARS

Approximately 20–30 percent of the adult population has significant fear of dentists and dental procedures. In 5–10 percent of the population, the fear is sufficiently strong to cause avoidance of routine dental care. Dental fears tend to increase during childhood and adolescence, reaching a peak in late adolescence and early adulthood and diminishing thereafter. Only a small proportion of children with dental fears continue to report fear later in life. Women report more dental fear than men. Observation of patient behavior and careful, sympathetic questioning will often identify many individuals with high levels of dental fears. Well-validated self-report questionnaires can also be used to screen individuals for dental fears.

People with dental fears are often concerned with pain, anesthetic injections, sounds, and other sensations that accompany dental assessment and treatment. In others, dental visits can induce claustrophobia, panic, or severe gagging. Patients may distrust dental personnel and the treatment plan for their care. Still others experience a perceived lack of control over the course of a visit.

Dental fears may develop in children or adolescents as a result of a perceived bad experience (e.g., poorly controlled pain) in a dental office, but a more likely source is modeling of dental fears by parents. Patients who develop dental fears in adulthood may have a higher likelihood of being diagnosed with other anxiety disorders. Patients with fears of injections or of health professionals may generalize those fears to a dental environment.

A variety of techniques have been developed to help fearful patients cope successfully with a dental visit. For example, the use of a stop signal will help many patients recover a sense of control over a visit. Use of breathing exercises, relaxation, and imagery can improve a patient's ability to cope with the sensations created by treatment or prophylaxis. The distraction provided by portable tape and CD players can help mask noises. Systematic desensitization and graduated exposure can help patients overcome fears of injections or a tendency to gag. Dentists themselves can manage fearful patients by providing up-to-date information regarding dental care.

The use of antianxiety agents for managing dental fear is common among many dentists. These agents may include nitrous oxide gas, tranquilizers (e.g., Valium), and intravenous sedation. Unfortunately, long-term follow-up studies show that patients who receive medication alone for managing fears do not experience reduction in fear and often fail to receive routine care. In contrast, behavioral interventions appear to produce good long-term results, as measured by the ability to receive continued, routine care by the patient (Milgrom et al., Getz, 1995).

ADHERENCE

Failure to remove plaque, a sticky biofilm containing bacteria, from the teeth causes gingivitis, an inflammation of the gums. Left untreated, gingivitis can progress to periodontitis (a more serious infection), loss of supportive bone, and eventually tooth loss. Thorough, effective brushing accompanied by flossing can disrupt and remove plaque, resulting in healthier gingiva and reduced numbers of carious lesions ("cavities").

The connection between oral care habits and oral health is more obvious and visible to patients than the connection between other disease and health care regimens (e.g., consumption of dietary fats and cardiovascular disease). Failure to brush teeth can result in gingivitis within 2–3 weeks. Treatment of gingivitis and periodontal disease patients can result in markedly reduced signs of infection (e.g., bleeding or pain with brushing and flossing, puffiness in the gums) within 2 weeks. Advertising by manufacturers of oral health care products such as mouthrinses and toothbrushes has increased public awareness of good oral health. The time needed to carry out oral health care is small. Thus, patient adherence to an oral health regimen should be greater than to programs in which the time and effort required from patients is greater and in which the connection between the regimen and an outcome is less obvious.

However, the first-ever Surgeon General's report on oral health (Public Health Service, 2000) identified a "silent epidemic" of dental and oral diseases that are disproportionately represented among members of racial and ethnic groups and among the poor and elderly. The report called the mouth a "mirror for general health and well-being" and noted how oral heath problems were frequently associated with other health problems, including cardiovascular diseases, premature/low term birth weight, and diabetes.

According to the Surgeon General's report, a major barrier to seeking and obtaining professional help is a general lack of public understanding and awareness of the importance of oral health. In some individuals, maintenance of oral health is not a high priority This may be due to the patient's low value for oral health, dental fears, or concerns about the financial cost of dental care. In some cases, a dentist's autocratic communication style does not encourage the shared responsibility that can increase patient compliance with oral care regimens.

A variety of approaches have been developed to encourage individuals to engage in oral health promotion behaviors. One set of strategies focuses primarily on parents. In this approach, parents are encouraged to introduce oral care activities at a very early age and to be good models for oral care. In addition, parents are encouraged to limit intake of sugary foods. For children with good motor control and for adolescents and adults, careful instruction in the techniques of brushing and flossing may improve these behaviors sufficiently so that the risk for gingivitis and carious lesions is reduced. The use of disclosing solutions or tablets that stain plaque can help patients identify areas on the teeth that need more careful brushing.

An ideal oral care regimen may require tooth and tongue brushing, flossing, and the use of a mouth rinse, but not all patients are willing to perform all these tasks. In this situation, techniques that reduce the risk for plaque build-up are preferable to a complicated oral care regimen that the patient does not follow. For example, it may be beneficial to recommend the use of an electric toothbrush alone when a patient is unwilling to brush and floss or when a patient's skill at either technique is marginal.

For those patients who need a more structured approach, adherence regimens based on operant models of behavior are used. These regimens emphasize successive approximation to the goal, careful monitoring by the patient (or other responsible party) of oral care behaviors, positive reinforcement for attainment of intermittent goals, and high levels of praise by dental personnel for success in maintaining good oral health.

Related Entry: Stressful Medical Procedures

BIBLIOGRAPHY

Crider, A. B., & Glaros, A. G. (1999). A meta-analysis of EMG biofeedback treatment of temporomandibular disorders. *Journal of Orofacial Pain, 13*, 29–37.

Dworkin, S. F., & LeResche, L. (1992). Research diagnostic criteria for temporomandibular disorder: Review, criteria, exams and specification, critique. *Journal of Craniomandibular Disorders, 6*, 301–355.

Milgrom, P., Weinstein, P., & Getz, T. (1995). *Treating fearful dental patients: A patient management handbook* (2nd ed., rev.). Seattle, WA: University of Washington, Continuing Dental Education.

Public Health Service. (2000). *Oral health in America: A report of the Surgeon General.* Washington, DC: U.S. Government Printing Office.

Alan G. Glaros

Depression

Depression is one of the most common psychiatric disorders and the fourth leading cause of disability worldwide. Depression can range in severity from mild disruptions of normal mood to disorders of psychotic intensity. Nearly everyone feels sad from time to time, but when these feelings last more than a few days and involve a number of other signs and symptoms that interfere with everyday life, we refer to it as a clinical disorder that can merit a formal psychiatric diagnosis. As a syndrome, depression typically involves negative affect, such as sadness, and a pervasive loss of interest in things that were previously enjoyed. Sometimes the predominant affect is irritability or boredom, especially among adolescents. These mood changes are often accompanied by a profound sense of pessimism (including thoughts of suicide) and negative beliefs about the self, such as "I am worthless or unlovable" or "I can't do anything right." The individual is often less energetic than usual, engages in fewer activities, withdraws socially, and is less productive. There also are often vegetative or physical symptoms, such as sleep problems (e.g., falling or staying asleep, sleeping too much), changes (decrease or increase) in appetite, and loss of interest in sex. If these signs and symptoms persist for at least 2 weeks and are of sufficient magnitude to interfere with everyday life, then the individual is considered to be in an episode of clinical depression. The field currently recognizes two different diagnostic entities relevant to depression. Major depressive disorder requires that these signs and symptoms be of sufficient severity for a period of

at least 2 weeks, dysthymia requires fewer signs, and symptoms that must be present for at least 2 years in adults and 1 year in youth. Some severe depressions can be chronic, and persons with persistent mild depression (dysthymia) are at elevated risk for episodes of major depression.

Most people who get depressed have depressions only. This is called unipolar disorder. However, some people who get depressed also have episodes of mania or hypomania (a milder version of mania). This is now called bipolar depression; it used to be referred to as manic–depression. As a syndrome, mania typically involves opposite changes in the same signs and symptoms as depression. Mood is typically elevated and often euphoric, energy and interests increase, and self-esteem can be inflated to the point of grandiosity. The individual takes on new ventures with reckless abandon and has little need for sleep. Appetites increase and buying sprees and sexual indiscretions are common. In addition to bipolar disorder (called bipolar I if it involves mania and bipolar II if only hypomania), the diagnostic nomenclature also recognizes a disorder called cyclothymia, a less severe version of bipolar disorder marked by mood swings in both directions.

Unipolar mood disorders are common, occurring in about 20 percent of women and about 10 percent of men, whereas bipolar disorders occur in only 1–2 percent of the population and affect the genders equally. Both unipolar and bipolar disorders recur at high rates and many people experience multiple episodes. These disorders are often chronic and even minimal symptoms are associated with increased risk for subsequent episodes and considerable functional impairment. Suicide is a major concern; about 2–4 percent of all depressed people will commit suicide and depression accounts for about 50 percent of all suicides. Moreover, other psychiatric or medical conditions often complicate the picture. About half of all persons with unipolar disorder also have significant problems with anxiety, and depression is a common cause and consequence of substance abuse. Many people become depressed in the face of serious medical illness, and the experience of depression is associated with increased risk for illnesses like heart disease and diabetes.

Depression can strike at any time, but its classic age of onset is in the late 20s for unipolar disorder and the late teens or early 20s for bipolar disorder. Recent evidence indicates that the rates of depressive disorders increase dramatically during ages 15–18 years, particularly in females. Many people who first get diagnosed with depression as adults describe experiencing episodes of depression starting in early adolescence that never came to clinical attention. Depression is rare in children but does occur, usually is short lived, and often is tied to ongoing stressful life events. Boys are as likely to be depressed as girls before the onset of puberty. Depression at this age often involves the appearance of lack of motivation and may be associated with acting-out behaviors. For reasons that are not understood, rates of depression significantly increase in girls during adolescence;

it is at this point that depression in girls begins to outnumber the rate in boys by two to one. Several possible mechanisms may be at work, including changes in hormones and sex-role stereotypes that limit options for women. Women are more likely than men to show an atypical symptom pattern marked by reactivity in mood linked to the ups and downs in relationships, sleeping more than usual, and an increase in appetite. Conversely, men and postmenopausal women are more likely to show a classic melancholic pattern of loss of interest, insomnia, and loss of appetite. This has led some to conclude that the presence of the sex-linked hormone estrogen may influence the expression of depression, if not its actual onset.

It is still not clear what causes depression (or mania), although there are several theories with at least some empirical support. Genetic factors appear to play a moderate role in unipolar depression, accounting for about one-third of the variance in risk in a manner related to severity. Genetic factors play an even larger role in bipolar disorder, which is one of the most heritable of the psychiatric disorders. It seems likely that anyone can become depressed, but that only people with a genetic predisposition can become manic. In either disorder, these genetic factors appear to function as an inherited predisposition (diathesis) that likely requires stressful life events to be expressed. Biological models of depression emphasize the role of neurotransmitter systems and endocrine processes that regulate mood and related vegetative processes like sleep, appetite, and sex. Although the exact mechanisms remain unclear, it is likely that these biological factors represent one way in which genetic propensities are expressed. Two major classes of stressful life events involve interpersonal loss and exposure to other kinds of uncontrollable negative outcomes. Beliefs and attitudes clearly play a role as well. People who have doubts about whether they are lovable or competent are at particular risk for depression. In both animals and humans, depression can be induced by at least three different means: biological depletion of necessary neurotransmitters, separation–loss of important interpersonal relationships, and exposure to uncontrollable stress.

Several types of interventions have been shown to be efficacious in the treatment of depression. Not surprisingly, these treatments correspond with the major theoretical perspectives. Antidepressant medications are widely used and are generally quite effective, but they do little to reduce risk once discontinued; patients with a history of recurrent or chronic depression are generally advised to stay on medications indefinitely. Although somewhat controversial, electroconvulsive therapy (ECT) remains the single most effective treatment for the most severe depressions, and is usually reserved for those patients who do not respond to medications. Mood-stabilizing medications like lithium and the anticonvulsant medications remain the core of treatment for bipolar disorder.

Traditional psychodynamic and experiential psychotherapies are widely practiced but rarely tested; there is little good evidence that they are effective in the treatment of depression. Nonetheless, a recent offshoot of dynamic therapy called interpersonal psychotherapy (IPT), which focuses on problems in current relationships, has been shown to be about as effective as medications in reducing acute distress and has a broader effect on the quality of interpersonal life. Similarly, the cognitive and behavior therapies (often referred to collectively as CBT) also appear to be about as effective as medications in reducing acute distress and have an enduring effect that reduces risks long after treatment is completed. Moreover, there is evidence that CBT also can be used to prevent the initial onset of depression in children and adolescents at risk. Both IPT and CBT appear to be viable alternatives to medication in the treatment of unipolar depression, and combinations with medications appear to be indicated for patients with more difficult-to-treat disorders. Although no one would advocate treating bipolar patients with psychotherapy alone, either IPT or CBT and especially family-focused therapy targeted at reducing conflict within the family can be useful adjuncts to medication treatment.

Despite the availability of efficacious interventions, many people still receive no specific treatment or inappropriate care. Undertreatment of mood disorders can be a consequence of societal stigma, lack of recognition by health care providers, or a failure to appreciate the potential benefits of treatment. The number of people receiving treatment for these disorders has increased over the past decade, particularly with respect to the use of medications, but undertreatment remains a serious problem.

Related Entries: Mood: The Relationship between Mood and Health, Negative Affect, Positive Affect, Postpartum Depression, Psychotherapy

BIBLIOGRAPHY

American Psychiatric Association. (1994). *Diagnostic and statistical manual of mental disorders* (4th ed.). Washington, DC: Author.

American Psychiatric Association. (2000). Practice guideline for the treatment of patients with major depressive disorder (revision). *American Journal of Psychiatry, 157*(Supplement 4).

American Psychiatric Association. (2002). Practice guideline for the treatment of patients with bipolar disorder (revised). *American Journal of Psychiatry, 159*(Supplement 4).

Angold, A., & Rutter, M. (1992). Effects of age and pubertal status on depression in a large clinical sample. *Developmental Psychopathology, 4*, 5–28.

Craighead, W. E., & Miklowitz, D. J. (2000). Psychosocial interventions for bipolar disorder. *Journal of Clinical Psychiatry, 61*(Supplement 13), 58–64.

Gillham, J. E., Shatte, A. J., & Freres, D. R. (2000). Preventing depression: A review of cognitive–behavioral and family interventions. *Applied and Preventive Psychology, 9*, 63–88.

Hankin, B. L., Abramson, L. Y., Moffitt, T. E., Silva, P. A., McGee, R., & Angell, K. E. (1998). Development of depression from preadolescence to young adulthood: Emerging gender differences in a 10-year longitudinal study. *Journal of Abnormal Psychology, 107*, 128–140.

Hollon, S. D., Thase, M. E., & Markowitz, J. C. (2002). Treatment and prevention of depression. *Psychological Science in the Public Interest, 3,* 39–77.

Judd, L. L., Akiskal, H. S., Maser, J. D., Zeller, P. J., Endicott, J., Coryell, W., et al. (1998). A prospective 12-year study of subsyndromal and syndromal depressive symptoms in unipolar major depressive disorders. *Archives of General Psychiatry, 55,* 694–700.

Murray, C. J. L., & Lopez, A. D. (1997). Global mortality, disability, and the contribution of risk factors: Global Burden of Disease Study. *Lancet, 349,* 1436–1442.

Nolen-Hoeksema, S., & Girgus, J. S. (1994). The emergence of gender differences in depression during adolescence. *Psychological Bulletin, 115,* 424–443.

Olfson, M., Marcus, S. C., Druss, B., Elinson, L., Tanielian, T., & Pincus, H. A. (2002). National trends in the outpatient treatment of depression. *Journal of the American Medical Association, 287,* 203–209.

Plomin, R., De Fries, J. C., McClearn, G. E., & Rutter, M. (1997). *Behavior genetics* (3rd ed.). New York: Freeman.

Young, A. S., Klap, R., Sherbourne, C. D., & Wells, K. B. (2001). The quality of care for depressive and anxiety disorders in the United States. *Archives of General Psychiatry, 58,* 55–61.

STEVEN D. HOLLON

JUDY GARBER

Diabetes Mellitus

Diabetes mellitus is a serious chronic illness. More than 17 million people in the United States have diabetes and at least 16 million have *prediabetes* (they are highly likely to develop the disease), and the numbers are growing fast. The number of adults with diabetes in the United States is expected to increase 165 percent over the next 50 years. Diabetes is the seventh leading cause of death, and due to the complications of the disease, is a major cause of blindness, amputations, heart disease, and stroke. Diabetes has become a major focus of health psychology because it has been shown that the course and outcome of the disease are strongly affected by how patients behave and take care of themselves. In order to understand the psychology of diabetes, one must first understand the biology.

BIOLOGY OF DIABETES

The cells of our bodies use the food that we eat for growth and energy by turning part of the food into glucose (sugar), which is found in the bloodstream. The pancreas (an organ in the abdomen) produces a hormone (insulin) that signals the cells to allow the glucose to enter them and be used and stored. Diabetes is a disorder of this metabolic process. There are two major types of diabetes. Type 1 diabetes occurs when the pancreas produces little, if any, insulin. People with Type 1 diabetes must give themselves insulin regularly, usually by injection, or they will get very sick and could die. About 5–10 percent of people with diabetes have Type 1; it usually appears suddenly and mostly in children and young adults. The remaining 90–95 percent have Type 2 diabetes, which is strongly linked to obesity. Type 2 diabetes usually develops gradually in older adults. However, there are growing numbers of children who are being diagnosed with Type 2 diabetes. Type 2 diabetes occurs when the body does not produce enough insulin and/or is not able to use the insulin that is made as well as it should. (Gestational diabetes is a third type of diabetes, it occurs during pregnancy and usually resolves after the baby's birth; however, one-third of women who have had gestational diabetes will later develop Type 2 diabetes.) In all types, the glucose does not get into the cells properly or sufficiently and builds up in the blood causing high blood sugar (*hyperglycemia*). People are diagnosed with diabetes when their blood sugars are very high; this usually causes symptoms of excessive thirst and hunger, frequent urination, and fatigue.

People with diabetes need to try to maintain normal blood glucose levels. Studies have clearly shown that when patients change their behavior to control their blood sugar they can prevent or delay the serious complications that often develop from the disease (i.e., eye disease, kidney damage, heart disease, nerve damage). A landmark study in 2001 also showed that when people who are at risk for diabetes lose weight and increase their activity level, they may even prevent the onset of the disease (Delamater et al., 2001). People with diabetes should do several things to manage the disease. The diabetes self-care regimen includes (1) frequent and regular blood glucose testing, (2) meal planning and dietary control, (3) exercise, and (4) taking prescribed medications.

PSYCHOLOGY OF DIABETES

One can see that the diabetes care regimen is all about self-care behaviors. People with the most common form, Type 2, are often overweight and live inactive, sedentary lives. When they are diagnosed, they have to make major lifestyle changes to closely watch and control what and when they eat, begin to exercise, and properly take medications (which may include regular insulin injections). There are several psychological factors that affect how well they make these changes and the quality of life they experience with this illness. The most well-studied are the influences of depression and stress.

Depression and Diabetes

Major depression is a mental illness that is twice as common in people with diabetes as in healthy people. People are diagnosed with major depression when they experience persistent feelings of sadness or lack of interest in previously pleasurable activities (*anhedonia*) as well as other symptoms, such as sleep, appetite, and concentration problems. Depression persists over time, it may not get better without treatment, and even when successfully treated, is likely to occur again. Depression is associated with poor blood glucose control as well as higher cholesterol levels (which also increase the risk of heart disease).

Why do individuals with diabetes get depressed? Depression may be physiological and be due to possible changes in brain chemicals and/or hormones that are common to both diabetes and depression, or it may be a biological response to chronic high, low, or variable blood sugar levels.

Living with diabetes also poses many emotional challenges that can overwhelm one's psychological resources and lead to depression. Patients need to control a basic activity of life, namely eating, which can lead to a feeling of loss of control over one's own body. Patients can feel ashamed of the stigma of having a chronic illness. Because diabetes is a hidden disease (one cannot tell if someone has diabetes just by looking at them), some people do not get enough emotional support from others. Also, patients often feel guilty about their less-than-perfect self-care. Finally, patients experience fear about the high likelihood that they will develop complications. They generally feel highly anxious when the first complication is diagnosed.

Serious complications of diabetes also add to the burden of the disease. Some people develop sexual dysfunction. For men, this may mean impotence; for women it may mean pain and decreased desire. Sexual dysfunction is very difficult to talk about; patients often do not even tell their doctors when it happens. Sexual dysfunction can affect how people feel about themselves, causing low self-esteem and feelings of shame. These problems and feelings can interfere with the relationship with one's partner, who may not understand why his or her sexual life has changed.

Another major complication can be kidney disease, which in some cases requires hemodialysis. This is a process in which the patient's blood is cleansed of impurities when the kidneys are not functioning properly and are unable to do so. It requires that the patient be hooked up to a dialysis machine three times per week, every week. One can imagine how much this would disrupt an individual's life and routines, interfering with work, recreation, and family activities. Thus, dealing with complications can also cause and increase depression. Research shows that the more complications an individual has, the poorer quality of life he or she experiences.

Depression can make diabetes self-care worse by affecting what one does and does not do. Someone who is depressed is less likely to take good care of himself or herself. The person feels hopeless and helpless, and may not even try to stick to a diet, exercise, or self-care regimen. Also, many people will overeat when they are depressed. This can cause weight gain and poor blood glucose control. Alcohol and illegal drug abuse are also

ways people try to cope with depression, and both will further impair the health and self-care regimen of the individual with diabetes.

Because depression can significantly interfere with optimal diabetes self-management and is a debilitating illness itself, it is important to diagnose and treat depression when it exists with diabetes. The two main ways to treat depression are with antidepressant medications and psychotherapy. These interventions with individuals with diabetes are only beginning to be studied. A 1997 study of antidepressants with depressed individuals with diabetes showed that, compared to patients treated with a placebo, the medication improved the depressive symptoms. It was less clear that it improved blood glucose control, but there was a trend in this direction. A 1998 study of cognitive–behavioral therapy (CBT; a form of psychotherapy that aims to help patients change their negative thoughts and behaviors) with a group of Type 2 diabetes patients also found that the depression improved. The blood sugar control of patients treated with CBT did not improve immediately, but was significantly improved compared to controls at 6 months follow-up. More research on the effect of treatment of depression on diabetes is needed.

Stress and Diabetes

When we are in situations that are new, challenging, or frightening, our bodies react by experiencing what is called the *stress response*. This has also been called the *fight-or-flight response*, as it is the body's way of getting ready to deal with the situation by running or getting away. In earlier times, this worked well when, for example, one had to deal with a tiger in the path. However, in modern times, the situations that cause people to react with the stress response are different; one often cannot run *or* fight. Examples of stressful situations might be having a talk with a teacher, taking an exam, or starting a new relationship.

Several studies of Type 2 diabetes patients showed that stress can negatively affect blood sugar control; this is less clear for those with Type 1 diabetes. This may happen in several ways. From a physical perspective, it is known that when a person experiences the stress response their body releases several hormones (e.g., epinephrine, cortisol) to mobilize the body's systems. This can result in higher blood glucose levels, which is normal, but a problem if one has diabetes and his or her blood glucose regulation system is already out of balance. From a behavioral perspective, it is known that when people experience stress it affects what they do and how well they take care of themselves. Stress may cause a diabetes patient to skip meals or overeat, pay less attention to the need for regular blood glucose testing, forget to take medications or attend doctor visits, and abuse alcohol or other drugs. These changes in self-care can also affect blood glucose levels and are thus considered indirect effects of stress on diabetes.

Stress management training is an intervention that aims to teach patients skills to help them cope with their high stress levels effectively. People cannot avoid stress but can learn to deal with it so that it does not negatively affect health. Examples of the skills taught in stress management training include progressive muscle relaxation (systematically relaxing all the muscles of the body), mental imagery (imagining a relaxing scene, like being at the beach), diaphragmatic breathing (taking deep, relaxing breaths), and cognitive restructuring (changing negative, anxiety-producing thoughts to positive, anxiety-decreasing thoughts). Several studies in which diabetes patients have been taught these skills demonstrated that learning to manage stress can improve blood sugar control. However, other studies did not support this conclusion, and more research needs to be done in this area.

REGIMEN ADHERENCE AND STRATEGIES FOR BEHAVIOR CHANGE

The self-management regimen that individuals with diabetes must adhere to requires significant behavior change. They must exercise and maintain strict dietary control, both to establish and maintain a healthy weight and to achieve normal blood glucose levels. They must test their blood glucose frequently and regularly, which involves multiple uncomfortable pinpricks, to monitor their levels and adjust meals, medications, and/or activity level accordingly. They must often take multiple medications; if it is insulin, this is usually by self- injection. They also need to check their feet daily for possible injuries and healing problems. How well an individual does all of this is called adherence to the diabetes self-care regimen.

There are many reasons that regimen adherence is very difficult. Some people do not have enough information about diabetes; one needs sound information to know what to do. They may not even know how important it is to take good care of themselves and that doing so will help them avoid complications. Some people have unrealistic goals, they try to change but get frustrated when the results are not fast enough. Some do not have the support of others; it is especially hard to change when no one is helping. Others do not have enough resources in their lives. For example, they do not have medical insurance to pay for their doctor visits or blood testing supplies. For others, life is already very stressful and adding the skills needed to deal with diabetes feels overwhelming, so they just avoid doing what they should.

Several psychological factors have been shown to relate to poor adherence. Patients with limited cognitive abilities and poor motivation often demonstrate poor adherence. Also, some patients have beliefs about diabetes that interfere with adherence. For example, patients who believe that the regimen that was prescribed for them by their doctor is unsuitable are less likely to follow that regimen. Those who minimize the seriousness of the disease are also less likely to adhere. A positive predictor of adherence is self-efficacy, or the confidence in one's ability to carry out the regimen tasks. A person who thinks he or she can do it is more likely to. The importance of social support has also been demonstrated, with those who feel emotionally supported by family and/or friends being more likely to adhere to the prescribed regimen.

Two areas of the self-care regimen that have been studied are adherence to blood glucose testing and adherence to diet and weight loss.

Weight loss and management are the most difficult aspects of the diabetes regimen. There are strategies for behavior change that have been demonstrated to improve adherence to weight loss. Interventions to teach these strategies have shown some success. First, patients are encouraged to set clear and reasonable goals. For weight management, this means aiming for a 2-lb, not a 10-lb, loss per week. Second, patients are encouraged to focus on changing their behaviors, not their numbers. This might mean switching to a low-fat diet rather than focusing on how many pounds they have lost. Third, they are urged to start with small, achievable steps and focus on one behavior at a time. This includes making small changes that help them make peace with food (e.g., trying to increase one's awareness of hunger and attention to taste). Fourth, patients are educated about the importance of social support and helped to take steps to identify a confidante and ask for help.

Weight loss programs that teach these principles can help overweight individuals lose weight; the average loss is about 10 percent of initial body weight. Even this modest weight loss can improve a patient's blood glucose control and also can improve blood pressure, lipid levels (fats in the blood), and quality of life. However, after 1 year most participants in these programs regain 30 percent of their weight, and after 5 years most have regained what they lost. Participants who increase their physical activity through exercise and those who consistently monitor their weight are the most likely to keep the weight off. It is clear that we need a better understanding of how to help people maintain the losses they achieve and establish stable weight management.

Regular and frequent blood glucose testing is also an important part of the self-care regimen and is difficult to maintain, as it involves taking time to perform uncomfortable pinpricks multiple times during the day. This allows patients to watch out for extreme high or low readings (hyper- and hypoglycemia), which can signal conditions that can make them very ill, and to adjust their medications, meals, and/or activity levels. Blood glucose fluctuations affect mood, making patients nervous, frustrated, and unhappy, and often interfere with life and may be embarrassing. As time passes with the disease, patients may become less sensitive to the physical signs that their blood sugar is too high or low, so regular and frequent testing becomes even more important. Daniel Cox and his colleagues (1995) have developed a program, called Blood Glucose Awareness Training (BGAT), to help. BGAT includes education and practice of skills to help patients identify the events that affect their blood sugar and to increase their sensitivity to bodily cues of low or high sugar so that they can quickly take appropriate steps.

DIABETES AND THE BIGGER PICTURE

Whereas much of the research has emphasized the psychological and social influences of the individual and family on diabetes self-management, there is also growing recognition that the larger context of one's life has a significant influence on self-care. This includes increased attention to the psychosocial influences of the patient's neighborhood and worksite and the overall health care system.

Most working-age adults spend the majority of their time at work. Factors in the working environment can either promote or interfere with good diabetes management. For example, when vending machines are stocked to offer water and sugar-free drinks, it helps diabetes patients limit their intake of sugar and maintain their dietary regimen. Similarly, many companies now have gyms available to employees so that they can incorporate exercise into their busy lives more easily. When individuals with diabetes work in a setting in which their schedules are rigid and inflexible, they have more difficulty managing their illness, as they cannot take the time to test themselves. Worksites and community settings are often places where programs can be offered to screen individuals for diabetes and provide health promotion programs. These activities are especially important for populations that are medically underserved, such as minorities and the poor.

Diabetes is a demanding and challenging disease. It requires that patients make many changes in how they live their lives. It affects their relationships with others and changes how the individual sees him/himself or herself. There is no vacation from diabetes; it is with the individual all day, every day, and frequently leads to more difficult and threatening problems in the future. However, most individuals with diabetes lead long and fulfilling lives. They learn to adapt, to cope with the ups and downs of the illness, and to turn to others for education and support when problems arise. An understanding of the illness, an appreciation of the pitfalls, and a knowledge base of positive ways to cope help the individual successfully manage the burdens of diabetes. Future efforts must lead to ways that larger communities and society can support those who have diabetes to ensure successful adaptation and better quality of life.

Related Entries: Cardiovascular System, Genetics and Health, Patient Adherence, Stressful Life Events

BIBLIOGRAPHY

Anderson, B. J., and Rubin, R. R. (Eds.). (2002). American Diabetes Association. www.niddk.nih.gov *Practical psychology for diabetes clinicians* (2nd ed.) Alexandria, VA: American Diabetes Association.

Cox, D. J., Gonder-Frederick, L., Polonsky, W., Schlundt, D., Julian, D., & Clarke, W. (1995). A multicenter evaluation of Blood Glucose Awareness Training–II. *Diabetes Care, 18*, 523–528.

Delamater, A. M., Jacobson, A. M., Anderson, B., Cox, D., Fisher, L., Lustman, P., et al. (2001). Psychosocial therapies in diabetes: Report of the Psychosocial Therapies Working Group. *Diabetes Care, 24*, 1286–1292.

Glasgow, R. E., Fisher, E. B., Anderson, B. J., LaGreca, A., Marrero, D., Johnson, S. B., et al. (1999). Behavioral science in diabetes: Contributions and opportunities. *Diabetes Care, 22*, 832–843.

National Institute of Diabetes and Digestive and Kidney Diseases (National Diabetes Information Clearinghouse). www.niddk.nih.gov

PAULA M. TRIEF

Diathesis–Stress Model

A diathesis–stress model describes a preexisting vulnerability that may be "triggered" by a stressful event. Most often these models focus on the development of psychopathology, but they have also focused on the development of short-term distress reactions (e.g., depressive adjustment) and medical disorder (e.g., phenylketonuria, PKU). The stress component of diathesis–stress models most often focuses on stressful life events and daily hassles, though any environmental factor (as opposed to genetic) may serve as a trigger (e.g., diet, occupational exposure, substance use).

Conceptualization of diathesis–stress models emerged out of a need for a model of human disorder that included both genetic and environmental factors. Irving Gottesman's model of schizophrenia describes a "genetic loading" for the disorder that is triggered by environmental stressors (e.g., familial conflict, poor resources). According to this model, the higher the diathesis or genetic load for schizophrenia, the less stress needed to develop schizophrenia. In other words, each person has a threshold for schizophrenia; most are very high, as only 1 percent of our population actually develops the disorder. Thus, conceptualizations of diatheses began as innate, genetic vulnerabilities. This concept has since expanded to describe a general preexisting vulnerability, which may be innate, learned, or of an unknown etiology.

General cognitive factors and more specific cognitive factors such as interpersonal beliefs are often studied as diatheses within depression research. General cognitive vulnerabilities represent the basis for Aaron Beck's well-known model of depression (Beck et al., 1979). Beck describes a "cognitive triad" of vulnerability to developing depression. This triad represents a worldview that consists of negative beliefs about the self, world, and future. Negative events are blamed on the self as opposed to external forces because the self is perceived as defective. World beliefs represent a preconceived negative view of the world and a tendency to interpret events in a negative fashion. Negative events are believed to extend into the future and are viewed as constant and never changing (e.g., "It will always be this way"). This triad of cognitive factors represents a vulnerability to develop depression when faced with a stressful event.

When faced with the stress of a chronic physical illness, some patients will develop a psychological disorder, but others will not. Why do only some patients experience difficulty adjusting and others adjust quickly or even find greater meaning in life? Many possible diatheses have received research attention, including distorted cognitions (e.g., Beck's model of depression), patients' general perception of control over adverse events (e.g., Seligman's model of hopelessness depression), and chronic negative mood (i.e., negative affect). A stressful event such as a diagnosis of chronic illness may trigger a preexisting vulnerability to psychological disorder. For example, patients who generally believe that events are out of their control may be vulnerable to developing a depressive disorder in response to a diagnosis of cancer.

Related Entries: Genetics and Health, Stressful Life Events

BIBLIOGRAPHY

Beck, A. T., Rush, A. J., Shaw, B., & Emery, G. (1979). *Cognitive therapy of depression.* New York: Guilford.

Gottesman, I. L., & Wolfgram, D. L. (1990). *Schizophrenia genesis: The origins of madness.* San Francisco: Freeman.

Seligman, M. E. P. (2000). The hopelessness theory of depression: A test of the diathesis–stress component in the interpersonal and achievement domains. *Cognitive Therapy and Research, 24,* 361–378.

SHAWNA L. EHLERS

Disclosure and Health

Disclosure is the act of revealing thoughts and emotions, often through language. Disclosure typically occurs in a social setting, with one or more individuals sharing thoughts and feelings with others. Such social sharing is neither recent nor rare; since the development of language, people have shared their stories with one another, across time, many cultures, and different situations. Evidence suggests that people feel a strong desire to share their experiences, and relatively few emotional experiences are kept private. Despite this longstanding and central role of disclosure to our lives, it is only relatively recently that there has been systematic study of the relation between disclosure and health.

Although historically not carefully studied, disclosure processes have long been a component in a variety of symbolic healing rituals. For example, confession and story telling have been used as a tool to promote health and well-being in both religious and secular settings for thousands of years. A central feature of most contemporary psychotherapeutic interventions is to translate thoughts and emotional experiences into language and to disclose them in a safe and supportive environment. With growing appreciation of the role that thoughts and emotions can have in influencing our physiological states, disclosure is one mechanism whereby psychological and social states might influence health and well-being. The cross-cutting theme addressed here is that disclosure of important and/or powerful thoughts and emotions may constitute an important component of a variety of therapeutic endeavors, and disclosure itself, regardless of the form it takes, may promote health and well-being.

Early investigation into the relation of disclosure to health and well-being provided a more complex picture. When examining the degree to which people disclosed, both in their natural lives and in therapeutic environments, rates of disclosure were often not related to health and well-being. In fact, there was some evidence that high rates of disclosure were associated with distress (e.g., depression, anxiety, fear, etc.), and higher disclosure rates during therapy were not associated with better psychotherapy outcomes. One explanation of this pattern is that people are more likely to disclose when they are psychologically distressed than when they are not distressed. Thus, if we examine people who are currently disclosing at high rates, we will (inadvertently) be observing them at times of high distress. A more important question is what is the relation of disclosure to health under more controlled circumstances, an issue we return to shortly.

There thus exists a bit of a contradiction—disclosure both represents a core and common social experience and perhaps also suggests distress. This view is reflected in common culture and language (the "folk model" of emotion and disclosure). Linguists, for example, have noted that cultural metaphors for strong emotions, such as anger, portray the body as a container for emotions. This metaphor is based largely on a hydraulic model, with contained emotion building up pressure unless it is let out via disclosure (e.g., "blowing off steam"). Overly contained ("bottled up") emotion can, in this metaphorical model, produce dangerous pressure and cause physiological and psychological damage. Thus, disclosure is often thought of as venting the accumulated build-up of strong (typically negative) emotion. It is important to note, however, that recent evidence suggests that raw emotional expression (lacking self-reflection) may not be very helpful. In fact, a number of studies have linked the persistent tendency to uncritically express negative emotions (e.g., anger) with increased stress, hopelessness, depression, and health problems.

NONDISCLOSURE AND INHIBITION

Accompanying the notion that disclosure is beneficial is the belief that *not* disclosing (or inhibiting) ones thoughts and feelings is a bad strategy that can lead to poor psychological and health outcomes. There are, in fact, many reasons why an individual might choose (or feel pressure to) not express his or her emotions. Inhibition may be promoted by limited emotional awareness, personal and cultural values (e.g., a stigma that keeps someone from sharing a problem, a desire to appear strong and independent), a lack of opportunity to disclose one's emotions (e.g., a lack of supportive listeners), or negative responses from others when disclosure is attempted. Ongoing and dynamic changes in social and cultural contexts also play a role in determining the balance between emotional disclosure and inhibition over time for an individual. In general, however, there is evidence that the persistent tendency to inhibit or conceal one's thoughts and strong emotions is related to negative outcomes.

Several studies have provided empirical evidence that inhibition may be associated with physiological burden and an increased risk of developing health problems. In the short term, the inhibition or suppression of strong emotions produces a much greater physiological response than not suppressing the emotions. For example, trying to suppress the emotional reaction of anger can produce a much greater increase in heart rate and blood pressure than would be produced without the need for such inhibition. Beyond these short-term effects, the suppression or inhibition of experiences or emotions over time can also be risky. For example, individuals who have experienced traumatic events but not disclosed them to others have more health problems than those who have disclosed more.

Other examples can be found in a variety of research studies. Results from the large Multi-center AIDS Cohort Study found that, among gay HIV+ (but otherwise healthy) men, those who concealed their sexual identity showed faster HIV progression than those who were open about their sexuality. Individuals with a chronic tendency to suppress negative emotions have been shown to have worse outcomes in response to malignant melanoma (skin cancer), whereas expressing emotions was related to positive immunological responses. In another study, holocaust survivors were interviewed about their personal experiences before and after World War II. Survivors who disclosed less during the interview and in the time since the war reported significantly worse health outcomes and more visits to their doctor 1 year later as compared to survivors who disclosed more. Similar findings have been observed in bereaved individuals: The more that surviving spouse talked about the death with others, the fewer the health problems he or she experienced following the loss. This and other accumulating evidence suggests that inhibiting thoughts and feelings about strong emotions or significant personal experiences may pose a risk for developing negative health outcomes.

In spite of this evidence, however, inhibition may be adaptive in some circumstances. There are times where disclosure might prove maladaptive or even harmful, particularly when disclosure would result in negative social or interpersonal consequences. The ability to moderate our emotional expression is an adaptive tool that enables us to determine when, to whom, and under what circumstances we share our personal experiences. There are many negotiations that take place both within and outside of an individual that modulate expression (e.g., how much, when, to whom), and appropriate inhibition is a useful and necessary social strategy. However, persistent and broadly applied inhibition, and a chronic tendency to not disclose, appears to pose a risk for negative psychological and physical health outcomes.

DISCLOSURE, HEALTH, AND WELL-BEING

As aforementioned, an important issue concerns what the effects of disclosure are under more controlled circumstances. Essentially all forms of talk therapy, regardless of theoretical orientation (e.g., psychoanalysis, cognitive–behavioral, etc.), recognize that the labeling of the problem and a discussion of its causes and consequences is an integral part of the therapeutic process. Such talk therapies have been shown to reduce psychological distress and promote both physical and mental well-being across a wide range of theoretical orientations, problems, and clientele. Much of the early work examining the effects of the structured disclosure entailed by talk therapies focused on mental health outcomes (such as reductions in depression). Only relatively recently, however, has disclosure been systematically examined in the context of health and well-being more broadly defined. Several significant clinical trials of psychosocial interventions suggested the important role that disclosure may have in the treatment of medical problems.

Dean Ornish and colleagues found that a healthy heart program that incorporated lifestyle, behavioral, and psychological change for individuals at high risk of heart disease significantly reduced their medical risk profiles. In fact, the Ornish program significantly *reversed* the severity of the heart disease. One important component of this program is to provide a safe, compassionate, and supportive group setting where patients are encouraged to disclose their thoughts and feelings about the stress and difficulties surrounding their disease and in their lives more broadly. Another pioneering study was conducted by David Spiegel and his colleagues for women with breast cancer. This study examined the effect of providing women diagnosed with breast cancer the opportunity to disclose to other women about their disease, again in a safe and supportive group environment. The women in the experimental group that were provided the opportunity to participate in the support groups lived, on average, about 17 months longer than women in the control group, who received no supportive interventions. Both of these studies suggested the important role disclosure may have in maintaining and promoting good physical health and reducing the mortality risk of certain diseases. Unfortunately, neither of these studies was able to confidently determine whether it was disclosure per se that resulted in the observed improvements or whether some other aspect of the experimental interventions contributed wholly or in part to the benefit received by participants. To better address this question, more careful experimental studies of disclosure and health needed to be conducted. Prior to presenting the effects of disclosure in carefully controlled experimental contexts, some of the forms disclosure can take are first examined.

MODES OF DISCLOSURE

Certainly the most typical mode of disclosure is to talk face to face with another person. Such disclosure may take the form of speaking with a friend, a family member, or a professional. However, there are a variety of circumstances that may arise that leave an individual without access to such a supportive listener. For this and a variety of other reasons (e.g., communication and computer technology), many other forms of disclosure have become popular. Interpersonal disclosure now occurs with great regularity from a distance, such as over the phone or by electronic mail. Support groups have grown in popularity, and exist both in traditional settings as well as "virtual" support groups conducted on the Internet via private chat rooms. Although these various modes of disclosure can differ in many ways (duration, content, expertise, etc.), they all share the feature of allowing individuals to disclose thoughts and feelings within an (ostensibly) safe and supportive environment.

A more recent line of enquiry examines whether disclosure can occur, and whether it is helpful, in the absence of an explicit audience. That is, is disclosure helpful if conducted by individuals on their own? In general, research supports the view that disclosure in a private setting, such as talking into a tape recorder, writing (or typing) about one's thoughts and feelings, or completing workbooks that involve disclosure, can each produce beneficial effects even without an explicit audience or listener. Although more work remains to be conducted in this important area, preliminary findings suggest that disclosure regardless of mode (e.g., interpersonal, verbal private, written private, etc.) can be beneficial, and no one mode shows clear superiority over the others (although there are undoubtedly individual differences in response to disclosure via different

modes). One recent line of research that examines the health effects of disclosure conducted in a private setting uses the administration of structured writing exercises that involve expressing thoughts and feelings about important (often stressful) events or topics.

DISCLOSURE THROUGH WRITING

Expressive writing has increasingly been used as an intervention to foster emotional disclosure while avoiding the potentially negative social interactions that might accompany interpersonal disclosure. The procedure, initially pioneered by James Pennebaker and colleagues (Pennebaker, 1995; Pennebaker & Beall, 1986), generally involves having participants come into a safe and private environment to write about their deepest thoughts and emotions about a stressful experience for 20–30 min, which they repeat for three to five sessions. In experimental settings, this writing is contrasted with writing about emotionally neutral topics. Such randomized designs for exploring the effects of disclosure are very important because they allow much clearer demonstration that any observed differences between the groups are due to disclosure. That is, such designs allow us to examine the effects of disclosure specifically and not confuse them with effects produced by a broader intervention, the context, or other uncontrolled factors. Early work utilizing this writing intervention found that individuals provided the opportunity to disclose in this manner showed reliable improvements in a wide array of health outcomes, including reports of physical health, psychological well-being, physiology (e.g., immune function), and measures of performance (e.g., academic performance) when compared to those individuals writing about emotionally neutral topics. Also important was that the benefits of written disclosure did not appear limited by age, race or ethnicity, education, gender, or language.

With the demonstration that disclosure via writing could promote health and well-being, researchers began to explore new domains in which to apply this novel intervention. A number of empirical studies have now demonstrated that such expressive writing can be a useful supplement to standard medical care for individuals with a range of physical illnesses. For example, individuals receiving medical care for chronic asthma or arthritis who completed a series of written disclosure exercises demonstrated clinically significant improvements in their disease (e.g., improved lung function, reduced pain) relative to patients who wrote about emotionally neutral topics. Related, although less dramatic, benefits have been observed in the context of cancer care and primary care settings. These studies, along with those discussed earlier, suggest that if patients with a physical illness are provided the opportunity to disclose in a safe and supportive way (whether interpersonally or via writing), they can experience health benefits beyond those attributable to their ongoing medical care.

HOW MIGHT DISCLOSURE IMPROVE HEALTH?

The accumulation of evidence that the disclosure of thoughts and feelings can make us feel better, both psychologically and physically, naturally leads to the question, "How does disclosure work?" Numerous theories have been proposed to explain the health benefits of disclosure. The theories vary in accordance with factors such as the theoretical orientation of a researcher or clinician (e.g., behavioral vs. psychodynamic), type of disclosure (interpersonal vs. written), and nature of the people under study (e.g., healthy vs. ill). A popular early explanation for the health effects of disclosure was that it removed the harmful effects of inhibiting, or not disclosing, thoughts and emotions surrounding an important event. More recently, however, other explanations have been offered, including exposure-based models, the acquisition of skills related to the recognition and regulation of emotion, increases in insight and processing of past experiences, and changes in the cognitive and/or linguistic representation of thoughts and emotions. Although some evidence consistent with each of these theories exists, continued research must examine the relative contribution of each of them to the health benefits of disclosure. Furthermore, it is likely the case that disclosure under different circumstances and for different individuals may operate through a variety of different pathways.

CONCLUSION

We are social beings, and appear to have strong tendencies to share our thoughts and feelings with others. Such disclosure has long been part of a variety of healing rituals, and scientific enquiry suggests that, under safe and supportive circumstances, disclosure may promote greater health and well-being. Examination of disclosure suggests it is most beneficial when it involves the expression of emotion along with self-reflection, rather than mere catharsis. Additionally, recent empirical evidence supports the view that disclosure can occur, and produce health benefit, even in the absence of an explicit audience (such as through writing). Disclosure interventions are useful tools for promoting both psychological and physical good health, and may represent a promising line of supplemental treatments for individuals with physical illness. A number of important questions about the health effects of disclosure, however, are open to further investigation. For example, what is the effect of the growing number of possible modes of disclosure, such as the telephone, the World Wide Web, or email? For whom will disclosure provide benefit, and under what circumstances? Through what mechanisms does disclosure improve health? Ongoing and future research into these and related questions will shed further light on the health effects of disclosure as well as aid in the design and implementation of disclosure as a therapeutic tool.

Related Entries: Coping, Psychotherapy, Stressful Life Events

BIBLIOGRAPHY

Consedine, N. S., Magai, C., & Bonanno, G. A. (2002). Moderators of the inhibition–health relationship: A review and research agenda. *Review of General Psychiatry, 6*(2), 204–228.

Kennedy-Moore, E., & Watson, J. C. (1999). *Expressing emotions: Myths, realities, and therapeutic strategies.* New York: Guilford.

Lepore, S. J., & Smyth, J. M. (Eds). (2002). *The writing cure: How expressive writing promotes health and emotional well-being.* Washington, DC: American Psychological Association.

Pennebaker, J. (1995). *Emotion, disclosure, and health.* Washington, DC: American Psychological Association.

Pennebaker, J. W., & Beall, S. K. (1986). Confronting a traumatic event: Toward an understanding of inhibition and disease. *Journal of Abnormal Psychology, 95,* 274–281.

Smyth, J. M., & Pennebaker, J. W. (1999). Sharing one's story: Translating emotional experiences into words as a coping tool. In C. Snyder (Ed.), *Coping: The psychology of what works.* New York: Oxford University Press.

Smyth, J., Stone, A., Hurewitz, A., & Kaell, A. (1999). Writing about stressful events produces symptom reduction in asthmatics and rheumatoid arthritics: A randomized trial. *Journal of the American Medical Association, 281,* 1304–1309.

JOSHUA SMYTH
DEBORAH NAZARIAN

Disease

Disease refers to an impairment in the normal state of an individual that interrupts or modifies the vital functioning of that individual and is in response to some combination of environmental factors (such as lead exposure), inherent defects (genetic abnormalities), or infective agents (viruses, bacteria, etc.). Although illness is often thought a synonym for disease, illness refers not to the symptoms defining a diagnosable disease, but rather to the subjective experience of ill health. Somatic or psychological symptoms accompany illness, and an individual may perceive himself or herself as suffering ill health, but these symptoms need not result from an underlying disease. Similarly, an individual with a disease need not perceive himself or herself as ill.

The terms chronic, acute, and infectious are often used to further classify disease types. Chronic indicates a lengthy duration and a slowly progressive course, whereas acute indicates a brief duration and a short course. Infectious refers to a disease caused by organisms entering and multiplying within the body, such as viruses or bacteria.

Related Entries:

MALI BUNDE

Double Blind

Double blind denotes a characteristic of experimental design in which neither experimenters nor participants are aware of which group of participants is receiving which treatment. Because beliefs and expectations can have a powerful influence on the behavior of participants and experimenters, it is important to use a double-blind procedure to eliminate these influences from experimental measures. Double-blind procedures are essential when evaluating the efficacy of medication treatments because researchers can make sure that the observed improvements (when present) are not due to self-fulfilling prophecies, placebo effects, or influence of the experimenters. In a study reported by Turner and his colleagues (1994), 98 percent of patients reported significant pain relief from ulcers after a certain treatment (gastric freezing). However, in a later double-blind procedure, this treatment was shown to be completely ineffective. Thus, double-blind studies enable us to examine the sole influence of a certain treatment by eliminating irrelevant psychological factors.

Related Entry: Placebo Effect

BIBLIOGRAPHY

Turner, J., Deyo, R. A., Loeser, J. D., Von Korff, M., & Fordyce, W. E. (1994). The importance of placebo effects in pain treatment and research. *Journal of the American Medical Association, 271,* 1609–1614.

ZLATAN KRIZAN

Drug Abuse

Drug abuse may be defined as the use of illicit substances or of federally approved substances that are used without a prescription of a medical provider. The abuse of substances may alter the cognition, mood, and behavior of an individual and, in some cases, alter brain structure and functioning. Drug abuse is a dependent behavior in that abusers continually need to administer the substance(s) to counter their experiences of withdrawal, which are characterized by physical and psychological cravings.

Drug abuse involves complex interrelated behaviors that may be difficult to modulate. The termination of drug abuse becomes complicated if the individual has developed a chemical dependence on the substance. For many of the drugs abused in the United States, the behavior often begins in adolescence. Numerous studies throughout the last several decades have indicated that drug abuse may provide a means of coping or a method to confront stressors, disinhibit and "feel good," and self-medicate an undiagnosed psychological problem. In the United States, drug abuse has had an enormous impact on society. Increasing at a rate of 5.9 percent each year from 1992 to 1998, the average cost of drug abuse was estimated at $143 billion dollars.

Common drugs of abuse are sedatives or central nervous system depressants (e.g., alcohol, barbiturates, and benzodiazepines), opioids (e.g., morphine, heroin, methadone), stimulants [e.g., cocaine, amphetamines, methamphetamines such as Ecstasy (methylenedioxy-n-methylamphetamine, MDMA)], hallucinogens (e.g., lysergic acid diethylamide, LSD; phencyclidine, PCP), cannabinoids (e.g., marijuana), inhalants (e.g., volatile solvents, nitrites, anesthetics), and anabolic steroids. One subset of abused substances known as "club drugs" [e.g., MDMA, gamma-hydroxybutyrate (GHB), ketamine, methamphetamine] have become more widely used particularly among younger individuals as well as gay and bisexual men and may result in serious health problems and even death. Furthermore, federally approved substances (e.g., Xanax, Valium, Oxycontin) and over-the-counter medications (e.g., cough syrup) have been abused by individuals. It is common for individuals to abuse more than one substance at a time. More than half of drug abusers admitted to substance abuse treatment programs reported polydrug abuse.

In the National Household Survey on Drug Abuse in 2000, patterns and prevalence of illicit drug demonstrated that men reported higher rates of use than women. However, similar rates of use of nonprescribed psychotherapeutic drugs (i.e., Oxycontin, Xanax, etc.) have been noted across gender. In addition, race/ethnicity, age, level of education, employment status, and geographical location have been related to rates of drug use. Specifically higher rates of use are reported among those in the developmental stage of late adolescence (ages 16–25 years), those with lower academic attainment, and those who are unemployed and who reside in metropolitan areas.

A variety of factors and theoretical models have been used to understand and explain drug abuse. The biological model posits that drug abuse is based on behavioral genetics, hereditary, and neurophysiology; and the personality or temperament model views drug abuse as the result of personality traits or psychodynamic influences such as the inadequacy of defense mechanisms and the developmental structure of an individual. The behavioral model focuses on drug abuse as a learned behavior; the cognitive model focuses on the importance of the interface of the individual and environment through observational learning. Other factors may influence drug abuse such as family, peers, race/ethnicity, gender, social class, and sexual orientation. From a biopsychosocial perspective, drug abuse is a behavior that permeates the biological, emotional, social, and cognitive domains of human life.

Intervention efforts regarding drug abuse have demonstrated that group treatment, multicultural therapeutic interventions, and the development of coping skills are essential in modulating drug abuse. Both harm-reduction and abstinence based programs have been used as a means of treating drug abuse.

Related Entry: Addiction

BIBLIOGRAPHY

Dowd, T. E., & Ruggle, L. (Eds.). (1999). *Comparative treatments of substance abuse.* New York: Springer.

Halkitis, P. N., Parsons, J. T., & Stirratt, M. (2001). A double epidemic: Crystal methamphetamine use and its relation to HIV prevention among gay men. *Journal of Homosexuality, 41*(2), 17–35.

Marlatt, A. G. (1998). *Harm reduction: Pragmatic strategies for managing high-risk behaviors.* New York: Guilford.

Office of National Drug Control Policy. (2001). *The economic costs of drug abuse in the United States, 1992–1998.* Washington, DC: Author.

Ott, P. J., Tarter, R. E., & Ammerman, R. T. (1999). *Sourcebook on substance abuse: Etiology, assessment, and treatment.* Needham Heights, MA: Allyn & Bacon.

U. S. Department of Health and Human Services. (1998). *The DASIS report: Polydrug use among treatment admissions: 1998.* Washington, DC: Author.

PERRY N. HALKITIS
LEO WILTON

Ee

Eating Disorders

Disturbances in eating behavior and attitudes severe enough to warrant a diagnosis affect perhaps some 6 percent of all adolescent and adult women in this country, making it one of the most common psychiatric disorders to affect this population. There are four categories of eating disorders recognized by the *Diagnostic and Statistical Manual of Mental Disorders,* fourth edition (*DSM-IV*) (American Psychiatric Association, 1994): Anorexia Nervosa (AN), Bulimia Nervosa (BN), Eating Disorder Not Otherwise Specified (EDNOS), and Binge Eating Disorder (BED).

AN and BN share many clinical features and this entry will be devoted primarily to these two eating disorders. EDNOS and BED and eating disorders in men are discussed separately at the end of this entry.

ANOREXIA NERVOSA

The term anorexia nervosa was coined by Sir William Gull in 1874, but many early reports of cases of self-starvation exist in the medical literature. AN affects about 0.5–1 percent of young women in the West. The main features of AN are emaciation (very low body weight), behavior aimed at producing weight loss (extreme dieting, purging, excessive exercise), and a morbid fear of becoming fat. Whereas the *DSM-IV* lists amenorrhea as one of diagnostic criteria, its value is being increasingly questioned because the absence or presence of amenorrhea does not materially alter the patient's response to treatment or the outcome. There are two types of individuals with AN: those who predominantly restrict their food intake and those who binge and purge.

AN typically begins in the teenage years in young women who have embarked on dieting to lose weight. After some initial weight loss the self-starvation becomes more rigorous, amenorrhea sets in, fear of becoming fat intensifies, and emaciation occurs. About 40 percent of these individuals then develop binge eating and purging while still emaciated. After a few years about one-third begin to recover and regain normal weight, although the period of recovery is often characterized by chaotic eating: periods of fasting interspersed by binge eating and sometimes vomiting (i.e., a period of Bulimia Nervosa). About one of four remains chronically ill with AN. AN is a psychiatric disorder that has a high mortality; those with AN are perhaps five times more likely to die than expected of the general population. Most of the premature deaths occur as a result of the emaciation and complications or of suicide.

Many medical complications can occur as a result of the self-starvation and severe weight loss. Among those who purge, severe metabolic abnormalities may cause cardiac arrest (leading to sudden death) and kidney failure. Fatigue, intolerance of cold, depression, anxiety, obsessive–compulsive behaviors, insomnia, preoccupation with eating and weight, and low self-esteem plague most patients with AN, who have hopes that maintaining a very low weight would be the answer to all their problems. For those with the bulimic subtype of Anorexia Nervosa, alcohol and substance abuse, shoplifting, sexual promiscuity, and self-mutilation may also occur.

Treatment consists of restoration of the malnourished state, correction of metabolic disturbances, normalization of the disturbed eating behaviors, restructuring of abnormal eating and self attitudes, and treatment of concommittant depression and anxiety. For those with very low body weight or severe metabolic disturbance, a period of inpatient treatment may be necessary. Osteopenia and osteoporosis may require more specialized treatment than just nutritional/weight restoration. A combination of psychotherapy, nutritional counseling, and medical treatment is almost always needed, whether the patient is treated in an inpatient or outpatient setting. For young patients living at home, family therapy focused initially on helping the family to help the patient normally and gain weight, and later to help the patient develop individuation and form an independent identity, is particularly helpful. Therapy aimed at increasing motivation for recovery may help those who are reluctant to give up their thinness. Antidepressant medications, particularly the serotonergic agents, may be useful in preventing relapse in AN restrictive subtype patients who have regained healthy weight, and in improving mood in those who have concommittant depression or anxiety or obsessive–compulsive features. In general, medications are not useful in helping AN patients to gain weight.

BULIMIA NERVOSA

Bulimia Nervosa (BN), a term coined by Gerard Russell in 1979, affects about 2 percent of young women in the West, although the figure approaches 5 percent if less severe cases are also included. Its main features are eating binges accompanied by a feeling of loss of control over eating, and purging behavior to get rid of the calories of the binge by self-induced vomiting and/or laxative abuse. Excessive exercising, abuse of diet pills to curb the urge to binge, abuse of diuretics to lose weight (although no calories are lost in this forced diuresis), and abuse of opecae to induce vomiting, which may cause muscle (and heart) damage, may also occur. Occasionally individuals with BN may chew large quantities of food when the urge to binge arises and then spit out instead of swallowing the food. In contrast to AN, patients with BN, by definition, have normal or high body weight. An emaciated patient with bulimic features would be diagnosed as AN, Bulimic subtype, not BN.

Onset of BN is typically in the late teens. After a period of dieting and weight loss and sometimes a phase of frank AN the urge to binge becomes overpowering. A sense of relief is soon followed by tremendous guilt during the binge, which, together with the discomfort of an overdistended stomach, compels the individual to purge. Cycles of binge, purge, and self-starvation develop and the individual becomes consumed with thoughts of weight and eating. Depression sets in and sometimes the abnormal eating behaviors occupy the majority of the waking hours of the individual's life. In a small proportion of individuals with BN, self-induced vomiting and self-starvation precede the onset of binging.

Perhaps because of the shame, depression, and feelings of loss of control, more individuals with BN than individuals with AN seek help. Perhaps about two-thirds recover in a few years, whereas one-third have periods of remission alternating with periods of relapse. Major complications such as cardiac arrest, esophageal or gastric bleeding, and severe electrolyte disturbances may occur.

Treatment consists usually of cognitive–behavioral therapy to change the individual's dysfunctional thoughts about weight and eating as well as self-concept and interpersonal relationships. Self-monitoring of eating behavior and attendant thoughts, identification of the antecedents to a binge/purge episode, and the restructuring of dysfunctional thoughts and behaviors to prevent binge/purge are some of the key components to this treatment. Also effective is interpersonal psychotherapy that focuses on issues such as role transition, loss, and interpersonal conflict. Treatment may be given in individual or group format. More recently self-help techniques that utilize treatment manuals and usually guided by a counselor have been found to be helpful and may be used as the first step of treatment, and cognitive–behavioral therapy or interpersonal therapy are used for those who failed to respond to self-help. Antidepressants, particularly the serotonergic agents, are sometimes useful in decreasing the dysphoria and the urges to binge. They are best used in combination with psychotherapy.

EATING DISORDERS IN NON-WESTERN CULTURES

As already mentioned, AN and BN are becoming more common in developed and developing Asian countries such as Japan, China, Taiwan, and Hong Kong. By and large, patients with BN in these non-Western countries demonstrate identical clinical features to their counterparts in the West. However, about 30 percent of individuals with AN in non-Western countries do not show the characteristic morbid fear of fatness that is considered to be a sine qua non of AN in the West. This suggests that reasons for the strive for thinness may be different for individuals with AN in different cultures, but the implications of this finding remain to be clarified.

BINGE EATING DISORDER

Binge eating was first described by Albert Stunkard in 1954 in the context of eating disturbances in obese individuals, along with night eating and eating without satiation. BED affects some 2–3 percent of adults in the general population and 8 percent of those who are obese. In contrast to the preponderance of females in AN and BN, BED affects men and women about equally. Other differences between BED and BN/AN are that BED is probably at least equally common among ethnic minorities as among Whites, the age at presentation is older (30–50 years vs. teens and late 20s), and most individuals with BED are overweight or obese. Although individuals with BED share many of the eating and self-attitude disturbances of individuals with BN, there is little "crossover" of individuals in these categories, that is, few people with BN develop BED or vice versa in longitudinal studies. Treatment consists of cognitive–behavior therapy which improves the eating behavior and attitudes, and in a small proportion of obese individuals with BED, this improvement is accompanied by some weight loss. BED seems to have a better prognosis than BN/AN, and individuals with BED seem to recover from their disorder in a few years, although the long-term outcome of BED remains unclear.

Eating Disorder Not Otherwise Specified

Currently, EDNOS is a category for all those individuals who have eating disturbances but do not meet specific criteria for AN, BN, or BED. For instance, an individual who has lost some weight but has not fallen below a body mass index (BMI) of 17 kg/m^2 would be given a diagnosis of EDNOS and not AN. Another example is an individual who binges and purges but not as frequently as twice a week or not for as long as 3 months will be given a diagnosis of EDNOS. Some studies have found that individuals with EDNOS may not have a more favorable prognosis than those diagnosed with AN or BN. It is certainly advisable that EDNOS individuals should get treatment for their eating disorder.

EATING DISORDER IN MEN

AN and BN affect many more women than men; the female-to-male ratio in the majority of studies is about 10:1. Men with AN/BN are more concerned about muscularity than thinness, more likely to have a comorbid alcohol/substance use disorder, and of course do not meet criteria for menstrual disturbance. In men with AN, loss of sexual appetite secondary to lowered testosterone, which occurs as a result of weight loss, is gradual and unlikely to be a spontaneous complaint. Aside from these differences, the clinical features of AN/BN in men are essentially the same as those in women.

Risk factors for pathogenesis of AN/BN in men are probably similar to those in women, although several studies have found that sexual orientation and premorbid obesity may be specific risk factors for men: about 20 percent of males with AN/BN have a homosexual orientation, and premorbid obesity affects about 50 percent of men with AN/BN. Treatment and outcome are essentially similar to those for women.

As mentioned, BED is almost as common in men as in women; most studies have found a female-to-male preponderance of 3:2. Again, the clinical features of BED between the genders are similar. Treatment for BED in men is similar to that for women, although there has been little systematic study.

There is little data on outcome of BED in men, but there is no obvious reason to expect that it would be different.

CAUSES OF AN AND BN

Epidemiologic studies have found that AN and BN occur much more commonly in young White females in industrialized and developed countries. Non-White immigrants in Western countries such as Arab college students in London or Chinese young women in Toronto are more likely to develop AN or BN than their counterparts in their country of origin. Many case reports also suggest that AN and BN are becoming much more common in developed, industrialized Asian countries such as Japan and Hong Kong. These evidences indicate that there is a sociocultural influence on the pathogenesis of AN and BN.

Family studies have found that AN and BN tend to run in families and that there is cross-transmission of AN and BN in families (i.e., relatives of individuals with AN are more likely to have BN and vice versa). Twin studies have found that the concordance rates of AN and BN (i.e., both twins having the disorder) are higher in monozygotic (identical) than dizygotic (fraternal) twins. Large-scale population twin studies have suggested that both environmental and genetic influences are probably equally important in the development of these eating disorders.

Efforts to locate the genes that may be involved in the development of AN and BN have focused on genes involved in the control of feeding and mood. Genes involved in control of neurotransmitters, particularly those involved in serotonergic neurotransmission, are also being studied. No definitive results have emerged from these efforts but the search continues.

Environmental factors point to the role of dieting behavior in precipitating the onset of the eating disorders. The population that is most often engaged in dieting to control or lose weight is also the population that is most commonly afflicted with AN and BN (i.e., young women in the West), and several longitudinal studies have found that young women who are dieting are much more likely to develop AN or BN at follow-up. Other factors that may be involved include an overabundance of easily available food, relaxation of rules governing eating behaviors, increasing prevalence of obesity and the attendant emphasis on dieting to control weight, increasingly complex roles for women in an industrialized society, and childhood sexual abuse.

Some studies have found that the risk factors for the development of AN and BN may be different. Personality traits such as perfectionism, obsessimality, low risk taking, and negative self-evaluation may be more relevant for the development of AN, whereas premorbid obesity, rigorous dieting, and family history of obesity are more important for BN. These findings await confirmation.

In summary, it seems likely that genetic factors predispose certain individuals to develop an eating disorder, and that environmental (such as dieting to control weight) and developmental (such as onset of puberty and attendant weight gain) factors may trigger the expression of such factors.

CONCLUSION

Although the prediction in the 1980s that the eating disorders may reach epidemic proportions has not materialized, these disorders nevertheless constitute a severe health hazard for a significant minority of women. There is also evidence to indicate that they are becoming more common in some developed and developing non-Western countries. Unfortunately, progress in treatment and prevention has been slow, AN patients have a high mortality, and many individuals with AN and BN become chronically ill. Meanwhile, obesity has become a real public health issue, and although obesity is not classified as an eating disorder, some of its underlying mechanisms such as those involved in eating and weight control, as well as the social and cultural context that breeds it, may have much in common with those that underlie the eating disorders. One can hope that a broad-based research program to better our understanding of the biopsychosocial factors associated with the eating disorders and with obesity will bring more effective prevention and treatment.

Related Entries: Body Image, Nutrition

BIBLIOGRAPHY

American Pyschiatric Association. (1994). *Diagnostic and statistical manual of mental disorders* (4th ed.) Washington, DC: Author.

Brumberg, J. J. (1989) *Fasting girls.* New York: Plume. A discussion of the social cultur.

Fairburn, C. G. & Brownell, K. D. (Eds.). (2002). *Eating disorders and obesity* (2nd ed.). New York: Guilford. A multiauthored volume that provides an up-to-date overview of many aspects of the eating disorders and obesity.

Hsu L. K. G. (1990). *Eating disorders.* New York: Guilford. A single-author review of anorexia and bulimia nervosa.

L. K. GEORGE HSU

Endocrine System

In complex animals the two principal systems of regulation are the endocrine system and the nervous systems. The endocrine system consists of the ductless endocrine glands, which secrete hormones directly into the bloodstream. The endocrine system and the autonomic nervous system both regulate most of the involuntary functions of the body, including circulatory functions (e.g., blood pressure and heart rate), energy and arousal levels, reproductive functions, and the immune system.

Another major function of endocrine hormones is to regulate tissue growth in young, developing organisms. For example, whether the brain of a developing human male fetus becomes masculinized depends on levels of circulating androgen hormones (e.g., testosterone) that are secreted by the testes of the fetus. One of the developing brain structures most affected by such circulating sex hormones is the hypothalamus, a brain structure that then becomes the major regulator of the entire endocrine system. Thus in many ways the endocrine system and the nervous systems regulate each other.

The cells of the body have receptors for some of the many kinds of endocrine hormones and/or for some of the many kinds of neural transmitters secreted by neurons. The receptors are structures on the cell membrane that are often compared to locks; the hormones (or neural transmitters) represent the keys. In contrast to neural transmitters, which are concentrated in tiny synapses between neurons, even minute concentrations of hormones must be able to affect target cells because hormones become extremely diluted after being secreted directly into the rich blood supply of the endocrine gland. However, distinctions between neural transmitters and endocrine hormones break down; several of the neural transmitters eventually enter the circulatory system and act as hormones. On the other hand, the sensitivity of neurons and of other target tissues to neural transmitters is affected by hormonal concentrations. Whether a hormone greatly affects several major organ systems or has very precise and limited effects depends on the distribution and density of the receptors for that hormone.

Whereas hormonal control of the endocrine glands is achieved through hormones secreted by the "master" pituitary gland, the pituitary itself is regulated by the hypothalamus. The hypothalamus is a nearby brain structure that plays a vital role in many kinds of motivation and in regulation of the body through its control of both the autonomic nervous system and the endocrine system. For endocrine control, in response to neural messages from other brain areas, the hypothalamus secretes hormones which flow into a closed (portal) circulatory system connecting the hypothalamus with the pituitary gland. The pituitary in turn secretes hormones directly into the blood; those pituitary hormones mainly regulate the hormonal output of the various endocrine glands.

This abbreviated summary of endocrine system responses to challenge and threat illustrates some of the ways that mind and body interact. When a situation is appraised as challenging (i.e., important and taxing, but likely to lead to success) energy is required. To meet that need the sympathetic–adrenal–medullary arousal system is activated when the hypothalamus causes the sympathetic branch of the autonomic nervous system to stimulate the medulla of the adrenal gland to secrete the hormone epinephrine (also called adrenaline) With other hormones, epinephrine causes increased blood circulation to vital areas (e.g., major muscles) and increases in blood sugar for energy for use by muscles and brain. The resultant feeling of energy is likely to affirm the appraisal that success is likely. Sympathetic–adrenal–medullary arousal can dissipate within minutes after the need for energy and arousal ceases.

On the other hand, if the same situation is appraised as threatening (i.e., important and taxing, but potentially disastrous), then besides the arousal of the sympathetic–adrenal–medullary system, the pituitary–adrenal–cortical arousal system is activated. The hypothalamus signals the pituitary by secreting a hormone, corticotropin-releasing hormone (CRH), into the portal system. Then CRH stimulates the pituitary to release adrenocorticotropic hormone (ACTH) into the blood system and ACTH signals the cortex of the adrenal gland to eventually release cortisol (typically at least 15 min after the crisis began). Although cortisol causes many positive changes in arousal, disadvantages of pituitary–adrenal–cortical arousal are that it dissipates in hours rather than minutes, long-term activation interferes with immune system and even brain (hippocampal) function, and feelings of energy are accompanied by feelings of tensions. The associated feelings of tension are likely to affirm the appraisal that disaster is likely.

Related Entry: Cortisol

BIBLIOGRAPHY

Dienstbier, R. A. (1989). Arousal and physiological toughness: Implications for mental and physical health. *Psychological Review, 96,* 84–100.

Folkman, S. & Lazarus, R. S. (1985). If it changes it must be a process: Study of emotion and coping during three stages of a college examination. *Journal of Personality and Social Psychology, 48,* 150–170.

Frankenhaeuser, M. (1979). Psychoneuroendocrine approaches to the study of emotion as related to stress and coping. In H. E. Howe, Jr., & R. A. Dienstbier (Eds.), *Nebraska Symposium on Motivation, 1978: Human Emotion* (Vol. 26, pp. 123–161). Lincoln: University Press of Nebraska.

O'Leary, A. (1990). Stress, emotion, and human immune function. *Psychological Bulletin, 108,* 363–382.

Tomaka, J. Blascovich, J. Kibler, J. & Ernst, J. M. (1997). Cognitive and physiological antecedents of threat and challenge appraisal. *Journal of Personality and Social Psychology, 73,* 63–72.

RICHARD A. DIENSTBIER

End-Stage Renal Disease

According to statistics reported in the U. S. Renal Data System for the year 2000,[*] just under 379,000 Americans suffered from end-stage renal disease (ESRD), which required renal-replacement therapy. The leading causes of ESRD in the United States are diabetes, which accounts for 35 percent of all American cases, and hypertension, which accounts for 23 percent of all American cases. Diseases of the kidneys (e.g., glomerulonephritis, polycystic kidney disease) can also lead to ESRD. Healthy kidneys perform many functions necessary for life: eliminating toxic metabolic wastes and excess fluids, maintaining normal blood chemistries, and producing hormones to control blood pressure and manufacture red blood cells. ESRD is the final stage of progressive kidney failure, when the extent of *nephropathy* (destruction of kidney cells) renders the kidneys unable to function at the minimum level necessary for life. Serious symptoms will then occur. Accumulation of fluid in the body causes high blood pressure, shortness of breath, and swelling. The build-up of metabolic waste products in the blood results in *uremia,* the symptoms of which include poor appetite, nausea and vomiting, and difficulties with mental capacities. Fatigue is common due to *anemia* (abnormally low levels of red blood cells). Other symptoms of ESRD include weight loss, weakness, changes in sleep patterns, itching, muscle twitching or cramps, and changes in skin color. If left untreated, ESRD leads to death.

Currently, ESRD can be treated (but not cured) with renal-replacement therapies that carry out some of the normal kidney functions: *dialysis* and *transplantation.* Two types of dialysis are available: *hemodialysis* and *peritoneal dialysis.* The majority of ESRD patients are treated with hemodialysis. This form of renal-replacement therapy involves connecting the patient to a hemodialysis machine, which then continuously circulates the blood outside of the body through a dialyzer (artificial kidney), a filter that removes wastes and excess fluid from the blood. This procedure takes 3–5 hr to complete and is usually performed three times a week. In continuous ambulatory peritoneal dialysis, a special solution is infused into the abdomen through an implanted catheter. The solution is left in the abdominal cavity for a period of approximately 4 hr to absorb toxins from the blood through the peritoneal membrane, which acts as a natural filter. The solution is subsequently drained out of the abdomen, and fresh solution is reintroduced. This procedure must be performed three to four times a day by the patient. Transplantation

---

[*] The data reported here were supplied by the U. S. Renal Data System (USRDS). The interpretation and reporting of these data are the responsibility of the authors and in no way should be seen as an official policy or interpretation of the U.S. government.

involves surgically implanting a healthy kidney obtained from a donor (a living relative or friend of the kidney recipient, or a *cadaveric* donor, a recently deceased person). In addition to renal-replacement therapies, patients must follow strict dietary and fluid-intake regimens as well as medication regimens to control blood chemistry changes, prevent dangerous fluid overload, and keep red blood cell counts within acceptable ranges. *Epoetin*, a synthetic version of a hormone, *erythropoeitin*, produced by the kidneys to stimulate red blood cell production, has led to improvements in ESRD patients' fatigue and capacity for physical activity.

ADJUSTMENT TO ESRD AND ITS TREATMENT

Renal-replacement therapies prolong survival in people with ESRD. Success in extending the duration of life with chronic kidney disease, though, has been met by an increasing emphasis on *quality of life* because the disease and its treatments are associated with medical and lifestyle challenges. Despite effective treatment, people continue to experience physical and medical problems. A number of people do not feel as well as they did before the onset of ESRD. The treatments also require major lifestyle changes. Maintenance hemodialysis, for example, requires a substantial amount of time for treatment sessions throughout the week. The strict dietary and fluid-intake restrictions can be difficult to maintain. Treatment side effects (e.g., fatigue, weakness) can reduce the capacity for active involvement in important areas of life. In addition, some of the psychosocial challenges facing people with ESRD can include changes in self-image as a result of being unable to live up to expectations at work, in the family, or in social relationships. Recreational activities can also be affected. A sense of helplessness and/or dependence on others can develop (e.g., on the medical team and often one's partner). Other stressors include changes in body image and the stigma of being a chronically ill person.

Despite these challenges, the majority of ESRD patients adjust well in terms of physical, psychological, and social outcomes, although some report poorer quality-of-life outcomes than healthy people. Elderly patients on dialysis often report better adjustment than do younger patients, who may view ESRD and its treatment as obstacles that make it more difficult to achieve valued life goals. People who are most likely to be distressed include those with more severe illness or those with additional illnesses beyond ESRD (e.g., diabetes, heart disease), a prior history of depression, or little social support. Emotional distress may be associated with fatigue and with feelings of uncertainty about one's future. However, some of the symptoms attributable to the biomedical disease process in ESRD (e.g., weakness, sleep disturbance, loss of libido) are similar to those associated with depression in physically healthy people. Such

symptoms could thus be due to the effects of the kidney disease, depression and distress, or both.

ILLNESS INTRUSIVENESS OF ESRD AND ITS TREATMENT

Although as many as 25 percent of ESRD patients experience clinically significant psychiatric problems, the majority of people continue to pursue important goals and lead meaningful lives. Adaptation to life with ESRD depends on the degree to which one can minimize the effects of *illness intrusiveness*, or illness- and treatment-induced disruptions to valued activities and interests in a person's life. ESRD can interfere with the relationship with one's partner, family roles and responsibilities, work and financial status, social relationships, recreational activities, and religious and community activities. The greater the extent of illness intrusiveness (i.e., the less able one is to participate in valued activities and interests because of ESRD and/or its treatment), the more distressed and dissatisfied a person will be about his or her quality of life.

The level of illness intrusiveness associated with ESRD depends in part on the type of renal-replacement therapy one receives. Compared to hemodialysis, for example, successful kidney transplantation is associated with fewer medical symptoms, physical limitations, and fluid and dietary restrictions, less fatigue, and more freedom. Transplant recipients are thus freer to engage in daily activities and to fulfill role responsibilities within the family and in work, social, and other areas of life. Consequently, although some transplant patients may report continuing anxiety and depressive symptoms long after the transplant, most indicate better health, less distress, and greater well-being and quality of life than those treated by hemodialysis.

In contrast, hemodialysis patients experience more physical limitations and lower emotional well-being, especially at the beginning of treatment, than do people on peritoneal dialysis or transplant recipients. Hemodialysis patients who subsequently receive a kidney transplant also reported better quality of life with the transplant. The strict dietary and fluid-intake restrictions associated with hemodialysis are difficult for many people to follow completely. Although the regimen associated with transplantation is less onerous, the procedure is not always associated with better outcomes. One study found that people on home hemodialysis reported better quality of life than transplant recipients, who required more hospitalizations than their counterparts on dialysis. Transplantation is also not without its complications. Transplant recipients are often concerned about side effects of medications, susceptibility to infections, transplant rejection episodes, and fear of losing the transplanted kidney. In general, ESRD patients' noncompliance with aspects of their treatment plans are of great concern to medical professionals because of their negative effects on health and posttransplant functioning. Much research has been devoted to finding ways to increase patients' compliance with their treatment plans, such as increasing their *self-efficacy*, their sense of being able to maintain compliance.

One important objective for people with ESRD is to maintain their capacity to continue or return to work. This is a key issue for rehabilitation for many reasons, including maintaining financial stability and engaging in productive activity. Involvement in work can also benefit self-image. Many people, though, may be unable to work due to fatigue, other functional disabilities, and the significant time demands associated with dialysis (9–15 hr weekly for the treatment, not including associated tasks). It has been estimated that only 10–50 percent of ESRD patients return to work after starting renal-replacement therapy. People who are more highly educated and those in white collar positions are more likely to return to work than those with lower levels of education or employed in positions with lower occupational prestige. However, blue collar workers can benefit from programs designed to increase occupational rehabilitation: In one study, blue collar workers who received such an intervention were almost three times as likely to return to work than those who did not.

The quality of interpersonal relationships and social support from family members and other important individuals (including medical caregivers) is also critical to adjustment in ESRD. Satisfaction with the care received from physicians and nurses has been found to be fairly high overall. The majority of people indicate that they receive high levels of support from family and friends. Familial and social support, in turn, is related to less physical dysfunction, better compliance with dietary restrictions, and better posttransplant adjustment. On the other hand, ESRD and its treatment can place a strain on a patient's partner and other family members. The healthy partner may be required to shoulder new responsibilities, including the dual roles of caretaker and family breadwinner when the patient is too ill to continue working. Sexual desire and sexual functioning can be affected by ESRD and its treatment, especially in men. Kidney transplantation can lead to improved sexual functioning, but even transplant recipients continue to experience difficulties. In general, how one's partner reacts to the illness influences a patient's adjustment. Patients and their partners typically show similar levels of adjustment. This, in turn, may affect the general psychosocial adjustment achieved by the family. If the patient's level of adjustment does not match the expectations held by family members or treatment staff, psychological adjustment can be negatively affected.

How people cope with the stresses of their illness and treatment has received some attention in recent research. Active, problem-solving coping strategies appear to be most effective in increasing psychosocial adaptation and adherence to the treatment regimen. These strategies involve addressing the underlying difficulty responsible for one's problems and taking steps to "solve the problem." Such coping tactics include (but are not limited to) acquiring information about the disease and its treatment, raising concerns with medical service providers, keeping up to date on one's health, and participating in the treatment. In addition to increased effectiveness in resolving problems that are indeed manageable, active problem-solving coping may help to cultivate a more general sense of control. Maintaining a sense of control over one's life, including one's illness and health, is related to better psychological adjustment and treatment outcomes. Some researchers have found, though, that adjustment and adherence to treatment regimens depend on whether the demands of the treatment "match" the ways that person typically copes with stress. For example, people who prefer to be actively involved in their treatment do better when they are allowed to control their treatment (e.g., home hemodialysis) than when they do not have such control (e.g., hospital hemodialysis, where medical staff conduct the treatment). In contrast, patients who prefer a low level of involvement in their treatment do better with hospital hemodialysis than home dialysis. In this respect, avoidant types of coping can be an effective means of coping for some patients when the treatment situation does not require active participation (Fricchione et al. 1992).

PSYCHOSOCIAL INTERVENTIONS FOR ESRD PATIENTS

In developing treatment plans for people with ESRD, adjunctive interventions can be included to improve psychosocial adjustment, physical functioning, and participation in important areas of life as much as possible. Interventions to help predialysis patients and patients already on dialysis to prepare for and adjust to the demands of ESRD and its treatments can be useful. Educational programs can increase knowledge about ESRD and alternative renal-replacement therapies. Skills-building programs can help people to develop skills needed to manage aspects of their treatment. Providing such information to ESRD patients can produce important benefits, at least in the short term. Benefits include increased illness-related knowledge, reduced distress and functional disabilities, extension of time before renal-replacement therapies are required, and increased likelihood of returning to work after the initiation of maintenance dialysis. In one study, dialysis patients who participated in regular support group meetings survived longer than those who did not!

Because ESRD and the various renal-replacement therapies exert a significant impact well beyond health, treatment planning must address the psychological, emotional, and social consequences of ESRD as well as the biomedical aspects. Multidisciplinary nephrology treatment teams include the physicians and nurses who provide direct medical care and allied health professionals such as dieticians, social workers, psychiatrists, psychologists, and occupational therapists. By reducing the illness intrusiveness of ESRD in all areas of the patient's life as much as possible, the goal is to maintain participation in meaningful activities and to substitute new interests when existing ones are incompatible with one's new life as an ESRD patient, maximizing long-term adaptation and preserving quality of life.

Related Entries: Chronic Illness, Organ Transplantation

BIBLIOGRAPHY

Binik, Y. M., Devins, G. M., Barre, P. E., Guttmann, R. D., Hollomby, D. J., Mandin, H. et al. (1993). Live and learn: Patient education delays the need to initiate renal replacement therapy in end-stage renal disease. *Journal of Nervous and Mental Disease, 181,* 371–376.

Binik, Y. M., & Mah, K. (1994). Sexuality and end-stage renal disease: Research and clinical recommendations. *Advances in Renal Replacement Therapy, 1,* 198–209.

Bremer, B. A. (1995). Absence of control over health and the psychological adjustment to end-stage renal disease. *Annals of Behavioral Medicine, 17,* 227–233.

Bremer, B. A., Haffly, D., Foxx, R. M., & Weaver, A. (1995). Patients' perceived control over their health care: An outcome assessment of their psychological adjustment to renal failure. *American Journal of Medical Quality, 10,* 149–154.

Chowanec, G. D., & Binik, Y. M. (1989). End-stage renal disease and the marital dyad: An empirical investigation. *Social Science and Medicine, 28,* 971–983.

Christensen, A. J., & Ehlers, S. L. (2002). Psychological factors in end-stage renal disease: An emerging context for behavioral medicine research. *Journal of Consulting and Clinical Psychology, 70,* 712–724.

Christensen, A. J., Smith, T. W., Turner, C. W., & Cundick, K. E. (1994). Patient adherence and adjustment in renal dialysis: A person by treatment interactional approach. *Journal of Behavioral Medicine, 17,* 549–566.

Christensen, A. J., Turner, C. W., Slaughter, J. R., & Holman, J. M. (1989). Perceived family support as a moderator psychological well-being in end-stage renal disease. *Journal of Behavioral Medicine, 12,* 249–265.

De-Nour, A. K. (1994). Psychological, social and vocational impact of renal failure: A review. In H. McGee & C. Bradley (Eds.), *Quality of life following renal failure* (pp. 33–42). Chur, Switzerland: Harwood.

Deniston, O. L., Luscombe, F. A., Bluesching, D. P., Richner, R. E., & Spinowitz, B. S. (1990). Effect of long-term epoetin beta therapy on the quality of life of hemodialysis patients. *ASAIO Transactions, 36,* M157–M160.

Devins, G. M. (1994). Illness intrusiveness and the psychosocial impact of lifestyle disruptions in chronic life-threatening disease. *Advances in Renal Replacement Therapy, 1,* 251–263.

Devins, G. M., Hollomby, D. J., Barre, P. E., Mandin, H., Taub, K., Paul, L. C., et al. (2000). Long-term knowledge retention following predialysis psychoeducational intervention. *Nephron, 86,* 129–134.

Devins, G. M., Hunsley, J., Mandin, H., Taub, K. J., & Paul, L., C. (1997). The marital context of end-stage renal disease: Illness intrusiveness and perceived changes in family environment. *Annals of Behavioral Medicine, 19,* 325–332.

Ferrans, C. E., Powers, M. J., & Kasch, C. R. (1987). Satisfaction with health care of hemodialysis patients. *Research in Nursing and Health, 10,* 367–374.

Franke, G. H., Heemann, U., Kohnle, M., Luetkes, P., Maehner, N., & Reimer, J. (2000). Quality of life in patients before and after kidney transplantation. *Psychology and Health, 14,* 1037–1049.

Frazier, P. A., Tix, A. P., Klein, C. D., & Arikian, N. J. (2000). Testing theoretical models of the relations between social support, coping and adjustment to stressful life events. *Journal of Social and Clinical Psychology, 19,* 314–335.

Fricchione, G. L., Howanitz, E., Jandorf, L., Kroessler, D., Zervas, I., & Woznicki, R. M. (1992). Psychological adjustment to end-state renal disease and the implications of denial. *Psychosomatics, 33,* 85–91.

Fukunishi, I. (1993). Anxiety associated with kidney transplantation. *Psychopathology, 26,* 24–28.

Gudex, C. M. (1995). Health-related quality of life in endstage renal failure. *Quality of Life Research, 4,* 359–366.

Hatchett, L., Friend, R., Symister, P., & Wadhwa, N. K. (1997). Interpersonal expectations, social support and adjustment to chronic illness. *Journal of Personality and Social Psychology, 73,* 560–573.

Hatchett, L. A. (2002). *Interpersonal expectations and adjustment to chronic illness: Testing the role of family demands and patients' self-concept.* Ann Arbor, MI: University Microfilms International.

Hener, T., Weisenberg, M., & Har-Even, D. (1996). Supportive versus cognitve–behavioral intervention programs in achieving adjustment to home peritoneal kidney dialysis. *Journal of Consulting and Clinical Psychology, 64,* 731–741.

King, K. (1994). Vocational rehabilitation in maintenance dialysis patients. *Advances in Renal Replacement Therapy, 1,* 228–239.

Klang, B., Björvell, H., Berglund, J., Sundstedt, C., & Clyne, N. (1998). Predialysis patient education: Effects on functioning and well-being in uraemic patients. *Journal of Advanced Nursing, 28,* 36–44.

Koch, U., & Muthny, F. A. (1990). Quality of life in patients with end-stage renal disease in relation to the method of treatment. *Psychotherapy and Psychosomatics, 54,* 161–171.

Kutner, N. G. (1994). Psychosocial issues in end-stage renal disease: Aging. *Advances in Renal Replacement Therapy, 1,* 210–218.

Kutner, N. G., & Brogan, D. (1990). Expectations and psychological needs of elderly dialysis patients. *International Journal of Aging and Human Development, 31,* 239–249.

Kutner, N. G., Brogan, D., & Kutner, M. H. (1986). End-stage renal disease treatment modality and patients' quality of life. *American Journal of Nephrology, 6,* 396–402.

Kutner, N. G., & Cardenas, D. D. (1982). Assessment of rehabilitation outcomes among chronic dialysis patients. *American Journal of Nephrology, 2,* 128–132.

Kutner, N. G. & Jassal, S. V. (2002). Quality of life and rehabilitation of elderly dialysis patients. *Seminars in Dialysis, 15,* 107–112.

Levenson, J. L., & Glocheski, S. (1991). Psychological factors affecting end-stage renal disease. A review. *Psychosomatics, 32,* 382–389.

Markell, M. S., DiBenedetto, A., Maursky, V., Sumrani, N., Hong, J. H., Distant, D. A., et al. (1997). Unemployment in inner-city renal transplant recipients: Predictive and sociodemographic factors. *American Journal of Kidney Diseases, 29,* 881–887.

McKevitt, P. M., Johnes, J. F., Lane, D. A., & Marion, R. R. (1990). The elderly on dialysis: Some considerations in compliance. *American Journal of Kidney Diseases, 16,* 346–350.

Moguilner, M. E., Bauman, A., & De-Nour, A. K. (1988). The adjustment of children and parents to chronic hemodialysis. *Psychosomatics, 29,* 289–294.

Neto, J. F., Ferraz, M. B., Cendoroglo, M., Draibe, S., Yu, L., & Sesso, R. (2000). Quality of life at the initiation of maintenance dialysis treatment—A comparison between the SF-36 and the KDQ questionnaires. *Quality of Life Research, 9,* 101–107.

Rao, V. K. (2002). Kidney transplantation in older patients: Benefits and risks. *Drugs and Aging, 19,* 79–84.

Rasgon, S., Schwankovsky, L., James-Rogers, A., Widrow, L., Glick, J., & Butts, E. (1993). An intervention for employment maintenance among blue-collar workers with end-stage renal disease. *American Journal of Kidney Diseases, 22*, 403–412.

Rodin, G. (1994). Depression in patients with end-stage renal disease: Psychopathoogy or normative response? *Advances in Renal Replacement Therapy, 1*, 219–227.

Rudman, L. A., Gonzales, M. H., & Borigda, E. (1999). Mishandling the gift of life: Noncompliance in renal transplant patients. *Journal of Applied Social Psychology, 29*, 834–851.

Schlebusch, L., Pillay, B. J., & Louw, J. (1989). Depression and self-report disclosure after live related donor and cadaver renal transplants. *South African Medical Journal, 75*, 490–493.

Siegal, B. R., Calsyn, R. J., & Cuddihee, R. M. (1987). The relationship of social support to psychological adjustment in end-stage renal disease patients. *Journal of Chronic Diseases, 40*, 337–344.

Steele, T. E., Baltimore, D., Finkelstein, S. H., Juergensen, P., Kliger, A. S., & Finkelstein, F. O. (1996). Quality of life in peritoneal dialysis patients. *Journal of Nervous and Mental Disease, 184*, 368–374.

Sutton, T. D., and Murphy, S. P. (1989). Stressors and patterns of coping in renal transplant patients. *Nursing Research, 38* , 46–49.

U.S. Renal Data System (2000). *USRDS 2002 annual data report: Atlas of end-stage renal disease in the United States.* Bethesda, MD: National Institutes of Health, National Institute of Diabetes and Digestive and Kidney Diseases.

KENNETH MAH
GERALD M. DEVINS

Epidemiology

Epidemiology is the study of disease patterns in the population and the risk factors that influence those patterns. Epidemiologists are concerned with the who, when, and where of disease occurrences. That is, epidemiologists investigate (1) whether persons who have a disease are different from persons who do not get the disease based on traits or characteristics of interest, (2) whether the occurrence of disease has increased or decreased over time, and (3) whether disease occurs more frequently in one geographic area than another.

Two hallmarks of epidemiologic studies are the focus on groups of people rather than individuals and the inclusion of a comparison group. Epidemiologic studies are either observational or experimental. In o*bservational* studies the epidemiologist does not have control over assignment to study groups. *Retrospective*, *cross-sectional*, and *prospective* studies are the three types of observational studies. Retrospective and cross-sectional studies are similar in that group membership is determined by the presence or absence of the disease in question and then information is obtained about characteristic(s) and/or exposure(s) of interest among group members. These types of studies differ in that retrospective studies obtain data on past exposures, whereas cross-sectional studies obtain information on current

exposures or characteristics. Prospective studies differ from both retrospective and cross-sectional studies in that groups are identified based on the presence or absence of the characteristic(s) or exposure(s) of interest and then are followed over time to determine who gets disease.

One example of a classic, prospective epidemiologic study is the Framingham Heart Study, a study of risk factors for cardiovascular disease (CVD) that was initiated in 1948 among residents of Framingham, Massachusetts. Residents between ages 30 and 62 years were eligible to participate and 6,500 persons were randomly selected from the community and invited to participate in the study. Assessments of factors thought to be related to heart disease (e.g., blood pressure, weight, cholesterol, smoking) were made every 2 years over a 20-year interval and new cases of and/or deaths from CVD were recorded. Investigators then examined the associations between the characteristics of interest and the risk of developing CVD among men and women during the follow-up period. The Framingham Heart Study is highly regarded for the important information about CVD risk factors that it provided. For example, it was this study that established that risk of CVD increases with increasing levels of total serum cholesterol.

In *experimental* studies the epidemiologist controls the assignment of study participants to the "exposed" or "unexposed" group. Community trials and clinical trials are the two types of experimental studies. In *community trials* (also called field experiments) the group as a whole is studied collectively and group assignment is not randomized (nor is randomization possible). A classic example of a community trial is the addition of flouride to the water supply of a city to examine whether flouride reduces the likelihood of getting dental caries. In this case, the comparison group is a community whose water supply is naturally low in flouride and is not supplemented. In *clinical trials*, individuals rather than communities are studied and participants are randomized either to receive the treatment of interest or to a control condition in which no active treatment is given. Experimental and control groups in clinical trials must be as similar as possible except with respect to the treatment of interest. This is accomplished through the randomization process, which makes it possible for the investigator to avoid introducing biases into the study and ensures that participants will be comparable on both known and unknown factors that could influence the outcomes of interest. Clinical trials can be *therapeutic* trials, which test the effectiveness of specific therapies in persons with disease; *intervention* trials, in which an intervention is given to persons who have not yet gotten the disease but are at increased risk of the disease because of certain characteristics they have; or *prevention* trials, which test the effectiveness of preventive therapies or procedures. The primary difference between clinical trials and prospective studies is that clinical trial participants are randomly assigned to the experimental or control group. This also is the greatest strength of clinical trials, which are often considered the "gold standard" by which to judge the effectiveness of treatments for numerous diseases.

SUSAN A. EVERSON-ROSE

Ethnicity and Health

Racial and ethnic differences in health care outcomes have become a recent target of scientific exploration. The term "race" has historically been used to distinguish major groups of people based their ancestry and physical characteristics. Today, race is most often used to distinguish a population based on biological factors such as genetics and common descent. The Caucasoid race is often characterized as pale, pinkish white to olive brown in skin color, of medium to tall stature, with a long or broad head. The Mongoloid race is often characterized as saffron to yellow or reddish brown in skin color, of medium stature, and with a broad head. The Negroid race is often characterized as brown to brown-black skin, usually with a longer head, of varying stature, and with thick, everted lips.

These racial groups vary on many other characteristics including hair color, texture, and length; nose bridge length and nostril width; and eye shape and color. Recently, the utility of "race" as a representative of distinct variance among groups of humans has grown into disfavor as having extremely limited utility, as not identifying unique intragroup genetic variance, and as having limited scientific value.

In contrast, the term "ethnicity" has grown into favor as primarily representing distinctions between groups of people based on behavior and cultural norms in addition to biological factors and physical characteristics. The term "ethnicity" is a derivation from the Greek word "ethnikos," which is translated literally as "gentile" or "heathen." This term was historically used to distinguish individuals other than the religious majority.

In the 19th century, the term ethnicity was first consistently used to refer to groups from a particular race or nation. Notably, several groups, primarily for the purpose of demonstrating superiority, introduced concepts such as Nordic supremacy, and the initial documented references to "racism" appeared. These individuals and groups asserted that certain cultures and nationalities were inherently inferior or superior to others. Unfortunately, these theories were also the foundation for later racially based atrocities in Nazi Germany, slavery in the United States, and a policy of segregation in South Africa (apartheid).

The modern meaning of "ethnic" is partially rooted in the historical description of "others" or the identification of those who may not be fully integrated into the majority culture. Ethnicity is most frequently used to distinguish groups of people based on their behaviors, cultural norms, historical experiences, ancestry, and beliefs as well as biology.

Immigrants and minorities in the United State face a range of cultural and psychological realities that challenge, facilitate, and undermine full participation in the health care system. The pressure to deny emotionality in the face of oppressive conditions, economic poverty, underemployment, lack of access to health care services, differential treatment in the health care system, and poor housing as a function of racism and cultural bias frequently fosters a sense of disenfranchisement and disconnection. Inadvertently, indifference within the health care system promotes the perception that it does not recognize or appreciate difference and is not responsive to or interested in presentations of illness that are not consistent with traditional American culture.

Unfortunately, immigrants and racial/ethnic minorities who are distressed or are ill may present their symptoms according to cultural idioms that are not valued in the U.S. health care system. For example, some Asian and African cultures are hesitant to complain with specificity about issues such as pain or mental distress in health care settings because of a belief that they might be deserving of such symptoms as punishment for wrong committed by their forefathers. In these cases, symptom presentation can be minimized and may differ from what most clinicians are trained to expect. This can lead to diagnostic and treatment errors. The impact of culture on idioms of distress, perceptions of the health care system in general, and symptom expression certainly deserves more attention from researchers, and sensitivities to such issues in clinical settings must be increased.

Research suggests that the psychological and physiological correlates and consequences of racism, or volitional disparities in outcomes as a function of race, are similar to those of better known stressors. Several laboratory studies have assessed the physiological and affective reactions of African Americans to discriminatory and racist vignettes and have found that such exposures are associated with increased cardiovascular and psychological reactivity. Other studies have demonstrated a positive relationship between self-reports of discrimination and blood pressure for African Americans. Yet others demonstrate that social support buffers the impact of racism on health outcomes. It appears that the perception of racial discrimination, in particular when evaluating ambiguous situations, has associated with it profound and negative affective consequences for Black men and women, and that ethnicity may moderate the effects of stress on activity of the hypothalamic–pitvitary–adrenal axis.

Racial and ethnic factors have also been shown to affect the health status of immigrant and refugee populations.

Acculturative stress represents the complex social and psychological sequelae of relocating and then attempting to assimilate into a new culture. For many, cultural migration is associated with societal disintegration, disruption of cultural norms, and identity confusion. In more severe forms, acculturative stress can be associated with elevated rates of suicide and symptoms such as anxiety, depression, feelings of marginality and alienation, and an overall decline in physical or psychological health status.

Significant variability exists in symptom severity for individuals experiencing acculturative stress. There appear to be several factors that may predispose individuals to greater impairment. These include pre-existing psychopathology, the cognitive appraisal of the relocation, the available coping skills repertoire, the attitudes toward the new culture, the degree of acceptance by the new culture of the immigrant, and the overall level of social support. Severe psychopathology or a history of recurrent moderate psychopathology, a negative appraisal of relocation, limited coping skills, a negative attitude toward the new culture, low levels of acceptance by the new culture, and limited or inadequate social support are all associated with increased negative reactions to the new culture and limited acculturative adjustment. In addition, younger age is associated with fewer consequences of cultural migration, and prior exposure to the new culture (positive or negative), familiarity with the language, and realistic expectations of the target culture can also increase acculturative adjustment.

Refugees represent a subset of immigrants that have been forced into relocation by political, cultural, or religious persecution. Refugees are more likely to have been victims of trauma prior to migration and suffer disproportionately from high rates of posttraumatic stress disorder and depression as compared to immigrants without refugee status. Lack of cultural cohesiveness, language barriers, economic hardship, and limited educational or employment opportunities can increase psychological distress and other adverse health outcomes in this population. Rates of psychological symptoms in refugee children appear inversely related to the mother's level of acculturation.

As the result of cultural differences in the presentation of symptoms associated with illness, unfamiliarity with the health care system, and a failure of many clinicians to recognize and integrate diversity into their conceptualization and treatment of immigrants, many of their psychological and physical symptoms are less likely to be recognized and appropriately diagnosed. This can lead to significant undertreatment of illness and more advanced disease when they do present for care.

In conclusion, terms such as "race" and "ethnicity" have been used as a mechanism for social, political, and other classifications independent of biological validity. Increasingly, it is being recognized that health and pathology are influenced by a cumulative interaction between biological, psychological/behavioral, cultural, and social factors including race and ethnicity. Better understanding and integration into conceptualization, interpretation, and treatment of these factors, their associated mechanisms, and their historical contexts (racism, discrimination, etc.) may result in the reduction of health disparities among racially, ethnically, and culturally diverse individuals.

Related Entries: Epidemiology, Illness Stereotypes, Public Health, Socioeconomic Status and Health

BIBLIOGRAPHY

Anderson, N. B., Myers, H. F., Pickering, T., & Jackson, J. S., (1989). Hypertension in Blacks: Psychosocial and biological perspectives. *Journal of Hypertension, 7*, 161–172.

Bennett, G. G., Merritt, M. M., Edwards, C. L., & Sollers, J. T. (in press). Affective responses to ambiguous interpersonal interactions among African Americans. *American Behavioral Scientist.*

Edwards, C. L., Fillingim, R. B., & Keefe, F. (2001). Race, ethnicity, and pain. *Pain, 94*, 133–137.

Gonzalez, H. M., Haan, M. N., & Hinton, L. (2001). Acculturation and the prevalence of depression in older Mexican Americans: Baseline results of the Sacramento area Latino study on aging. *Journal of the American Geriatrics Society, 49*, 948–953.

Hovey, J. D. (2000a). Acculturative stress, depression, and suicidal ideation in Mexican immigrants. *Cultural Diversity and Ethnic Minority Psychology, 6*, 134–151.

Hovey, J. D. (2000b). Acculturative stress, depression, and suicidal ideation among Central American immigrants. *Suicide and Life-Threatening Behavior, 30*, 125–139.

Hovey, J. D., & King, C. A. (1996). Acculturative stress, depression, and suicidal ideation among immigrant and second-generation Latino adolescents. *Child and Adolescent Psychiatry, 35*, 1183–1192.

James, S. A., LaCroix, A. Z., Kleinbaum, D. G., & Strogatz, D. S. (1984). John Henryism and blood pressure differences among Black men. II. The role of occupational stressors. *Journal of Behavioral Medicine, 7*, 259–275.

Krieger, N., & Sidney, S. (1996). Racial discrimination and blood pressure: The CARDIA study of young Black and White adults. *American Journal of Public Health, 86*, 1370–1378.

McNeilly, M. D., Anderson, N. B., Armstead, C. A., Clark, R., Corbett, M., Robinson, E. L., et al. (1996). The perceived racism scale: A multidimensional assessment of the experience of White racism among African Americans. ethnicity and Disease, 6, 154–166.

McNeilly, M. D., Robinson, E. L., Anderson, N. B., Pieper, C. F., Shah, A., Toth, T. S., et al. (1995). Effects of racist provocation and social support on cardiovascular reactivity in African Americans. *International Journal of Behavior Medicine, 2*, 321–338.

Mghir, R., Freed, W., Raskin, A., & Katon, W. (1995). Depression and posttraumatic stress disorder among a community sample of adolescent and young adult Afghan refugees. *Journal of Nervous and Mental Disease, 183*, 24–30.

Miller, A. M., & Chandler, P. J. (2002). Acculturation, resilience, and depression in midlife women from the former Soviet Union. Nursing Research, 51, 26–32.

Morris-Prather, C. E., Harrell, J. P., Collins, R., Leonard, K. L., Boss, M., & Lee, J. W. (1996). Gender differences in mood and cardiovascular responses to socially stressful stimuli. *Ethnicity and Disease, 6*, 123–131.

Nwadiora, E., & McAdoo, H. (1996). Acculturative stress among Amerasian refugees: Gender and racial differences. *Adolescence, 31*, 477–487.

Sack, W. H., Clarke, G. N., & Seeley, J. (1996). Multiple forms of stress in Cambodian adolescent refugees. *Child Development, 67,* 107–116.

Shapiro, J., Douglas, K., de la Rocha, O., Radecki, S., Vu, C., & Dinh, T. (1999). Generational differences in psychosocial adaptation and predictors of psychological distress in a population of recent Vietnamese immigrants. *Journal of Community Health, 24,* 95–113.

Sundquist, J., Bayard-Burfield, L., Johansson, L. M., & Johansson, S. E. (2000). Impact of ethnicity, violence and acculturation on displaced migrants: Psychological distress and psychosomatic complaints among refugees in Sweden. *Journal of Nervous and Mental Disease, 188,* 357–365.

Thompson, V. L. (1996). Perceived experiences of racism as stressful life events. *Community Mental Health, 32,* 223–233.

Williams, C. L., & Berry, J. W. (1991). Primary prevention of acculturative stress among refugees: Application of psychological theory and practice. *American Psychologist, 46,* 632–41.

CHRISTOPHER L. EDWARDS
KATHERINE L. APPLEGATE
ELWOOD ROBINSON

Euthanasia and Physician-Assisted Suicide

As advances in medical technology enable terminally ill individuals to prolong life, a growing number of individuals have sought to actually hasten death, either through refusing life-sustaining interventions or, more recently, ending their life by taking a lethal medication. Although many of these issues have existed for decades or even centuries, the 1990s brought interest in the methods, legality, and morality of hastened death to the forefront of medicine, politics, philosophy, and psychology. The center of these debates has concerned euthanasia and physician-assisted suicide as options for individuals diagnosed with a terminal illness. Euthanasia refers to the administration of a medication or other toxic substance, typically (but not necessarily) by a physician, with the specific intent of causing the death of the individual. Physician-assisted suicide (PAS), on the other hand, involves providing information and/or medication that the individual will use to end his or her life but without actually administering the lethal medication. Although PAS has been the center of most debates in the United States, euthanasia has been the focus in Europe and Australia.

In fact, the practice of euthanasia has been ongoing in the Netherlands for more than 20 years, despite only having been officially legalized in 2001. In the United States, two 1997 Supreme Court decisions (*Vacco v. Quill* and *Washington v. Glucksberg*) cleared a path for legalization, despite asserting that no "right to die" exists for terminally ill individuals (i.e., laws prohibiting assisted suicide were not unconstitutional despite the well-established right to refuse life-sustaining interventions). Shortly afterward, Oreon enacted the Death with Dignity Act (DWDA), establishing the nation's first legally sanctioned practice of PAS. The controversy around these laws has spurred the interest of researchers around the country to help develop an understanding of why medically ill and terminally ill individuals would want to hasten death.

A number of research studies have emerged in the past decade, studying both patients who have requested and/or received euthanasia and PAS and those who might be interested were these options legal in their region. Several similarities have emerged from studies of patients who seek euthanasia or assisted suicide, typically demonstrating the importance of psychological and social factors in driving decisions to seek euthanasia and PAS whereas pain and symptom burden have been much less prominent. However, significant differences have also emerged between studies in the United States and Netherlands, such as the dramatic disparity in the frequency with which these end-of-life options are utilized. Whereas 3–5 percent of Netherlands deaths are attributed to euthanasia and PAS (the vast majority being euthanasia), only less than 0.1 percent of Oregon deaths result from PAS (20–30 cases annually).

However, because of the limitations in studying actual patient requests for assisted suicide, researchers have increasingly focused on the desire for hastened death among medically ill and terminally ill populations. Research on the desire for hastened death, unlike studies of patient requests for PAS and euthanasia, has consistently identified hopelessness and major depression as the primary reasons why a more rapid death might be desired. These studies have further bolstered the growing evidence that, despite the frequent reliance on intolerable physical symptoms as a moral justification for PAS and euthanasia, psychosocial factors are much more prominent in driving patient interest in hastened death. This growing literature has fueled a new set of end-of-life questions such as whether decisions to hasten death, when driven by psychological factors such as depression and hopelessness, can nevertheless be "rational." Issues of decision-making competence, which are a prerequisite for any health care decision making, are difficult to resolve and poorly understood in the context of euthanasia and hastened death. Nonetheless, the importance of these and other questions related to end-of-life decisions will undoubtedly foster continued interest and empirical study over the coming decades.

Related Entry: Hospice Care

BIBLIOGRAPHY

Rosenfeld, B. (2000). Assisted suicide, depression and the right to die. *Psychology, Public Policy and Law, 6,* 529–549.

Sullivan, A. D., Hedberg, K., & Fleming, D. W. (2000). Legalized physician-assisted suicide in Oregon—The second year. *New England Journal of Medicine, 342,* 598–604.

Van der Maas, P. J., van Delden, J. J. M., Pijnenborg, L., & Looman, C. W. N. (1991). Euthanasia and other medical decisions concerning the end of life. *Lancet, 338,* 669–674.

BARRY ROSENFELD

Exercise, Effects and Benefits

Physical activity is bodily movement produced by the contraction of skeletal muscle that increases energy expenditure above the basal level. In contrast, exercise denotes a subcategory of physical activity that is planned, structured, repetitive, and purposive in the sense that improvement or maintenance of one or more components of physical fitness is the objective. Physical fitness, generally considered a product of both genetics and physical activity, is the ability to carry out daily tasks with vigor and alertness, without undue fatigue, and with ample energy to enjoy leisure-time pursuits and to meet unforeseen emergencies. The most commonly used measure of physical fitness is the ability of the circulatory and respiratory systems to supply oxygen during sustained physical activity, and is referred to as cardiorespiratory or cardiovascular fitness. Physical activity, then, is the more general category that encompasses exercise and largely determines physical fitness.

PHYSICAL ACTIVITY AND PHYSICAL HEALTH

Physical fitness and physical activity are undeniably beneficial for physical health. Both men and women with higher levels of cardiovascular fitness have a decreased risk of dying from all causes (see Figure 1), from cardiovascular disease, and from cancer, and a similar relationship has been found between physical activity and mortality from all causes, cardiovascular disease, and cancer.

Physical activity also has positive effects on several chronic health conditions, namely, obesity, Type 2 diabetes, and osteoporosis. As the most variable component of energy expenditure, physical activity can influence the development of obesity as well as success in achieving both initial and long-term weight loss. Physical activity also reduces the likelihood that a person at risk for Type 2 (adult-onset) diabetes will develop the disorder and enhances blood glucose regulation in those with the disease. With respect to osteoporosis, the National Institutes of Health recommends that physical activity should be encouraged during childhood and adolescence to promote optimal bone growth and reduce the risk of osteoporosis later in life, whereas those with osteoporosis should engage in physical activity both to slow down bone loss and to lower the risk of falls.

PHYSICAL ACTIVITY AND PSYCHOLOGICAL WELL-BEING

Many people believe that physical activity improves psychological well-being, and a large number of studies have sought to demonstrate that physical activity elevates mood, reduces depression, and alleviates anxiety. A review of the evidence reveals a strong consensus among researchers that mood enhancement is a primary benefit of physical activity. Similarly, physical activity has been useful in ameliorating mild to moderate depression. Some studies also have shown that physical activity reduces anxiety, defined as a feeling of aprehension or fear that lingers, though the evidence for this link is less consistent.

HOW MUCH PHYSICAL ACTIVITY IS ENOUGH?

Knowing that more active individuals are healthier than less active individuals brings up two related questions:

1. How much physical activity is enough?
2. What type of physical activity is most effective?

In terms of the benefits of physical activity for physical health, the single most important factor may be total energy expenditure. Among sedentary, unfit adults, the accumulation of 30 min of walking per day (or the equivalent energy expenditure in other activities) is likely to result in clinically significant health benefits. This approach to physical activity, in which the emphasis is on accumulation of moderate-level activity, has been described in terms of promoting *lifestyle activity*. Some evidence suggests that among adults lifestyle activity may bring about positive health effects comparable to those of a programmed exercise regimen, and that individuals may be more likely to maintain the former than the latter.

These recommendations have been generated in reaction to the public health issue posed by the great number of adults in the United States who engage in little or no activity beyond that required for daily living. Thus, an emphasis has been placed on motivating these sedentary persons to engage in at least a minimal level of activity that would bring about meaningful health improvements. Moreover, the greatest differential in health outcomes is between adults who engage in virtually no activity and those who engage in activity equal to at least 30 min of brisk walking per day (see Figure 1). Combined with evidence that improvements in cardiovascular fitness may be achieved through accumulated short, intermittent bouts of activity, the result has been a shift away from earlier recommendations that emphasized continuous bouts (i.e., 30 min or more) of relatively vigorous activity. It is likely, however, that the frequency, duration, intensity, and type of activity that will

groups in men and women.

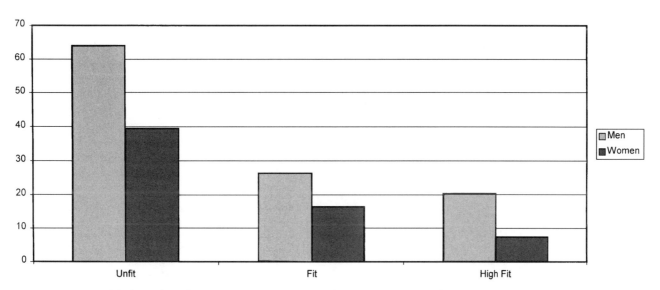

Figure 1. Age-adjusted death rates from all causes per 10,000 person-years of follow-up (1970–1985) by fitness groups in men and women. Fitness was determined by treadmill test time and grouped into quintiles. Individuals scoring in the lowest quintile were categorized as unfit, those in the 2–3 quintiles were categorized as fit, and those in the 4–5 quintiles were categorized as high fit. Figure is adapted from data in Blair et al. (1989).

promote optimal health will vary from person to person and across different health outcomes. For example, the amount and type of activity that promotes optimal bone health may differ from the amount and type of activity that promotes optimal psychological well-being.

An additional level of complexity is introduced when focusing on the psychological benefits of physical activity. Although some psychological benefits of physical activity may be related to underlying changes in physiology that occur in response to exercise, it is generally believed that benefits also may derive from nonphysiological aspects of physical activity, such as social interaction, distraction, or simple enjoyment of the activity. Moreover, the likelihood that an individual will adhere to an activity prescription must be considered. Because adherence is critical to achieving health benefits, the choice of activity thus becomes an essential consideration in any exercise prescription.

COMMON STRATEGIES TO PROMOTE PHYSICAL ACTIVITY

A number of strategies have been employed to promote physical activity in individuals and/or communities. Approaches that have shown evidence of being effective include the following:

1. *Point-of-decision prompts* are signs placed by elevators and escalators to motivate people to use nearby stairs.

2. *Community-wide campaigns* typically involve many sectors of the community, combine multiple intervention approaches, and employ a highly visible communication campaign linking all elements into an integrated program.

3. *School-based physical education* involves modifying school curricula and policies to increase the amount of time that students spend in moderate or vigorous activity while in physical education classes.

4. *Social support interventions in community settings* focus on changing physical activity behavior by encouraging supportive relationships for behavior change; for example, programs may set up a "buddy" system or set up walking groups.

5. *Individually adapted health behavior change programs* are tailored to the individual, and teach participants behavioral skills that enable them to incorporate physical activity into daily routines.

EXERCISE PROMOTION IN SPECIAL POPULATIONS

Because physical activity has important health benefits in youth and many young people are not meeting established guidelines, improving the physical activity levels of youth is an important public health challenge. Recommended levels of activity for youth range from 30 to 60 min per day of moderate-to-vigorous activity. Unfortunately, social and economic forces have restricted opportunities for children and adolescents to be physically active while trends in leisure-time activities have increased time spent in sedentary activities such as watching television and playing video games. In reaction to these trends, programs have been designed to enhance access to facilities for activity, bolster participation in school-based physical education, and reduce television watching.

The elderly also stand to benefit considerably from increased physical activity both in terms of quality of life and health outcomes. Physical activity typically declines with age, and age-associated illness further contributes to a decline in activity among the elderly. In addition to the demonstrated benefit of physical activity for reducing all-cause mortality, participation in physical activity has shown promise among the elderly for ameliorating several age-associated declines in function, including cognitive function, cardiovascular fitness, and muscle and bone strength. Importantly, exercise that is initiated in late life, even after a sedentary middle age, may result in substantial gains in life expectancy.

In sum, physical activity is consistently and strongly related to multiple dimensions of health and offers an effective means of reducing morbidity and mortality. Physical activity is valuable in the prevention and treatment of obesity, diabetes, osteoporosis, depression, and heart disease. Because of the large proportion of the U.S. population that is sedentary, the promotion of physical activity has huge potential for enhancing public health. Moreover, meaningful health benefits may be realized by accumulating as little as 30 min per day of moderate activity, though more and/or more intense activity may be required to bring about specific improvements such as enhanced cardiovascular fitness or weight loss. The benefits are particularly evident among youth and the elderly, both of whom stand to gain enormously from adopting and maintaining an active lifestyle.

Related Entry: Prevention

BIBLIOGRAPHY

Berger, B., & Motl, R. (2000). Exercise and mood: A selective review and synthesis of research employing the Profile of Mood States. *Journal of Applied Sport Psychology, 12*, 69–92.

Blair, S., Cheng, Y., & Holder, J. S. (2001). Is physical activity or physical fitness more importnat in defining health benefits? *Medicine and Science in Sports and Exercise, 33*(6 Supplement) S379–S399.

Blair, S., Kohl, H., Gordon, N., & Paffenbarger, Jr., R. (1992). How much physical activity is good for health? *Annual Review of Public Health, 13*, 99–126.

Blair, S., Kohl, H., Paffenbarger, R., Clark, D., & Cooper, K. (1989). Physical fitness and all-cause mortality; A prospective study of healthy men and women. *Journal of the American Medical Association, 262*, 2395–2401.

DeBusk, R., Stenestrand, U., Sheehan, M., & Haskell, W. (1990). Training effects of long versus short bouts of exercise in healthy subjects. *American Journal of Cardiology, 65*, 1010–13.

Dunn, A., Trivedi, M., & O'Neal, H. (2001). Physical activity dose–response effects on outcomes of depression and anxiety. *Medicine and Science in Sports and Exercise, 33*(6 Supplement), S587–S597.

Kahn, E. B., Ramsey, L. T., et al. (2002). The effectiveness of interventions to increase physical activity: A systematic review. *American Journal of Preventive Medicine, 22*(4S), 73–107.

Kelley, D., & Goodpaster, B. (2001). Effects of exercise on glucose homeostasis in Type 2 diabetes mellitus. *Medicine and Science in Sports and Exercise, 33*(6 Supplement), S495–S501.

King, A., & Tribble, D. (1991). The role of exercise in weight regulation in nonathletes. *Sports Medicine, 11*, 331–349.

National Institutes of Health. (2000). *Osteoporosis prevention, diagnosis, and therapy* [NIH Consensus Statement 17(1)]. Bethesda, Md: Author.

Sallis, J. F., Prochaska, J. J., & Taylor, W. C. (2000). A review of correlates of physical activity of children and adolescents. *Medicine and Science in Sports and Exercise, 32*, 963–975.

U.S. Department of Health and Human Services. (1996). *Physical activity and health: A report of the surgeon General*. Atlanta, GA: Centers for Disease Control and Prevention.

Wagner, E. H., LaCroix, A. Z., Buchner, D. M., & Larson, E. B. (1992). Effects of physical activity on health status in older adults I: Observational studies. *Annual Review of Public Health, 13*, 451–468.

MARGARET SCHNEIDER JAMNER

Ff

Fear Appeals

Fear appeals or fear-arousing communications originated from the fear-drive reduction model advanced by Dollard and Miller (1950). A central tenet of that model is that fear motivates individuals to engage in a recommended behavior, which reduces the unpleasant fear state. Fear communication appeals consist of a fear-arousing message and a recommendation for a specific behavior, which, if followed, will reduce the fear state. The general assumption was that high levels of fear would be related to attitude and behavioral change.

One of the first experimental studies to test this hypothesis was conducted by Janis and Feshbach (1953). Junior high school students received recommendations for oral hygiene (i.e., brushing one's teeth three times a day) coupled with three different fear appeals. The high-fear condition consisted of pictures of decaying teeth and gums. The mild-fear condition consisted of less vivid pictures, and the no-fear condition omitted pictures of decaying teeth. Contrary to expectations, students in the no-fear condition were more likely to change their dental hygiene compared to students in either the mild- or high-fear conditions. Janis and Feshbach attributed these findings to defensive avoidance among students exposed to the high-fear message. They argued that messages with too much or too little fear-arousing content are ineffective compared to messages with medium-fear content.

An overwhelming majority of subsequent studies, however, have not confirmed these initial results or its interpretation. Following Janis and Feshbach's basic study design, higher levels of fear were consistently associated with greater intentions for behavior or actual behavior change. One such study exposed students to three levels of fear-arousing information about the failure of obtaining a tetanus shot. Intentions for and actual inoculation behavior correlated linearly with increased fear arousal, that is, students with a higher fear level were much more likely to obtain a tetanus shot. This basic pattern of results has been confirmed using a number of paradigms, such as safe driving, dental hygiene, and smoking.

Another consequence of these studies was the realization that fear appeals were transient and short lived and that intentions could best be translated into behavior if the individual received an action plan. An action plan is a detailed instruction on how to perform the recommended behavior. For example, in one of the studies, students received a campus map that highlighted the health center where they could obtain the recommended tetanus inoculation. With an action plan, students exposed to both high- and low-fear messages obtained tetanus shots. However, an action plan alone was not enough to motivate behavior.

These later studies led to the formulation of a new theoretical framework, called the parallel processing model. In contrast to the fear-drive model, which assumes serial processing (i.e., the processing of cognitive information followed by emotional reactions), this framework postulates the parallel processing of fear messages (i.e., the simultaneous processing of the threat stimulus on a cognitive and an emotional level). Both levels of processing can trigger coping and appraisal responses designed to deal with the threat and its emotional impact.

Related Entries: Health Promotion, Message-Framing Effects, Prevention

BIBLIOGRAPHY

Dabbs, J. M., Jr., & Leventhal, H. (1966). Effects of varying the recommendations in a fear-arousing communication. *Journal of Personality and Social Psychology, 4,* 525–531.

Dollard, J., & Miller, N. E. (1950). *Personality and psychotherapy.* New York: McGraw-Hill.

Janis, I. L. (1967). Effects of fear arousal on attitude change: Recent developments in theory and experimental research. In L. Berkowitz (Ed.), *Advances in experimental social psychology* (Vol. 3, pp. 00–00). New York: Academic.

Janis, I. L., & Feshbach, S. (1953). Effects of fear-arousing communications. *Journal of Abnormal and Social Psychology, 48,* 78–92.

Leventhal, H. (1970). Findings and theory in the study of fear communications. *Advances in Experimental Social Psychology, 5,* 119–186.

Leventhal, H., & Niles, P. (1965). Persistence of influence for varying durations of exposure to threat stimuli. *Psychological Review, 16,* 223–233.

Leventhal, H., & Singer, R. (1966). Affect arousal and positioning of recommendation in persuasive communications. *Journal of Personality and Social Psychology, 4,* 137–146.

Leventhal, H., Singer, R., & Jones, S. (1965). Effects of fear and specificity of recommendations upon attitudes and behavior. *Journal of Personality and Social Psychology, 2,* 20–29.

Leventhal, H., & Trembly G. (1968). Negative emotions and persuasion. *Journal of Personality, 36,* 154–168.

Leventhal, H., & Watts, J. C. (1966). Sources of resistance to fear-arousing communications on smoking and lung cancer. *Journal of Personality, 34,* 155–175.

Rogers, R. W., & Deckner, C. W. (1975). Effects of fear appeals and physiological arousal upon emotion, attitudes and cigarette smoking. *Journal of Personality and Social Psychology, 32,* 222–230.

Rogers, R. W., & Thistlethwaite, D. L. (1970). Effects of fear arousal and reassurance upon attitude change. *Journal of Personality and Social Psychology, 15,* 227–233.

Sutton, S. R. (1982). Fear-arousing communications: A critical examination of theory and research. *Social Psychology and Behavioral Medicine, 13,* 303–337.

MICHAEL DIEFENBACH

Fetal Alcohol Syndrome

Fetal alcohol syndrome (FAS) is a set of birth defects that occur because of prenatal exposure to alcohol. A diagnosis of FAS requires three criteria, each addressing a constellation of symptoms or deficits. First are facial abnormalities, including small eye openings (short palpebral fissures), a thin upper lip without the typical ridges between nose and lip (flattened philtrum), and flat midface with a low nasal bridge. Second is evidence of retarded growth, such as low birth weight and a low weight-to-height ratio. Third are structural brain abnormalities (e.g., small head circumference) with corresponding neurological signs such as impaired fine motor skills or poor hand–eye coordination. Individuals with FAS demonstrate a range of behavioral and cognitive problems that manifest in specific learning deficits, poor school performance, and problems with attention, memory, judgment, and impulse control. These problems often affect mental health and social adjustment.

FAS is the most severe form of a constellation of disorders related to prenatal alcohol exposure. Alcohol-related birth defects (ARBD) include congenital defects of the skeletal or other organ systems. These defects are not always present in the context of full FAS. Alcohol-related neurodevelopmental disorder (ARND) describes neurodevelopmental abnormalities such as small head size, neurological problems, and behavioral and cognitive deficits, without facial anomalies or growth retardation. FAS affects up to 12,000 infants each year, or between 0.5 and 2 per 1,000 births. FAS is the leading known cause of mental retardation in the United States.

There is no known safe level of alcohol consumption during pregnancy. When a pregnant woman drinks alcohol it gets into her bloodstream, which travels through the placenta and circulates through her baby. Alcohol is a teratogen, which means that it is toxic to the developing baby. However, not every woman who consumes alcohol when pregnant gives birth to a child with FAS. The likelihood of alcohol exposure causing harm to the fetus depends on several factors.

One is the mother's drinking pattern. Binge-type drinking, characterized by high blood alcohol concentrations (BACs), is the drinking pattern most associated with fetal damage. A given number of ounces of alcohol consumed in small amounts over several days is less likely to harm a baby's development than the same number of ounces consumed on a single occasion. Why high BACs are associated with FAS is not fully understood. A critical level of alcohol may be required to cause fetal damage. Alternatively, high BACs may simply result in longer exposure of the fetus to alcohol.

Another factor affecting the likelihood and type of fetal alcohol effects is when during the pregnancy alcohol exposure occurs. Organ systems are most vulnerable to damage during periods of rapid cell division, and organ systems mature at different rates in the human fetus. The varied forms of FAS, ARBD, and ARND likely arise as a function of individual differences in the timing and intensity of alcohol exposure.

FAS is completely preventable if a woman abstains from alcohol during pregnancy. If a woman is trying to conceive or thinks she may be pregnant, she should stop drinking.

Related Entries: Alcoholism, Addiction, Denial, Reproductive System, Pregnancy, Postpartum Depression

BIBLIOGRAPHY

Maier, S. E., & West, J. R. (2001). Drinking patterns and alcohol-related birth defects. *Alcohol Research and Health, 25,* 168–174.

May, P. A., & Gossage, J. P. (2001). Estimating the prevalence of fetal alcohol syndrome. *Alcohol Research and Health, 25,* 159–167.

Warren, K. R., & Foudin, L. L. (2001). Alcohol-related birth defects—The past, present, and future. *Alcohol Research and Health, 25,* 153–158.

KATE B. CAREY

Fibromyalgia

Fibromyalgia syndrome (or fibromyalgia) is a chronic disorder characterized by widespread pain and persistent fatigue. Rheumatologists and pain management specialists typically treat fibromyalgia; however, patients also seek the care of family practice physicians and neurologists. According to the American College of Rheumatology, fibromyalgia is defined by widespread muscle and soft tissue pain and tenderness in all four quadrants of the body for a minimum of 3 months, and sharp pain when pressure is applied to at least 11 of 18 specified "tender points" on the patient's body (Wolfe et al., 1990). Patients have difficulty sleeping and concentrating, feel fatigued, and wake up in the morning feeling stiff and unrefreshed. They may experience headaches, tingling or numbness, weakness, irritable bowel syndrome (constipation, diarrhea, and abdominal pain), temporomandibular joint dysfunction syndrome (or TMJ), multiple chemical sensitivity syndrome, and depression. There are no laboratory tests to diagnose fibromyalgia, and other illnesses are ruled out before a diagnosis is made.

Fibromyalgia is not life threatening, nor does it cause deformity. The course of fibromyalgia waxes and wanes. Flare-ups are particularly common following times of physical or emotional stress. Fibromyalgia can be disabling and may severely interfere with a patient's regular activities and work.

The definite cause of fibromyalgia is unknown. Certain factors may place a person at increased risk for developing fibromyalgia, such as having a parent with fibromyalgia, another rheumatologic disorder (such as rheumatoid arthritis), an infectious disease (such as Lyme disease), chronic fatigue syndrome, or a psychiatric condition (such as major depression). Women are more likely to be diagnosed with fibromyalgia than men. Fibromyalgia can occur at any age. Roughly 1–4 percent of the population may be afflicted with this disease.

There are many theories of the etiology, or cause, of fibromyalgia. It may be caused by an imbalance in the brain chemicals (particularly serotonin, norepinephrine, and substance P) that control mood and the sleep cycle. Fibromyalgia may result from sleep cycle abnormalities or growth hormone imbalances. Based on functional magnetic resonance imaging (fMRI) studies, fibromyalgia patients may be overly sensitive to pain, perhaps due to increased sensitivity of pain receptors in the spinal cord and brain. For many years, fibromyalgia was thought to be a psychological condition, but there is little research support for this notion.

Although there is no cure for fibromyalgia, there are some effective treatments. Doctors commonly prescribe medications (such as antidepressants) to improve sleep and mood and block pain signals. The physician may also inject trigger points with an anesthetic or prescribe muscle relaxants. Physical therapy, gentle exercise, education, and counseling are often included. Promising new research shows that growth hormone injections might be able to reduce patient's pain and stiffness. Cognitive–behavioral therapy may be effective for pain control as well.

A variety of other alternative and complementary treatments are often used to treat fibromyalgia; however, few of these therapies have been examined in controlled research studies. These include biofeedback, acupuncture, meditation, transcutaneous electrical nerve stimulation (TENS), massage therapy, dietary supplements, and chiropractic therapy.

Related Entries: Arthritis, Chronic Fatigue Syndrome, Pain

BIBLIOGRAPHY

American College of Rheumatology. Available from http://www.rheumatology.org

Bradley, L. A., & Alarcon, G. S. (1997). Fibromyalgia. In W. J. Koopman (Ed.), *Arthritis and allied conditions: A textbook of rheumatology* 13th ed., pp. 00–00). Baltimore: Williams & Wilkins.

Clauw, D. J. (2001). Fibromyalgia. In S. Ruddy, E. D. Harris, Jr., & C. B. Sledge (Eds.), *Kelley's textbook of rheumatology* (6th ed., pp. 00–00). Philadelphia: Saunders.

Simons, D. G., Travell, J. G., & Simons, L. S. (1998). *Travell & Simons' myofascial pain and dysfunction: The trigger point manual.* Baltimore: Lippincott, Williams & Wilkins.

Wolfe, F., Smythe, H. A., Yunus, M. B., et al. (1990). The American College of Rheumatology 1990 criteria for the classification of fibromyalgia: Report of the multicenter criteria committee. *Arthritis and Rheumatism, 33,* 160–172.

SUZANNE C. LECHNER

Fight-or-Flight Response

The designation of the fight-or-flight response is commonly attributed to Walter Cannon. In the early 20th century Cannon wrote extensively about the arousal of the body due to situations involving fear and the resulting response of aggression or flight. For obvious reasons, the fight-or-flight response is of survival benefit to the individual. When faced with imminent danger (e.g., a tiger in the forest) a person is afforded two primary options; fight or run away. The fight-or-flight response prepares the body for rapid action to cope with the threat by quickly increasing the supply of oxygen and sugar (glucose) to the bloodstream, accelerating metabolism, releasing natural painkillers (endorphins), and increasing the sensitivity of all five senses.

In addition, the fight-or-flight response is associated with a hypothalamic–pituitary–adrenocortical (HPA) axis response, which triggers both sympathetic nervous system and endocrine activity as a result of exposure to fear, anxiety, or stress. Sympathetic arousal includes increases in heart rate, blood pressure, and sweating; alterations in blood flow from the periphery toward muscles; activation of the adrenal medulla; and reductions in digestive processes. The endocrine response includes the release of corticotrophin-releasing factor, stimulating the pituitary gland to release adrenocorticotropic hormone, which then triggers the release of glucocorticoids, including cortisol, from the adrenal cortex.

The work of two additional scientists guided much of the early research on fight-or-flight and stress. Hans Selye believed that all people responded to stressful situations in basically the same manner with a series of three stages, the alarm reaction, the resistance stage, and the exhaustion stage. In contrast, Richard Lazarus believed that stressful interactions are dynamic and apt to change quickly. Therefore, individuals constantly appraise and reappraise stressful situations. In Lazarus's view, the individual's appraisal of a stressful situation (e.g., is this dog a threat to my safety or is it a friendly dog?) was of the utmost importance because it guides the individual's coping strategies (i.e., fighting or fleeing). Lazarus believed that people made an initial appraisal of a stressful situation, but also reappraised situations as their environment changed. In doing so, people could continue to react appropriately to an ever-changing environment.

Much research has been devoted to effects of enduring long-term stress. Selye's research suggested that excessive long-term production of glucocorticoids had detrimental effects on the body, including high blood pressure, steroid diabetes, inhibition of growth, inhibition of the inflammatory response, damage to muscle tissue, infertility, and suppression of the immune system. These effects have been associated with such health concerns as heart attack, slow healing of injuries, cancer, and stunted growth in children. Some research has shown that individuals who are providing long-term care for relatives, a situation known to cause stress, demonstrate a slowed healing response to lab-induced punch biopsy wounds. Also, a group of elderly patients who had increased levels of glucocorticoids (a hormone that has been shown to increase with greater levels of stress) in their blood demonstrated greater difficulties in learning a maze. The researchers concluded that long-term exposure to stress increases the release of glucocorticoids and destroys neurons in the brain.

Related Entries: General Adaptation Syndrome, Nervous System, Psychophysiology, Stressful Life Events

BIBLIOGRAPHY

Cannon, W. (1929). *Bodily changes in pain, hunger, fear and rage* (2nd ed.). New York: Appleton.

Kiecold-Glaser, J. K., Marucha, P. T., Malarkey, W. B., Mercado, A. M., & Glaser, R. (1995). Slowing of wound healing by psychological stress. *Lancet, 346,* 1194–1196.

Lazarus, R. (1984). Puzzles in the study of daily hassles. *Journal of Behavioral Medicine, 7,* 375–389.

Lupien, S., Lecours, A. R., Schwartz, G., Sharma, S., Hauger, R. L., Meaney, M. J., et al. (1996). Longitudinal study of basal cortisol levels in healthy elderly subjects: Evidence for subgroups. *Neurobiology of Aging, 17,* 95–105.

Selye, Hans. (1956). *The stress of life.* New York: McGraw-Hill.

SCOTT ENGEL
DAVID A. WITTROCK

Five-Factor Model of Personality

Throughout most of the 20th century, psychologists debated which traits are central to human personality. After decades of largely fruitless controversy, a widespread consensus emerged during the late 1980s that the five-factor model (FFM) provides a simple, basic, and highly informative scheme for understanding personality. The FFM consists of five largely independent dimensions: Neuroticism versus Emotional Stability (being distressed, dissatisfied, and moody vs. being calm and relaxed), Extraversion versus Introversion (being friendly, assertive, and enthusiastic vs. being reserved, timid, and aloof), Openness or Intellect (being intellectually curious, imaginative, and eager to try new experiences vs. being unimaginative, narrow, and inflexible), Agreeableness vs. Antagonism (being polite, cooperative, and kind vs. being rude, aggressive, and selfish), and Conscientiousness vs. Undependability (i.e., being cautious, disciplined, and reliable vs. being impulsive, disorganized, and careless).

The FFM has its origins in the 1930s, when Gordon W. Allport and Henry S. Odbert constructed a set of 4,504 terms that represented all of the personality traits described in the English language. From the 1940s through the mid-1960s, trait researchers reduced this initial pool to a much smaller set of terms by (1) eliminating words that were archaic or obscure and (2) grouping closely related terms into clusters that appeared to reflect a common underlying characteristic. Various studies of reduced sets of these terms eventually led to the recognition that they could be reduced to the five core traits defining the FFM. The final step in the evolution of the model came in the 1980s, when Costa and McCrae demonstrated that these same five traits also could be identified in most of the most popular self-report personality inventories.

The widespread acceptance of the FFM reflects three basic considerations. First, because of the original work of Allport and Odbert, it can be claimed that these five characteristics are firmly rooted in our very language. Consequently, unlike competing models, the FFM appears to be intrinsic to human nature and is not the product of some arbitrary theory. Second, the FFM has a robustness and replicability that is unmatched by any other model; that is, the same five dimensions have been identified in (1) in studies of children, adolescents, and adults and (2) across a wide range of cultures. Third, the FFM contains traits that are very general with an extremely broad range of applicability. Accordingly, it allows researchers to study personality in a very simple, efficient, but reasonably comprehensive manner.

The FFM traits also have important connections to health. Conscientiousness has emerged as a particularly strong predictor of general health and overall longevity. In addition, low levels of Agreeableness have been linked to the Type A personality pattern and to the subsequent development of cardiovascular problems. Finally, Neuroticism is broadly related to the reporting of physical symptoms such as headaches, nausea, and chest pain. Although this trait is associated with certain health problems, it also has been established that neurotic individuals tend to overreport symptoms and to exaggerate the magnitude of these problems.

Related Entries: Conscientiousness, Neuroticism

BIBLIOGRAPHY

Friedman, H. S. (2000). Long-term relations of personality and health: Dynamisms, mechanisms, tropisms. *Journal of Personality, 68*, 1089–1107.

John, O. P., & Srivastava, S. (1999). The big five trait taxonomy: History, measurement, and theoretical perspectives. In L. A. Pervin & O. P. John (Eds.), *Handbook of personality: Theory and research* (2nd ed., pp. 00–00). New York: Guilford.

McCrae, R. R., & Costa, P. T., Jr. (1999). A five-factor theory of personality. In L. A. Pervin & O. P. John (Eds.), *Handbook of personality: Theory and research* (2nd ed., pp. 00–00). New York: Guilford.

Smith, T. W., & Williams, P. G. (1992). Personality and health: Advantages and limitations of the five-factor model. *Journal of Personality, 60*, 395–423.

DAVID WATSON

Folkman, Susan (1938–)

Susan Folkman is professor of medicine, director of the Osher Center for Integrative Medicine, and the Osher Foundation Distinguished Professor in Integrative Medicine at the University of California, San Francisco (UCSF). She is best known for her theory and research on coping. This work has had special influence in the fields of psychology, behavioral medicine, and nursing.

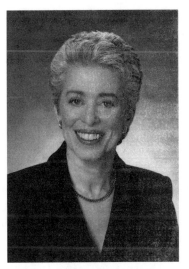

Folkman, Susan

Folkman received her BA in history from Brandeis University in 1959 and then, after four children, returned to school in 1972 to earn an MEd in counseling psychology from the University of Missouri, St. Louis, in 1974 and a PhD in educational psychology from the University of California, Berkeley, in 1979. While at the University of California, Berkeley, she worked with Prof. Richard S. Lazarus doing community-based research on stress and coping. She coined the terms "emotion-focused coping" and "problem-focused coping" in her dissertation research with Lazarus to describe the two major functions of coping—the management of stress-related emotion and the management of the problem causing the emotion. She and Lazarus elaborated a theory of stress and coping and developed a measure, The Ways of Coping, that subsequently became widely used by researchers in the United States and around the world. The research on stress and coping that she and Lazarus conducted provided fundamental information about coping, including the definition of distinct types of coping, the identification of situational factors that influence coping, and the relationship between coping and mood.

Folkman remained at Berkeley as a research psychologist working in collaboration with Lazarus until 1987, when she moved to UCSF. There she focused her research on the ways people cope with severe and enduring health-related stress. She conducted a series of studies with the caregivers of people with HIV/AIDS and other chronic illnesses, which showed that even under the most dire circumstances people still experience positive emotions. This observation led to an interest in the adaptive functions of positive emotions in the stress process and the kinds of coping processes that generated positive emotions. The kinds of coping that are used to generate positive emotions are often focused on positive meaning, defined in terms of the individual's goals, beliefs, and values.

In 1997 she received an honorary doctorate from the University of Utrecht in the Netherlands in recognition of her contributions to the psychology of stress and coping.

SUSAN FOLKMAN

BIBLIOGRAPHY

Fordyce, W. E. (1976). *Behavioral methods for chronic pain and illness.* St. Louis: Mosby.

WILBERT E. FORDYCE

Fordyce, Wilbert E. (1923–)

Wilbert Evans Fordyce was born January 3, 1923, in Sunnyside, Washington, the youngest son of a physician father and RN mother. He is professor emeritus of the University of Washington School of Medicine, Department of Rehabilitation Medicine and Pain Service. He is a fellow of the American Psychological Association (APA) and of Divisions 12, 22, 25, and 38. He received his PhD in clinical psychology from the University of Washington in 1953. He has served as president of APA's Division 22 (Rehabilitation Psychology), the American Congress of Rehabilitation Medicine, and the American Pain Society. He is a founding member, honorary member, and former councilor of the International Association for the Study of Pain.

In collaboration with Roy S. Fowler, Jr., PhD, in the mid 1960s he devised the rudiments of a behaviorally based approach to chronic pain: the "operant pain program." The essentials were to conceptualize chronic illness in behavioral terms, that is, to analyze symptoms potentially as operants subject to modification by contingency management. The core of the ensuing program included time-contingent analgesics delivered on a fading schedule to eliminate physician-prescribed medication addiction, a common occurrence prior to the behavioral approach. The program also included working to quota rather than to tolerance in exercise and activity programs to promote reactivation, thereby using rest as a reinforcer contingent on performance. Methods were also devised to modify social/environmental contingencies to "sick" and "well" behavior. These procedures are now somewhat standard practice in pain management worldwide. The overall program often included, as needed, short-term psychotherapy, family counseling, and vocational counseling. These methods were spelled out in his book, *Behavioral Methods for Chronic Pain and Illness* (Fordyce, 1976).

Conceptualizing symptoms as behavior was a paradigm shift. Analysis of symptom patterns to determine whether systematic environmental contingencies were present has broadened our understanding and moved us away from a too heavy reliance on psychodynamic notions of symptom control in the management of chronic illness.

Framingham Heart Study

CONTRIBUTIONS TO HEALTH PSYCHOLOGY

The Framingham Heart Study (FHS) is one of the leading prospective, longitudinal studies of cardiovascular disease (CVD) in the world. This study was initiated in 1948 with support from the National Heart Institute (now the National Heart, Lung and Blood Institute). The three major objectives were to (1) obtain data on arteriosclerotic and hypertensive CVD, (2) determine prevalence of all forms of CVD, and (3) test the efficiency of various diagnostic procedures. The objectives encompassed the desire to identify risk factors leading to CVD and to understand how to modify and prevent them. The term "risk factors" was coined by Framingham investigators.

Cardiovascular diseases and events included coronary deaths, heart attacks (*myocardial infarction*), congestive heart failure, heart pain (*angina pectoris*), coronary artery diseases, and stroke. Common biological CVD risk factors of concern include high blood pressure (*hypertension*), diabetes, obesity, high cholesterol, family history of CVD, genetic disposition to CVD, smoking, and age. Diseases of the brain (including vascular disease, dementias, and Alzheimer's disease) became a target of investigation as the study progressed.

The study is in its 55th year. Most persons were free of CVD when they joined the study at the first time (baseline) of data collection. Data collection was repeated approximately every 2 years. For those initially free of CVD, data were collected before CVD developed (*prospective* data collection). Thus it was possible to determine the role these risk factors played in the emergence and progression of CVD.

As early as 1978, the Framingham epidemiologists began to describe the role of psychosocial variables as risk factors for CVD. As just an example, Type A (aggressive, overly ambitious, hostile, and cynical) behavior, anxiety, and worry are associated with the development of CVD, even when biological risk factors such as hypertension, diabetes, high cholesterol, and obesity are taken into account.

Cognitive function has been studied in relation to CVD. The cognitively debilitating effects of stroke were described in 1998. A series of studies of the relationships between biological risk factors for CVD and cognitive functioning were initiated in 1990 using data collected between 1954 and 1978. The reasoning was as follows. Biological risk factors for CVD have adverse effects on brain function. They should be associated with lowered performance on neuropsychological tests.

These hypotheses were confirmed. Risk factors present in midlife, high blood pressure, diabetes, obesity, and smoking, were related to modest deficits in cognitive functioning years later. Moreover, modestly lowered cognitive functioning in midlife, particularly on tests of memory, was related to a higher likelihood of developing dementia in old age.

By 2003, two major findings of importance had emerged from studies with cognitive functioning outcomes: (1) biological CVD risk factors are associated with a lowering of cognitive functioning that is proportional to the number of risk factors present, and (2) in some individuals, mild cognitive dysfunction may herald the development of dementia in very old age and many years after it is first detected.

As early as 1971 a new prospective longitudinal study with the children of the FHS participants (the Offspring Cohort) began. The neuropsychological battery was expanded and an important diagnostic tool was added, *magnetic resonance imaging* (MRI). The brain images resulting from MRI allowed a quantification of specific types of brain injuries related to CVD risk factors. These studies with the Offspring Cohort have already begun to lead to a better understanding of the mechanisms by which CVD risk factors lead to brain injury and, in turn, to lowered cognitive functioning.

Finally, in 2003 prospective longitudinal investigations of the children of the Framingham Offspring Cohort began. Among other contributions, these multigenerational studies with the offspring are expected to lead to a better understanding of the role of genetic factors in the progression from poor cognitive functioning to dementia.

Related Entries: Cardiovascular System, Cholesterol, Coronary Heart Disease

BIBLIOGRAPHY

Eaker, E. D., Pinsky, J., & Castelli, W. P. (1992). Myocardial infarction and coronary death among women: Psychosocial predictors from a 20-year follow-up of women in the Framingham Study. *American Journal of Epidemiology, 135*, 854–864.

Elias, M. F., Elias, P. K., Robbins, M. A., Wolf, P. A., & D'Agostino, R. B. (2001). Cardiovascular risk factors and cognitive functioning: An epidemiological perspective. In S. Waldstein & M. F. Elias (Eds.), *Neuropsychology of cardiovascular disease* (pp. 83–104). Hillsdale, NJ: Erlbaum.

Haynes, S. G., Feinleib, M., Levine, S., Scotch, N., & Kannel, W. B. (1978). The relationship of psychosocial factors to coronary heart disease in the Framingham Study. *American Journal of Epidemiology, 107*, 384–402.

Kase, C. S., Wolf, P. A., Kelly-Hayes, M., Kannel, W. B., Beiser, A., & D'Agostino, R. B. (1998). Intellectual decline after stroke. The Framingham Study. *Stroke, 29*, 805–812.

Markovitz, J. H., Matthews, K. A., Kannel, W. B., Cobb, J. L., & D'Agostino, R. B. (1993). Psychological predictors of hypertension in the Framingham Study: Is there tension in hypertension? *Journal of the American Medical Association, 270*, 2439–2443.

Seshadri, S., Beiser, A., Selhub, J., Jacques, P. F., Rosenberg, I. H., D'Agostino, R. B., et al. (2002). Plasma homocysteine as a risk factor for dementia and Alzheimer's disease. *New England Journal of Medicine, 346*, 476–483.

MERRILL F. ELIAS
RALPH B. D'AGOSTINO
MICHAEL A. ROBBINS
PHILIP A. WOLF

Friedman, Howard S.

Howard S. Friedman, born in New York City, received his AB in 1972 from Yale University and his PhD from Harvard in 1976. He is currently Distinguished Professor of Psychology at the University of California, Riverside.

Friedman's research spans several important conceptual and empirical areas within health psychology, including expressivity and nonverbal communication, emotion and health, and psychosocial predictors of longevity. Friedman is well known for his innovative work in opening such areas as a health psychology approach to the prevention of skin cancer, depression as a risk factor for heart disease, and the idea of a disease-prone personality, which he demonstrated through meta-analysis. Over the past quarter-century he has authored or coauthored dozens of influential health psychology articles and was named a Most Cited Author by the Institute for Scientific Information.

Known as a pioneer in shaping the emergence of the health psychology discipline, Professor Friedman has developed new courses and authored, coauthored, or edited many influential health psychology books, including *Social Psychology and Medicine* (1982), *Interpersonal Issues in Health Care* (1982), *Personality and Disease* (1990) (translated into Japanese), *The Self-Healing Personality* (1991/2000) (translated into many languages), *Hostility, Coping, and Health* (1992), and *Health Psychology*, second edition (2002). He is editor-in-chief of the *Encyclopedia of Mental Health* (1998), which emphasizes the links between mental and physical health.

Despite these achievements, Friedman is probably best known for his groundbreaking studies of psychosocial predictors of health and lifespan mortality risk. This project, an archival prospective study of predictors and mediators of health and longevity, was begun by Friedman in 1991, when he brought together a multidisciplinary research team to study the lives of 1,528 men and women first assessed by Lewis Terman in

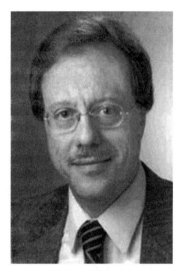

Friedman, Howard S.

1921. Early findings from this project indicated that childhood personality (especially conscientiousness) predicted longevity, whereas the psychosocial stress of parental divorce was related to increased mortality risk across the life span. The focus of this ongoing project is to uncover mechanisms underlying pathways to health and longevity. The picture of health that is emerging embodies prudence and impulse control, stable family relations, and social integration. An award-winning teacher, Friedman is also well known in the fields of social psychology and communications, and is editor of the *Journal of Nonverbal Behavior.*

BIBLIOGRAPHY

Friedman, H. S. (Ed.). (1990). *Personality and disease.* New York: Wiley.

Friedman, H. S. (Ed.). (1991). *Hostility, coping, and health.* Washington, DC: American Psychological Association.

Friedman, H. S. (Ed.). (1998). *Encyclopedia of mental health.* San Diego, CA: Academic.

Friedman, Howard S. (2000). *The self-healing personality: Why some people achieve health and others succumb to illness.* New York: iUniverse.com.

Friedman, H. S. (2002). *Health psychology* (2nd ed.). Upper Saddle River, NJ: Prentice Hall.

Friedman, H. S., & Booth-Kewley, S. (1987). The "disease prone personality": A meta-analytic view of the construct. *American Psychologist, 42,* 539–555.

Friedman, H. S., & DiMatteo, M. R. (Eds.). (1982a). *Social psychology and medicine.* Cambridge, MA: Oelgeschlager, Gunn, & Hain.

Friedman, H. S., & DiMatteo, M. R. (Eds.). (1982b). *Interpersonal issues in health care.* New York: Academic.

Friedman, H. S., Tucker, J. S., Schwartz, J. E., Tomlinson-Keasey, C., Martin, L. R., Wingard, D. L., et al. (1995). Psychosocial and behavioral predictors of longevity: The aging and death of the "Termites." *American Psychologist, 50,* 69–78.

Friedman, H. S., Tucker, J. S., Tomlinson-Keasey, C., Schwartz, J. E., Wingard, D. L., & Criqui, M. H. (1993). Does childhood personality predict longevity? *Journal of Personality and Social Psychology, 65,* 176–185.

LESLIE R. MARTIN

Friedman, Meyer (1910–2001)

Meyer Friedman received his AB from Yale University (1931) and his MD from Johns Hopkins Medical School (1935). He devoted his career to the prevention of heart attacks, first as director of the Harold Brunn Institute of Cardiovascular Research in San Francisco (1939–1984), then as the director of the Meyer Friedman Institute, established in his honor (1984–2001).

Meyer Friedman and his colleagues were the first to notice type A behavior (TAB), to investigate it, and to successfully modify it. TAB persons are always in a rush (time urgency and hurry sickness), become angry easily, and feel insecure (Type B persons do or feel none of these things). Friedman found 33 distinct signs of TAB; TAB persons may exhibit one or more of them. They may, for example, draw back one corner of the mouth or nod continuously while speaking, or blink more than 40 times a minute. Friedman videotaped his interviews with such patients, and was later able to document which signs of TAB might be present.

After an initial pilot project, published in 1959, which suggested that TAB might be a risk factor for heart attack, he conducted two large, well-designed randomized controlled trials that proved TAB was significant, and later that it could even be modified.

The first, the Western Collaborative Group Study, involved 3,154 healthy, middle-aged men, who were followed for $8\frac{1}{2}$ years. The results showed that men with TAB were twice as likely to get heart attacks as a control group, a conclusion supported by a 75-member review panel assembled by the Heart, Lung and Blood Institute.

To find out whether modifying TAB could help prevent heart attacks, researchers at the Harold Brunn Institute and Stanford, Harvard, and Yale Universities began a second trial, the Recurrent Coronary Prevention Project, involving 1,013 people who had already had a heart attack. After $4\frac{1}{2}$ years, an analysis of the results showed that those persons who had successfully modified TAB (by changing lifelong habits and belief systems) were having 44 percent fewer heart attacks than the control group. Learning of this, the National Heart, Lung and Blood Institute ordered the study stopped. The results had already proved that appropriate behavior modification could save many lives.

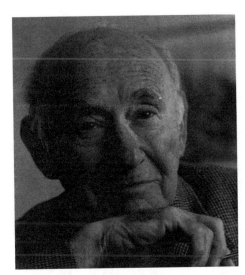

Friedman, Meyer

In 1993 Friedman received the Upjohn Award from the International Society for Behavioral Medicine.

BIBLIOGRAPHY

Friedman, M. (1996). *Type A behavior: Its diagnosis and treatment* (1996). New York: Plenum.

Friedman, M., & D. Ulmer. (1984) *Treating Type A behavior and your heart.* New York: Ballentine.

GERALD W. FRIEDLAND

Functional GI Disorders

Functional gastrointestinal disorders (FGID) include a set of 25 illnesses concentrated in one of five anatomic regions in the GI tract. They are called functional disorders because the locus of the problem is in how the gut functions, not the physical structure of the GI tract. Although benign (i.e., not medically dangerous), FGIDs are serious illnesses and account for approximately 17 million physician visits annually, making them some of the most common conditions encountered by gastroenterologists and general internists. FGIDs are associated with diminished quality of life, work absenteeism, and psychological distress. The functional GI disorder called irritable bowel syndrome (IBS) alone costs the U.S. health care system up to an estimated $30 billion annually in direct and indirect costs. Generally speaking, FGIDs strike women in larger numbers than men, usually first appear in the second and third decades of life, and decrease with age. The course of FGIDs is variable, with symptoms waxing and waning over time. Research evidence suggests that FGIDs might run in families, although it is unclear whether this finding reflects the influence of genetic, social learning, or combined factors.

The most common FGIDs include irritable bowel syndrome (IBS), functional or nonulcer dyspepsia (FD), functional constipation, and gastrointestinal reflux disease (GERD). IBS, the most common FGID, is characterized by lower abdominal pain/discomfort, bloating, and bowel dysfunction. Bowel dysfunction can alternate among diarrhea, constipation, and normal bowel function even though diagnostic testing shows no evidence of physical pathology. In patients with FD, on the other hand, pain is concentrated in the upper abdomen and is associated with abdominal fullness often after meals; bloating; and nausea. Patients with functional constipation pass small amounts of hard, dry bowel movements typically less than three times per week. There is substantial overlap among FGIDs. For example, approximately 40 percent of individuals with IBS have reflux symptoms and 45 percent have dyspepsia. Patients' symptom pattern can transition between disorders such they that have symptoms of one disorder (e.g., IBS), which in turn are replaced by symptoms of another (e.g., dyspepsia). There is a higher prevalence of FGIDs in patients whose organic GI disorders (e.g., Crohn's disease and ulcerative colitis) are in remission. Functional GI symptoms may also occur with medical disease (e.g., esophegitis, peptic ulcer) in a way that complicates medical diagnosis. In comparison to controls, FGID patients report more nongastrointestinal symptoms, including sexual dysfunction, insomnia, fibromyalgia, facial pain, chronic pelvic pain, and chronic fatigue. Diagnoses of FGIDs are based on characteristic bowel patterns, the nature, location, and quality of any accompanying symptoms (e.g., pain), and exclusion of other organic GI disease processes (e.g., infection or colon cancer) through physical examination and routine diagnostic tests.

Because of the benign nature of FGIDs, physical abnormalities cannot be detected or, if present (e.g., motility disturbance), correlate weakly or inconsistently with symptoms (e.g., pain). Because symptoms of FGIDs mimic other diseases whose symptoms correspond with physical abnormalities, patients with IBS often undergo extensive work-ups before obtaining a correct diagnosis. Although each of these diagnostic tests has utility in evaluating certain GI problems, their routine is not typically necessary to establish a diagnosis of a FGID. Because there is no "objective" marker of FGID symptoms, establishing a diagnosis, recognizing clinical features, and excluding other medical disorders that may have a similar clinical presentation can be problematic. The old view that FGID should be viewed as a "diagnoses of exclusion" has given way to an empirically validated symptom-based diagnostic system known as the "Rome" criteria.

The exact cause of FGIDs is not well established, but research suggests that they are best understood from the perspective of a biopsychosocial model. The biopsychosocial model holds that individual biology (e.g., genetic predisposition, GI physiology), behavior, and higher order cognitive processes (coping, illness beliefs, abnormal central processing of gut stimuli) influence FGIDs through their interaction with each other, with early life factors (e.g., trauma, modeling), and with the individual's social and physical environments (e.g., reinforcement contingencies).

At the heart of the model is the belief that FGIDs involve a dysregulation in interactions among the central nervous system (CNS) and the enteric nervous system (ENS). This neural network is referred to as the brain–gut axis. The neural transmission lines of the brain–gut axis are bidirectional and reciprocal, with the CNS (brain–spinal cord) receiving information from the digestive tract and modulating the ENS (gut). Normal GI function involves a high degree of coordination between the brain and the gut. In FGID patients, however, there is a persistent disruption in the interaction of the brain–gut axis, which is manifested in enhanced sensitivity of the GI tract to common stimuli such as food, stress, and stool passage; disturbances in contractions of the GI tract (i.e., motility); and, at least among more severely affected patients, psychological dysfunction.

Research based on the biopsychosocial model has pointed to three main pathways through which psychological factors influence IBS. The first key pathway is directly through physiological systems. Psychological factors (e.g., stress, negative emotional states) can normatively induce changes in gut function, but their effect is particularly pronounced in IBS patients. Psychological factors (e.g., negative mood states, expectation, attention) can also contribute to FGIDs by influencing pain perception. The second pathway is through the adoption of illness behaviors that can exacerbate IBS symptoms, prolong recovery following diagnosis, obscure symptom profile, and compromise function. Health behaviors are strongly influenced by one's psychological health. FGID patients, particularly the more severely affected, show higher levels of psychological distress and higher rates of psychiatric comorbidity than non-treatment-seeking patients and patients seen in primary care. Anxiety, mood, and somatization disorders are the most common cormorbid psychiatric disorders seen in FGID patients. A third pathway by which psychological factors (e.g., early abuse, interpersonal stressors, family reinforcement of illness behaviors) influence FGIDs is by mediating the risk for onset. This line of research has focused extensively on the high rates of abuse in treatment-seeking patients. For example, severely affected IBS patients with a positive history of abuse are more likely to have refractory symptoms and consume greater health care resources. Psychological factor (e.g., stress) may also increase the probability that a patient

who develops an organic GI disorder will subsequently develop a FGID.

Because there is no biological marker for symptoms, the goals of medical treatment are normalization of bowel function, decreased pain/discomfort, and improvement in quality of life through a combination of pharmacologic agents, behavioral self-change interventions, and lifestyle modification. The exact constellation of treatment strategies is not prescriptive, but is based on the nature (e.g., predominant bowel habit) and severity of symptoms (mild, moderate, severe) of the individual patient. There is a general belief that patients whose symptoms are more severe have more complicated clinical profiles, which require a combination of pharmacologic agents, lifestyle change, and psychological treatments. By the same token, less severely affected patients typically respond to lifestyle modification (e.g., dietary change) and limited medication, if at all. The type of pharmacologic agent is based on the most predominant symptoms. For patients whose FGID involves diarrhea, a therapeutic trial of loperamide (trade name Imodium), diphenoxylate (Lomotil), psyllium (Metamucil), methylcellulose (Citrucel), or a low-dose tricyclic antidepressant may be pursued. Patients with constipation often undergo a trial of increased dietary fiber, supplemental fiber, an osmotic laxative (e.g., milk of magnesia, lactulose), or a stool softener if symptoms are not relieved by dietary fiber alone. Patients with pain/gas/bloating symptoms may benefit from a trial of an antispasmodic agent, such as dicyclomine (Bentyl) or hyoscyamine with Phenobarbital (Levsin), or a low-dose antidepressant.

With respect to psychological treatments, most research has focused on IBS. Four different classes of psychological treatments (brief psychodynamic psychotherapy with relaxation, hypnotherapy, cognitive–behavioral therapy, and cognitive therapy) have each been shown to be superior to symptom monitoring or routine medical care in reducing IBS symptoms. Treatments featuring cognitive therapy and hypnotherapy have been replicated and have been found to be superior to attention-placebo control conditions. Hypnotherapy has arguably the best empirical support in that its therapeutic benefits have been independently replicated by two different research groups and maintained over time. Hypnosis is a procedure that in the context of FGID patients uses suggestions for relaxation, calmness, and well-being and specific instructions called hypnotic inductions to alter patients' gut sensations. The psychological treatment with the second-most-consistently positive track record is cognitive therapy. Cognitive therapy is a specific psychological treatment designed to reduce excessive emotional or physiological reactions associated with GI symptoms by modifying or eliminating negatively skewed thinking patterns (e.g., jumping to conclusions) and belief systems (perfectionism) that underlie these reactions. A related goal of cognitive therapy is to provide patients with a general set of problem–solving or coping skills to manage a wide range of situations associated with GI symptoms. Cognitive therapy techniques are often combined with behavioral interventions (e.g., structured muscle relaxation exercises, biofeedback training, social skills instruction), which are designed to alter maladaptive patterns of behaviors that influence illness experience. Data based on a series of smaller scale clinical trials with IBS patients indicate that psychological treatments are effective in reducing IBS symptoms in comparison to control conditions (waiting list control, symptom monitoring), although it is not know what type of treatments are most effective for what type of patients. Although IBS has been the target of most psychologically oriented clinical trials, there are a limited number of clinical trials showing that psychological treatment that features either psychodynamic psychotherapy or cognitive–behavioral therapy may be useful in reducing symptoms of nonulcer dyspepsia.

BIBLIOGRAPHY

Blanchard, E. B., & Scharff, L. (2002). Psychosocial aspects of assessment and treatment of irritable bowel syndrome in adults and recurrent abdominal pain in children. *Journal of Consulting and Clinical Psychology, 70*, 725–738.

Camilleri, M., & Prather, C. M. (1992). The irritable bowel syndrome: Mechanisms and a practical approach to management. *Annals of Internal Medicine, 116*, 1001–1008.

Clouse, R. (2001). Therapy of functional gastrointestinal disorders. *Journal of Functional Syndromes, 1*, 61–68.

Drossman, D. A., Richter, J. E., Talley, N. J., et al. (Eds.). (1994). *Functional gastrointestinal disorders: Diagnosis, pathophysiology and treatment [Rome II]*. McLean, VA: Degnon Associates.

Lynn, R. B., & Friedman, L. S. (1993). Irritable bowel syndrome. *New England Journal of Medicine, 329*, 1940–1945.

JEFFREY LACKNER

Gg

Gate Theory of Pain

The gate control theory of pain, published by Melzack and Wall in 1965, proposes that the transmission of nerve impulses from the body to the brain is modulated by a gating mechanism in the spinal cord. This gating mechanism is influenced by the pattern of activity in incoming sensory fibers as well as by nerve impulses that descend from the brain. When the output of the spinal cells exceeds a critical level, it activates brain areas that produce pain.

The theory's emphasis on the modulation of inputs in the spinal dorsal horns and the dynamic role of the brain in pain processes had a clinical as well as a scientific impact. Psychological factors, which were previously dismissed as "reactions to pain," were now seen to be an integral part of pain processing and new avenues for pain control by psychological therapies were opened. Similarly, neurosurgical procedures such as cutting nerves and pathways have been gradually replaced by a host of methods to modulate the sensory input. Physical therapists and other health care professionals now use a multitude of modulation techniques for the treatment of chronic and acute pain.

The gate control theory has been extended by proposing that specialized systems in the brain are selectively involved in the sensory–discriminative, motivational–affective, and cognitive–evaluative dimensions of subjective pain experience. The McGill Pain Questionnaire, which taps into subjective experience, was developed and is widely used to measure pain.

Recent studies describe severe pains in the phantom body of paraplegics with verified total sections of the spinal cord, and Melzack has proposed the concept of a "neuromatrix"—a widely distributed, parallel processing neural network in the brain—which holds that pain can be generated by brain mechanisms in the absence of sensory input from the body area that is perceived as painful.

Related Entries: McGill Pain Inventory, Nervous System, Pain, Placebo Effects

BIBLIOGRAPHY

Melzack, R. (1975). The McGill pain questionnaire: Major properties and scoring methods. *Pain, 1*, 277–299.

Melzack, R. (1987). The short-form McGill pain questionnaire. *Pain, 30*, 191–197.

Melzack, R. (1990). Phantom limbs and the concept of a neuromatrix. *Trends in Neuroscience, 13*, 88–92.

Melzack, R., & Casey, K. L. (1968). Sensory, motivational and central control determinants of pain: A new conceptual model. In D. Kenshalo (Ed.), *The skin senses* (pp. 423–443). Sprinfield, IL: Thomas.

Melzack, R., & Loeser, J. D. (1978). Phantom body pain in paraplegics: Evidence for a central "pattern generating mechanism" for pain. *Pain, 4*, 195–210.

Melzack, R., & Wall, P. D. (1965). Pain mechanisms: A new theory. *Science, 150*, 971–979.

Melzack, R., and Wall, P. D. (1996). *The challenge of pain* (Updated 2nd ed.). London: Penguin.

RONALD MELZACK

General Adaptation Syndrome

Hans Selye, one of the pioneers in the field of stress research, studied the effects of long-term, severe stress on physical health. He suggested that the body responds to stress in three sequential stages. These stages constitute the general adaptation syndrome.

118

Selye investigated the effects of a wide variety of physical stressors on laboratory animals. He observed that exposure to many kinds of severe stress resulted in the same pattern of physical symptoms in rats. Based on his experience as a physician, he concluded that this discovery was relevant to human illness.

After further study, Selye came to believe that he could describe the stages of the body's reaction to a wide variety of stressors. Selye called the process of reaction the general adaptation syndrome (GAS), which he broke down into three stages: alarm, resistance, and exhaustion.

Alarm occurs when an animal or person is first subjected to an acute stressor. The body responds by mobilizing its defenses in the fight-or-flight emergency response. At this point, the individual may successfully combat the stressor and survive, or the stressor may overpower the individual, resulting in death. If the individual survives and yet the stressor continues, the body continues to experience an extreme state of arousal. This heightened state of arousal taxes the body's resources and cannot be maintained. At this point, the body moves from the alarm stage to the resistance stage.

In the *resistance* stage, the body attempts to adapt to chronic stress. Although the organism may appear to be functioning normally, its resources are being exceptionally taxed. As a result, the organism becomes more vulnerable to what Selye called *diseases of adaptation*. Stress is not the sole cause of these diseases; they result from a combination of factors, one of which is the depletion of the body's resources due to the need to adapt to chronic stress. Diseases of adaptation include cardiovascular disease, hypertension, ulcers, asthma, and diseases that result from compromised immune function.

If severe stress continues, the body's resources may become so depleted that the stage of *exhaustion* ensues. At this point, the organism is so weak that death can occur.

Selye's theory of the GAS has had a lasting impact on the field of stress research. It marked an important milestone in the understanding of the impact of stress on physical health. Further research later established that, contrary to Selye's theory, the body does react differently to different stressful situations. Selye's work has also been criticized for focusing heavily on the physical reaction to stress and not taking into account the emotional or cognitive reaction. In human beings, stressful events in and of themselves do not determine the nature of the reaction they precipitate. Emotional responses and cognitive appraisal both play a role in determining the impact of an event on an individual. Researchers have built on Selye's initial contribution by adding a consideration of these factors to the analysis of the impact of stress on health and disease.

Related Entry: Stressful Life Events

BIBLIOGRAPHY

Sarafino, E. (2002). *Health psychology: Biopsychosocial interactions* (4th ed.). New York: Wiley.
Selye, H. (1956). *The stress of life*. New York: McGraw-Hill.
Selye, H. (1976). *Stress in health and disease*. Woburn, MA: Butterworth.

ALIZA WEINRIB

Genetics and Health

Genetics affects virtually everything about living organisms. Psychology's greatest involvement with genetics concerns genetic differences among people, and books such as Plomin et al.'s (2003) *Behavioral Genetics in the Postgenomic Era* embody that emphasis. In *A Holistic Conceptualization of Stress and Disease*, Newberry et al. (1991) detail the numerous pathways linking psychological variables to disease and note the broad role of genetics in questions relevant to health psychology.

GENETICS BACKGROUND

Table 1 explains genetics terms, which are italicized on first use in this entry. Texts such as Klug and Cummings's (2002) *Essentials of Genetics* provide more detail. *Genes* are *DNA* segments providing instructions for the production of proteins, and proteins direct virtually all aspects of organism structure and function. Protein production from a gene (*gene expression*) normally occurs only when the protein is needed. Genetic variation reflects *mutations*. Variants of individual genes are termed *alleles*, and the set of genes and alleles possessed by any organism is its *genotype*. Human genes are on 23 *chromosome* pairs, and with few exceptions we have two copies of each gene. *Recessive* alleles are not seen in the *phenotype* unless two copies are present.

Genetic influences are often subtle. The idea that there is "a" gene "for" a trait is extremely misleading. When traits are *polygenic* no single gene necessarily has a large influence. In *gene–gene interaction* (epistasis) a particular allele's impact depends on the alleles of other genes. Moreover, genes can act quite indirectly: A "genetic effect" on television watching might really be an effect on shyness or athleticism.

One must also recognize that genetics and environment are often entangled. In *gene–environment interaction*, a genetic predisposition may produce the trait only under particular environmental conditions. Genes and environment can be correlated even when they are not causally related. For example, a seeming genetic influence on food preference could reflect

Table 1. Some Genetics Terminology[a,b]

Allele: Any of several variants of a *gene*, especially variants that can influence *phenotype*.

Chromosomes: Bodies in cell nuclei that contain *DNA* combined with proteins. Humans have 23 matched pairs of chromosomes, one member of each pair coming from each parent. Therefore, except for *genes* on the sex chromosomes, humans and most other animal species ordinarily have two copies of each gene. The two copies can be different *alleles*.

DNA: Deoxyribonucleic acid. DNA is the molecule that specifies the genetic information. The order of "bases" (abbreviated A, C, G, T) on this molecule carries the genetic code.

Gene: A stretch of *DNA* that specifies a protein. Each triplet of bases identifies one amino acid to be added to the protein chain. Genes make up only a small fraction of human DNA.

Gene expression: Refers to whether a *gene* is "turned on" or not. When a gene is expressed, its *DNA* is transcribed into messenger RNA and the protein is produced. Gene expression is controlled by complex sets of specialized proteins and regulatory DNA sequences.

Gene–environment interaction: Occurs when the effect of *genotype* depends upon environmental circumstances. A genetic predisposition for alcoholism, for example, may not be realized unless the individual's environment is stressful.

Gene–gene interaction (also called epistasis): A situation in which the effect of one *allele* depends upon which alleles of other *genes* are present. For instance, the sickle cell hemoglobin allele may have much reduced effects if a mutation involving the gene for fetal hemoglobin allows fetal hemoglobin to be produced into adulthood.

Genome: The entire order of *DNA* bases in an individual or species. Sometimes restricted to signifying an individual's set of *genes* and *alleles*.

Genomics: The study of the entire *genome*, or of large numbers of *genes* simultaneously.

Genotype: An individual's set of *genes* and *alleles* (see *genome*). Term may be limited to those genes or alleles involved in the context under consideration.

Heterozygous: Having, for the *gene* under consideration, two different *alleles* rather than two copies of the same allele. (Because persons receive one copy of each *chromosome* from each parent, they ordinarily have two copies of each gene.)

Mutation: A genetic modification, usually produced by a basically random event. Mutations can be as small as a single base change or as large as duplication of an entire *chromosome*. Small mutations produce new *alleles*.

Phenotype: The observed characteristics of an individual (as opposed to *genotype*, which refers to the *genes* themselves).

Polygenic: Influenced by multiple *genes*. The larger the number of genes affecting a particular attribute, the smaller the average effect per gene must be. *Gene–gene interaction* implies polygenic influences.

Polymorphism: The existence in a population of two or more possible base sequences at a particular site in *DNA*.

Quantitative genetics (QG): An approach to genetic research that, in human investigations, relies upon calculating estimates of heritability and environmental effects from data on such things as the similarities of twins to each other and the similarities of adoptees to their biological and adoptive parents. It is the genetics approach most familiar to psychologists. QG must make more assumptions than methods that attempt to study specific *chromosome* regions and *genes* directly.

Recessive: Referring to a trait produced only when the individual receives two copies of the pertinent *allele*, one from each parent (cystic fibrosis and phenylketonuria are examples of recessive disorders). As opposed to a dominant trait, which is seen in the *phenotype* with just one copy of the pertinent allele.

---

[a] In the text, the first use of these terms is italicized. They are also italicized in this table the first time they appear in the description of other terms.

[b] Different writers use these terms in somewhat different ways, and the explanations given here are intended to be helpful, not technically definitive.

distinctions between cultures whose members just happen to differ genetically.

These intricacies vastly complicate efforts to understand human genetics. Few if any analyses have yet been able to deal adequately with all of the factors that operate in polygenic inheritance. Many claims about genetic effects, particularly if based upon simple *quantitative genetics* (QG) results, are decidedly preliminary. Still, much is known about relatively simple situations. Important initial evidence on more complex issues and new technology stemming from the Human Genome Project promise rapid progress.

GENETICS AND DISEASE

For hundreds of diseases, certain genotypes confer increased susceptibility. [Table 2 lists some genetic disorders. Massimini (2000) provides a thorough treatment in *Genetic Disorders Sourcebook*.] Genetic contributions may be of many types. Sometimes, as in cystic fibrosis and sickle cell disease, sin-gle abnormal alleles more or less directly produce the condition. Other disorders (e.g., Type 2 diabetes and some heart diseases) are polygenic and/or involve indirect genetic influences. One potential indirect genetic influence involves stress reactivity. Some rat strains with genetically low stress hormone levels cannot combat inflammatory diseases such as arthritis. (Those strains may also differ in the sickness response that accompanies immune activation.) The molecular genetic abnormalities causing cancer (e.g., abnormal cell division signals) can represent mutations resulting from exposure to environmental carcinogens. Such genetic influences are acquired, not inherited.

Reactions to medications are another way in which geneotype influences disease. Both therapeutic benefits and side effects can be affected. Increased toxicity occurs with genetic deficiencies in the enzymes that metabolize the anticancer drug mercaptopurine, for example. The anticlotting drug warfarin can cause bleeding when its primary "detoxifying" enzyme is produced at a low level. As an example from the benefit side, positive response to lipid-lowering medications called "statins" has been associated with polymorphisms predicting

Table 2. Examples of Genetic Diseases[a]

Disease Resulting from Mutation of One Gene	Complex Diseases that May Have Genetic Components
Amyotrophic lateral sclerosis (Lou Gehrig's disease) (D)*	Alzheimer's disease*
Congenital deafness*	Asthma*
Cystic fibrosis (R)	Atherosclerosis*
Duchenne muscular dystrophy (R)	Cancers (breast and ovary, Burkitt lymphoma, chronic myeloid leukemia, colon,
Familial hypercholesterolemia (D)	lung, malignant melanoma, pancreatic, prostate)*
Gaucher disease (a fat-metabolizing enzyme deficiency) (R)	Crohn's disease (an inflammatory bowel disease)*
Hemophilia A (R)	Diabetes mellitus Type 1 (formerly called "juvenile onset")*
Huntington disease (D) (lethal degenerative nerve disease)	Diabetes mellitus Type 2 (formerly called "adult onset")*
Marfan syndrome (D) (connective tissue disorder; long extremeties)	Epilepsy*
Neurofibromatosis (D) (disfiguring nervous system tumors)	Obesity*
Osteogenesis imperfecta (D)	
Phenylketonuria (R)	
Polycystic kidney disease (D)	
Severe combined immunodeficiency ("bubble boy" disease)	
Sickle cell anemia (R)	
Tay–Sachs disease (fatal neurologic disease of early childhood)	

(D), Dominant gene; (R), recessive gene; an asterisk indicates a condition that may also occur as a noninherited disease and/or to which environmental contributions are thought to be important.

atherosclerosis risk. Such effects are complex, but pharmacogenomics should eventually allow tailoring drug therapy to individual patients, providing improved treatment and, of particular significance to health psychology, improved patient compliance.

Even when diseases have clear genetic bases, environmental influences and psychological factors can modify outcomes. A genetic predisposition to Type 2 diabetes, for instance, need not produce disease in persons whose circumstances require high activity levels and preclude overeating; genotype and environment interact. The present epidemic of obesity and the increased Type 2 diabetes among American youth are not surprising.

GENETICS AND HEALTH-RELEVANT PSYCHOLOGICAL/BEHAVIORAL VARIABLES

As Plomin and colleagues stress, and QG studies support, it is reasonable to suspect that many major psychological individual differences (in skills/abilities and personality/temperament) are genetic to some degree. However, all of the complexities regarding genetic effects apply. Attempts to identify specific genes have been disappointing, though there are good leads. Genes coding for proteins that regulate the actions of the neurotransmitters serotonin and dopamine have been associated with anxiety, depression, and change seeking, though the results are not consistent. There are some data suggesting that gene–gene interactions may contribute to the inconsistencies.

Like all behavior, health behavior (e.g., diet choices, exercise, health care utilization) is probably genetically influenced, perhaps via personality and abilities. Thus behavior can be an indirect means by which genotype leads to disease. To the ex-

tent that culture/subculture is affected by—not merely associated with genetics, genetic effects on health behavior could be produced through social influences.

The health belief model, described in texts such as Taylor's (1999) *Health Psychology*, provides a useful perspective. In this view, practicing a particular health behavior depends on perceived personal health threat (risk and severity) and judgment that a health behavior will be effective. Those who believe that they are at risk, that a particular health behavior will work, and that they can change their behavior are most likely to engage in that health behavior. Because people tend, often incorrectly, to equate "genetic" with "unmodifiable," they are particularly likely to see genetic risks as insurmountable.

GENETIC TESTING

Genetic testing is an increasingly important means of assessing health risks. DNA tests exist for many disorders, and more are becoming available. When a disorder has a simple monogenetic basis, the tests are quite predictive. When multiple genes and/or environmental effects are involved, or when the critical gene is recessive, they are necessarily less predictive and may not offer the hoped-for reduction in uncertainty. Tests for *BRCA1/BRCA2* are currently receiving much attention. Alleles of these genes rather strongly predict early-onset breast and ovarian cancer.

Psychological considerations in testing for disease risk include decisions to get testing and reactions to test results. These issues may be understood, in part, via health beliefs. The thought that one has a family history of a particular disease should increase perceived health threat and therefore the motivation for such health behaviors as seeking testing. A study by Shaw and Bassi (2001) generally supports the health belief model. However, knowledge can be distressing, and some persons may cope with the stress of possible genetic disease by avoiding information about their risk. This disengagement strategy is associated with genetically influenced personality variables and, consistent with the health belief model, with the absence of effective interventions.

Reactions to positive tests reflect some of the same factors as decisions to undergo testing. Positive results, especially for serious, genetically simple conditions must almost automatically be stressful. From the health belief perspective, once risk is established, coping becomes the issue. Whether an individual takes action or slips into fatalistic thinking should depend upon the person's perception that their behavior could alter the threat, by belief that they can perform the necessary behaviors, and by individual psychological differences.

Another issue regarding genetic testing is the possibility that risk information will be accessed by employers or insurers, resulting in discrimination. That possibility further increases the worry some feel about testing, as Shaw and Bassi (2001) note, and creates a sense in the medical community that the risks of testing need to be considered carefully.

GENETIC COUNSELING

Genetic counseling helps people understand genetic conditions. Counselors serve parents who might pass traits on to children and persons concerned about their own status. Much of the counseling involves explanation of the genetic "odds," but counselors also deal with patient distress (including helplessness that may stem from seeing genetic risk as uncontrollable), refer them to support services, and serve as patient advocates. Weil's (2000) *Psychosocial Genetic Counseling* provides a general introduction to psychological issues in the field.

Genetic counselors have specialized graduate degrees and have studied both medical genetics and counseling practice. They come to the field from many undergraduate backgrounds, including psychology.

CONCLUSIONS

Genetic effects are complex as well as extensive. For health psychology, one consequence of genetic effects is their implication for research results. The relationships of stress, coping, personality, and health behavior to each other and to disease will be affected by genetics. For clinical health psychology practice, the issues also include the relevance of particular assessments and interventions for particular patients. It is easy, for instance, to imagine collaborations between clinical health psy-

chologists and genetic counselors. Furthermore, health psychology can make significant contributions to the study of human genetics/*genomics* by identifying important variables for investigation and by contributing to the interpretation of research findings.

Related Entries: Alcoholism, Biomedical Model, Cancer, Hypertension, Smoking Cessation, Smoking Prevention

BIBLIOGRAPHY

Gould, S. J. (1981). *The mismeasure of man.* New York: Norton.
Hamer, D. (2002). Rethinking behavior genetics. *Science, 298,* 71–72.
Harper, P. S. (1998). *Practical genetic counselling.* Oxford: Oxford University Press.
Klug, W. S., & Cummings, M. R. (2002) *Essentials of genetics.* Upper Saddle River, NJ: Prentice Hall.
Massimini, K. (2000). *Genetic disorders sourcebook.* Detroit, MI: Omnigraphics.
National Center for Biotechnology Information. *Genes and disease.* Available from www.ncbi.nlm.nih.gov
National Society of Genetic Counselors. Available from *www.nscg.org*
Newberry, B. H., Jaikins-Madden, J. E., & Gerstenberger, T. J. (1991). *A holistic conceptualization of stress and disease.* New York: AMS.
Plomin, R., & Crabbe, J. (2000). DNA. *Psychological Bulletin, 126,* 806–828.
Plomin, R., DeFries, J. C., Craig, I. W., & McGuffin, P. (Eds.) (2003). *Behavioral genetics in the postgenomic era.* Washington, DC: American Psychological Association.
Shaw, J. S. III, & Bassi, K. L. (2001). Lay attitudes toward genetic testing for susceptibility to genetic diseases. *Journal of Health Psychology, 6,* 405–423.
Taylor, S. E. (1999). *Health psychology.* Boston: McGraw-Hill.
Weil, J. (2000). *Psychosocial genetic counseling.* New York: Oxford University Press.

BENJAMIN H. NEWBERRY
JULIE K. CREMEANS-SMITH
DAVID B. FRUEHSTORFER
DEBORAH L. NEWBERRY

Kiecolt-Glaser, Janice, and Glaser, Ronald

Janice Kiecolt-Glaser, PhD, professor of psychiatry, and Ronald Glaser, PhD, professor of molecular virology, immunology, and medical genetics, both in the Ohio State University College of Medicine and the Ohio State Institute for Behavioral Medicine Research, initiated their collaborative research program in psychoneuroimmunology (PNI) in 1982; at that time the scant literature on humans addressed immunological changes in response to extreme and novel events. They began by looking at very ordinary events like examinations; for example,

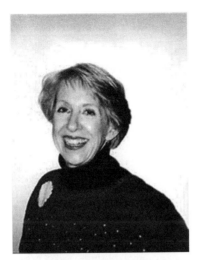

Kiecolt-Glaser, Janice

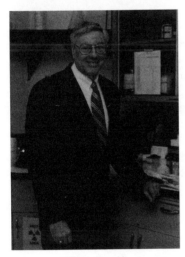

Glaser, Ronald

medical students showed adverse immunological changes during academic examinations compared to lower stress periods when they were not scheduled to take tests. Subsequently these researchers have shown that psychological stress can have significant consequences for health—it can impair one's ability to fight off an infections; to respond to vaccines including hepatitis B, influenza, and pneumococcal pneumonia; and to heal wounds. Much of this work has been focused within a context of aging; older adults are a particularly important group in this regard because immune function declines with age, and these age-related decrements are thought to be associated with the greatly increased morbidity and mortality from infectious illness in the elderly. Furthermore, older adults show greater immunological impairments related to depression or stress than younger adults. Thus, their studies with older adults have provided particularly important population-related data for PNI research.

In addition, their programmatic work has focused on the ways in which close personal relationships influence immune and endocrine function and health. For example, lonelier medical students had poorer immune function than students who were not as lonely. Medical students who reported greater social support mounted a stronger immune response to hepatitis B vaccine than those with less support. Spousal caregivers of dementia sufferers who reported lower levels of social support on entry into their longitudinal study and who were most distressed by dementia-related behaviors showed the greatest and most uniformly negative changes in immune function 1 year later. Men and women who had recently undergone a marital separation or divorce had poorer immune function than demographically matched married individuals. Laboratory studies on the physiological consequences of marital discord demonstrated pervasive differences in autonomic, endocrine, and immune function reliably associated with hostile behaviors during marital conflict. These studies have provided a window on the pathways through which close personal relationships affect physiological functioning and health, key mechanistic data that complement epidemiologic studies of social relationships.

In 2001 Kiecolt-Glaser was elected to the Institute of Medicine of the National Academy of Sciences. This honor, among the very highest for a scientist, was a recognition of the impact of their interdisciplinary collaborative work.

Related Entries:

BIBLIOGRAPHY

Glaser, R., & Kiecolt-Glaser, J. K. (Eds.). *Handbook of human stress and immunity.* San Diego, CA: Academic.

Kiecolt-Glaser, J. K., McGuire, L., Robles, T., & Glaser, R. (2002). Psychoneuroimmunology: Psychological influences on immune function and health. *Journal of Consulting and Clinical Psychology, 70,* 537–547.

JANICE KIECOLT-GLASER
RONALD GLASER

Glass, David C. (1930–)

David C. Glass was born on September 17, 1930. He did his PhD and postdoctoral training at New York University. He is professor emeritus of psychology at the University at Stony Brook (New York), where he was also vice provost for research and dean of the Graduate School.

The essential characteristic underlying Dr. Glass's contributions to health psychology is a systematic effort to integrate

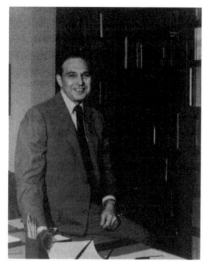

Glass, David C.

biological and social bases of behavior. An important outcome of this effort is a set of testable theoretical hypotheses aimed at identifying mechanisms linking behavior and physical disease. Experimental social psychology methods typify his work, beginning with studies on noise stress and its effects on behavioral and physiological processes.

One of the key variables in this research is a perception of lack of control over the stressor. If an individual believes he or she can neither escape nor avoid aversive noise, stressful post-noise effects (e.g., lowered frustration tolerance) are more severe than if the perception is one of control. Dr. Glass pursued potential mechanisms whereby perceived control ameliorates the stress response. One experiment led into an entirely new area, later subsumed under the field of health psychology.

An individual-difference variable, the Type A coronary-prone behavior pattern, was included in the study for possible associations with perceived uncontrollability. The behavior pattern includes excessive achievement striving, time urgency, and competitive hostility. The results revealed a significant interaction between Type A and uncontrollability. Subsequent research indicated that Type A individuals, in contrast to less driven Type Bs, exhibit enhanced efforts to master uncontrollable stressful events (hyperresponsiveness). However, such efforts decline after prolonged stress exposure (hyporesponsiveness). These data formed the basis of a biobehavioral model that led to work on how Type A behavior potentiates physiological processes (e.g., catecholamine release) that may be associated with cardiovascular pathology.

The hyporesponsiveness part of the model is akin to the notions of helplessness and depression. Clinical depression has been linked to the onset of new coronary events in several studies. Accordingly, Dr. Glass speculated about associations between hyporesponsiveness, depression, and myocardial infarction. This led to studies exploring linkages between uncontrollability and depression. Some support was obtained for the idea that perceived lack of job control and resultant frustration of achievement striving may generate feelings of failure, and eventually professional burnout and depressive symptomatology.

Dr. Glass's research has won him several honors, including the Socio-Psychological Prize of the American Association for the Advancement of Science in 1971, and the Outstanding Contribution to Health Psychology Award (American Psychological Association) in 1988. He is past president of the Academy of Behavioral Medicine Research.

Related Entries:

BIBLIOGRAPHY

Glass, D. C. (1977). *Behavior patterns, stress and coronary disease.* Hillsdale, NJ: Erlbaum.

Glass, D. C., and Contrada, R. J. (1984). "Type A behavior and catecholamines: A critical review." In M. G. Ziegler and C. R. Lake (Eds.), *Frontiers in clinical neuroscience: Norepinephrine* (pp. 00–00). Baltimore: Williams and Wilkins.

Glass, D. C., and McKnight, J. D. (1996). Perceived control, depressive symptomatology and professional burnout: A review of the evidence. *Psychology and Health, 11,* 23–48.

Glass, D. C., and Singer, J. E. (1972). *Urban stress: Experiments on noise and social stressors.* New York: Academic.

DAVID GLASS

Hh

Hardiness

Early in psychologists' study of the relationship between stress and health, a question arose about people who experience high levels of stress in their lives but do not suffer negative health consequences: What is it that enables some people not to get sick and even thrive under stress? Suzanne C. Kobasa (now Ouellette) proposed that peoples' personalities make a critical difference for how they perceive and respond to stressful life events. Concerned that stress researchers painted a too-passive picture of people as victims of stress, she sought to understand individuals' distinctive experiences and attempts to find meaning in the face of stress. She drew from existential philosophy and psychology and adult development research to propose the personality construct of hardiness as a buffer of the health-damaging effects of stressful life events. Kobasa characterized hardiness as having three components: commitment, control, and challenge. Commitment represents engagement in life and a view of experiences as meaningful, purposeful, and interesting; control is an individual's effort to maintain some influence over what life brings; challenge is an orientation toward change as an inevitable and even rewarding part of life that is matched by an ability to be cognitively flexible and tolerant of ambiguity.

In several studies with male telephone company executives contending with the formidable work stress of the divestiture of American Telephone and Telegraph (AT&T) alongside general life stressors, Kobasa and colleagues observed that the executives who reported high levels of hardiness under high stress were significantly less likely to report negative changes in health than executives characterized by low hardiness. In the more than 20 years of research that followed, there has been continuing support for the general connection between hardiness and better health. In addition, other related aspects of personality such as sense of coherence, optimism, explanatory style, and control and self-efficacy have been found to protect and enhance well-being.

Researchers from a variety of disciplines including psychology, nursing, education, and social work have identified the effectiveness of hardiness to enhance both physical and mental health and minimize outcomes like burnout in a number of groups faced with distinctive stresses. The groups have included immigrants, patients with serious illness, caregivers, elementary school teachers, nurses, disaster workers, and army recruits. How does hardiness work? Research as summarized in several reports, including that by Maddi (1999), one of the original investigators, shows that hardiness influences how people perceive and what they do about stressful life events. People who report hardiness are less likely to appraise life events as threatening, see themselves as capable of responding effectively, and are more likely to engage in particular kinds of coping such as the direct problem-solving coping and mobilization of social support observed by Florian and colleagues (1995).

Issues to be developed include the measurement of hardiness. Research has relied almost exclusively on paper-and-pencil questionnaire measures and both psychometric and conceptual critiques by Funk (1992), Ouellette (1998), and others have pointed out their limitations. Also, researchers have identified some physiological and biological mechanisms associated with hardiness, but results are inconsistent. Finally, cultural questions about how hardiness develops and has its effect in particular social and ideological settings have only begun to be raised.

Related Entries: Coping, Optimism and Health, Stressful Life Events

BIBLIOGRAPHY

Florian, V., Mikulincer, M., & Taubman, O. (1995). Does hardiness contribute to mental health during a stressful real-life situation? The roles of appraisal and coping. *Journal of Personality and Social Psychology, 68*, 687–695.

Funk, S. C. (1992). Hardiness: A review of theory and research. *Health Psychology, 11*, 335–345.

Kobasa, S. C. (1979). Stressful life events, personality, and health: An inquiry into hardiness. *Journal of Personality and Social Psychology, 37*, 1–11.

Kobasa, S. C. (1982). The hardy personality: Toward a social psychology of stress and health. In G. Sanders & J. Suls (Eds.); *Social psychology of health and illness* (pp. 00–00). Hillsdale, NJ: Erlbaum.

Kobasa, S. C., Maddi, S. R., & Kahn, S. (1982). Hardiness and health: A prospective study. *Journal of Personality and Social Psychology, 42*, 168–177.

Maddi, S. R. (1999). The personality construct of hardiness: I. Effects on experiencing, coping, and strain. *Consulting Psychology Journal, 51*, 95–105.

Ouellette, S. C. (1998). The relationship between personality and health: What self and identity have to do with it. In R. Contrada & R. Ashmore (Eds.), *Self, social identity, and physical health* (pp. 00–00). Oxford: Oxford University Press.

Ouellette, S. C. & DiPlacido, J. (2001). Personality's role in the protection and enhancement of health: Where the research has been, where it is stuck, how it might move. In A. Baum, T. A. Revenson, & J. Singer (Eds.), *Handbook of health psychology* (pp. 00–00). Mahwah, NJ: Erlbaum.

SUZANNE C. OUELLETTE

Health Belief Model

INTRODUCTION

The health belief model (HBM) emerged from the work of U.S. public health researchers Godfrey Hochbaum, Stephen Kegels, Howard Leventhal, and Irwin Rosenstock, who were attempting to develop models to explain why individuals fail to engage in preventive health measures. Early studies by Hochbaum concerned why people seek diagnostic x-rays for tuberculosis. In 1956 Hochbaum published a paper on this topic, which contained references to factors that would later become part of the HBM, such as perceived personal susceptibility and perceived benefits of engaging in the preventative behavior. The first clear formulation of the HBM appeared in a paper by Rosenstock in 1966, and was later refined by Marshall Becker in 1974. Today, the HBM is one of the most widely used social cognition models in health psychology. This entry describes the model, defines the various components within the model, and summarizes how the HBM has been used to predict and explain health behaviors. Finally, ways in which the HBM has been used to help design health interventions are discussed.

COMPONENTS OF THE MODEL

The model contains two main components, (1) perceptions of the threat of illness and (2) evaluations of the effectiveness of behaviors aimed at counteracting the threat of illness (see Figure 1). Threat perceptions result from beliefs about the perceived susceptibility to the illness and the perceived severity of the consequences of the illness. Perceived susceptibility refers to an individual's assessment of his or her personal risk of contracting a condition. Perceived severity is concerned not just with medical consequences, but also with the potential effects of an illness on an individual's job, family life, and social relations. Whether an individual engages in a health-related behavior is determined by the combined effect of these two variables. An individual will decide on the particular action to be taken by evaluating the possible alternatives. Health behaviors will be evaluated in terms of their perceived benefits or efficacy and also by their perceived costs or barriers. Examples of perceived benefits are the reduction of susceptibility to an illness or the reduced severity of an illness. Examples of perceived barriers are the health behavior being painful, inconvenient, unpleasant, or expensive. Therefore, according to the HBM, individuals are likely to follow a particular health action if they believe that they are susceptible to a particular condition or illness that they consider to be serious, and believe the benefits of the action taken to counteract the condition or illness outweigh the costs.

Although Hochbaum discussed cues to action in some of his early publications, they were not added to the HBM until later. Health motivation was also not an original part of the model, but in 1974 Becker published an influential paper suggesting that it should be added to the model. According to Janz and Becker (1984), cues to action include a diverse range of triggers to the individual taking action and are commonly divided into factors that are internal (e.g., physical symptom) or external (e.g., mass media campaign, advice from others such as physicians) to the individual. Becker defined health motivation as readiness to be concerned about health matters and argued for its inclusion in the model as certain individuals may be predisposed to respond to cues to action because of the value they place on their health.

Other influences on the performance of health behaviors include demographic factors such as age, gender, ethnicity, socioeconomic status, and education. Psychological characteristics such as personality, peer pressure, and perceived control over behavior are also thought to play a role. Both these groups of factors are assumed to exert their influence indirectly by influencing the other six components of the HBM. Evidence, however, to support this contention is mixed. For example, a study by Orbell et al. (1996) found that HBM components did mediate the effects of social class on uptake of cervical screening, but did not mediate the effects of marital status or sexual experience.

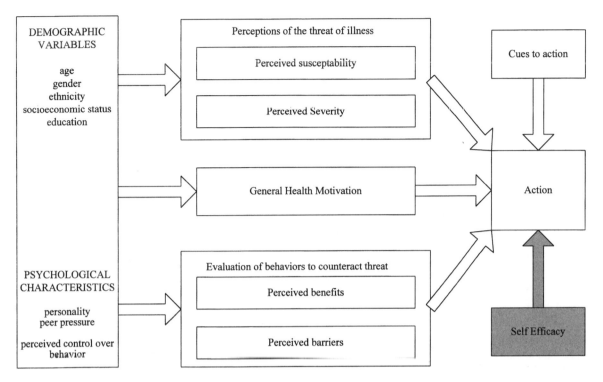

Figure 1.   The health belief model [the model with self-efficacy represents the modified HBM suggested by Rosenstock et al. (1998)].

APPLICATIONS OF THE HBM

The HBM has been applied to a wide range of populations and health behaviors. Sheeran and Abraham (1996) distinguished three broad areas of research: (1) preventative health behaviors, (2) sick role behaviors, and (3) clinic use. They noted that the preventative health behaviors to which the HBM have been applied include smoking, alcohol use, diet, exercise, genetic screening, health screening, vaccination, breast self-examination, contraceptive use, and dental behaviors. Sick role behaviors include compliance with professionally recommended medical regimens in response to illness. Sheeran and Abraham described how the HBM has been used to study adherence to a wide range of regimens such as those concerned with hypertension, diabetes, and renal disease. Examples of how the HBM has been applied to clinic use include physician visits for preventative, psychiatric, and parent and child conditions. According to Sheeran and Abraham, there is no strong evidence that the HBM has been more predictive of behavior in any one of these areas compared to any other.

The HBM has also been used to inform health interventions. For example Willamson and Wardle (2002) employed the HBM when designing an intervention aimed at increasing participation with colorectal cancer screening. The study placed particular emphasis on seven barriers that have been identified with respect to colorectal cancer screening. The barriers were presented in a series of cartoons that also offered solutions to the barriers and provided professional advice. Other such interventions include that by Gilliam et al. (2001), who drew upon the HBM when designing a HIV prevention program for adolescents. Such interventions have reported reasonable levels of success in changing behavior, demonstrating the practical utility of the model.

EFFECTIVENESS OF THE MODEL

In 1984 Janz and Becker carried out a review of research that had employed the HBM. They reviewed 46 studies and found that in 89 percent of them, the barriers component had a significant relationship with health behavior, susceptibility was significant in 81 percent of the studies, benefits in 78 percent, and severity in 65 percent. A later study by Harrison et al. (1992) went a step further and examined the strength of the relationships between the constructs. These researchers identified 234 studies that had employed the HBM, although only 16 of these were found to measure each of the components adequately. In line with Janz and Becker, Harrison and his colleagues found that the barriers component had the highest average correlation with health behavior ($r = -0.21$), followed by the susceptibility ($r = 0.15$), benefits ($r = 0.13$), and severity ($r = 0.08$) components. Although the predictive power of individual components is relatively modest (each only accounts for between 0.5 and 4 percent of variance in behavior), it is the combined effects of the six health beliefs that is generally of interest.

CRITICISMS OF THE MODEL

Despite the popularity of the HBM, it suffers from a number of weaknesses compared to other similar social cognition models. The manner in which the variables within the model combine to produce behavior has not been precisely specified and this has resulted in the HBM being frequently tested as six independent predictors of behavior. There are also frequent variations in the manner in which the six constructs are employed. Important social cognitive variables found to be highly predictive of behavior in other models are not incorporated in the HBM. For example, social pressure and intentions to perform a behavior are key components of the theory of reasoned action and theory of planned behavior but do not appear in the HBM. Self-efficacy (i.e., an individual's belief that he or she is capable of performing a specific behavior to attain a desired outcome) is also a powerful predictor of behavior in models based on social cognitive theory but were not originally included in the HBM. Rosenstock et al. (1988) have, however, since published a paper that incorporates self-efficacy into the model.

The HBM does not specify a causal ordering among the variables, as is done in other models. Such information might allow for more powerful analysis of data and clearer indications of how interventions may have their effects. It is possible that threat is better viewed as a more distal predictor of behavior. The model also does not distinguish between a motivational stage dominated by cognitive variables and a volitional phase where action is planned, performed, or maintained. Such distinctions are thought to be important in understanding various health behaviors. There is clearly much scope for the model to be refined and improved upon.

In summary, the HBM has been very widely used and provides a useful framework for examining health behaviors and identifying key health beliefs. It has met with moderate success in predicting a range of health behaviors. One appealing characteristic of the HBM is that it was developed by public health researchers working directly with health behaviors. This has resulted in the model containing constructs that possess face validity to those working in the health promotion and disease prevention areas. The model's popularity may in part be due the commonsense operationalization of a number of relevant cognitive variables.

Related Entries: Self-Efficacy, Theory of Reasoned Action and Planned Behavior, Transtheoretical Model

BIBLIOGRAPHY

Becker, M. H. (1974). The health belief model and personal health behavior. *Health Education Monographs, 2*(4).

Gilliam, G. A., Eke, A., Aymer, F., & O'Neil, C. (2001). Developing a theory-based, culturally sensitive intervention for adolescents: The Antigua School Project. In B. A. Dicks (Ed.), *HIV/AIDS and children in the English speaking Caribbean* (pp. 105–126). New York: Haworth.

Harrison, J. A., Mullen, P. D., & Green, L. W. (1992). A meta-analysis of studies of the health belief model with adults. *Health Education Research, 7*, 107–116.

Hochbaum, G. M. (1956). Why people seek diagnostic x-rays. *Public Health Reports, 71*, 377–380.

Hochbaum, G. M. (1958). *Public participation in medical screening programs: A sociopsychological study* (Public Health Service Publication No. 572). Washington, DC: U.S. Government Printing Office.

Janz, N. K., & Becker, M. H. (1984). The health belief model: A decade later. *Health Education Quarterly, 11*, 1–47.

Orbell, S., Crombie, I., & Johnston, G. (1996). Social cognition and social structure in the prediction of cervical screening uptake. *British Journal of Health Psychology, 1*, 35–50.

Rosenstock, I. M. (1966). Why people use health services. *Millbank Memorial Fund Quarterly, 44*, 99–124.

Rosenstock, I. M. (1974). The health belief model and preventative health behavior, *Health Education Monographs, 2*, 354–386.

Rosenstock, I. M., Strecher, V. J., & Becker, M. H. (1988). Social learning theory and the health belief model. *Health Education Quarterly, 15*, 175–183.

Sheeran, P. & Abraham, C. (1996). The health belief model. In M. Conner & P. Norman (Eds.), *Predicting health behavior: Research and practice with social cognition models* (pp. 23–61). Buckingham, UK: Open University Press.

Williamson, S. & Wardle, J. (2002). Increasing participation with colorectal cancer screening: The development of a psycho-educational intervention. In D. Rutter & L. Quine (Eds.), *Changing health behavior: Intervention and research with social cognition models* (pp. 105–122). Buckingham, UK: Open University Press.

MARK CONNER
BRIAN McMILLAN

Health Promotion

At the beginning of the 20th century acute diseases, including tuberculosis, pneumonia, and other infectious diseases, were the primary causes of death in the United States. By the end of the 20th century this pattern had undergone a major shift. According to Centers for Disease Control and Prevention (CDC) statistics, chronic and preventable diseases, including heart disease, cancer, stroke, and diabetes, account for 7 of every 10 deaths in the United States. Although multiple factors contribute to these chronic diseases, a survey of the actual causes of these deaths by McGinnis and Foege (1993) identified tobacco, diet and activity patterns, alcohol, microbial agents, toxic agents, firearms, sexual behavior, motor vehicles, and illicit use of drugs as the top 10 contributors. These contributors not only cause death (mortality) but cause illness (morbidity) and compromise positive functioning and well-being. The majority of these contributors involve behavioral choices, and behavior is central to the maintenance of health and prevention of disease.

Health promotion was defined by Green and Kreuter (1991) as "any combination of health education and related organizational, economic, and environmental supports for behavior of individuals, groups or communities conducive to health" and by O'Donnell (1989) as "the science and art of helping people change their lifestyle to move toward a state of optimal health." The practice of health-promoting and preventative behaviors and the avoidance of health-compromising behaviors are at the core of health promotion.

A key component of health promotion is an understanding of health. At its founding in 1948, the World Health Organization (WHO) offered a landmark definition of health as "a complete state of physical, mental, and social well-being and not merely the absence of disease or infirmity." This definition moved the focus beyond a negative definition of health as the absence of disease to include positive well-being, and included not only physical health, but also mental and social aspects of health.

Health promotion interventions focus on a wide variety of health behaviors, including smoking prevention and cessation, diet and nutrition, physical activity, weight control, sexual behavior, accidental injury prevention (e.g., seat belt use, bicycle helmet use, firearm safety), alcohol and drug use, stress management, social support, disease screening (e.g., cancer, blood pressure, and human immunodeficiency virus [HIV] screening), vaccinations, dental hygiene, and preventive skin care (e.g., sunscreen use). The majority of these specific health behaviors affect multiple health disease outcomes and pathways (e.g., heart disease, cancer, diabetes, metabolic syndrome, hypertension, hyperlipidemia), both directly and indirectly. For example, physical inactivity directly increases the risks for heart disease, cancer, and stroke, and also indirectly impacts these diseases through its associations with risk factors such as obesity and hypertension.

Many of these deleterious health behaviors occur in significant segments of the American population. Health promotion interventions often target these behaviors at an individual level. Yet because individual health behaviors are influenced by social and environmental factors, health promotion interventions also focus on higher-level efforts to impact health behaviors through environmental changes, systemic interventions, and public policy. On a national level, the U.S. Public Health Service and the Department of Health and Human Services have developed initiatives to define measurable health goals, including Healthy People 2000 and Healthy People 2010. Health promotion interventions are guided by these goals, such as the Healthy People 2010 objectives to increase the quality and years of healthy life and eliminate health disparities, with a focus on 28 specific areas, including cancer, nutrition and overweight, and tobacco use. These goals also provide a measure of the success of healthy promotion interventions. The final report on Healthy People 2000 showed mixed results in meeting similar health objectives, with success in some areas (e.g., reducing cancer deaths) but significant challenges remaining in others (e.g., tobacco use).

MODELS OF HEALTH BEHAVIOR AND HEALTH BEHAVIOR CHANGE

Models and theories of health behavior guide scientific understanding of these behaviors and provide direction for how to effect behavior change. Although a comprehensive discussion of all models and theories of health behavior and health behavior change is beyond the scope of this entry and several are discussed in other entries in this encyclopedia, a few key models and theories are highlighted here.

The WHO definition of health is consistent with a biopsychosocial model of health, which defines health or illness as a consequence of biological, psychological, and social processes, rather than a biomedical model of illness, which explains illness in terms of somatic, biochemical, and neurophysiological processes. This biopsychosocial model underpins health promotion efforts that focus not only on biological mechanisms, but also on psychological, social, and environmental factors that influence health behavior.

Traditional learning theories, including classical conditioning described by Ivan Pavlov in the 1920s and operant conditioning described by B. F. Skinner in the 1930s, help explain a variety of behaviors, including health behaviors, and form the early basis on which health promotion has subsequently developed. These theories emphasize the unidirectional impact of the environment on behavior and learning, and do not include cognitive factors. Subsequent theories have emphasized the importance of individual cognitive and social factors. Social cognitive theory, a version of social learning theory developed by Albert Bandura in the 1980s, has been one of the most influential theories guiding research. Social cognitive theory emphasizes the reciprocal relationship among behavior, environment, and personal factors (including cognitive processes related to self-efficacy and outcome expectations, i.e., beliefs that one can successfully undertake a behavior change and that doing so will result in valued outcomes or benefits).

Other models include the health belief model developed by Irwin Rosenstock and colleagues in the 1950s. This model defines four beliefs that influence the likelihood of engaging in a health behavior: (1) the perceived susceptibility to a disease, (2) the perceived severity of the disease, (3) the perceived benefits to action, and (4) the perceived barriers to action. The transtheoretical model developed by James Prochaska and Carlo DiClemente in the 1970s and 1980s describes the stages and processes of change that people may move through when changing a health behavior. The five stages are precontemplation (not intending to change behavior), contemplation (thinking about changing behavior), preparation (beginning to make behavior changes), action (actively changing a behavior), and maintenance (maintaining a successful behavior change). These models and theories—and others, including the relapse prevention model, the self-determination theory, and the updated theory of reasoned action and planned behavior—focus on intrapersonal, behavioral, and microenvironmental processes.

In addition, health promotion draws upon meso- and macroenvironmental and community approaches. For example, social ecology models focus on the macroenvironment, specifically on transactional interactions between people and their physical, social, institutional, and cultural environments. Applying these macroenvironmental models to health promotion emphasizes environmental factors that contribute to health behaviors and provides an opportunity to intervene at these macro levels (i.e., through urban planning and neighborhood design).

TARGET POPULATIONS AND SETTINGS

The prevalence of specific diseases and the practice of health behaviors often vary according to sociodemographic characteristics (e.g., age, education, income level, ethnicity). For example, according to the CDC, low-income adults are more likely to be overweight and older adults are more likely to be injured by accidental falls than those in other age groups. As a result health promotion interventions often target specific populations, making use of tailored approaches to effectively meet their needs.

Where do health promotion interventions take place? This question is intricately tied to the issue of the target population. To reach a wide variety of audiences from the general healthy population to specific high-risk populations, health promotion interventions typically occur in a variety of settings, including health care settings, schools, work sites, communities, state and local legislatures, and the consumer marketplace. Depending on the intervention setting, different behavior change theories, models, and intervention strategies drive successful health promotion interventions. For example, a work site intervention may rely on a social ecology model, a community approach may use mass media campaigns, and an individual counseling

approach in a health care setting may use specific behavior modification techniques such as behavioral self-monitoring or individualized goal setting.

CONTRIBUTIONS OF HEALTH PROMOTION INTERVENTIONS AND EVIDENCE FOR EFFECTIVENESS

Health promotion interventions have focused on a range of risk and protective behaviors that contribute to disease and health, especially smoking prevention and cessation, diet and nutrition, physical activity, weight control, sexual behavior, and accidental injury prevention. In addition to excellent reviews of the literature and meta-analyses, several national panels have convened in the past decade to examine the evidence and propose national guidelines (e.g., the National Heart, Lung, and Blood Institute's 1998 Clinical Guidelines on the Identification, Evaluation, and Treatment of Overweight and Obesity in Adults). These evaluation efforts have been enhanced by efforts to obtain representative national data (e.g., the Behavioral Risk Factor Surveillance System [BRFSS] and the National Health and Nutrition Examination Survey [NHANES]), not only on disease prevalence, but also on preclinical conditions (e.g., blood pressure) and specific health behaviors.

Smoking Prevention and Cessation

Mass consumption of tobacco began in the 1920s in the United States and increased until the 1960s. Following the release of the first Surgeon General's report on the health consequences of smoking in 1964, the percentage of smokers began to decline. This decline lasted until 1991, when smoking prevalence failed to decrease. In 2000 over 23 percent of U.S. adults smoked cigarettes. Tobacco use remains the leading cause of preventable morbidity and mortality, contributing to more than 450,000 deaths annually from a variety of diseases including heart disease and cancer. Both psychosocial and physiological mechanisms are involved in the initiation of regular smoking, active continued smoking, smoking cessation, and cessation maintenance.

Smoking cessation and prevention interventions utilize both clinical and public health approaches. National panels (e.g., the Surgeon General's report on reducing tobacco use and tobacco cessation guidelines) have concluded that intensive clinical intervention programs, including psychosocial interventions, have demonstrated efficacy. Meta-analyses have revealed that success of psychosocial interventions is associated with time spent in counseling, social support (both in treatment and outside treatment), problem solving (including skills training, relapse prevention, and stress management), and aversive smoking procedures.

The vast majority of smokers who quit do so on their own or with minimal assistance. As opposed to intensive clinical interventions that may be costly and reach a smaller percentage of people, public health approaches target the broad population. Because the majority of smokers begin smoking in their teens, early prevention efforts are critical. As evidenced by the decline in smoking spurred by the initial Surgeon General's report, public health efforts can have a definitive impact. Public health approaches are employed in a variety of domains; both work site and community-level interventions have demonstrated some efficacy. Health-care setting interventions, such as having a primary health care provider ask about smoking and advise quitting, are efficacious but not necessarily widely adopted. Other multipronged public health approaches, including directed advertising, tobacco taxes, and legislation banning smoking in particular settings (e.g., restaurants), appear to be effective in decreasing the prevalence of smoking.

Diet and Nutrition

Poor diet is a risk factor for heart disease and cancer and is central to weight control and eating disorders. For example, high saturated fat intake is associated with increased serum cholesterol levels. On the other hand, increased consumption of fruits and vegetables protects against multiple cancers including colon and breast cancer. Thus dietary change is a primary target of health promotion interventions. The first Surgeon General's recommendations for nutrition were published in 1988. Guidelines from the National Academy of Sciences suggest that adults should consume 45–65 percent of their calories from carbohydrates, 20–35 percent from fat, and 10–35 percent from protein, and 21–38 g of fiber daily. Dietary guidelines also suggest consuming at least five servings of fruits and vegetables per day. Few Americans, however, comply with these guidelines. For example, according to the BRFSS, less than 25 percent consume the recommended number of fruits and vegetables.

Health promotion interventions targeting individuals can successfully impact dietary composition. Individual and group counseling approaches often involve self-monitoring (e.g., keeping food diaries) and receiving regular feedback on progress. Less intensive community interventions (e.g., providing self-help materials in health care centers) have also shown a significant though usually smaller impact. The National Cancer Institute has sponsored a number of community interventions as part of the "5 A Day" program to increase consumption of fruits and vegetables, including mass media campaigns and the use of lay advocates in churches. Work site interventions have shown some effectiveness in reducing dietary composition through the use of multiple strategies, including health education and environmental changes in food availability or nutritional composition. Finally, several states have undertaken legislative approaches similar to those used with tobacco through the use of so-called "fat taxes" to tax less nutritious, "snack" foods.

Physical Activity

Although physical activity affects multiple health and disease outcomes including heart disease, cancer, hypertension, and diabetes, and the benefits of engaging in regular physical activity are generally accepted, the first Surgeon General's report documenting the health benefits was not published until 1996. The CDC and American College of Sports Medicine recommend that adults accumulate 30 min or more of at least moderate-intensity physical activity on 5 or more days a week, and the National Academy of Sciences suggests 60 min of daily moderate-intensity physical activity to prevent weight gain and realize other health benefits. Yet, according to the Surgeon General, more than 60 percent of Americans are not active enough to get health benefits, and more than 25 percent are completely sedentary. Several target groups have an even greater percentage of sedentary behavior, including women, ethnic minorities, and low-educated, low-income, and older adults.

Because physical activity habits often begin in childhood, youth are frequently targeted for intervention. Successful youth interventions have been implemented in school environments and have included an active physical activity or physical education curriculum. Adult interventions have used a variety of approaches including structured group-based activities, home-based activities supervised through periodic face-to-face or mediated approaches (e.g., the telephone), interventions that target routine activities undertaken throughout the day, and environmental interventions. Interventions using behavior modification principles have been shown to have significant effects on physical activity, at least during the period when the intervention was being actively delivered. Tailored telephone and print-mail interventions have also proven effective for increasing physical activity.

Weight Control

Obesity rates rose dramatically over the second half of the 20th century. Based on 1999 NHANES data, 61 percent of U.S. adults are overweight or obese, and these rates are even higher in specific sociodemographic groups such as African–American and Mexican–American women. Since the late 1970s obesity rates have doubled in adults and children and tripled in adolescents. Overweight and obesity are associated with an increase in risk factors for cardiovascular disease and diabetes such hypertension, hyperlipidemia, and physical inactivity. In fact, weight is intricately linked to both diet and physical activity, and health promotion interventions targeting diet and/or physical activity often target weight control as well.

In 2001 the Surgeon General issued a call to action to prevent and decrease overweight and obesity in the United States. Behavioral weight-loss interventions, specifically group-based interventions using behavior-modification principles and focusing on improving eating (e.g., type and amount of food eaten) and physical activity behaviors (e.g., frequency, duration, and types of activity), have proven to be effective in facilitating weight loss. In children, family-based behavioral treatments can produce long-term weight reductions. Although weight losses can be achieved in adults, weight losses are typically not maintained over time, with weight increasing over longer term follow-up. Traditionally, weight-loss treatments sought to reach ideal weights; however, panels have suggested the importance of losing and maintaining more modest weight losses (e.g., 5–15 percent of body weight) that can still confer significant health benefits. Indeed, in addition to promoting weight loss, weight control interventions also target maintenance of weight losses and prevention of weight gain, although much work remains to be done in these areas.

Because obesity is such a prevalent problem, large-scale interventions, including the school, community, and legislative dietary and physical activity interventions, have produced some results. Although these results are typically smaller than those seen in more intensive, clinical approaches, they have the potential to have a significant impact on weight at a population level. More research is needed on the effectiveness of these interventions for weight control.

Sexual Behavior

Twelve million American are infected with sexually transmitted diseases (STDs) every year, and 800,000–900,000 people are infected with HIV. In 2001 the Surgeon General issued a call to action to promote sexual health and responsible sexual behavior. Unsafe sexual practices increase the risk for contracting multiple STDs including HIV. Health promotion interventions in this area are aimed at preventing and altering high-risk sexual behaviors (e.g., having sex without using a condom) and maintaining these changes over time. Intervention involves accurately educating individuals about the mechanisms of contraction, increasing motivation for change, and changing social norms. The success of these specific approaches often depends on the target population. Among youth, regular school attendance and community-based youth development programs have a proven effect on sexual behavior. Some clinic- and school-based programs have also been effective. Targeting adolescents and adults, a number of community curriculum-based prevention programs, in addition to some clinic-based programs, have shown success in preventing infection.

Accidental Injury Prevention

In 1999 accidents were the fifth leading cause of death in the United States. Health promotion interventions have targeted behaviors to minimize both the prevalence and the adverse impact of accidental injury and include individual, community, and legislative approaches. Motor vehicle accidents are the most common cause of accidental injury, and alcohol is often involved in these accidents. Legislative approaches requiring mandatory seat belt use and limiting legal blood alcohol content have been effective in reducing motor vehicle fatalities. Because specific types of accidental injuries are more common in different age groups, interventions often target specific populations. Parents are usually targeted to decrease accidental injuries in children. For example, communitywide interventions using mass media advertising and health-care provider interventions aimed at encouraging increased bicycle helmet use in children have had success. Injurious falls are a major cause of accidental injury among the elderly, due in part to high rates of osteoporosis along with other aging-related risk factors (e.g., increasing difficulties with vision and motoric balance). In another example of the interconnection between health behaviors, the development of bone loss and osteoporosis has been linked with inadequate diet and physical activity behaviors, and can be impacted by interventions in these areas.

CONCLUSIONS

This entry provides an overview of the breadth of impact health promotion interventions can have on a range of diseases and conditions across the life span. Although research aimed at intervention development and evaluation has been reasonably promising, it is clear that expanded scientific as well as public health efforts will be required if national public health goals are to be reached. Among the areas that deserve future attention to reach these goals are building theories that continue to include a broader transdisciplinary perspective (i.e., discussion and interaction among a greater number of scientific, health, and environmental disciplines); emphasizing multilevel approaches to intervention that recognize the interplay among individual, organizational, environmental, and policy domains; tailoring preventive interventions to meet the needs of population segments at particular risk; evaluating methods for systematically combining health behaviors to facilitate physical and behavioral synergy; exploring technological advances in the delivery of health promotion interventions in greater depth; and attending to methods for translating and disseminating successful health promotion interventions to a broader segment of the American public. Given the significant health challenges that Americans face, systematic attention to all of these areas will likely be necessary to achieve population-wide successes.

Related Entry: Public Health

BIBLIOGRAPHY

Baum, A., Revenson, T. A., & Singer, J. E. (Eds.). (2001). *Handbook of health psychology.* Mahwah, NJ: Erlbaum.

Behavioral Risk Factor Surveillance System. Available at http://www.cdc.gov/brfss/

Centers for Disease Control and Prevention. Available at http://www.cdc.gov/

Dietary Guidelines Advisory Committee. (2000). *Report of the Dietary Guidelines Advisory Committee on the dietary guidelines for americans, 2000.* Washington, DC: U.S. Department of Agriculture. Available at http://www.ars.usda.gov/dgac

Glanz, K., Lewis, F. M., & Rimer, B. K. (Eds.). (1997). *Health behavior and health education: Theory, research, and practice* (2nd ed.). San Francisco: Jossey-Bass.

Green, L. W., & Kreuter, M. W. (1991). *Health promotion and planning: An educational and environmental approach* (2nd ed.). Mountain View, CA: Mayfield.

Healthy People 2010. Available at http://www.health.gov/healthypeople/

Kaplan, R. M., Sallis, J. F., & Patterson, T. L. (Eds.). (1993). *Health and human behavior.* New York: McGraw-Hill.

McGinnis, J. M., & Foege, W. H. (1993). Actual causes of death in the United States. *Journal of the American Medical Association, 270,* 2207–2212.

National Academy of Sciences, Institute of Medicine. *Dietary reference intakes for energy, carbohydrate, fiber, fat, fatty acids, cholesterol, protein, and amino acids.* Available at http://www.iom.edu/

National Center for Health Statistics. *Healthy People 2000 final review.* Available at http://www.cdc.gov/nchs/products/pubs/pubd/hp2k/review/highlightshp2000.htm

National Center for Health Statistics. *National health and nutrition examination survey.* Available at http://www.cdc.gov/nchs/nhanes.htm

National Heart, Lung, and Blood Institute. *Clinical guidelines on the identification, evaluation, and treatment of overweight and obesity in adults.* Available at http://www.nhlbi.nih.gov/guidelines/obesity/ob_home.htm

O'Donnell, M. P. (1989). Definition of health promotion: Part III: Expanding the definition. *American Journal of Health Promotion, 3,* 5.

Office of Disease Prevention and Health Promotion. Available at http://odphp.osophs.dhhs.gov/

Office of the Surgeon General. Available at http://www.surgeongeneral.gov/sgoffice.htm

Office of the Surgeon General. *Physical activity and health: A report of the Surgeon General.* Available at http://www.cdc.gov/nccdphp/sgr/sgr.htm

Office of the Surgeon General. *Reducing tobacco use: A report of the Surgeon General.* Available at http://www.cdc.gov/tobacco/sgr_tobacco_use.htm

Pate, R. R., Pratt, M., Blair, S. N., et al. (1995). Physical activity and public health: A recommendation from the Centers for Disease Control and Prevention and the American College of Sports Medicine. *Journal of the American Medical Association, 273,* 402–407.

Smith, T. W., Kendall, P. C., & Keefe, F. J. (Eds.). (2002). Behavioral medicine and clinical health psychology [Special issue]. *Journal of Consulting and Clinical Psychology, 70*(3).

Wing, R. R., Voorhees, C. C., & Hill, D. R. (Eds.). (2000). Maintenance of behavior change in cardiorespiratory risk reduction [Special issue]. *Health Psychology, 19*(Supplement 1).

World Health Organization. Available at http://www.who.int/about/overview/en/

Jennifer Hoffman Goldberg
Abby C. King

Helplessness

Helplessness refers to maladaptive passivity in situations where an active response can alleviate negative conditions or produce positive ones. Helplessness entails not just a deficit in activity, but also a lack of motivation, aversive feelings—notably anxiety and depression—and cognitive difficulties in recognizing that certain behaviors indeed affect what happens. Helplessness has been explained from theoretical perspectives ranging from psychoanalytic accounts of symptom formation through sociological accounts of alienation, but perhaps its best-known contemporary explanation has emerged from studies by psychologists of what has come to be known as learned helplessness. These studies have investigated the causes and consequences of helplessness and led to effective strategies of treatment and prevention.

LEARNED HELPLESSNESS

Learned helplessness was first described several decades ago by investigators studying animal learning. Researchers immobilized a dog and exposed it to a series of electric shocks that could be neither avoided nor escaped. Twenty-four hours later, the dog was placed in a situation in which electric shock could be terminated by a simple response. The dog did not make this response, however, and passively endured the shock. This behavior was in contrast to dogs in a control group who reacted vigorously to the shock and learned readily how to turn it off.

These investigators proposed that the dog had learned to be helpless: When originally exposed to uncontrollable shock, it learned that nothing it did mattered. The shocks came and went independently of the dog's behaviors. Response–outcome independence was represented by the dogs as an expectation of future helplessness that was generalized to new situations to produce motivational, emotional, and cognitive difficulties. The deficits that follow in the wake of uncontrollability are known as the learned helplessness phenomenon, and the associated cognitive explanation as the learned helplessness model.

Much of the early interest in learned helplessness stemmed from its clash with traditional stimulus–response theories of learning. Alternative accounts of learned helplessness were proposed that did not invoke mentalistic constructs, and many of these alternatives emphasized an incompatible motor response learned when animals were first exposed to uncontrollable shock. This response was presumably generalized to the second situation, where it interfered with performance at the test task. For example, perhaps the dogs learned that holding still when shocked somehow decreased pain. If so, then they held still in the second situation as well because this response was previously reinforced. Studies testing the learned helplessness model versus the incompatible motor response alternatives showed that expectations were critical in producing helplessness following uncontrollable events.

Support for a cognitive interpretation of helplessness also came from studies showing that an animal could be immunized against the debilitating effects of uncontrollability by first exposing it to controllable events. The animal learns during immunization that events can be controlled, and this expectation is sustained during exposure to uncontrollable events, precluding learned helplessness. In other studies, learned helplessness deficits were undone by forcibly exposing a helpless animal to the contingency between behavior and outcome. So, the animal was compelled to make an appropriate response at the test task, by pushing or pulling it into action. After several such trials, the animal notices that escape is possible and begins to respond on its own. Again, the process at work is cognitive. The animal's expectation of response–outcome independence is challenged during the therapy experience, and hence learning occurs.

HELPLESSNESS AND HUMAN PROBLEMS

Psychologists interested in humans, and particularly human problems, were quick to see the parallels between learned helplessness as produced by uncontrollable events in the laboratory and maladaptive passivity as it exists in the real world. Thus, researchers began several lines of research on learned helplessness in people.

In one line of work, helplessness in people was produced in the laboratory much as it was in animals, by exposing them to uncontrollable events and observing the effects. Unsolvable problems usually were substituted for uncontrollable electric shocks, but the critical aspects of the phenomenon remained: Following uncontrollability, people show a variety of deficits. In other studies, researchers documented further similarities between the animal phenomenon and what was produced in the human laboratory, including immunization and therapy.

In another line of work, researchers proposed various failures of adaptation as analogous to learned helplessness and investigated the similarity between these failures and learned helplessness: depression; physical illness; academic, athletic, and vocational failure; worker burnout; deleterious psychological effects of crowding, unemployment, noise pollution, chronic pain, aging, mental retardation, and epilepsy; and passivity among ethnic minorities.

ATTRIBUTIONAL REFORMULATION

As research ensued, it became clear that the original learned helplessness explanation was an oversimplification. The model failed to account for the range of reactions that people display in response to uncontrollable events. Some people show the hypothesized deficits across time and situation, whereas others do not. Furthermore, failures of adaptation that the learned helplessness model was supposed to explain, such as depression, are often characterized by a striking loss of self-esteem, about which the model is silent.

In an attempt to resolve these discrepancies, Lyn Abramson, Martin Seligman, and John Teasdale reformulated the helplessness model as applied to people. They explained the contrary findings by proposing that people ask themselves why uncontrollable (bad) events happen. The nature of the person's answer then sets the parameters for the subsequent helplessness. If the causal attribution is stable ("it's going to last forever"), then induced helplessness is long-lasting; if unstable, then it is transient. If the causal attribution is global ("it's going to undermine everything"), then subsequent helplessness is manifest across a variety of situations; if specific, then it is correspondingly circumscribed. Finally, if the causal attribution is internal ("it's all my fault"), the person's self-esteem drops following uncontrollability; if external, self-esteem is left intact.

These hypotheses comprise the attributional reformulation of helplessness theory. This new theory left the original model in place because uncontrollable events were still hypothesized to produce deficits when they gave rise to an expectation of response–outcome independence. The nature of these deficits, however, was now said to be influenced by the causal attribution offered by the individual.

In some cases, the situation itself provides the explanation made by the person. In other cases, the person relies on his or her habitual way of making sense of events that occur: explanatory style. People tend to offer similar explanations for disparate bad (or good) events. Explanatory style is therefore a distal, although important, influence on helplessness and the failures of adaptation that involve helplessness. An explanatory style characterized by internal, stable, and global explanations for bad events can be described as pessimistic, and the opposite style—external, unstable, and specific explanations for bad events—can be described as optimistic.

INTERVENTIONS

One practical implication of these ideas is that helplessness and its consequences can be alleviated by changing the way people think about response–outcome contingencies and how they explain the causes of bad events. Cognitive therapy for depression is effective in part because it changes these sorts of beliefs and provides clients with strategies for viewing future bad events in more optimistic ways.

Another practical implication is that helplessness and its consequences can be prevented in the first place by teaching clients cognitive–behavioral skills before the development of problems. One protocol based on these tenets, designed for group administration to middle-school students, is the Penn Resiliency Program (PRP). PRP is a 12-session curriculum administered by school teachers and guidance counselors. The program contains two main components, one cognitive and the other based on social problem-solving techniques.

In the cognitive component, five core cognitive techniques are translated, through the use of cartoons and skits, into a language that adolescents can understand and apply to their own lives. Group facilitators begin by teaching students about the link between thoughts and feelings. In the second lesson, students learn how to evaluate the beliefs they learned to recognize in the first lesson. Skits are used to help find differences between the beliefs of fictitious characters who are thriving and those who are not. By the end of the lesson, students have learned that "me" (it's my fault), "always" (it's going to be this way forever), and "everything" (it affects everything I do) beliefs about bad events are more likely than others to result in undesirable outcomes.

In the third lesson, two detectives are contrasted: one good and one bad. The good detective makes a list of many possible suspects (beliefs) and chooses the one most supported by the evidence. The bad detective always chooses the first suspect that pops into his head. Students are taught to evaluate their beliefs as if they were the good detective. In the fourth lesson, students learn to decatastrophize, or to evaluate the accuracy of their first and often erroneous belief. In the fifth lesson, students intensively practice a technique called the hot seat, which helps transition the cognitive skills from the classroom into the real world by providing an opportunity for rapid-fire disputation of negative beliefs.

Through the cognitive component, students learn to evaluate the accuracy of their interpretations of the world. In the social-problem-solving component, students learn seven skills that help them better interact with this world: assertiveness, negotiation, relaxation, procrastination, social skills, decision making, and problem solving. The PRP has been successfully evaluated in school and managed care settings in both the United States and China. Results indicated that prevention participants reported fewer depressive symptoms and were less likely to report symptoms in the moderate to severe range through 2 years of follow-up. At 2 years, 22 percent of the prevention participants compared to 44 percent of controls reported symptoms in the moderate to severe range.

Related Entries: Coping, Depression, Optimism and Health, Stressful Life Events

BIBLIOGRAPHY

Abramson, L. Y., Seligman, M. E. P., & Teasdale, J. D. (1978). Learned helplessness in humans: Critique and reformulation. *Journal of Abnormal Psychology, 87,* 49–74.

Buchanan, G. M., & Seligman, M. E. P. (Eds.). (1995). *Explanatory style.* Hillsdale, NJ: Erlbaum.

Cardemil, E. V., Reivich, K. J., & Seligman, M. E. P. (2002). The prevention of depressive symptoms in low-income minority middle school students. *Prevention and Treatment, 5*(8). Available at http://journals.apa.org/prevention/volume5/pre0050008a.html

Freres, D. R., Gillham, J. E., Reivich, K. J., & Shatté, A. J. (2002). Preventing depressive symptoms in middle school students: The Penn Resiliency Program. *International Journal of Emergency Mental Health, 4,* 31–40.

Garber, J., & Seligman, M. E. P. (Eds.). (1980). *Human helplessness: Theory and applications.* New York: Academic.

Gillham, J. E., Reivich, K. J., Jaycox, L. H., & Seligman, M. E. P. (1995). Prevention of depressive symptoms in schoolchildren: Two-year follow-up. *Psychological Science, 6,* 343–351.

Gillham, J. E., Shatté, A. J., & Freres, D. R. (2000). Preventing depression: A review of cognitive–behavioral and family interventions. *Applied and Preventive Psychology, 9,* 63–88.

Jaycox, L. H., Reivich, K. J., Gillham, J., & Seligman, M. E.P. (1994). Prevention of depressive symptoms in school children. *Behaviour Research and Therapy, 32,* 801–816.

Maier, S. F., & Seligman, M. E. P. (1976). Learned helplessness: Theory and evidence. *Journal of Experimental Psychology: General, 105,* 3–46.

Peterson, C. (1991). Meaning and measurement of explanatory style. *Psychological Inquiry, 2,* 1–10.

Peterson, C., & Bossio, L. M. (1991). *Health and optimism.* New York: Free Press.

Peterson, C., Maier, S. F., & Seligman, M. E. P. (1993). *Learned helplessness: A theory for the age of personal control.* New York: Oxford University Press.

Peterson, C., & Seligman, M. E. P. (1984). Causal explanations as a risk factor for depression: Theory and evidence. *Psychological Review, 91,* 347–374.

Seligman, M. E. P. (1975). *Helplessness: On depression, development, and death.* San Francisco: Freeman.

Seligman, M. E. P. (1991). *Learned optimism.* New York: Knopf.

Seligman, M. E. P., Castellon, C., Cacciola, J., Schulman, P., Luborsky, L., Ollove, M., et al. (1988). Explanatory style change during cognitive therapy for unipolar depression. *Journal of Abnormal Psychology, 97,* 13–18.

Seligman, M. E. P., Reivich, K. J., Jaycox, L. H., & Gillham, J. (1995). *The optimistic child.* New York: Harper Perennial.

Yu, D. L., & Seligman, M. E. P. (2002). Preventing depressive symptoms in Chinese children. *Prevention and Treatment, 5*(9). Available at http://journals.apa.org/prevention/volume5/pre0050009a.html

CHRISTOPHER PETERSON
DEREK R. FRERES

HIV/AIDS

HIV (human immunodeficiency virus) is the virus that causes AIDS (acquired immunodeficiency syndrome). AIDS, the final stage of the infection process, is characterized by severe immunodeficiency. During this stage, an infected person's immune system loses its ability to fight off "opportunistic" infections (e.g., pneumonia) that can lead to death.

EPIDEMIOLOGY

In the United States, 850,000 people are estimated to be infected with HIV. This estimate is imprecise because not all states require test providers to report HIV to their health departments, and not all infected persons have been tested. Better surveillance data are available for AIDS (because all states do require reporting of AIDS cases), and indicate that 793,026 cases of AIDS have been reported to the Centers for Disease Control and Prevention (CDC) through June 2001. AIDS cases are seen disproportionately among economically disadvantaged persons in urban settings, especially among ethnic and racial minorities. African Americans, in particular, have been especially vulnerable to HIV and account for approximately 40 percent of all AIDS cases in the United States.

Improved antiretroviral treatments for HIV, first developed in 1995, led to a decline in AIDS-related mortality in the United States and other nations with access to modern medicine. However, despite improvements in health among some who are infected with HIV, there is still no cure, and AIDS-related illnesses continue to claim many lives. During 2000, for example, AIDS was the fifth leading cause of death among young adults in the United States.

Global estimates of HIV and AIDS indicate that as many as 40 million people worldwide are now living with HIV or AIDS. The total number of deaths since the beginning of the epidemic is estimated at 22 million. The epidemic does not appear to have slowed, with an estimated 5 million new infections in 2000. Globally, the primary mode of transmission is heterosexual intercourse. Women account for 48 percent of HIV cases worldwide. The majority of people with HIV live in the developing world, with nearly 28.5 million cases on the continent of Africa, 6.1 million cases in south and southeast Asia, and 1.4 million cases in Latin America.

TRANSMISSION AND DISEASE COURSE

HIV transmission occurs when HIV-infected blood, semen, vaginal secretions, or breast milk enters the blood stream of an uninfected person. Once infected, a person experiences an acute illness that may pass unnoticed. Next, there is a extended phase during which the person has few symptoms, but remains infectious to others. After several years, an untreated person may begin to develop symptoms suggestive of HIV disease, such as enlarged lymph glands, fever, weight loss, diarrhea, and fatigue. The immune system has become much less effective, as indicated by reduced CD4 lymphocyte levels; if untreated, infected persons become vulnerable to opportunistic infections, many of which can be life threatening. Treatment of HIV disease can interrupt the natural history of the disease and delay immunocompetence for extended periods.

HIV ANTIBODY TESTING

Diagnosis of HIV infection occurs through HIV antibody testing. In the United States it is possible to receive testing at most health departments or through private medical providers. Testing can be anonymous or confidential. Anonymous testing does not require the person seeking testing to provide his or her name. Confidential testing does require the use of a name. The CDC recommends and many states require both pre- and posttest counseling by a trained health professional.

The most commonly used diagnostic test for HIV is the enzyme-linked immunoassay (ELISA) test. This screening test determines whether antibodies to HIV are present in the blood. A positive result does not necessarily mean that the person is infected with HIV because there are other conditions that may lead to a false positive result. For this reason, a positive ELISA test is usually followed by a second ELISA and then by a confirmatory test called the Western blot test. A positive Western blot is generally interpreted as conclusive for an HIV infection. Negative tests do not rule out HIV infection because there is a time interval between HIV infection and the appearance of measurable antibodies (this interval is called the window period). Therefore, if an individual is suspected of being infected with HIV but is thought to be in the window period, testing may need to be repeated at a later date.

Getting tested is important for anyone who believes that she or he may have been exposed to HIV. This allows one to seek medical, psychological, and social services, as appropriate; in addition, testing positive signals the need to avoid behaviors that might inadvertently transmit the virus to others. Although testing is often portrayed as a prevention strategy, it has limited effectiveness for this purpose. Overall, based on a meta-analysis of the scientific literature, HIV counseling and testing tends to lead to risk reduction for those persons who test positive but does not alter risky sexual behavior among those who test negative. However, there have been a number of prevention programs that have been more effective.

PREVENTION OF HIV

Several prevention strategies have been implemented, with varying degrees of success. These strategies target the transmission mode, and are designed to prevent, or at least reduce, the likelihood of the transfer of infected bodily fluids between an infected (HIV+) and an uninfected (HIV−) person.

BLOOD PRODUCTS

Efforts to prevent transmission through blood transfusions is the United States have been very successful. Since 1985, all donated blood has been tested for HIV antibodies, and potential blood donors with high-risk histories have been strongly discouraged from donating blood. Outside of the United States, however, many developing countries cannot afford to screen all blood products, and transmission via this mechanism continues. Transmission through blood transfusions and accidental exposures (e.g., occupational needle sticks) are relatively rare in the developed world but continue to occur in the developing world.

OCCUPATIONAL AND ACCIDENTAL EXPOSURES

Accidental and occupational exposures (e.g., needle sticks among health care workers) are rare. Prevention efforts involve the use of "universal precautions," procedures that begin with the assumption that all patients could be infected with HIV; therefore, emergency medical personnel, health care workers, and others likely to come into contact with bodily fluids are required to protect themselves by wearing latex gloves and other protective coverings when caring for their patients. In addition, health care workers are required to dispose of uncapped needles and syringes in specially made, puncture-resistant containers. Universal precaution procedures also involve the incineration (and careful discarding) of medical waste, trash, and linens in hospitals and other health care settings.

A second strategy to reduce occupational or accidental transmission involves the use of "postexposure prophylaxis" or PEP. This strategy is used only when a person is exposed to an infected bodily fluid. In such cases, the use of PEP reduces the odds of HIV infection occurring by as much as 81 percent. Therefore, the CDC recommends PEP for health care workers who are accidentally exposed to HIV-infected body fluids.

Limited resources in many poorer countries make it difficult for these countries to implement such strategies to reduce accidental and occupational exposures.

MATERNAL–CHILD TRANSMISSION

Maternal–child transmission can occur through the placenta before birth, during delivery, and through breast feeding. The likelihood of perinatal transmission without medical intervention is estimated to be 25 percent. The risks of such transmission can be reduced to less than 10 percent if a pregnant woman takes zidovudine (AZT) during pregnancy followed by brief treatment of the newborn infant. The risk of transmission through breast feeding is approximately 10 percent. Therefore, in the United States and other developed countries, HIV-infected mothers are discouraged from breast feeding and advised to use commercially prepared formula instead.

However, in countries where clean water is not available and where infectious diseases and malnutrition cause significant infant mortality, the World Health Organization and other organizations recommend breast feeding.

INTRAVENOUS DRUG USE

Intravenous drug use (IDU) is associated with HIV transmission primarily because drug users often share their drug-injection equipment or "works" with one another. Needles and syringes often have small amounts of HIV-infected blood, which can mix with the next users' blood and lead to infection. If infected blood is present in a syringe that is shared, the likelihood of transmission is high. In the United States, sharing of unsterilized drug injection needles accounted for 27 percent of the new infections in 2001.

To reduce the risk of HIV infection resulting from IDU, several strategies have been used. One involves exchanging clean needles for used (potentially contaminated) needles. Research completed in the United States has found that HIV incidence was reduced by such needle exchange programs. If needle exchange is not available, then drug users are discouraged from sharing needles with other users and taught how to clean their works prior to use. Perhaps the best strategy is to provide drug abuse treatment. Research reveals that persons who reduce or stop their drug use are less likely to engage in HIV-related risk behavior.

SEXUAL TRANSMISSION

Most cases of HIV in the United States and globally result from sexual transmission. In the United States, unprotected anal and vaginal intercourse are responsible for nearly three-fourths of new infections.

The most effective way to eliminate the sexual transmission of HIV is to abstain from all penetrative sexual activities. Research with adolescents suggests that abstinence programs can have short-term benefits. For example, one study compared the effects of (1) an abstinence-oriented program (2) a safer-sex program, and (3) a health promotion control group implemented with African-American adolescents from middle schools serving low-income, inner-city communities. At the 3-month follow-up, students in the abstinence intervention were less likely to report having had sexual intercourse than were control group participants; however, this effect weakened at the subsequent follow-up evaluations. As expected, students in the safer-sex intervention reported a higher frequency of condom use at all follow-ups. Among adolescents who reported sexual experience at baseline, the safer-sex intervention group reported less sexual intercourse at 6- and 12-month follow-ups than did the control and abstinence intervention groups, and less unprotected intercourse at all follow-ups than did the control group. The results indicate that both abstinence and safer-sex interventions reduced HIV sexual risk behaviors, but that safer-sex interventions have longer lasting effects and are more effective for sexually experienced adolescents.

For adults and adolescents who remain sexually active, prevention efforts tend to encourage "safer sex," a term which refers to a set of risk reduction strategies, including reducing the number of sexual partners, engaging in a mutually monogamous relationship with an uninfected partner, using condoms consistently and correctly, shifting from higher risk to lower risk sexual activities, and reducing the frequency of unprotected intercourse. These strategies provide different levels of protection against HIV, depending on the circumstances, partner characteristics, and behavioral practices. Most prevention programs tend to emphasize condom use, which provides the best protection for sexually active persons.

There is now a large literature devoted to evaluating the efficacy of a variety of HIV prevention programs. Such programs have been evaluated in a wide range of settings, including clinics that provide services for sexually transmitted disease (STD), family planning, and other sexual health needs; primary, secondary, and higher educational environments; prisons; military facilities; and a range of community-based settings. Programs have been tailored to address the unique needs of men who have sex with men, heterosexual women, adolescents, alcohol and drug users, persons living with mental illness, and other populations.

Two large studies demonstrate that behavioral intervention programs can lead to reduced risk behavior and lowered incidence of new STDs. The National Institute of Mental Health Multisite HIV Prevention Trial Group investigated the efficacy of a group-based intervention with 3,706 high-risk men and women who were recruited from 37 medical clinics across the United States. The intervention evaluated was based on a social-skills-training approach. Patients who received the intervention reported fewer unprotected sexual acts, had higher levels of condom use, and were more likely to use condoms consistently over a 12-month follow-up period. In addition, those men who were recruited from an STD clinic also had a gonorrhea reinfection rate that was one-half that of the control group.

A second study investigated an individualized intervention and was conducted in STD clinics. For this trial, men and women seeking care at such a clinic were randomly assigned to one of three conditions: (1) a four-session counseling program lasting 200 min, (2) a two-session counseling program lasting 40 min, or (3) standard care. Compared with patients receiving standard care, participants in both counseling interventions reported more condom use at 3 and 6 months postintervention. After 6 months, 30 percent fewer participants in both counseling interventions had new STDs, and after 12 months,

20 percent fewer participants had new STDs. Benefits were similar for men and women.

Scholarly reviews of the research literature consistently identify several characteristics of effective HIV prevention programs. First, such programs follow theoretical models that identify multiple determinants of sexual risk behavior. The most prominent models are derived from social cognitive theory and recognize the influence of intrapersonal, interpersonal, dyadic, and other environmental factors. Second, successful interventions usually have a behavioral skills component, which helps program recipients to strengthen self-management, condom use, and interpersonal negotiation skills while becoming better informed about HIV transmission and prevention and more aware of personal vulnerability to HIV infection.

Evaluation of existing prevention programs has also identified some limitations. One concern involves the transfer of research-based interventions to community-based providers. Some transfer is occurring but this tends to happen slowly, and there is concern about whether the adoption of science-based programs is true to the original (tested) intervention. A second concern involves the durability or sustainability of risk reduction. Most research studies follow participants for 1 year or less. Because the need for behavior change is lifelong, research is needed to determine whether the risk reduction benefit persists over longer time intervals.

LIVING WITH HIV DISEASE

Men and women living with HIV disease face numerous challenges, including coping with the stress of a life-threatening illness, adhering to a complex medical regimen, and adopting safer sexual practices.

Coping with HIV Disease

Although the nature and severity of psychological distress resulting from HIV varies from person to person, there is agreement that several phases of the illness are associated with increased anxiety and depressive symptoms. Initial notification of an HIV+ test result, the initial onset of physical symptoms or a sudden decline in CD4 counts, diagnosis of AIDS, and a first hospitalization all represent potent stressors during the course of HIV illness.

Regardless of illness stage, all persons living with HIV must cope with the challenge of living with a chronic, life-threatening disease. Even among those who respond well to treatment, long-term survival is not assured. Sustained viral suppression requires strict adherence to complex drug regimens, and the treatment itself can cause serious and, in some instances, intolerable side effects. Also, because HIV is a stigmatized illness, patients may experience discrimination and rejection from family, friends, partners, and employers. In addition, many HIV-infected individuals must also cope with other life stressors, including social marginalization, unemployment, mental illness, and substance abuse difficulties.

There has been considerable interest in understanding whether psychosocial factors influence HIV disease progression. Studies linking psychosocial variables longitudinally with disease progression in HIV have yielded somewhat contradictory results, but several have provided evidence to suggest that positive psychological adjustment can be associated with improved clinical outcomes. Other investigators have sought to evaluate the impact of stress-reduction interventions on mental health functioning and, in some instances, HIV disease course. For example, cognitive–behavioral stress management programs have shown promise as an approach to reducing psychological distress and improving health-related outcomes among persons living with HIV. This and other studies provide evidence that stress management and supportive interventions can reduce distress and contribute to improved quality of life for people living with HIV.

Adhering to HIV Medications

Successful treatment results in almost total suppression of HIV viral load to "undetectable levels." However, patients who are unable to take their medications as prescribed are likely to develop drug resistance and may experience poor clinical outcomes. HIV treatment regimens are demanding; they often require patients to take medications throughout the day and night, often at varying intervals. Given the demanding nature of these regimens and the frequent occurrence of unpleasant side effects, it is perhaps not surprising that many patients experience difficulties with taking their medication as prescribed. Studies indicate that suboptimal adherence is reported by between one-third and one-half of patients taking complex HIV treatments.

Research investigating factors that contribute to HIV treatment adherence difficulties point to the challenges of developing interventions to improve adherence. Risk factors that characterize individuals who are at elevated risk for contracting HIV—poverty, social marginalization, substance abuse, and mental illness—are also likely to impair HIV treatment adherence. Psychosocial factors, including social support, psychological distress, and self-efficacy beliefs, also appear to be important factors contributing to combination therapy adherence. Patients report many reasons for missed doses, including simple forgetting, confusion about the treatment regimen, concerns about side effects, and difficulties in fitting complicated pill-taking regimens into a daily routine. Many patients also raise concerns about the psychological impact of being reminded frequently of one's disease and fear that others will find out that they are HIV+. Finally, aspects of the treatment itself, including patients' knowledge about treatments, influence adherence.

For example, a recent study found that patients who did not understand the relationship between missed doses and the development of drug resistance were more likely to report poor adherence.

Interventions to promote HIV medication adherence have only recently begun to appear in the scientific literature. Nonetheless, several strategies have emerged, and are often used in practice settings. Initially, many patients benefit from provider-based education regarding the drug regimen and the consequences of poor adherence. Patients need to understand that even slight deviations from prescribed regimens can result in treatment failure. Patients also benefit from having clear expectations regarding medication side effects. Once it is clear that patients understand the importance of taking medications as prescribed, clinicians can then suggest personalized strategies to promote adherence, such as the use of multiple reminders (e.g., daily pill boxes, daily checklists, watch alarms) and the use of problem solving to facilitate integration of pill taking into daily activities. Interventions should also help patients to use social support networks, especially family members and partners, to reinforce patients' efforts to follow treatment plans.

Adopting Safer Sex Behaviors

Although many persons living with HIV refrain from risky sexual behaviors, studies indicate that at least 30 percent of persons living with HIV engage in risky behaviors. Continued sexual risk behavior among persons living with HIV may inadvertently transmit the virus to uninfected partners, and can lead to more rapid disease progression if such encounters result in coinfections with another STD or "superinfection" with a more virulent HIV strain.

Paradoxically, the availability of improved HIV treatments have eroded commitment to safer sex due to the belief that AIDS is no longer the dire health threat it had been. In a study involving HIV+ and HIV-negative gay men in Chicago, 27 percent of respondents expressed reduced concern about HIV due to new treatments. In addition, reduced HIV concern was strongly associated with unprotected anal sex.

HIV risk-reduction interventions involving persons living with HIV have been quite limited. Research on HIV counseling and testing suggests that posttest counseling promotes short-term reductions in HIV risk behavior among newly infected men and women, but other research reveals that HIV+ persons often revert to high-risk behavior, perhaps due to safer sex fatigue or burnout. Thus, more intensive interventions may be needed to bring about sustained risk reduction and behavior change.

Several studies have investigated such intensive programs, using two different strategies. One strategy focuses on helping HIV+ persons to adjust emotionally and cope with HIV infection. An initial study evaluated a stress management program for HIV+ men that included relaxation training, systematic desensitization, physical exercise, and self-management training. Although risk reduction was not a primary goal of the intervention, participation in the program was associated with a reduction in participants' number of partners. A second study corroborated the value of an emotion-focused intervention, and reported similar effects using a support group for depressed HIV+ men.

An alternative strategy focuses more directly on sexual risk reduction. Research testing this approach with HIV+ men and women evaluated the benefits of exercises designed to increase disclosure of serostatus to sexual partners and to identify strategies for maintaining safer sex. Compared to participants in a control condition, participants who received this risk reduction intervention reported fewer occasions of unprotected sex at 3- and 6-month follow-up assessments. These studies suggest that interventions that provide emotional support and skills-building exercises can help HIV+ people to reduce risky sexual behavior.

CONCLUSIONS

The past two decades have witnessed many advances in the scientific understanding of HIV prevention and care. Health psychologists have played, and will continue to play, an active role in the development, evaluation, and implementation of innovative risk reduction and prevention interventions; they will also continue to help people infected with HIV to adjust to the disease and benefit from new, but increasingly demanding medical treatments. Research gains from this rapidly changing specialty promise continued benefits for our understanding of many other infectious and chronic illnesses.

Related Entries: Chronic Illness, Contraception, Coping, Human Sexuality, Patience Adherence, STD Prevention, Stressful Life Events

BIBLIOGRAPHY

Antoni, M. H., Cruess, D. G., Cruess, S., Lutgendorf, S., Kumar, M., Ironson, G., et al. (2000). Cognitive–behavioral stress management intervention effects on anxiety, 24-hr urinary norepinephrine output, and T-cytotoxic/suppressor cells over time among symptomatic HIV-infected gay men. *Journal of Consulting and Clinical Psychology, 68*, 31–45.

Chesney, M. A., Ickovics, J. R., Chambers, D. B., Gifford, A. L., Neidig, J., Zwickl, B., et al. (2000). Self-reported adherence to antiretroviral medications among participants in HIV clinical trials: The AACTG adherence instruments. *AIDS Care, 12*, 255–266.

Coates, T. J., McKusick, L., Kuno, R., & Stites, D. P. (1989). Stress reduction training changed number of sexual partners but not immune function in men with HIV. *American Journal of Public Health, 79*, 885–887.

Jemmott, J. B., Jemmott, L. S., & Fong, G. T. (1998). Abstinence and safer sex HIV risk-reduction interventions for African American adolescents: A randomized controlled trial. *Journal of the American Medical Association, 279*, 1529–1536.

Kalichman, S. C., Rompa, D., Cage, M., DiFonzo, K., Simpson, D., Austin, J., et al. (2001). Effectiveness of an intervention to reduce HIV transmission risks in HIV+ people. *American Journal of Preventive Medicine, 21*, 84–92.

Kamb, M. L., Fishbein, M., Douglas, J. M., Rhodes, F., Rogers, J., Bolan, G., et al. (1998). Efficacy of risk-reduction counseling to prevent human immunodeficiency virus and sexually transmitted diseases—A randomized controlled trial. *Journal of the American Medical Association, 280*, 1161–1167.

Kelly, J. A., Murphy, D. A., Bahr, G. R., Kalichman, S. C., Morgan, M. G., Stevenson, L. Y., et al. (1993). Outcome of cognitive–behavioral and support group brief therapies for depressed, HIV-infected persons. *American Journal of Psychiatry, 150*, 1679–1686.

National Institute of Mental Health Multisite HIV Prevention Trial Group. (1998). The NIMH multisite HIV prevention trial: Reducing HIV sexual risk behavior. *Science, 280*, 1889–1894.

Vanable, P. A., Ostrow, D. G., McKirnan, D. J., Taywaditep, K. J., & Hope, B. A. (2000). Impact of combination therapies on HIV risk perceptions and sexual risk among HIV+ and HIV-negative gay and bisexual men. *Health Psychology, 19*, 134–145.

Weinhardt, L. S., Carey, M. P., Johnson, B. T., & Bickham, N. L. (1999). Effects of HIV counseling and testing on sexual risk behavior: A meta-analytic review of the published research, 1985–1997. *American Journal of Public Health, 89*, 1397–1405.

MICHAEL P. CAREY
PETER A. VANABLE

Homeostasis

In the course of the evolution of our species, the internal fluid environment of the human body evolved to immerse cells with the substances necessary for life. Regulatory mechanisms associated with the nervous system, endocrine system, immune system, and organ systems (e.g., cardiovascular and respiratory systems) developed to maintain an internal state of physiological balance or equilibrium so as to provide cells with the substances necessary for living in a changing environment. This lifelong task of maintaining balance while dealing with a dynamic environment is called homeostasis. When the brain detects an imbalance of the inner environment, regulatory mechanisms are enlisted to reinstate balance. Such stressors as infections, physical injury, excessive work demands, and interpersonal problems (e.g., divorce or social isolation) can disrupt this equilibrium. Chronic or intense stressors may contribute to a failure of reinstating homeostasis through biological, behavioral, cognitive, and/or affective adjustments, which may then foster tissue damage or even death.

Related Entries: Allostatic Load, General Adaptation Syndrome

RANDALL S. JORGENSEN

Hospice Care

The hospice has it roots in early Christendom, as a place of respite for weary travelers. These refuges spread throughout the Byzantine and Roman cultures, and the Latin term *hospitium* came into use. Through the Middle Ages and during the Crusades, hospices proliferated and expanded their role to provide care for the sick and dying, but then virtually disappeared during the Reformation. Then, in 19th-century Ireland and France, hospices were established specifically to provide terminal care. It was her experiences in these settings, witnessing the benefits of around-the-clock analgesics for pain control in patients with far advanced cancer, that prompted Dame Cecily Saunders to promote the modern-day hospice, beginning at St. Christopher's in London.

The concept of the hospice migrated to the United States in the 1970s, beginning with small grassroots programs and demonstration projects, followed by rapid proliferation in the 1980s, largely as a result of legislation that created a defined Medicare Hospice Benefit. Subsequent decades have seen continued modernization and rapid expansion of hospice services, mostly in the home environment, concurrent with the growing acceptance of palliative medicine as a credible and much-needed specialty and domain of the health care continuum to improve end-of-life care. During this time, the hospice concept has broadened in scope from a service almost entirely dedicated to cancer patients, to the care of all patients with life-limiting illnesses such as end-stage cardiac or pulmonary disease and advanced dementia (e.g., Alzheimer's disease).

The essential philosophy of hospice care is to focus on comfort, dignity, and personal growth at life's end. This encompasses biomedical, psychosocial, and spiritual aspects of the dying experience, emphasizing quality of life and healing or strengthening interpersonal relationships, rather than prolongation of the dying process at any and all costs. To reach these goals requires expertise in pain and symptom management as well as intra- and interpersonal dynamics at this unique time in the human life cycle. Additionally, hospice care supports the well-being of those (usually family members) who are in primary caregiving roles and provides bereavement care for survivors.

Modern hospice care is a team effort, with the typical hospice interdisciplinary team consisting of medical providers (physician, nurse, nursing assistant), psychosocial care providers (social worker), spiritual care providers (minister, rabbi, etc), and other supportive care professionals as needed (nutritionist, physical therapist, pharmacist, speech therapist, etc.). A hallmark of current hospice care, and a requirement under the provisions of the Medicare Hospice Benefit, is the involvement of volunteers, who provide visitation, companionship, housekeeping help, errands, and many other types of needed assistance.

In thes United States, most hospice care is provided in the home, but it can be rendered in any environment, including inpatient settings, long-term care facilities (nursing homes, assisted living centers), or anywhere else the patient resides. There are more than 3,000 hospice programs operating within the United States. Most are small programs with fewer than 30 patients, with budgets bolstered by charitable giving to provide needed services. There is a trend toward growth and consolidation to form larger multisite programs, creating operating efficiencies through economies of scale and innovative information systems. This allows more effective use of limited resources to reach far more patients from all social spheres, with the ability to provide more and more advanced palliative services for symptom control and optimization of quality of life. As a result, we are beginning to witness a blending of the humanistic patient- and family-centered philosophy that characterizes traditional hospice with the myriad innovations that have been derived through scientific advances of modern medicine. Coupled with and supported by sophisticated management systems, significant improvements in quality of life at the end of life, with reductions in health care expenditures, can been realized by patients who elect modern-day hospice care.

BIBLIOGRAPHY

American Academy of Hospice and Palliative Medicine. Available at www.aahpm.org

American Hospice Foundation. Available at www.americanhosice.org

Berger, A. M., Portenoy, R. K., & Weissman, D. E. (Eds.). (2002). *Principles and practice of palliative care and supportive oncology* (2nd ed.). Philadelphia: Lippincott Williams & Wilkins.

Doyle, D., Hanks, G. W. C., & MacDonald, N. (Eds.). (1998). *Oxford textbook of palliative medicine* (2nd ed.). New York: Oxford University Press.

National Hospice and Palliative Care Organization. Available at www.nhpco.org

PERRY G. FINE

Hostility and Health

Historically, hostility is among the most widely and thoroughly investigated psychosocial risk factors for health. From the investigation of Type A behavior pattern (TABP), hostility has emerged as a multidimensional construct involving affect, behavior, and cognition. In general, *anger* refers to negative affect ranging from feelings of irritation and annoyance to rage and may be conceptualized as an acute emotional state or an enduring trait. *Aggression* refers to overt attacking or destructive behavior. *Hostility* refers to a set of negative attitudes, beliefs, and appraisals of the worth, intent, and motives of others. These related though distinct facets are often collectively referred to with the umbrella term *hostility*.

Hostility is assessed with self-report and structured interviews. Perhaps because of its origins in basic personality research, the Cook–Medley Hostility (Ho) Scale is the most widely used self-report measure of hostility. This 50-item scale was derived from the larger Minnesota Multiphasic Personality Inventory. Higher scores are associated with greater interpersonal difficulties, lower social support, more difficulties at work, and more conflict within marriages. In addition, Cook–Medley hostility is associated with a variety of health outcomes and serves as the cornerstone in hostility–cardiovascular disease research. The Aggression Questionnaire (AQ) is a more recent self-report measure, which measures the hostility spectrum of cognitions (hostility), affect (anger), and behavior (physical, verbal aggression). The AQ is demonstrated to have reliable construct validity and is associated with cardiovascular reactivity (CVR) during social stress in the laboratory. The most widely researched interview is the Interpersonal Hostility Assessment Technique (IHAT). With the IHAT interview, emphasis is on how the person responds rather than the content of his or her response. The IHAT yields four subscales, which contribute to the total score, referred to as the Hostile Behavior Index (HBI). Higher HBI scores are associated with disease severity in coronary artery disease (CAD) patients and predict the magnitude of change in blood pressure during experiences of anger.

Substantial evidence links hostility and trait anger to increased risk of cardiac disease morbidity and mortality. These conclusions are based on increasingly well designed prospective studies, which show a predictive relationship between hostility and later acute cardiac events such as myocardial infarction (MI; heart attack), sudden cardiac death, and stroke. For example, Kawachi and colleagues (1996) found that trait anger predicted incidence of MI over a 7-year follow-up. In addition, hostility and anger are also predictive of progression or worsening of atherosclerosis, the build-up of fatty plaques in the arteries that underlies coronary heart disease. Finally, hostility may play a role in triggering acute cardiac events, through the experience of anger. Episodes of anger are more common in the 2 hr prior to a coronary event (e.g., MI) than during control periods, suggesting that the arousal of anger can trigger acute myocardial infarction. In the laboratory, arousal of anger evokes ischemia in patients with coronary artery disease, which may confer increased risk of acute MI. Hence, the literature supports hostility as a significant risk factor for the development and progression of cardiac disease as well as acute cardiac events that may be triggered by hostility through the tendency to experience episodes of anger.

Cardiovascular reactivity is one proposed pathway linking psychosocial risk factors such as hostility to cardiovascular disease (CVD). The "reactivity hypothesis" suggests that larger, more frequent, and more prolonged cardiovascular responses (e.g., heart rate, blood pressure, and associated physiological changes) initiate and promote the development of CAD. Studies have shown these physiological responses are associated with atherosclerosis and myocardial ischemia in the laboratory and during daily life.

Laboratory and ambulatory studies demonstrate a reliable relationship between hostility and larger and more frequent cardiovascular responses. In particular, research suggests that individuals higher in hostility experience greater cardiovascular reactivity during experiences of anger than do less hostile individuals. For example, several laboratory investigations have demonstrated that more-hostile individuals display larger changes in blood pressure, heart rate, and other markers of cardiovascular and neuroendocrine functioning during harassment in the laboratory. Hence, CVR may mediate the relationship between hostility and experiences of psychological distress and increased disease risk.

In addition to individual risk, researchers are increasingly aware of the interactive effects between hostility and the social context. For example, in several studies hostile persons report larger changes in anger and demonstrate greater physiological reactivity to stressful interpersonal situations than less hostile persons. In addition, hostile persons appraise the actions of others as intentionally aggressive and less friendly, process negative information about others more readily, behave in less friendly ways during interactions with family members, and experience discord and conflict in personal relationships. The resulting interplay suggests that hostile individuals not only may respond to their environment in maladaptive ways, but also transactionally create increased frequency, intensity, and duration of interpersonal stress. Not surprisingly, evidence suggests that more-hostile individuals have lower levels of social support and experience more frequent episodes of interpersonal stress at home and at work. Moreover, recent evidence suggests that when faced with a stressful situation, more-hostile individuals show less psychological and physiological benefit from their social support than do less hostile individuals. These findings suggest that hostility may confer greater risk for cardiovascular disease through increased psychosocial vulnerability.

In summary, hostility is increasingly recognized as a robust psychosocial risk factor for cardiovascular disease. Future research will likely continue to focus on examining both the psychosocial and psychophysiological mechanisms involved in the relationship between hostility and health. In addition, experts in complementary areas of behavioral medicine have begun to search for suspected interpersonal and genetic determinants of hostility. Finally, although interventions tailored at managing anger are well proven, more work is needed to demonstrate that such interventions can influence health outcomes such as future MI and early cardiovascular mortality.

Related Entries: Cook–Medley Hostility Scale, Type A Behavior Pattern

BIBLIOGRAPHY

Brownley, K. A., Light, K. C., & Anderson, N. B. (1996). Social support and hostility interact to influence clinic, work, and home blood pressure in Black and White men and women. *Psychophysiology, 33,* 434–445.

Christensen, A. J., & Smith, T. W. (1993). Cynical hostility, self-disclosure, and cardiovascular reactivity. *Psychosomatic Medicine, 55,* 532–537.

Davis, M. C., Matthews, K. A., & McGrath, C. E. (2000). Hostile attitudes predict elevated vascular resistance during interpersonal stress in men and women. *Psychosomatic Medicine, 62,* 17–25.

Everson, S. A., Kauhanen, J., Kaplan, G., Goldberg, D., Julkunen, J., Tuomilehto, J., et al. (1997). Hostility and increased risk of mortality and myocardial infarction. The mediating role of behavioral risk factors. *American Journal of Epidemiology, 146,* 142–152.

Fredrickson, B. L., Maynard, K. E., Helms, M. J., Haney, T. L., Siegler, I. C., & Barefoot, J. C. (2000). Hostility predicts magnitude and duration of blood pressure response to anger. *Journal of Behavioral Medicine, 23,* 229–243.

Guyll, M., & Contrada, R. J. (1998). Trait hostility and ambulatory cardiovascular activity: Responses to social interaction. *Health Psychology, 17,* 30–39.

Hemingway, H., & Marmot, M. (1999). Psychosocial factors in the aetiology and prognosis of coronary heart disease: Systematic review of prospective cohort studies. *British Medical Journal, 318,* 1460–1467.

Ironson, G., Taylor, C. B., Boltwood, M., Bartzokis, T., Dennis, C., Chesney, M., Spitzer, S., & Segall, G. M. (1992). Effects of anger on left ventricular ejection fraction in coronary disease. *American Journal of Cardiology, 70,* 281–285.

Julkunen, J., Salonen, R., Kaplan, G. A., Chesney, M. A., & Salonen, J. T. (1994). Hostility and the progression of carotid atherosclerosis. *Psychosomatic Medicine, 56,* 519–525.

Kawachi, I., Sparrow, D., Spiro, A., III, Vokonas, P., & Weiss, S. C. (1996). A prospective study of anger and coronary heart disease: The Normative Aging Study. *Circulation, 94,* 2090–2095.

Lepore, S. J. (1995). Cynicism, social support, and cardiovascular reactivity. *Health Psychology, 14,* 210–216.

Linden, W., Gerin, W., & Davidson, K. (2003). Cardiovascular reactivity: Status quo and a research agenda for the new millennium. *Psychosomatic Medicine, 65,* 5–8.

Miller, T. Q., Smith, T. W., Turner, C. W., Guijarro, M. L., & Hallet, A. J. (1996). A meta-analytic review of research on hostility and physical health. *Psychological Bulletin, 119,* 322–348.

Mittleman, M. A., Maclure, M., Sherwood, J. B., Mulry, R. P., Tofler, G. H., Jacobs, S. C., et al. (1995). Triggering of acute myocardial infarction onset by episodes of anger. *Circulation, 92,* 1720–1725.

Smith, T. W. (1992). Hostility and health: Current status of a psychosomatic hypothesis. *Health Psychology, 11,* 139–150.

Smith, T. W., & Ruiz, J. M. (2002). Psychosocial influences on the development and course of coronary heart disease: Current status and implications for research and practice. *Journal of Consulting and Clinical Psychology, 70,* 548–568.

Williams, J. E., Paton, C. C., Siegler, I. C., Eigenbrodt, M. L., Nieto, F. J., & Tyroler, H. A. (2000). Anger proneness predicts coronary heart disease risk: Prospective analysis from the Atherosclerosis Risk in Communities (ARIC) study. *Circulation, 101,* 2034–2039.

JOHN M. RUIZ

Human Sexuality

The term human sexuality, although sometimes narrowly used to mean sexual behavior, refers to a wide array of topics as well as a dimension of personality. Sexuality includes, but is not limited to, the physiology of sexual functioning and the genetic, neurological, and hormonal systems involved; emotional and interpersonal relationships, love, and intimacy; gender identity (male, female) and gender roles; and sexual orientation (heterosexual, bisexual, or homosexual). Sexuality in general and sexual activity for reproduction, pleasure, and intimacy are positive and important determinants of quality of life for many people. Conversely, factors that interfere with sexual functioning can cause emotional distress and negatively impact a person's sense of self-worth. Furthermore, feeling that one's sexual behaviors or desires are abnormal or stigmatized because they are not consistent with those of others people can cause significant stress and anxiety. What is considered normal sexuality and sexual behavior is to some extent culture specific. In many societies, open discussion of sexuality is considered taboo, a situation that can result in misconceptions about what constitutes normal sexual functioning and sexual health.

PHYSIOLOGY OF SEXUALITY

The human sexual response cycle has four distinct phases: excitement, plateau, orgasm, and resolution, although the progression from one phase to the next can vary widely among people and within the same person across time. The physiology of sexuality and progression through the sexual response cycle are affected by psychological and social factors. For example, what is sexually arousing to an individual is thought to result from an interaction of genetic predisposition, experiences during sexual development, and the impressions made by cultural and social environments, all of which may lead to particular thoughts and feelings during a specific sexual encounter that either increase or decrease arousal.

SEXUAL DYSFUNCTION

Although much past research attempted to classify problems of sexual functioning as "psychological" versus "organic" or physical, current thinking is that sexual problems are usually the result of biological, social, and psychological factors interacting. Sexual dysfunctions are typically classified as involving problems with desire, arousal, or orgasm. Sexual dysfunction is more prevalent for women than men, and is related to poor physical and emotional health and to negative experiences in sexual relationships. Stress, anger, depression, and anxiety are among the specific psychological factors that can impede optimal sexual functioning, and sexual functioning is also affected by the dynamics of the interpersonal relationship in which sex occurs.

HEALTH, ILLNESS, AND SEXUALITY

Physical effects and stress resulting from illness can impact sexual functioning. The experience of cardiovascular illness, diabetes, cancer, chronic obstructive pulmonary disease, and chronic pain have been found to interfere with sexual functioning. For example, vascular and neurological abnormalities resulting from diabetes can lead to erectile disorder; however, the common misconception that diabetes typically leads to erectile "impotence" can unnecessarily increase anxiety among men newly diagnosed with diabetes. The resulting anxiety may impact sexual functioning independently from physical effects of diabetes.

Finally, sexual activity can result in acute and chronic health effects from sexually transmitted infections, such as HIV/AIDS and hepatitis, as well as unintended pregnancy. Such problems not only can affect the physical health of the individual, but can have a broad impact on future social and psychological functioning.

Related Entries: Contraception, HIV/AIDS, Infertility, Pregnancy, STD Prevention

BIBLIOGRAPHY

Abramson, P. R., & Pinkerton, S. D. (2002). *With pleasure: Thoughts on the nature of human sexuality* (2nd ed.). Oxford: Oxford University Press.

Bancroft, J. (1989). *Human sexuality and its problems* (2nd ed.). New York: Churchill Livingstone,

Masters, W., Johnson, V. E., & Kolodny, R. (1995). *Human sexuality* (5th ed.). New York: Harper Collins.

Shover, L., and Jensen, S. B. (1988). *Sexuality and chronic illness.* New York: Guilford.

LANCE S. WEINHARDT

Hypertension

Hypertension is a condition characterized by higher than normal blood pressure within the arteries. Blood pressure is usually expressed as systolic over diastolic pressure (e.g., 120/80). Systolic pressure refers to the highest pressure reached when the heart beats, and diastolic pressure refers to the lowest pressure achieved while the heart is relaxed between beats. For adults, normal blood pressure exists when systolic blood pressure is less than 130 mm Hg and diastolic blood pressure is less than 85 mm Hg. Hypertension exists if resting blood pressure exceeds either 140 mm Hg systolic or 90 mm Hg diastolic (or blood pressure is normalized while the person is taking antihypertensive medication).

Resting blood pressure levels typically vary with each beat of the heart, and can be increased temporarily by a variety of factors including excitement, nervousness, or use of substances such as caffeine or nicotine. Therefore, a diagnosis of hypertension is not made on the basis of a single blood pressure measurement. According to recent clinical guidelines (Anonymous, 1997), a diagnosis of hypertension should be based on at least three sets of seated, resting blood pressure readings obtained over a period of several weeks. In addition, the patient should not have smoked or consumed any caffeine in the 30 min before the readings are obtained. Because the goal is to obtain the best estimate of a person's usual blood pressure, measurements of typical blood pressure at home or at work can be useful in making a diagnosis of hypertension or guiding treatment decisions.

Approximately 15 percent of all cases of hypertension can be linked to specific cause, such as kidney disease or hormonal disturbance. The remaining 85 percent of all cases, often referred to as primary or essential hypertension, cannot be related to a single, specific cause. Instead, research suggests that multiple factors contribute to essential hypertension, including genetics, diet (high calories, high sodium, low potassium, excessive alcohol), sedentary lifestyle, and stress.

Efforts to control hypertension are important because elevated blood pressure within the arteries can lead to damage in a variety of organs including the heart, the brain, the kidneys, and the eyes. In fact, as blood pressure increases above normal levels, so does one's risk for heart disease and stroke. Thus, individuals with high-normal blood pressure (e.g., 135/85) are at increased risk for cardiovascular disease even though they do not meet the criteria for a diagnosis of hypertension. Similarly, among those with hypertension, more severe blood pressure elevations (e.g., 180/110) are associated with greater risk for cardiovascular disease. When high blood pressure is combined with other cardiovascular disease risk factors, such as smoking, diabetes, and a diet high in fat and calories, overall risk becomes even higher. Thus, whereas the primary treatment for hypertension is medication, additional lifestyle modification efforts may be directed toward weight loss, reducing alcohol intake, increasing exercise, and stress management, depending on the needs of the individual patient.

Related Entry: Blood Pressure

BIBLIOGRAPHY

Anonymous. (1997). The sixth report of the Joint National Committee on prevention, detection, evaluation, and treatment of high blood pressure. *Archives of Internal Medicine 157,* 2413–2446.

CHRISTOPHER R. FRANCE

Hypnosis

Hypnosis has been defined in numerous ways varying in specificity from "an altered state of consciousness" to "a relaxed state"; However, no single definition has been universally accepted. Likewise, several competing theories to account for the phenomena associated with hypnosis have been devised. Some theorists stress the importance of the biological and physiological aspects of hypnosis, whereas others stress the emotional and psychological characteristics. Therefore, to enhance understanding of the nature of hypnosis, it is necessary to examine procedural aspects and the contexts in which this technique is used.

The experience of hypnosis begins with an induction designed to foster relaxation and concentration. Although many techniques exist, one popular method, eye fixation, involves instructing the participant to concentrate on a specific point, become increasingly relaxed, eventually close his or her eyes, and follow the hypnotist's suggestions. After proper training, some choose to self-induce hypnosis, following a script designed for their purposes, whereas others are induced by a trained professional. Induction can occur in group or in individual settings, depending on the desired purpose.

People vary in their susceptibility to hypnosis. Therefore, susceptibility tests such as the Stanford Hypnotic Susceptibility Scale (SHSS; Weitzenhoffer & Hilgard, 1962) are often used to assess the likelihood of hypnosis' effectiveness with the individual. People are classified as low, moderate, or high in susceptibility according to their performance on measures of susceptibility to hypnotic suggestions.

Hypnosis has been used in a variety of settings, with numerous types of participants, for multiple purposes. As a technique in psychotherapy, hypnosis has been found to be effective in the treatment of stress, anxiety, depression, post-traumatic stress disorder, and eating disorders and for purposes of behavior modification (i.e., smoking cessation and weight loss). Hypnosis can also be used to manage pain during and after surgery, labor/delivery, and various medical and dental procedures (e.g., lumbar punctures, dialysis, and root canals). Support for the efficacy of hypnosis as a pain management technique varies from study to study and differs according to the specific application in question. However, the general consensus in the literature provides support for its use in pain management across a wide range of medical and dental procedures. Hypnosis, biofeedback training, and relaxation/imagery techniques have also been used in the treatment of cancer, heart disease, and other chronic illnesses. Again, there is no definitive conclusion regarding the efficacy of hypnosis and the related techniques mentioned with chronic illnesses; however, there is at least moderate support for its effectiveness.

It should be noted that hypnosis is by no means a cure-all. Neither should it be used without guidance and training from a skilled professional. Dangers of misusing hypnosis include the possibility of precipitating a psychiatric illness, worsening a mental or medical illness, masking illness, and other hazards. However, when used responsibly, hypnosis can be an effective intervention for a wide variety of psychological, medical, and behavioral problems.

Related Entries: Biofeedback, Relaxation Response

BIBLIOGRAPHY

Crasilneck, H. B., & Hall, J. A. (1985). *Clinical hypnosis: Principles and applications* (2nd ed.). Orlando, FL: Grune & Stratton.
Weitzenhoffer, A. M., & Hilgard, E. R. (1962). *Stanford Hypnotic Susceptibility Scale, Form C.* Palo Alto, CA: Consulting Psychologists.
Wester, W. C., & Smith, A. H. (Eds.). (1984). *Clinical hypnosis: A multidisciplinary approach.* Philadelphia: Lippincott.

TRACY E. MORAN

Hypochondriasis

Hypochondriasis is a clinical syndrome characterized by the persistent fear that one has a serious medical illness despite reassurance to the contrary from medical experts. Although many people experience occasional anxiety about their health, these feelings are usually short lived. To receive a diagnosis of hypochondriasis, the fear must persist for at least 6 months and cause severe emotional distress or significant impairment such as difficulties with work performance or social relations, often because of repeated medical visits.

Research suggests that the misinterpretation of either normal fluctuations in bodily sensations or minor physical symptoms is central to the development of hypochondriasis. For example, an individual with hypochondriasis might interpret a headache as evidence of having a brain tumor, despite negative medical tests and reassurance from his or her doctor. It is not clear why these misinterpretations occur, but the disorder often develops during stressful life events that involve death or illness.

Additionally, hypochondriacal tendencies may be learned from family members during childhood.

Related Entry: Medical Student's Disease

BIBLIOGRAPHY

Starcevic, V., & Lipsitt, D. R. (Eds.). (2001). *Hypochondriasis: Modern perspectives on an ancient malady.* London: Oxford University Press.

PAULA G. WILLIAMS

Ii

Illness Stereotypes

People have a rich set of knowledge about many health problems; they know what may cause an illness, what its symptoms are, how long it lasts, and what its outcome is likely to be. In many cases, they also have beliefs about the groups of people who are likely to develop particular illnesses. People may associate health problems with specific genders, ages, and/or race or ethnic groups. For example, cardiac disease is associated with middle-age men, eating disorders are associated with young White women, and HIV/AIDS often is associated with gay men.

Associations between health problems and social groups are known as illness stereotypes or illness schemas. These stereotypes are based on information acquired from a number of sources, including formal education, the media, acquaintances, and personal experience. Because these beliefs can come from both medical and nonmedical sources, they vary in how consistent they are with clinical and epidemiologic data about the actual occurrence of health problems across social groups.

Illness stereotypes are important to health psychology because they influence how people think about and respond to potential health problems in themselves and others. Many symptoms, such as fatigue and loss of appetite, are ambiguous and may be associated with several illnesses. When people try to interpret these symptoms, they may take into account their stereotypes about the groups that are likely to develop particular illnesses. When an individual's characteristics match an illness stereotype, that is, when he or she belongs to a group that is associated with a specific illness, symptoms are likely to be interpreted in terms of that illness. In contrast, when an individual's characteristics do not match an illness stereotype, that is, when his or her group is not associated with a particular illness, people may look for different ways to explain the symptoms, such as other illnesses or environmental causes. For example, research by René Martin and her colleagues (1998) has shown that when a man has chest pains, people readily interpret them as signaling a heart attack. However, when a woman has identical pains, people are sensitive to information suggesting that they may be due to stress rather than cardiac disease.

Illness stereotypes influence judgments made by both lay people and medical professionals. Illness stereotypes may influence the likelihood that lay people will engage in preventative health behaviors as well as seek medical treatment for their symptoms. For example, a heterosexual man may decide not to engage in safer-sex behaviors because he associates HIV/AIDS with gay individuals. In a similar manner, illness stereotypes may lead medical professionals to misdiagnose symptoms or underestimate illness severity in patients who do not match their expectations for a particular illness. A follow-up study by Martin and Lemos (2002) found that, similar to lay people, practicing physicians are less likely to suspect cardiac disease when a patient is female, particularly if she has high levels of stress. Thus, due to their influence on both lay people and medical professionals, illness stereotypes are likely to influence health decision making at several points in the journey from initial symptoms to medical diagnosis and treatment.

Related Entry: Cognitive Representations of Illness

BIBLIOGRAPHY

Catania, J. A., Coates, T. J., & Kegeles, S. (1994). A test of the AIDS risk reduction model: Psychosocial correlates of condom use in the AMEN cohort study. *Health Psychology, 13*, 548–555.

López, S. R. (1989). Patient variable biases in clinical judgment: Conceptual overview and methodological considerations. *Psychological Bulletin, 106,* 184–203.

Martin, R., Gordon, E. I., & Lounsbury, P. (1998). Gender disparities in the attribution of cardiac-related symptoms: Contribution of common sense models of illness. *Health Psychology, 17,* 346–357.

Martin, R., & Lemos, K. (2002). From heart attacks to melanoma: Do common sense models of somatization influence symptom interpretation for female victims? *Health Psychology, 21,* 25–32.

JENNIFER S. HUNT

Immune System: Structure and Function

The immune system is engaged in a constant surveillance of the body for pathogens or tumors. Whether disease develops depends on the virulence of the pathogen and the competence of the immune system. To prevent disease, the immune system must recognize, attack, and remember substances that threaten health, either foreign pathogens or mutations of the body's own cells. To do so, it must be able to distinguish self from nonself substances called antigens (meaning "antibody generators"). To efficiently eliminate antigens, the immune system must respond as quickly and as strongly as possible to kill abnormal cells or infectious agents. At the same time, it must be tightly regulated to avoid destroying healthy tissues. When immune regulation breaks down, excessive inflammation can cause collateral damage resulting in autoimmune and allergic diseases. Conversely, immunosuppression can result in increased susceptibility to infection, and malignant tumors can arise when there is unchecked growth of mutant cells.

COMPONENTS OF THE IMMUNE SYSTEM

All of the cells of the immune system are derived from stem cells in the bone marrow. These cells give rise two classes of progenitor cells: (1) lymphoid progenitors are precursors to antigen-specific T and B lymphocytes and (2) myeloid progenitors are the precursors for the nonspecific macrophages, monocytes, dendritic cells, mast cells, and granulocytes (neutrophils, eosinophils, basophils). B cells remain in the bone marrow during development, selection, and maturation, whereas T cells migrate to the thymus to mature. Once mature, T and B cells emerge from these primary immune organs to reside in secondary immune organs (e.g., lymph nodes, spleen, tonsils, and lymphoid mucosa). T and B cells circulate from lymphoid organs to the tissues through lymphatic and blood vessels, monitoring sites where pathogens are likely to invade the body (airways, gastrointestinal tract, reproductive tract, skin). Pathogens are normally taken up by antigen-presenting cells (macrophages and dendritic cells), which process and transport the antigen to secondary lymphoid organs, where they induce T and B cell responses. Macrophages are widely distributed throughout the body, where they act as a first line of defense to engulf and digest antigens, a process known as phagocytosis. They are derived from circulating precursor cells known as monocytes, which differentiate into macrophages once they enter tissues. Immature dendritic cells also circulate in the blood until they migrate into the tissues and mature after ingesting pathogen. Once mature, dendritic cells migrate to the lymph nodes to present antigens. Mast cells also differentiate in the tissues, where they are located near small blood vessels and act to alter vascular permeability during allergic reactions. Neutrophils, eosinophils, and basophils are collectively known as granulocytes. They normally circulate in the blood until they are recruited to sites of infection and inflammation. Neutrophils play an important role in controlling bacterial infections, whereas eosinophils and basophils are involved in parasitic infections and allergic inflammation.

FUNCTIONS OF THE IMMUNE SYSTEM

The functions of the immune system can be divided into two systems: (1) innate or nonspecific immunity and (2) specific or adaptive immunity. These interacting systems differ in terms of the timing and specificity of their responses. Innate immunity provides an immediate but relatively nonspecific response to contain pathogens at the site of entry into the body. Innate immune defenses include inflammatory and acute-phase responses as well as the anatomical and chemical barriers provided by the skin and mucous membranes. Specific immunity is characterized by antigen specificity through T and B lymphocytes. It also exhibits immunological memory, where heightened responses occur upon subsequent exposure to the same antigen, but this is not an immediate response. Although specific immunity is more selective and adaptive than innate immunity, it is a slow and complex process and occurs over several days to weeks. Conversely, innate immunity provides an immediate front-line response, but it lacks memory and can damage healthy tissue due to its nonspecific nature.

INNATE IMMUNITY

Inflammation

Inflammation is a local response designed to limit pathogen invasion and tissue damage. Phagocytes such as macrophages and neutrophils play a central role in the inflammatory response. They recognize foreign invaders through nonspecific receptors that identify common features of pathogens. Because a large pool of phagocytic cells is readily available, inflammatory responses can be observed within 1–2 hr after infection. During this time, macrophages use several mechanisms to contain infection. First, they release toxic enzymes and ingest the invading cells. Activated macrophages also synthesize and release nitric oxide, a gas that interferes with the proliferation of bacteria and other pathogens. In addition, activated macrophages release substances called cytokines, which are chemical messengers secreted by one cell that communicate with other cells. Cytokines act locally to facilitate the inflammatory response and to attract other immune cells that promote healing at the site of infection or injury. For example, neutrophils, which normally flow freely in the blood stream, are recruited out of the circulation to the site of infection by cytokines such as interleukin-1 (IL-1) that are released by activated macrophages. A similar mechanism is used to recruit all leukocytes (white blood cells, including monocytes, granulocytes, and lymphocytes) to the site of infection or inflammation.

Natural Killer Cells

Natural killer cells (NK cells) are nonspecific lymphocytes that specialize in destroying tumor cells and virus-infected cells. Although they lack specific antigen receptors, they are able to recognize and kill some abnormal cells. NK cells secrete perforins, chemical bullets that blow holes in the pathogen's cell membrane, allowing granzymes to enter the cell. Granzymes signal the target cell to commit suicide, a process known as apoptosis.

Acute-Phase Response

Whereas inflammation begins as a local response designed to contain infection, a systemic reaction known as the acute-phase response or sickness syndrome will occur if the infection spreads to other parts of the body. This response is triggered when high concentrations of inflammatory cytokines (e.g., tumor necrosis factor alpha, IL-1, and IL-6) enter the circulation to initiate a series of physiological and behavioral changes that help fight infection and promote healing. The acute-phase response involves the release of proteins by the liver, which migrate to the site of infection. Interestingly, some of these acute-phase proteins act like nonspecific antibodies, which bind a broad range of pathogens. Other physiological changes include fever, increased slow wave sleep, and increased leukocyte production and circulation. Behavioral changes are also observed during the acute-phase response, including decreased feeding, physical activity, exploration, social interaction, sexual activity,

and aggression. Other psychological changes include increased pain sensitivity, depressed mood, and memory impairments. The highly conserved nature of these sickness behaviors, which are even observed in invertebrates, suggests that they evolved to help fight infection and enhance survival. Indeed, recent research indicates that sickness syndrome is an adaptive motivational state coordinated by the brain rather than a collection of reflexive responses reflecting the pathological consequences of infection or injury. Finally, activation of the hypothalamic–pituitary–adrenal (HPA) axis is part of the acute-phase response. Cytokines released during infection activate the HPA axis to release glucocorticoids, hormones that help to mobilize energy and decrease inflammation. The latter negative feedback mechanism acts to counterregulate the inflammatory cytokines to prevent damage to normal tissues. However, when HPA-axis activity is blunted, excessive inflammation can result in immunopathology and contribute to the development of autoimmune diseases.

SPECIFIC IMMUNITY

The T and B cells use antigen-specific receptors to recognize and destroy antigens. To recognize antigen, part of the antigen must be presented to T cells by an antigen-presenting cell (APC), such as macrophages and dendritic cells. After engulfing and processing the antigen, the APC displays specific parts of the antigen on its surface. The T cell interacts with an antigenic site on the displayed piece of antigen. T cells have receptors that allow them to recognize and bind to specific antigenic sites. Thus, a large repertoire of T cell receptors must be produced to adequately cover the large range of pathogens that will be encountered over the life span. When a T cell receptor recognizes an antigenic site, it triggers proliferation and differentiation processes, which normally occur in the lymphoid tissues. The T cell rapidly divides to yield an army of T cells with antigen-specific receptors that perform different tasks. Two classes of T cells, helper and cytotoxic T cells, are distinguished by CD4+ and CD8+ molecules on their surface, respectively. Both types of T cells act to contain intracellular pathogens, but they also perform distinct tasks. T helper cells coordinate the immune response by assisting in antigen recognition and by secreting cytokines that activate other T and B cells to increase their numbers. Cytotoxic T cells are able to kill virus-infected cells or tumor cells and thus play a major role in antiviral and antitumor activity. Another class of T cells, known as suppressive T cells, can actively inhibit the actions of other T cells through the secretion of suppressive cytokines. In the case of B cells, they differentiate into plasma cells that secrete antibody. This process is normally triggered by antigen-binding and helper T cell activity. These plasma cells rapidly divide and secrete antibodies, immunoglobulin molecules that act as receptors for antigen. These are soluble molecules that circulate in the blood, where they can inactive antigen through binding or mark it to be destroyed.

Thus far we have described the primary immune response that is initiated when the immune system does not have prior experience with the antigen. During the primary response, a subset of lymphocytes differentiates into memory T and B cells and remain in circulation for many years to provide immunity from diseases. Upon exposure to the antigen, memory T and B cells respond quickly to eliminate the antigen, a process known as the secondary immune response.

IMMUNE-RELATED DISEASES

Immunodeficiency and autoimmune diseases illustrate the importance of the immune system. Persistent infection of the immune system by human immunodeficiency virus (HIV) leads to acquired immune deficiency syndrome (AIDS). HIV evades detection by hiding in immune cells. It destroys helper T cells through its direct cytotoxic effects and by triggering cytotoxic T cells. When helper T cell counts plummet, susceptibility to opportunistic infections increase, leading to AIDS and eventual death. In autoimmune diseases, normal immune responses are directed against a self-antigen. For example, T cells may lose their ability to distinguish between self and non-self due to the development of autoreactive receptors that bind self-antigen. Such self-reactive T cells attack healthy tissues of the body, causing diseases such as multiple sclerosis, Type I diabetes, lupus, and rheumatoid arthritis. Other work suggests that suppressor T cells may lose their ability suppress the actions of cytotoxic T cells in autoimmune disease. By understanding the mechanisms mediating these diseases, research may lead to the development of innovative strategies for disease prevention and treatment.

Related Entries: Arthritis, Cancer: Biopsychosocial Aspects, HIV/AIDS, Psychoneuroimmunology

BIBLIOGRAPHY

Janeway, C. A., Travers, P., Walport, M., & Schlomchik, M. (2001). *Immunobiology: The immune system in health and Disease* (5th ed.). New York: Garland.

Maier, S. F., & Watkins, L. R. (1998). Cytokines for psychologists: Implications of bidirectional brain communication for understanding behavior, mood, and cognition. *Psychological Review, 105*, 83–107.

Parkin, J., & Cohen, B. (2001). An overview of the immune system. *Lancet, 375*, 1777–1788.

MARY W. MEAGHER

Incidence

Incidence is defined as the number of new cases of a disease or disorder reported in a particular time period, generally 1 year, for a given population. In epidemiologic research, this number is an indication of the change in reported cases across time periods. In other words, incidence provides an indicator of rise or decline in reported cases and can be used to demonstrate disease or disorder trends. For example, according to the U.S. Renal Data System, the incidence of end-stage renal disease, or loss of kidney function, in the United States was approximately 70,100 in 1995 and approximately 92,600 in 2000. These data suggest that the number of cases of end-stage renal disease in the United States is on the rise. Incidence, the number of new cases of a disorder in a particular population, can be compared to prevalence, the number of total cases of a disorder in a given population.

Related Entries: Epidemiology, Prevalence

JAMIE A. CVENGROS

Infertility: Causes, Consequences, and Treatments

Infertility is defined as the inability to obtain and sustain a pregnancy after 12 months of regular, unprotected intercourse. Based on the number of people who turn to medical specialists when they are having trouble getting pregnant, infertility is estimated to affect 10–12 percent of North American couples at all stages of their reproductive lives, irrespective of their race, ethnicity, or income. Issues related to the woman's reproductive capacity account for approximately 35–40 percent of fertility problems, whereas issues related to the adequate delivery and production of a man's sperm account for 30–35 percent. In 15–20 percent of infertility cases problems are diagnosed in both members of the couple. For about 10 percent of those who seek treatment, no medical diagnosis can be found to account for their inability to produce a child. Factors commonly associated with an increased incidence of infertility include a family history of fertility problems, increased age, certain childhood traumas such as physical or sexual abuse, congenital and genetic abnormalities, eating disorders, exposure to toxins in the workplace, chemotherapy and radiation treatments, and excessive drug and alcohol use.

Becoming a parent is considered by most people to be one of the most significant events in adulthood. Parenthood socially and personally marks a major transition in people's lives and in their relationships. Consequently, it is extremely difficult for couples to learn that they are infertile. Most people assume their fertility is under their control and are shocked when they decide it is time to begin their families but find that, without medical assistance, they may not be able to have children. Couples often wonder why they are unable to produce a child when most of their friends appear to have no difficulty getting pregnant. They ask themselves what they might have done to cause their infertility, and are often surprised to find themselves experiencing a range of powerful emotions, including sadness, grief, anger, inadequacy, and depression. Although infertile women tend to express these feelings more openly than men, men also find it very difficult and challenging to cope with a diagnosis of infertility. Being unable to produce a child together puts tremendous pressure on a couple's relationship, particularly in terms of their intimate and sexual lives, as sex for pleasure is replaced by sex for procreation and couples fail to achieve a pregnancy each month in spite of their best efforts. The medical process of diagnosing and treating fertility problems is very time consuming as well as being emotionally and physically invasive, focusing as it does on the most intimate and private aspects of a couple's lives and bodies. Treatment is also very expensive, particularly the advanced reproductive technologies, thereby adding even more stress to the experience of trying to produce a child.

Fortunately, as medical science continues to unravel the mysteries of human reproduction more is being learned about the causes of infertility, making it possible for physicians to better advise their patients about the timing of parenthood in their lives and to better diagnose fertility problems when these arise. Also, since the 1978 birth of the first baby through the advanced reproductive technology of *in vitro* fertilization, significantly more successful treatments have been and are continuing to be discovered and refined each year to help infertile couples realize their dreams of producing a child. Currently, approximately 50–70 percent of infertile couples who are able to access expert medical care eventually achieve a viable pregnancy. Those for whom treatment is not successful usually pursue other parenting options such as adoption, although some couples go on to construct very satisfying lives without children.

Related Entries: Aging, Coping, Human Sexuality, Pregnancy, STD Prevention, Stressful Life Events

BIBLIOGRAPHY

Daniluk, J. C. (2001). *The infertility survival guide: Everything you need to know to cope with the challenges while maintaining your sanity, dignity, and relationships.* Oakland, CA: New Harbinger.

Deveraux, L. L., & Hammerman, A. J. (1998). *Infertility and identity: New strategies for Treatment.* San Francisco: Jossey-Bass.

Hammer-Burns, L. H., & Covington, S. N. (Eds.). (1999). *Infertility counselling: A comprehensive handbook for clinicians.* New York: Parthenon.

Leiblum, S. R. (Ed.). (1997). *Infertility: Psychological issues and counseling strategies.* New York: Wiley.

JUDITH C. DANILUK

Irrational Health Beliefs Scale

The Irrational Health Belief Scale (IHBS) is a 20-item self-report measure designed to assess differences in the tendency of individuals to view or appraise health-related information or experiences in a distorted or irrational manner. Alan Christensen and his colleagues developed the IHBS with the belief that health behaviors and decisions are influenced not only by the knowledge an individual has about a health-related situation or decision, but by irrational health beliefs or appraisals as well. For example, patients prone to making overgeneralizations about health-related experiences might be more likely to perceive their physician's advice as unnecessary given a past experience that may be objectively irrelevant (e.g., "This advice was not useful when my friend tried it, therefore it is not useful for anyone"). Similarly, patients prone to making irrational inferences about common but unpleasant treatment side effects might be more likely to discount the value of a recommended treatment should side effects arise (e.g., "A medication that makes me feel tired can't be good for me").

Christensen and his colleagues believe that simply educating patients about their health and health recommendations is not sufficient for some individuals because of a tendency of these individuals to distort the information that they receive. Research findings from two studies were consistent with this premise. In a study involving 392 college students, a greater degree of distorted thinking as defined by the IHBS was uniquely and significantly associated with a less positive pattern of health practices (e.g., poorer nutrition, less exercise, greater alcohol and tobacco use). In a second study involving 107 individuals with Type 1 (insulin-dependent) diabetes, IHBS scores were associated with how successful patients were in maintaining blood sugar control as well as with self-reported adherence to the diabetic self-care regimen (e.g., blood glucose monitoring, insulin injections). Higher scores reflecting a greater tendency to view one's health irrationally were associated with poorer adherence and poorer glucose control. These findings may have implications for the design of psychoeducational approaches to health behavior change because they suggest that psychological intervention programs that help patients to identify and modify maladaptive, distorted thinking may be an important addition to more traditional health education approaches that rely solely on the provision of information to patients.

BIBLIOGRAPHY

Christensen, A. J., Moran, P. J., & Wiebe, J. S. (1999). Assessment of irrational health beliefs: Relation to health practices and medical regimen adherence. *Health Psychology, 18,* 169–176.

ALAN J. CHRISTENSEN

Jj

Jenkins Activity Survey

The Jenkins Activity Survey (JAS) was developed by C. David Jenkins, Stephen Zyzanski, and Ray Rosenman to measure Type A behavior, which consists of excessive achievement striving, competitiveness, time urgency, and hostility. Type A behavior had previously been implicated as a risk factor for coronary heart disease (CHD) when measured using a structured interview. Beginning with an initial pool of 50 questionnaire items, statistical analyses identified a subset of 21 items that best predicted Type A interview assessments. These include questions about being hard driving and competitive, setting quotas and deadlines for oneself, becoming impatient when others talk slowly, being quick and punctual, and having a high activity level. As a self-administered questionnaire, the JAS has practical advantages over the structured interview. Administration and scoring are more easily standardized and trained interviewers are not needed.

Research by David Glass provided evidence to support the construct validity of the JAS. Behavioral observation indicated that individuals identified as Type A on the basis of high JAS scores differed as expected from their Type B counterparts, individuals whose low JAS scores reflect a more relaxed, easy-going style. Type As were more likely to work hard to succeed, to suppress internal states (e.g., fatigue) that might interfere with achievement, to pace their activities rapidly, to become impatient when interrupted, and to express hostility when harassed. Research by Glass also supported a theoretical model in which Type A behaviors reflect a style of coping with environmental stressors that threaten personal control.

Other work has focused on measurement issues. For example, scoring systems have been developed in which subsets of JAS items are used to assess individual components of Type A separately. These include speed and impatience, job involvement, and hard-driving competitiveness. Although originally designed for research on coronary-prone behaviors, measures derived from the JAS have been used in a wide range of investigations in psychological and health science.

Cumulative findings have revealed that the JAS only partially captures Type A behaviors reflected in structured interview assessments, and does not reliably predict CHD. Various elements of Type A behavior are not as closely interrelated as was originally hypothesized, and not all confer coronary risk. JAS scores reflect time urgency and a pressured drive to succeed, but not the hostile, antagonistic style that largely accounts for associations between structured interview assessments and CHD. It also has been found that, compared with structured interview assessments, JAS scores are less consistently associated with physiologic activity thought to reflect mechanisms whereby Type A behaviors influence cardiovascular health. Because it does not appear predictive of CHD, some researchers have questioned the utility of continued use of the JAS in health research. However, as noted by Kenneth Hart, it is possible that the JAS identifies individuals at risk for general ill health, rather than detecting a specific vulnerability to coronary disease. Hart cites studies such as that of Jerry Suls and Christine Marco that indicate a predictive association between JAS scores and illness measures derived from medical charts.

Related Entry: Type A Behavior Pattern

BIBLIOGRAPHY

Glass, D. C. (1977). *Behavior patterns, stress, and coronary disease.* Hillsdale, NJ: Erlbaum.

Hart, K. E. (1997). A moratorium on research using the Jenkins Activity Survey for Type A behavior? *Journal of Clinical Psychology, 53*, 905–907.

Jenkins, C. D., Zyzanski, S. J., & Rosenman, R. H. (1971). Progress toward validation of a computer-scored test for the Type A coronary-prone behavior pattern. *Psychosomatic Medicine, 33*, 193–202.

Suls, J. M., & Marco, C. A. (1990). Relationship between JAS- and FTAS-Type A behavior and non-CHD illness: A prospective study controlling for negative affectivity. *Health Psychology, 9*, 479–492.

Richard J. Contrada

Kk

Kaplan, Robert M. (1947–)

Robert M. Kaplan was born in San Diego, California, on October 26, 1947. He is professor and chair of the Department of Family and Preventive Medicine at the University of California, San Diego (UCSD). He is a past president of several organizations, including the American Psychological Association Division of Health Psychology, Section J of the American Association for the Advancement of Science (Pacific), the International Society for Quality of Life Research, and the Society for Behavioral Medicine. He is chair of the Behavioral Science Council of the American Thoracic Society and president of the Academy of Behavioral Medicine Research. Dr. Kaplan is the editor-in-chief of the *Annals of Behavioral Medicine*, associate editor of the *American Psychologist*, and consulting editor of four other academic journals. Selected additional honors include APA Division of Health Psychology Annual Award for Outstanding Scientific Contribution (for a junior scholar in 1987 and for a senior scholar in 2001); Distinguished Research Lecturer (1988) and Health Net Distinguished Lecturer (1991); University of California 125 Anniversary Award for Most Distinguished Alumnus, University of California, Riverside; American Psychological Association Distinguished Lecturer; and the Distinguished Scientific Contribution Award from the American Association of Medical School Psychologists.

His public service contributions include various National Institutes of Health (NIH), Agency for Healthcare and Quality, and Veterans Administration grant review groups, and service on the local American Lung Association board of directors and the regional research committee for the American Heart Association. He has served as cochair of the Behavioral Committee for the NIH Women's Health Initiative and as a member of both the National Heart, Lung, and Blood

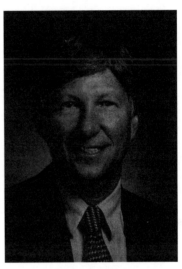

Kaplan, Robert M.

Institute (NHLBI) Behavioral Medicine Task Force and the Institute of Medicine National Academy of Sciences Committee on Health and Behavior. In addition, he is the chair of the Cost/Effectiveness Committee for the NHLBI National Emphysema Treatment Trial. Dr. Kaplan is the author or coauthor of more than a dozen books and more than 350 articles or chapters.

Over the past 30 years, Kaplan and his colleagues have developed a General Health Policy Model. The model is used to quantify the health status of populations, and combines measures of mortality, morbidity, and preference for health states. Measures based on the model are now used in research studies worldwide. The UCSD group introduced the concept of a quality-adjusted life year (QALY). When the U.S. Department of Health and Human Services set health objectives for the year 2010, the first overall objective was to increase QALYs for the U.S. population. The concept and model also served as the basis for a controversial policy in the state of Oregon to allocate health care resources according to their cost/utility.

ROBERT M. KAPLAN

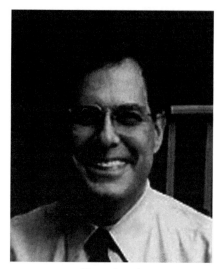

Krantz, David

Krantz, David

Dr. David Krantz is professor and chairman of the Department of Medical and Clinical Psychology at the Uniformed Services University (USUHS) in Bethesda, Maryland. He also holds appointments as professor of psychiatry and medicine (cardiology) at Georgetown University Medical Center. He received his BS from the City College of New York in 1971 and a PhD in psychology from the University of Texas at Austin in 1975, where he worked under the guidance of his mentor, Prof. David C. Glass. During the course of his graduate education, he also had the opportunity to interact with and learn from an unusually gifted cohort of fellow students who have since gone on to become noted health psychologists, including Karen Matthews, Sheldon Cohen, Michael Scheier, James Pennebaker, and Charles Carver.

Dr. Krantz has authored more than 160 scientific publications, including five books. The focus of his research has been on problems relating to the role of behavior in cardiovascular disorders and on other issues regarding the effects of psychological stress on human health. Early in his career, he worked on social-psychological and psychological aspects of the Type A behavior pattern. He also became interested in applications of personal control to health care and developed the Krantz Health Opinion Survey, an instrument for measuring preferences for information and self-treatment in health care.

Since the mid-1980s his research has focused on understanding the role of behavior, stress, and psychosocial factors as triggers of cardiac events such as myocardial ischemia (inadequate blood flow to heart tissue) and sudden cardiac death in heart patients. This work, which has been published regularly in both cardiology/medical and behavioral science journals, began with a series of collaborative studies with nuclear cardiologist Alan Rozanski, the first of which was published in the *New England Journal of Medicine*. This study demonstrated that acute mental stress could induce ischemia in more than 50 percent of cardiac patients, and that mental stress-ischemia was usually asymptomatic or "silent." Subsequent studies showed that mental stress could cause abnormal constriction in diseased coronary arteries, and studies done with James Blumenthal at Duke University and with colleague Willem Kop at USUHS showed that the presence of mental stress ischemia was an important predictor of subsequent cardiac health outcomes in coronary patients. Dr. Krantz's current work has expanded to look at electrocardiogram-derived markers of vulnerability to sudden cardiac death (t-wave alternans) that are responsive to mental stress in vulnerable patients with implantable cardiac defibrillators. Dr. Krantz's work has contributed toward increasing our understanding of how psychological stress affects cardiac physiology in vulnerable patients and has built important linkages between psychology and cardiology.

For his work, Dr. Krantz has twice received the American Psychological Association (APA) Annual Award for Outstanding Contributions to Health Psychology; he received the APA Early Career Scientific Award in 1982. He is a past president of the Academy of Behavioral Medicine Research and served as editor-in-chief of the APA journal *Health Psychology* from 1995 to 2000.

DAVID KRANTZ

Ll

Lay Referral Network

A lay referral network consists of friends, family, and others in a person's social context that may influence an individual's response to symptoms or perceived health threats. It may aid an individual in labeling symptoms, identifying their etiology, or improving symptom management. If one's lay referral network includes people with disease, one may be sensitized to certain symptoms. For example, individuals with a family history of heart disease may be more vigilant about recognizing symptoms of chest pain or shortness of breath. Surprisingly, consultation with others may result in either being encouraged or delayed in seeking medical attention. Delays in entering the medical treatment setting may be due to (1) the time-consuming nature of seeking out others and discussing symptoms, (2) reduced anxiety about one's well-being following discussion with a strong social support network, and (3) encouragement from others to continue to fulfill one's normal responsibilities and not seek medical care.

Related Entry: Social Support

NAN E. ROTHROCK

Lazarus, Richard S. (1922–2002)[1]

Lazarus obtained his BA in 1942 from the City College of New York. After military service in World War II, he returned to

---

[1] Dr. Lazarus passed away on November 24, 2002, in Walnut Creek, California.

graduate school in 1946, and obtained his doctorate at Pittsburgh in 1948. Afterward, he taught at Johns Hopkins and Clark University (where he directed clinical training), then came to Berkeley in 1957, where he remained until becoming an emeritus in 1991. In addition to lectures after retirement and an informal faculty–student colloquy that he organized with a colleague, he continued to write articles and books on psychological stress, coping, the emotions, and health issues.

Lazarus has been honored in many ways for his scholarly contributions. Among the most important are the 1989 Distinguished Scientific Contribution Award of the American Psychological Association (APA) and two honorary doctorates, one in 1988 from Johannes Gutenberg University in Mainz, Germany, the other in 1995 from Haifa University in Israel. The Division of Health Psychology of the APA presented him with its annual award in 1989 for outstanding contributions to health psychology. He is listed as the 80th of the 100 most eminent psychologists of the 20th century.

He has published more than 200 scientific articles and more than 20 books, both monographs and textbooks in personality and clinical psychology. In 1966, he published *Psychological Stress and the Coping Process*, which is regarded as a classic. He published *Stress, Appraisal, and Coping* with Susan Folkman in 1984, which continues to have worldwide influence. In 1991, he published *Emotion and Adaptation*, which extended his cognitive–motivational–relational theory of stress to the emotions.

Lazarus maintained that there are two main routes whereby psychological stress can affect health. One is through stress hormones that affect every organ of the body. The second is through the coping process. If you cope effectively, stress can be satisfying and under control rather than debilitating or dysfunctional. He has also written that how we manage our stress is a key factor in health and well-being. In effect, coping is an essential target of research on health outcomes.

In 1994, he and his wife, Bernice, published *Passion and Reason: Making Sense of Our Emotions.* His autobiography appeared in 1998, along with *Fifty Years of the Research and Theory of R. S. Lazarus: An Analysis of Historical and Perennial Issues.* This was followed in 1999 by *Stress and Emotion: A New Synthesis,* which extended and expanded his earlier views. A historically focused bird's-eye view of his pioneering work on stress, coping, and the emotions appeared in his chapter in a 2001 book edited by Scherer, Schorr, and Johnstone, *Appraisal Processes in Emotion.*

When Lazarus began his research and writing in 1948 there was little interest in stress except on the part of the military. By the 1970s, it had become apparent that stress, coping, and the emotions are inevitable features of daily life and play an important role in health and illness. He freely admitted that his own highly stressful childhood greatly influenced his interests in that subject. When asked whether his research helped him manage his own life stress, he responded that he is much better at giving advice to others than in following it himself.

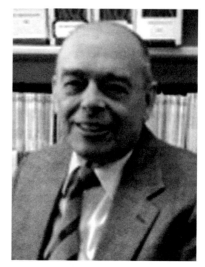

Leventhal, Howard

BIBLIOGRAPHY

Lazarus, R. S. (1966). *Psychological stress and the coping process.* New York: McGraw–Hill.

Lazarus, R. S. (1991). *Emotion and adaptation.* New York: Oxford University Press.

Lazarus, R. S. (1998a). *Fifty years of the research and theory of R. S. Lazarus: An analysis of historical and perennial issues.* Mahwah, NJ: Erlbaum.

Lazarus, R. S. (1998b). *The life and work of an eminent psychologist.* New York: Springer.

Lazarus, R. S. (1999). *Stress and emotion: A new synthesis.* New York: Springer.

Lazarus, R. S. (2001). Relational meaning and discrete emotions. In K. R. Scherer, A. Schorr, & T. Johnstone (Eds.), *Appraisal processes in emotion: Theory, methods, research* (pp. 37–67). Oxford: Oxford University Press

Lazarus, R. S., & Folkman, S. (1984). *Stress, appraisal, and coping.* New York: Springer.

Lazarus, R. S., & Lazarus, B. N. (1994). *Passion and reason: Making sense of our emotions.* New York: Oxford University Press.

RICHARD S. LAZARUS

Leventhal, Howard (1931–)

Howard Leventhal received his PhD in psychology from the University of North Carolina at Chapel Hill. He is the Board of Governors Professor of Health Psychology at Rutgers, the State University of New Jersey, and held previous faculty appointments at Yale University and the University of Wisconsin at Madison. Leventhal is best known for his research on commonsense models of illness and self-regulation in response to health threats.

Leventhal's early research challenged the assumption that simply exposing people to alarming information about health threats would elicit preventive health behaviors. Instead, in a 1965 study with Singer and Jones, Leventhal found that a frightening message about the risks of tetanus was ineffective in persuading students to be vaccinated. However, inoculation behavior was facilitated when that same appeal was accompanied by an action plan. The action plan merely asked students to consult their schedules and a campus map to anticipate how they could efficiently go about attaining their vaccines. The action plan was essential in allowing people to cope with the fearful emotions triggered by the threatening message.

Leventhal's fear appeal research presaged the development of his dual-process model of health and illness coping. The model's premise is that laypeople function as active problem solvers in the self-management of somatic threats. The model proposes that perceived threats are processed via parallel and semi-independent cognitive and affective routes.

The cognitive pathway involves commonsense models or representations of illness, which incorporate lay symptom labels, temporal expectations, and personal beliefs about etiology, consequences, and treatment. Illness representations prompt coping behaviors (e.g., gathering information); coping effectiveness is evaluated on an ongoing basis and such feedback may modify the individual's understanding of the health threat. Leventhal and colleagues Safer, Tharps, and Jackson characterized the person suffering symptoms as a sort of lay diagnostician who, before entering the health care delivery system, evaluated whether he or she was ill (appraisal delay), whether the illness warranted professional intervention (illness delay), and whether the benefits of treatment were likely to outweigh its costs (utilization delay).

Meyer, Leventhal, and Gutmann found that hypertension patients were more likely to be compliant in taking their prescribed medications when they believed that they could detect symptoms of elevated blood pressure—even though hypertension is an asymptomatic disorder and the patients' medications had no objective effects on their mislabeled symptoms. This study is a classic example of how lay conceptualizations of illness determine behavior, even when those representations would be viewed as inaccurate by health care providers.

In addition to coping directly with symptoms or other health threats, people also must deal with accompanying unpleasant emotions such as fear or anger. The affective path of Leventhal's dual-process model also involves coping, appraisal, and feedback, but here the coping efforts are directed toward affect regulation and may involve strategies such as distraction and relaxation. The early fear appeal research described in the foregoing illustrates how negative emotion can inhibit health-relevant behaviors unless the individual is provided with a strategy that allows fear reduction. Along related lines, Johnson and Leventhal (1974) found that patients undergoing endoscopy were less distressed and less likely to gag during the procedure if they first were given information about typical sensations and coping strategies such as deep breathing. Other important work includes Leventhal and Cleary's multiple-regulation model of smoking, which posits that physiologic factors alone cannot explain smoking behavior. Smoking also has cognitive and emotional underpinnings that contribute to persistent cravings even after nicotine has be cleared from the individual's metabolism.

In 1984, Leventhal received the Senior Investigator Award for Outstanding Contributions to Health Psychology from Division 38 of the American Psychological Association. He is a member of the Institute of Medicine of the National Academy of Science.

Related Entries: Cognitive Representations of Illness, Fear Appeals, Self-Regulation, Treatment Delay

BIBLIOGRAPHY

Johnson, J. E., & Leventhal, H. (1974). Effects of accurate expectations and behavioral instructions on reactions during a noxious medical examination. *Journal of Personality and Social Psychology, 29*, 710–718.

Leventhal, H., & Cleary, P. S. (1980). The smoking problem: A review of the research and theory in behavioral risk modification. *Psychological Bulletin, 88*, 370–405.

Leventhal, H., Leventhal, E. A., & Cameron, L. (2001). Representations, procedures, and affect in illness self-regulation: A perceptual–cognitive model. In A. Baum, T. A. Revenson, & J. E. Singer (Eds.), *Handbook of health psychology* (pp. 19–47). Mahwah, NJ: Erlbaum.

RENÉ MARTIN

Life Orientation Test

The Life Orientation Test (LOT) provides a measure of dispositional optimism. The LOT was used in early studies examining the effects of optimism and pessimism in health-related domains. Subsequently, the LOT was superseded by a modified version called the Life Orientation Test–Revised (LOT–R). The LOT–R consists of six coded items plus four filler items. Half the coded items are worded in an optimistic way, half in a pessimistic way, and respondents indicate the degree of their agreement or disagreement with each item on a 5-point scale. The LOT–R has good internal consistency and is reliable over time. Because of item overlap, the correlation between the LOT and the LOT–R is extremely high. Both scales provide continuous distributions of scores, which tend to be positively skewed, but not greatly so. There is no empirical criterion to use to categorize people as optimistic or pessimistic.

Related Entries: Coping, Hardiness, Optimism and Health, Stressful Life Events

BIBLIOGRAPHY

Scheier, M. F., & Carver, C. S. (1985). Optimism, coping and health: Assessment and implications of generalized outcome expectancies. *Health Psychology, 4*, 219–247.

Scheier, M. F., Carver, C. S., & Bridges, M. W. (1994). Distinguishing optimism from neuroticism (and trait anxiety, self-mastery, and self-esteem): A reevaluation of the Life Orientation Test. *Journal of Personality and Social Psychology, 67*, 1063–1078.

MICHAEL F. SCHEIER

Mm

Managed Mental Health Care

The generic term managed care refers to various administrative and financial arrangements to regulate the site, cost, and utilization of health services. As health care costs began to escalate in the early 1960s, insurance companies, purchasers, and consumers became increasingly concerned, and different delivery models were developed with the intention of controlling costs and increasing efficiency. More than 160 million people in the United States are now covered by some form of managed care, with numbers continuing to grow.

In the United States, the most notable forms are health maintenance organizations (HMOs) and preferred provider organizations (PPOs). HMOs are "Health care systems that finance and deliver comprehensive health care services. Services are provided to an enrolled group of people for a prepaid fixed sum of money." PPOs are "Companies that organize their own network of providers to deliver services and establish fees. . . . The PPO arranges for services to be provided, but does not provide the services" (Tuttle & Woods, 1997, pp. 127–128). In the last decade, versions of the HMO model have predominated and largely incorporated the PPO model.

Within HMOs, there are also important distinctions, including for-profit versus not-for profit, staff/group model versus network model, and single specialty (e.g., psychiatry) versus comprehensive (e.g., full medical) services. Independent studies repeatedly show that top ratings for quality and patient satisfaction go to nonprofit, staff-model organizations (in which providers are salaried employees within a comprehensive system rather than private practitioners being paid piecemeal to see individual patients). Most mental health care is provided by separate ("carve-out") companies, however, as Sanchez and Turner (2003) note, although there are considerable pressures for mental health services to be part of integrated ("carve-in") comprehensive programs.

Cutting across different delivery systems, ideally there are eight characteristics common to psychotherapy and behavioral health services under managed care: (1) specific problem solving, (2) rapid response and early intervention, (3) clear definition of patient and therapist responsibilities, (4) flexible use of time, (5) interdisciplinary cooperation, (6) multiple formats and modalities, (7) intermittent treatment or a "family practitioner" model, and (8) a strong orientation toward results and accountability (Hoyt, 2000). Important nuances for diverse cultural, ethnic, and socioeconomic groups must also be considered.

The espoused meta-goals of managed care are (1) increased access, with universal access being the ideal, (2) increased effectiveness and an emphasis on accurate outcomes assessment and doing what works, and (3) benefits preservation and maintaining coverage for treatments having clinical/medical necessity.

So far, however, efforts toward cost containment have been primary. Managed mental health care (sometimes called managed behavioral health care) has been through several generations since the early 1960s, each adding different ways to control costs. Total cost is the product of the per-session price times the number of sessions. Managed care has developed various mechanisms to hold down both. Primary mechanisms to reduce utilization include (1) requiring pretreatment authorization or certification, (2) carefully limiting the range of diagnoses and treatments that will be covered, (3) designing benefit plans to encourage use of efficient providers, and (4) requiring patients to make copayments to share costs. Primary mechanisms to control the price per session include (1) setting a limited payment for a defined group of beneficiaries, (2) offering lower fee-for-service payments to providers, (3) presetting the payment for certain diagnostic groups, (4) reviewing claims, and (5) extending insurance coverage to supposedly equally (or at least adequately) effective treatment alternatives (e.g., groups instead of one-to-one meetings, medications instead of counseling). Different managed care organizations use different combinations of these methods, and clinicians and patients need to know the different rules as they wend their way through what is sometimes formidable paperwork.

Kaiser Permanente Health Plan, which continues to receive high ratings for quality and satisfaction, was the first large not-for-profit staff-model HMO. Kaiser was also the first, beginning in the late 1950s, to include mental health coverage as part of its comprehensive benefits package (Cummings, 2002). Until then, it was feared that including psychotherapy would drastically increase costs. Research showed, however, just the opposite, that providing focused psychiatric services actually helped to control and reduce overall costs. This finding, which is called the medical utilization offset phenomenon, has been replicated in various settings numerous times. Many patient visits to medical doctors do not involve any "objective" findings, and other seemingly "medical" problems, such as diabetes, asthma, and headaches, often have a large psychosocial component (e.g., emotional stress, interpersonal conflict, and noncompliance with medical regimens). One of the results of research demonstrating the positive impact of focused psychological intervention on medical utilization has been the development of health psychology and the breaking down of the false dichotomy of mind–body dualism in favor of movement toward the integration of primary care and behavioral health care. The provision of mental health services in the context of general medical/surgical practice highlights the importance of interdisciplinary collaboration, including the training of health psychologists in the areas of medicine and psychopharmacology as well as the training of physicians and nurses to be able to detect and accurately diagnose psychiatric conditions such as depression, anxiety disorders, and alcohol and substance abuse.

Managed care, especially within the for-profit and carve-out sector, has generated much controversy and criticism. By definition, managed care involves someone other than the particular clinician and client managing or regulating the type and length of services to be provided and paid for. Although some (especially not-for-profit) companies have made significant achievements (including some attention toward prevention and early detection and treatment), numerous complaints have been made, some with documentation, that some patients have been denied needed and covered services. In addition to possible undertreatment and patient abandonment, other concerns involve the continuing likelihood and autonomy of health care professionals, issues of provider competence, dual relationships and potential conflicts of interest, confidentiality and privacy, the balancing of responsibilities toward individuals and the larger society, and conflicts between managed care and various models of psychotherapy. Problems remain of what to do (and

how to pay for it) regarding patients with chronic conditions, including those with persistent and debilitating mental illness and severe personality disorders. The various issues, physical and mental, presented by an aging population are also a continuing and growing concern.

The ethical, clinically appropriate, and fiscally viable realization of the principles and promises of managed care are continuing challenges. It will be important that those who care to manage must manage to care—about people *and* profits. The alternative will be "mangled care," not "managed care."

BIBLIOGRAPHY

Aronson, J. (1997). *The dictionary of managed behavioral health care.* Washington, DC: Brunner/Mazel.

Chiles, J., Lambert, M. J., & Hatch, A. L. (1999). The impact of psychosocial interventions on medical cost offset: A meta-analytic review. *Clinical Psychology: Science and Practice, 6,* 204–220.

Cummings, N. A. (2002). The founding of the Kaiser Permanente Mental Health System: How the first comprehensive psychotherapy benefit was written. In *The collected papers of Nicholas A. Cummings: Vol. 2. The entrepreneur in psychology* (pp. 1–18). Phoenix, AZ: Zeig, Tucker & Theisen.

Cummings, N. A., Cummings, J. L., & Johnson, J. N. (Eds.). (1997). *Behavioral health in primary care: A guide for clinical integration.* Madison, CT: Psychosocial Press.

Cummings, N. A., & Follette, W. T. (1968). Psychiatric services and medical utilization in a prepaid health plan setting: Part 2. *Medical Care, 6,* 31–41.

Cummings, N. A., O'Donohue, W., Hayes, S. C., & Follette, V. (Eds.). (2001). *Integrated behavioral healthcare: Positioning mental health practice with medical/surgical practice.* San Diego, CA: Academic.

Dea, R. A. (2000). The integration of primary care and behavioral healthcare in Northern California Kaiser Permanente. *Psychiatric Quarterly, 71,* 17–29.

Follette, W. T., & Cummings, N. A. (1967). Psychiatric services and medical utilization in a prepaid health plan setting: Part 1. *Medical Care, 5,* 25–35.

Hersch, L. (1995). Adapting to health care reform and managed care: Three strategies for survival and growth. *Professional Psychology: Research and Practice, 26,* 16–26.

Hoyt, M. F. (1995). *Brief therapy and managed care: Readings for contemporary practice.* San Francisco: Jossey-Bass.

Hoyt, M. F. (2000). *Some stories are better than others: Doing what works in brief therapy and managed care.* Philadelphia: Brunner/Mazel.

Miller, I. J. (1996). Managed care is harmful to outpatient mental health services: A call for accountability. *Professional Psychology: Research and Practice, 27,* 349–363.

Mumford, E., Schlesinger, H., Glass, G., Patrick, C., & Cuerdon, R. (1984). A new look at evidence about reduced cost of medical utilization following mental-health treatment. *American Journal of Psychiatry, 141,* 1145–1158.

Sanchez, L. M., & Turner, S. M. (2003). Practicing psychology in the era of managed care: Implications for practice and training. *American Psychologist, 58,* 116–129.

Simon, R. (2001). Psychotherapy soothsayer: Nick Cummings foretells your future. *Psychotherapy Networker, 25*(4), 34–39, 62.

Sturm, R., & Wells, K. B. (1995). How can care for depression become more cost-effective? *Journal of the American Medical Association, 273,* 51–58.

Tuttle, G. McC., & Woods, D. R. (1997). *The managed care answer book for mental health professionals.* Bristol, PA: Brunner/Mazel.

VandenBos, G. R., Cummings, N. A., & DeLeon, P. H. (1992). A century of psychotherapy: Economic and environmental influences. In D. K. Freedheim (Ed.), *History of psychotherapy: A century of change* (pp. 65–102). Washington, DC: American Psychological Association.

Weitz, R. D. (Ed.). (2000). *Psycho-economics: Managed care in mental health in the new millennium.* New York: Haworth.

MICHAEL F. HOYT

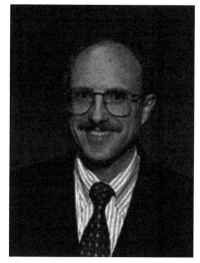

Manuck, Stephen B.

Manuck, Stephen B. (1948–)

Stephen B. Manuck was born on December 3, 1948, in San Francisco, California. He is currently a professor in the Department of Psychology at the University of Pittsburgh, where he is also chair of the Graduate Program in Biological and Health Psychology and directs the Behavioral Physiology Laboratory. Before moving to Pittsburgh in 1980, Manuck taught at the University of Virginia and the Bowman Gray School of Medicine (now Wake Forest University School of Medicine). He is a graduate of the University of California at Davis (BA, 1970) and Vanderbilt University (PhD, 1974). Over much of his career, Manuck has studied cardiovascular reactions to psychological stress and their role in the development of heart disease. Research conducted in his laboratory demonstrates that stress-induced cardiovascular responses vary appreciably among individuals. These differences are stable over time, have both genetic and environmental determinants, and are correlated with personality factors that confer risk for ischemic heart disease. In addition, people who respond to stress with the largest cardiovascular reactions are more likely than others to exhibit preclinical vascular pathology or to have a history of coronary disease. Other work in Manuck's laboratory shows that exposure to acute psychological stress also suppresses aspects of cellular immunity.

With Jay R. Kaplan of Wake Forest University School of Medicine, Manuck also studies biological mechanisms underlying the behavioral exacerbation of coronary artery disease in nonhuman primates. This work has shown that socially dominant (high-status) male cynomolgus monkeys develop coronary atherosclerosis of greater severity than subordinate (low-status) animals, but only among monkeys living in unstable, or stressful, social conditions. This worsening of atherosclerosis in dominant males was found to be mediated by activation of the sympathetic nervous system. Among females, on the other hand, socially subordinate animals develop the greatest atherosclerosis. This results from the chronic suppression of ovarian function that characterizes subordinated female mammals generally, and can be mitigated by estrogen supplementation with contraceptive steroids. Finally, Manuck and Kaplan have shown that, like

humans, monkeys vary greatly in the magnitude of their cardiac reactions to stress and that among both males and females, animals exhibiting the largest psychophysiologic responses also develop the most extensive coronary atherosclerosis. Together, these studies provide a basis in experimental pathobiology for analogous observations in the social epidemiology of humans.

Currently, Manuck's laboratory is studying neurobiological factors that may underlie multiple sources of behavioral and biological risk for cardiovascular disease and the application of neurogenetics to health psychology. Manuck is a past president of the Academy of Behavioral Medicine Research (1993–1994), chaired the Task Force on Behavioral Research in Cardiovascular, Lung, and Blood Health and Disease for the National Heart, Lung, and Blood Institute (1998), and represents health psychology on the National Advisory Committee for the Decade of Behavior.

STEPHEN B. MANUCK

McGill Pain Questionnaire

The McGill Pain Questionnaire (MPQ) was developed by Melzack in 1975 to assess different components of perceived, subjective pain. Respondents are required to choose the words that best describe their pain from a list of 78 adjectives. The adjectives are grouped into 20 subclasses describing different aspects of pain. There are three major categories of pain descriptors in the MPQ—sensory, affective, and evaluative—and separate scores for each can be derived. In addition, the Present Pain Intensity (PPI) score is obtained by asking the patient,

"Which word describes your pain right now?" and presents five descriptors that range from 1 (*mild*) to 5 (*excruciating*).

Melzack (1987) also introduced a short form of the MPQ (SF–MPQ). This takes only a couple of minutes to complete, correlates highly with the standard version, and is sensitive to treatment-related changes in pain report. It is frequently employed in clinical trials of new analgesic drugs. The MPQ, in standard and short forms, has been translated into many languages and is the most widely used method for the measurement of subjective pain experience.

Related Entries: Gate Theory of Pain, Pain

BIBLIOGRAPHY

Melzack, R. (1975). The McGill Pain Questionnaire: Major properties and scoring methods. *Pain, 1,* 277–299.
Melzack, R. (1987). The short-form McGill Pain Questionnaire. *Pain, 30,* 191–197.
Melzack, R., and Katz, J. (2001). The McGill Pain Questionnaire: appraisal and current status. In D. Turk and R. Melzack (Eds.), *Handbook of pain assessment* (pp. 35–52). New York: Guilford.

RONALD MELZACK

Medical Anthropology

Medical anthropology has traditionally been concerned with how people in non-Western societies explain the causes of ill health, how their disease categories and etiologies differ from Western nosologies, and how specific cultural practices may either protect people from, or make them more vulnerable to, disease. There are three dominant approaches in medical anthropology: ecological, interpretive, and critical.

The ecological approach examines human–environment interaction and how these interactions may put sectors of the population at differential risk of disease and injury. Well-known examples include the study of cultural adaptations to malaria and the increase in schistosomiasis as a result of development projects that increase irrigation. Some ecological medical anthropologists also examine how population health status has changed throughout human history, examining, through skeletal remains, for example, how the Neolithic revolution, in which humans changed from being foragers to agriculturalists, led to increases in parasite load and decreases in nutritional status.

The symbolic or interpretive paradigm in medical anthropology grew out of the study of non-Western religions, specifically the analysis of rituals intended to restore the health of the individual or group, and is concerned with analyzing non-biomedical understandings of sickness in both Western and non-Western contexts. Central to the interpretive approach has been the distinction between "disease"—abnormalities in the functioning of biologic organs and systems—and "illness"—the cultural understandings of and responses to such malfunctioning. This distinction has been useful to medical anthropologists who encounter societies with quite elaborate systems of illness classification that do not correspond to Western biomedical nosologies.

The critical perspective in medical anthropology examines how the global capitalist economy and (neo)colonial histories have put people at increased risk for poor health through shaping the environments people live in, their access to biomedical care, the labor structures that rupture communities, and the erosion of indigenous medical systems. Critical perspectives have also critiqued biomedicine as a system that locates disease within individuals rather than within inequitable social relations, thereby obscuring ultimate causes of disease.

All three paradigms have addressed issues of mental health. Medical anthropologists have posed such questions as the following. Do all societies exhibit similar incidences of depression or schizophrenia? Is psychopathology manifested similarly cross-culturally, or is illness behavior governed by cultural rules which shape the expression of symptoms? Can we assess mental illness in other societies by using the theoretical constructs of Western psychiatry, or are the DSM and other nosologies of psychopathology problematic in contexts that differently interpret deviations from normal behavior? For example, dissociative states are widely found in human societies; however, this behavior is not universally medicalized, and in some world areas it is interpreted as indicating a "patient's" special access to the divine. Through posing such questions, medical anthropologists have consistently challenged generalizations about health psychology premised on Western understandings of "normal" behavior and based solely on research with Western populations.

BIBLIOGRAPHY

Baer, H., Singer, M., & Susser, I. (1997). *Medical anthropology and the world system: A critical perspective.* Westport, CT: Bergin & Garvey.
Brown, P. (1981). Cultural adaptation to endemic malaria in Sardinia. *Medical Anthropology, 5,* 311–339.
Brown, P. (1998). Understanding medical anthropology: Biocultural and cultural approaches. In P. Brown (Ed.), *Understanding and applying medical anthropology* (pp. 00–00). Mountain View, CA: Mayfield.
Cohen, M., & Armelagos, G. (Eds.). (1984). *Paleopathology at the origins of agriculture.* New Haven, CT: Yale University Press.
DesJarlais, R., & Kleinman, A. (Eds.). (1995). *World mental health: Problems, priorities and responses in low-income countries.* New York: Oxford University Press.

Gaines, A. (1992). *Ethnopsychiatry: The cultural construction of professional and folk psychiatries.* Albany, NY: State University of New York Press.

Hahn, R. (1995). *Sickness and healing: An anthropological perspective.* New Haven, CT: Yale University Press.

Heyneman, D. (1974). Dams and disease. *Human Nature, 2,* 50–57.

Hughes, C. (1990). Ethnopsychiatry. In T. Johnson and C. Sargent (Eds.), *Medical anthropology: Contemporary theory and method* (pp. 00–00). New York: Praeger.

Kleinman, A., Eisenberg, L., & Good, B. (1978). Culture, illness and care: Clinical lessons from anthropologic and cross-cultural research. *Annals of Internal Medicine, 88,* 251–258.

Rubel, A. (1964). The epidemiology of a folk illness: *Susto* in Hispanic America. *Ethnology, 3,* 268–283.

Scheper-Hughes, N. (1979). *Saints, scholars and schizophrenics: Mental illness in rural Ireland.* Berkeley: University of California Press.

Taussig, M. (1980). Reification and the consciousness of the patient. *Social Science and Medicine, 14B,* 3–13.

Turshen, M. (1984). *The political ecology of disease in Tanzania.* New Brunswick, NJ: Rutgers University Press.

Wardlow, H. (1996). 'Sympathy for my body': Breast cancer and mammography at two Atlanta clinics. *Medical Anthropology, 16,* 319–340.

Wardlow, H. (2002). Giving birth to *Gonolia*: 'Culture' and sexually transmitted disease among the Huli of Papua New Guinea. *Medical Anthropology Quarterly, 16,* 151–175.

Wiley, A. (1992). Adaptation and the biocultural paradigm in medical anthropology: A critical review. *Medical Anthropology Quarterly, 6,* 216–236.

HOLLY WARDLOW

Medical Student's Disease

Medical student's disease is the phenomenon that occurs when medical students develop groundless concerns about their own bodily sensations and falsely connect their symptoms to an illness with a known disease label. These reactions are often transient and are associated with a disease being studied at the time. Medical student's disease is a source of considerable emotional distress, which can interfere with success in medical school. To reduce their anxiety, students may seek reassurance from instructors and physicians, or they may pursue an extensive study of the disease in question. The process of matching personal symptoms to illness has been suggested to affect 70–80 percent of medical students. However, more recent studies have failed to find a prevalence of hypochondrial fears in medical students as compared with other student groups. Medical student's disease has also been termed "hypochondriasis of medical students," "nosophobia," or "medical studentitis."

Related Entry: Hypochondriasis

HEATHER WADE

Medication Event Monitoring System

Medication event monitoring (mem) is a method for quantifying ambulatory patients' exposure to prescription drugs. It compiles patients' drug-dosing histories with time-stamping electronic microcircuitry incorporated into pharmaceutical packages. Integral microswitches or optical sensors detect one or more predefined maneuvers made with the package that are required for removal of a dose of drug. The microcircuit automatically records the time and date whenever the microswitches/sensors indicate the occurrence of those maneuvers, which constitute the "medication event." No special action by the patient is required. The mem principle is adaptable to any type of package and thus far has been applied to cup-type packages for solid oral dosage forms, aerosol dispensers for inhaled drugs, unit-dose "blister" packages, and eyedrop dispensers. Each type of package has its own medication event.

Why compile patients' dosing histories? It is basic to understanding the clinical and economic consequences of commonly occurring deviations from prescribed drug regimens. The need for such understanding has grown in direct relation to the ever-growing interventional power of prescription drugs. All drug actions depend on both the size and the timing of doses. When prescribed drug treatment fails, as often occurs, the dosing history rules in or out inadequate dosing as the reason. Thus, a reliable dosing history is a form of diagnostic test, with much more information than most diagnostic tests, as it is a running record, over weeks or months, rather than a measurement made at a single point in time. Using the dosing history as input to a suitable pharmacokinetic model, one can compute the entire time–history course of a drug's concentration in plasma.

A mem record is interpreted as a dosing history on the assumption that the patient took the correct dose at each recorded time and date. This assumption is widely accepted as correct, but not flawless, by the authors of over 600 scientific papers, reviews, editorials, and book chapters that describe clinical research based on mem system monitoring. This periodically updated bibliography is at www.aardex.ch/.

Events can, of course, be entered into the memory at times when no medication is taken, for example, when the package is opened for refilling by a pharmacist, or if the customary sequence of medication event and dose taking is interrupted, or if a patient seeks to compile a false record of dosing. Falsification is difficult because the package must be entered at each scheduled dosing time for weeks or months—not impossible, but demanding. Occasional extraneous events have little impact on data interpretation in long-term treatment, but in short treatments care is needed to avoid extraneous events.

The data generated by mem include the length of the interval between each dose. For many drugs, the lengths of these intervals provide the greatest statistical explanatory power for drug actions and pharmaceutical outcomes. To help patients execute prescribed drug regimens correctly, a computer-generated display of their dosing history is useful for pinpointing dosing errors and when they occurred. Several widely used graphical formats can be seen at www.aardex.ch/.

Related Entry: Patient Adherence

BIBLIOGRAPHY

Cramer, J. A. (1995). Microelectronic systems for monitoring and enhancing patient compliance with medication regimens. *Drugs, 49,* 321–327.

Kastrissios, H., & Blaschke, T. F. (1997). Medication compliance as a feature in drug development. *Annual Review of Pharmacology and Toxicology, 37,* 451–475.

Urquhart, J., & de Klerk, E. (1998). Contending paradigms for the interpretation of data on patient compliance with therapeutic drug regimens. *Statistics in Medicine, 17,* 251–267.

JOHN URQUHART

Meditation

In both religious and nonreligious contexts, people have practiced a variety of forms of meditation for thousands of years. The shifting of mental focus and awareness is a common theme shared across types of meditation that otherwise differ in procedures and psychological objectives. These procedures and psychological objectives are highly influenced by cultural outlook. In this entry, Western and Eastern philosophical views of meditation are discussed, followed by a survey of research. To illustrate how meditation defies a singular definition, the entry leads off with a brief presentation of some differing perspectives on this phenomenon. The entry closes with a call for the integration of Eastern and Western perspectives as a means of shedding light on meditation and its effects.

WHAT IS MEDITATION?

Meditation has been characterized, for example, as (1) one of the many procedures that elicit a salubrious state of restorative relaxation (namely, relaxation response), (2) a means to gain enhanced self-awareness through inner reflection, (3) a method of ritualized prayer or reciting of holy verses designed to unify the practitioner with God, or (4) a means of unifying with the true way of nature through disciplined mental exercises designed to unfetter the mind of illusory conceptions of reality. That is, objectives range from the spiritual unity with God characteristic of Judeo-Christian and Islamic practices; to the development of a higher, cosmic consciousness associated with yogic-based practices (e.g., Transcendental Meditation, TM); to the Zen cultivation of pure seeing or perception as a way of coping with universal suffering; to the induction of the relaxation response to reduce the damaging effects of the stress of modern living that is characteristic of the Western tradition. In short, the characterization and objectives of meditation vary as a function of cultural and sociological developmental milieus.

AMELIORATION OF STRESS: THE WESTERN INTEREST

With advances in industrialization and technology (e.g., improved sanitation, housing, and medical care), diseases of lifestyle (e.g., heart disease, high blood pressure, diabetes, and some cancers) have replaced the chief causes of death prior to 1900 (namely, infectious diseases and trauma). Unhealthy aspects of the modern Western lifestyle include a chronic sense of (1) "hurry–worry" triggered by the demands of a fast-paced, competitive society, (2) poor nutrition, (3) increased substance abuse, (4) pollution, (5) lack of exercise, and (6) loss of social support. Our modern ways appear linked to behavioral and psychological processes that are discordant with the Stone Age biology we inherited through evolution. For decades researchers have posited and reported evidence supporting the notion that a frequent and excessive induction of the fight-or-flight response contributes to stress-related diseases.

Briefly, our body is constantly working at striking a balance between energy conservation (rest and restoration) and energy expenditure (physiological adaptations for exercise, or for attack or defensive maneuvers). Rest and restoration are the domain of the parasympathetic nervous system (PSNS), whereas adaptation to states of physical exertion, threat, and emergency are the domain of the sympathetic nervous system (SNS), which is linked to the fight-or-flight response. The brain's registering of threatening or crisis situations triggers the SNS and reduces PSNS activity and also sets in motion a cascade of events inducing the release of stress hormones (bodily created substances that are released into the blood stream for regulation of the body's responses). The relaxation response, with its decreased respiration, muscle tension, and cardiovascular activation characteristic of PSNS dominance, has been conceptualized as a "hypometabolic state" associated with a quieting and calming of both the mind and the body and, thus, rest and restoration.

Given these considerations, Western researchers have focused on examining the attenuation of fight-or-flight-induced arousal as a means of investigating the psychological and physical benefits of meditation.

ANXIETY DISTRESS

Anxiety, or the experience of worry, tension, and/or bodily arousal (e.g., cold, sweaty hands), is though to reflect high levels of arousal. Meditators have been reported to self-report lower anxiety and depressed mood levels than nonmeditators. Studies randomly assigning persons without prior meditation experience to either a meditation group or a nonmeditation control group showed that the greatest decreases in anxiety occurred for those taught meditation. The effects of meditation on the frequent and across-situation experience of anxiety (trait anxiety) was examined using meta-analysis, which combines statistics testing differences between groups (e.g., meditators vs. nonmeditators) across studies to yield an average statistic showing the strength of the treatment effect. The meta-analysis showed that TM displayed the strongest effect of all the relaxation techniques. Moreover, concentration meditation (i.e., focusing on an external object like a vase) showed the weakest effect. However, studies exist showing no effects of meditation on levels of anxiety, and that the effects of meditation do not necessarily generalize to behavioral or physiological markers of anxiety. Furthermore, it has been reported that prospective meditators high in trait anxiety appear more likely to not complete the study and to benefit less from the intervention. Finally, studies of short duration (i.e., less than 3 months) often did not reveal meditation effects.

MARKERS OF PHYSICAL HEALTH

One randomized study of older African Americans with mildly elevated blood pressure showed TM to be more effective at lowering blood pressure than either progressive muscle relaxation or education only. In a study of people at high risk for cardiovascular disease (high blood pressure, high cholesterol, and/or tobacco use), persons randomized to meditation/relaxation plus health education, relative to those randomized to a health education only group, showed lower blood pressure and cholesterol levels, thereby suggesting reduced risk for heart disease; the blood pressure results were maintained 4 years postintervention, and the cholesterol differences were present at 8 months postintervention. Similarly, for a group of adolescents with blood pressure elevated for their age and gender, those randomly assigned to TM, relative to those randomly assigned to a health education control group, showed decreases

in resting systolic blood pressure and reduced cardiovascular reactivity to psychological stress. Relative to patients randomized into a control group, a meditation/mindfulness group (i.e., passive nonjudgmental awareness of thoughts, feelings, breathing, and bodily sensations) showed a more rapid response to the medical treatment for psoriasis (skin disorder). In a longitudinal study of elderly participants, those randomly assigned to a TM condition showed improved memory function, lower systolic blood pressure, and greater longevity than persons not taught TM. Other studies report meditation to reduce stress hormones (chemical messengers activating bodily responses via the blood stream; e.g., cortisol) and foster adjustment to chronic pain.

SUMMARY AND CONCLUSIONS

Even though a corpus of evidence indicates that meditation positively affects the affective, psychological, and physical functioning of practitioners, our current state of knowledge is still quite limited, despite decades of research. Studies typically deploy small samples. Moreover, there is a paucity of randomized group studies examining the impact of factors such as (1) expectancy and demand characteristics (e.g., placebo effects or rituals designed to cultivate a positive expectation of change), (2) duration of treatment, (3) amount of meditation (how many times per day and how much time per meditation), (4) type of meditation (e.g., sitting with eyes open while counting breaths vs. eyes closed while silently repeating a mantra), (5) the critical elements of meditation (e.g., focusing and refocusing attention on a single object vs. allowing attention to flow, in a nonjudgmental manner, with the changing contents of consciousness), (6) amount of time as a practitioner, (7) religious- versus non-religious-affiliated meditation (e.g., Sufi meditation practices vs. Benson's secular approach), and (8) the mechanisms distinguishing different types of meditation from each other as well as from other types of relaxation procedures. Although comparing meditators to nonmeditators (i.e., case–control studies) have yielded some differences (e.g., trait anxiety, blood pressure, and pulse rate), these differences can result from the drawing of samples from two different groups (those who chose to meditate versus those who did not). Recall that persons who meditate tend to manifest a profile of low reported psychological symptoms, and highly anxious people tend to drop out of meditation training. These studies of anxiety are consistent with the notion that case–control studies cannot separate pre-existing group differences involving a myriad of psychological, biological, demographic, and lifestyle factors from the effects of meditation.

Whether the effects of meditation are unique or simply represent a general relaxation response or states of simple rest has been debated. For example, it has been reported that the peripheral changes associated with increased PSNS (e.g., reductions in respiration, heart rate, or sweat glands) are equivalent to simply resting. Studies incorporating brain waves (electroencephalogram) and behavior (slow, rolling eye movements or gross bodily jerks) indicated that experienced meditators lapsed into sleep episodes or hovered between drowsiness and wakefulness; some argue that, like the studies of peripheral responses, this shows meditation is merely a state of rest or low arousal, whereas others argue that such hovering reflects the ability to shift attention to maintain a state between sleep and wakefulness. Again, most of the evidence relates to case–control studies or studies of a handful of meditators (e.g., five persons of the Sufism), making it difficult to separate the effects of the meditation from the characteristics of the persons meditating.

In sum, there is a body of evidence indicating the salubrious effects of meditation. However, methodological shortcomings obfuscate the mechanisms of how meditation affects physical and psychological well-being. Likewise, failure to obtain clear results may result from the disconnection of the Western, behavioral methods from the objectives of mediation practices developed in non-Western cultures. For example, some Zen practices are oriented to a nonjudgmental awareness of the ebb and flow of thoughts, emotions, bodily sensations, and images to develop perceptions less biased by emotional needs. How is a measure of trait anxiety or heart rate on one or more occasions going to address this phenomenon? For research in this area to progress substantially, it is important to recognize that conceptual views of meditation vary widely, and to work at developing methods and procedures that reflect these views and objectives rather than attempting to make the phenomenon fit our available and convenient Western methods. It is time to go beyond viewing meditation as primarily a tool for reducing stress-induced arousal, particularly because it is known that patterns of arousal vary among people (e.g., some people may primarily react through the cardiovascular system, others through the gastrointestinal system). In other words, it is time to undertake a biopsychosocial integrative approach, in which cognitive measures of attention and memory, measures of brain function, patterns of SNS and PSNS responding, markers of freedom from disturbing cognition (e.g., use of palm-held computers to record occurrence of disturbing ruminations versus the occurrence of feeling joy over feeling connected to surrounding events and people), measures of individual differences (e.g., openness to experience or optimism), lifestyle (nutrition and substance use), and social functioning (e.g., healthy assertion versus hostile, agonistic behavior) are integrated into a multidimensional profile of the successful meditators. Additional randomized, prospective studies are essential to examine the direct effects of meditation.

Related Entries: Coping, Hypnosis, Pain, Relaxation Response, Stressful Life Events

BIBLIOGRAPHY

Alexander, C. N., Langer, E. J., Newman, R. I., Chandler, H. M., & Davies, J. L. (1989). Transcendental Meditation, mindfulness, and longevity: An experimental study with the elderly. *Journal of Personality and Social Psychology, 57*, 950–964.

Austin, J. H. (1998). *Zen and the brain.* Cambridge, MA: MIT Press.

Barnes, V. A., Treiber, F. A., & Davis, H. (2001). Impact of Transcendental Meditation on cardiovascular function at rest and during acute stress in adolescents with high normal blood pressure. *Journal of Psychosomatic Research, 51*, 597–605.

Benson, H. (1976). *The relaxation response.* New York: Avon.

Eppley, K. R., Abrams, A. I., & Shear, J. (1989). Differential effects of relaxation techniques on trait anxiety: A meta-analysis. *Journal of Clinical Psychology, 45*, 957–974.

Kabat-Zinn, J., Wheeler, E., Light, T., Skillings, A., Scharf, M. J., Cropley, T. G., et al. (1998). Influence of mindfulness mediation-based stress reduction intervention on rates of skin clearing in patients with moderate to severe psoriasis undergoing phototherapy (UVB) and photochemotherapy (PUVA). *Psychosomatic Medicine, 60*, 625–632.

Seeman, T. E., Dubin, L. F., & Seeman, M. (2003). Religiosity/spirituality and health: A critical review of the evidence for biological pathways. *American Psychologist, 58*, 53–63.

West, M. A. (Ed.). (1987). *The psychology of meditation.* New York: Oxford University Press.

RANDALL S. JORGENSEN

Mental Status Examination

A mental status exam is a systematic examination of cognitive and emotional functioning to assist in determining potential causes of behavioral or psychological symptoms. Thorough examination of mental status is preceded by assessment of the patient's current and past medical, psychiatric, educational, and family history. Observations of the patient's current appearance, mood, and alertness are noted. The patient's orientation to time, place, and person is assessed. In general, a mental status examination includes assessment of current level of consciousness, attention, language, and higher cognitive functions such as memory, constructional ability, and abstract reasoning.

After obtaining historical information and current concerns, a mental status examination might begin with assessment of attention. Briefly, attention is the patient's ability to concentrate on a stimulus without becoming distracted. Patients may exhibit impaired attention following brain injury, stroke, or dementia. Additionally, psychological problems including depression, anxiety, and attention-deficit/hyperactivity disorder may compromise a patient's attentional abilities.

Assessment of language articulation, production, comprehension, and vocal inflection is important in the mental status exam. Language should be assessed in the oral, auditory, and written formats. Brain damage, particularly to the dominant hemisphere of the brain, can compromise language abilities. Additionally, psychotic disorders may result in incomprehensible language. In the assessment of language abilities, it is important to consider the functioning of organs critical in the production of speech. For example, dysfunction of the larynx can result in speech deficits.

Current memory functioning is also assessed in a mental status examination. Immediate recall, memory for day-to-day events, memory for events from the past, and the ability to learn new information are assessed in a mental status evaluation. Memory dysfunction is a hallmark symptom of many forms of dementia. Traumatic brain injury is also frequently associated with memory dysfunction. Depression, anxiety, and dissociative disorders may impair memory functioning. Finally, numerous medications (psychotropics, beta blockers, anticonvulsants, steroids), alcohol, and recreational drugs may cause decreased memory performance.

A mental status evaluation should assess a patient's ability to draw or construct two- and three-dimensional figures. Lesions to the parietal lobes of the brain frequently result in constructional ability dysfunction. Additionally, a dementing disorder, such as Alzheimer's disease, may affect functioning on these tasks.

Lastly, higher cognitive functions should be assessed. Functions that may be assessed include basic knowledge, abstract thinking, social awareness, and calculation. These functions rely on intact cortical functioning. Diseases involving large portions of the cortex, traumatic brain injury to significant portions of the cortex, or severe psychiatric disorders (e.g., schizophrenia) often affect functioning on these tasks.

Human behavior may be affected by numerous factors (mood, medication, brain damage, and disease). Thorough mental status evaluations provide critical information for explaining the origin of atypical human behavior.

Related Entries: Dementia, Neuropsychology

BIBLIOGRAPHY

Strub, R. L., & Black, F. W. (2000). *The mental status examination in neurology* (4th ed.). Philadelphia: Davis.

Trzepacz, P. T., & Baker, R. W. (1993). *The psychiatric mental status examination.* New York: Oxford University Press.

CARISSA NEHL

Message-Framing Effects

The design of persuasive, information-based interventions to promote healthy behavioral practices involves many decisions. These challenges include specifying what information to include and how the information should be presented. One important decision is whether to develop a message that emphasizes the benefits of adopting the advocated behavior (e.g., "If you get a mammogram, you are taking advantage of the best available method for detecting breast cancer early") or one that emphasizes the costs of failing to adopt the advocated behavior (e.g., "If you do not get a mammogram, you fail to take advantage of the best available method for detecting breast cancer early"). These two messages reflect the use of a gain- or loss-framed appeal, respectively.

Does the frame of a message influence its impact on behavioral decisions? During the last decade or so, researchers have systematically examined the influence of gain- and loss-framed appeals on a broad range of health practices (e.g., mammography, HIV testing, use of sun screen, Pap testing, use of mouth rinse, clinical skin examinations). The relative effectiveness of the two frames has been shown to depend on how people construe a particular health behavior. Consistent with a framework set forth by Rothman and Salovey (1997), gain-framed appeals are more effective when people are deciding whether to adopt a behavior that affords a relatively safe or certain outcome, whereas loss-framed messages are more effective when people are deciding whether to adopt a behavior that affords a risky or uncertain outcome. Furthermore, Rothman and Salovey showed that the distinction between detection and prevention behaviors can be used as a heuristic to predict the relative impact of gain- and loss-framed appeals. Because detection behaviors are designed to detect the presence of a health problem, people typically construe being screened as a risky endeavor, one runs the risk of finding a health problem. In this context, loss-framed appeals are more effective. In contrast, prevention behaviors are designed to forestall illness and maintain a person's current health. Because these behaviors are risky only to the extent that one chooses not to adopt them, deciding to use them is the safe option. Hence, here, gain-framed appeals are more effective.

Although the distinction between prevention and detection behaviors has served as an effective heuristic to guide predictions as to whether a gain- or a loss-framed appeal will be more persuasive, investigators need to recognize that any ancillary factors that influence how individuals construe a given behavior can affect their response to a framed message (Rothman et al., 2002). For example, after receiving a consistent series of clear, healthy exams, a woman might begin to consider obtaining a mammogram as a health-affirming behavior that elicits minimal feelings of risk or uncertainty. In light of this new representation, a gain-framed appeal that emphasized the benefits of screening mammography might be the most effective way to promote subsequent screening. However, women who continue to construe the behavior as involving psychological risk or uncertainty may be more responsive to a loss-framed appeal.

Related Entry: Fear Appeals

BIBLIOGRAPHY

Rothman, A. J., Kelly, K. M., Hertel, A., & Salovey, P. (2002). Message frames and illness representations: Implications for interventions to promote and sustain healthy behavior. In L. D. Cameron and H. Leventhal (Eds.), *The self-regulation of health and illness behavior* (pp. 278–296). London: Routledge.

Rothman, A. J., & Salovey, P. (1997). Shaping perceptions to motivate healthy behavior: The role of message framing. *Psychological Bulletin, 121,* 3–19.

ALEXANDER J. ROTHMAN
PETER SALOVEY

Minnesota Multiphasic Personality Inventory-2

The Minnesota Multiphasic Personality Inventory-2 (MMPI-2) is the most widely used and researched objective personality inventory in the world. It consists of 567 true–false items that examinees complete based on their experience of their emotions, behavior, interpersonal preferences, and psychiatric symptoms. The instrument was designed as an initial screening instrument to detect the presence of psychopathology. It also aids clinicians in making diagnostic decisions about mental illness and personality structure.

Over the years, new uses have been found for the MMPI-2. Human resources personnel use it to make employment decisions. Clinicians use it to enhance their treatment planning by tailoring interventions to patients' emotional needs and personality style. The test facilitates the evaluation of change over the course of psychotherapy. Alternatively, it serves as a therapeutic intervention when clinicians provide patients with test feedback that will help them make positive changes in their lives.

Starke Hathaway and J. C. McKinley developed the original MMPI in 1942 by using the empirical scale-construction strategy. First, they compiled a large pool of potential test items based on their experience with psychiatric patients. Then, they administered these items to groups of patients whose diagnoses were well established and to a group of controls. Finally, they compared the responses to determine which items would discriminate best between the controls and specific patient groups. These items were retained for the final version of the instrument.

Eventually, the original MMPI needed to be revised. The test made use of diagnostic nosology that had become outdated. Many of its items had become obsolete or objectionable. Furthermore, the original normative sample was not a good representation of the diverse population of the United States. Therefore, James N. Butcher and others completed a revision and restandardization of the instrument, publishing the MMPI-2 in 1989. The new norms for the instrument were based on a sample of 2,600 people who provide a more relevant comparison group for today's patients.

The MMPI-2 has many strengths as an evaluation tool. It is practical, cost-effective, and objectively interpreted. It is written in simple language (eighth-grade reading level) and is easy to administer and score. There is strong evidence for the instrument's good psychometric properties. The variables that are measured in an MMPI-2 profile are generally familiar to clinicians. Finally, the test includes a set of validity scales that can be used to assess the test-taking attitudes of the examinee.

Critics of the MMPI-2 point out that the names of the clinical scales are archaic and no longer in common use. They caution that when an examinee has limited education and a lower socioeconomic occupation, the validity of the MMPI-2 profile must be monitored more closely. Also, they point out that the setting in which the instrument is administered can have a significant impact on profile elevations.

The MMPI-2 must be used cautiously with medical patients so that psychiatric norms are not misapplied. However, the instrument has much utility in answering questions about medical patients' willingness to express physical symptoms, their distress or discomfort about their illness, and their general coping skills, level of tension, and depressive symptoms.

BIBLIOGRAPHY

Bombardier, C. H., Divine, G. W., Jordan, J. S., Brooks, W. B., & Neelon, F. A. (1993). Minnesota Multiphasic Personality Inventory (MMPI) cluster groups among chronically ill patients: Relationship to illness adjustment and treatment outcome. *Journal of Behavioral Medicine, 16,* 467–484.

Butcher, J. N. (1990). *MMPI-2 in psychological treatment.* New York: Oxford University Press.

Butcher, J. N., & Williams, C. L. (1992). *Essentials of MMPI-2 and MMPI-A interpretation.* Minneapolis: University of Minnesota Press.

Greene, R. L. (2000). *The MMPI-2: An interpretive manual* (2nd ed.). Boston: Allyn & Bacon.

HEIDI T. BECKMAN

Modeling

Modeling, or observational learning, can occur simply by observing the behavior of someone else. This learning process is efficient because it helps to avoid extensive trial and error. Although modeling is an effective way to learn desirable responses, it can also result in undesirable learning of aggressive behaviors and more subtle responses such as fears, prejudices, and positive or negative reactions to people, situations, or objects. For instance, aggressive behaviors seen on television or in movies can increase the probability of such behavior in the viewer. Childrens' observations of their parents' behavior toward each other often creates a model of what marriage is like and may ultimately influence the children's own behavior toward a romantic partner.

Albert Bandura was a pioneer in the scientific study of observational learning. Prior to his work it was assumed that learning required both activity and reinforcement of that activity. However, Bandura viewed learning as a cognitive process consisting of four basic steps including attention, retention, reproduction, and motivation. By this he meant that to learn from the behavior of others it is necessary to notice the behavior, remember it, have the skills available to reproduce it, and want to behave in that way. He emphasized that observation of the behavior need not lead to its immediate repetition. The learning might be stored away until some similar situation occurs.

Although people may learn from observation, they do not imitate every behavior they see. Imitation is likely if the outcome of the model's behavior results in a positive rather than negative outcome for the model and also if it results in something the observer values. The greater the similarity of the model to the observer, the more likely the behavior is to occur. Observational learning is also more likely if the model is viewed as a high-status person. Entertainment celebrities and sports heroes are examples of effective, high-status models and are often used by advertisers for that reason.

Emotional responses are also affected by modeling. Disabling levels of anxiety can often be traced to exposure to models who are extremely fearful. Even specific fears, such as the fear of dogs, often develop not from a negative experience with a dog, but from observing someone else's fright at an encounter with a dog or even from hearing a vivid description of such an encounter.

Although modeling may create anxiety, it can also be an effective treatment approach to reducing fears or anxiety.

Watching a live or videotaped model deal effectively with an anxiety-provoking situation can significantly reduce fears. Such modeling is more effective if the model initially appears somewhat fearful but is able to use effective coping methods that the viewer can learn through observation. Bandura points out that modeling not only results in learning, but it can also increase the observer's feelings of self-efficacy by encouraging the belief that, "If they can do it, so can I."

Modeling is also effective as a long-term behavior-change technique. Membership in organizations such as Alcoholics Anonymous provides both examples of others who can change their behavior and access to information about coping methods that have helped others. Modeling is also used as a health promotion technique, for instance, in motivating improved dietary or exercise behavior.

Related Entries: Operant Conditioning, Secondary Gain

BIBLIOGRAPHY

Bandura, A. (1977). *Social learning theory.* Englewood Cliffs, NJ: Prentice Hall.
Bandura, A. (1986). *Social foundations of thought and action: A social cognitive theory.* Englewood Cliffs, NJ: Prentice Hall.

BARBARA R. SARASON

Momentary Assessment

As the field of self-report advanced and investigators recognized that recall was prone to distortion by cognitive processes and memory limitations, alternative assessment methodologies were developed. Recording experiences at the moment they occur in order to reduce recall bias was one such technique. Often called ESM (the experience sampling method) or EMA (ecological momentary assessment) (Stone et al., 1999), these methods have subjects record their immediate experience in their natural environments as they go about their everyday lives. Subjects typically make from 3 to 20 recordings per day. These qualities increase the ecological validity of the resulting data and allow for a detailed description of everyday life. In addition to self-reported experiences (ESM), EMA extended these sampling methods to the recording of physiological states.

Depending on the goals of a research project, momentary data may be aggregated or examined in a more fine-grained manner. For instance, a researcher studying pain might want to describe the pain patients were experiencing before and after an intervention. As an alternative to a recall pain measures, momentary reports of pain could be collected several times a day and averaged pre- and postintervention. A detailed description of the dynamic effects of the intervention might also be of interest and analysis of the momentary pain reports taken just after the intervention would show the temporal course of the intervention effect.

There are three primary ways of collecting momentary data: event contingent (where event occurrence prompts for a recording), interval contingent (where recordings are made at regular intervals), and random recordings (where individuals are signaled to make a recordings according to an predetermined schedule). A study's goal determines the type of sampling schedule used, and often two or more schedules are combined; a common momentary study design is random recording and event contingent. In terms of signaling subjects to make random recordings, early research used pagers and programmed wrist watches, but the advent of handheld computers has made possible complex sampling schemes. Because high levels of compliance are necessary for momentary research protocols, electronic data capture with handheld computers (which allow data entry via touch-sensitive screens and time–date mark entries) is highly desirable.

Momentary research is becoming an important tool for health psychology research. For example, the search for mechanisms underlying some of the basic associations discovered in this field can be profitably examined with momentary techniques. One example concerns the association between social relationships and physiological states, which has been demonstrated in laboratory analogue experiments, although little is known about how supportive relationships operate in the real world. Investigators are sampling relationship experiences with electronic diaries and associating those data with those from other in-field devices such as ambulatory blood pressure monitors for blood pressure and portable peak flow meters for lung function.

A large volume of data is produced by momentary paradigms, which require skillful data management. Analysis of these data can also be challenging because the usual unit of the analysis is not the person, which is typical in behavioral science research, but the momentary experience. It is optimally analyzed with multilevel models that explicitly adjust for this and other characteristics of momentary data. In addition, momentary studies require considerable investigator resources and are relatively high in subject burden.

Related Entry: Self-Report Methods

BIBLIOGRAPHY

Schwartz, J., & Stone, A. A. (1998). Data analysis for EMA studies. *Health Psychology, 17*, 6–16.

Shiffman, S. (2000). Real-time self-report of momentary states in the natural environment: Computerized ecological momentary assessment. In A. Stone, J. Turkkan, J. Jobe, et al. (Eds.), *The science of self-report: Implications for research and practice* (pp. 00–00). Mahwah, NJ: Erlbaum.

Stone, A. A., Shiffman, S., & DeVries, M. (1998). Rethinking our self-report assessment methodologies: An argument for collecting ecological valid, momentary measurements. In D. Kahneman, E. Diener, & N. Schwarz (Eds.), *Foundations of hedonic psychology: Scientific perspectives on enjoyment and suffering* (pp. 26–39). New York: Russell Sage Foundation.

Wheeler, L., & Reis, H. (1991). Self-recording of everyday life events: Origins, types, and uses. *Journal of Personality, 59*, 339–354.

ARTHUR A. STONE

Mood: The Relationship Between Mood and Health

Researchers typically refer to affect as the umbrella term encompassing various feeling states, including moods and emotions. Moods differ from emotions, however, in important ways. For one, moods last longer and are less intense than emotions. For instance, the emotion of fear may be extremely intense but might last for only a few seconds or minutes. An anxious mood, on the other hand, will be more subdued compared to fear, but may last for a few hours or more. Also, whereas emotions are response systems to external events, moods are influenced by internal as well as external events. Thus, moods are connected to internal biological processes such as daily biological rhythms. In fact, research has shown that positive moods show a consistent circadian pattern; people tend to report experiencing more positive moods at certain times of the day.

Related Entries: Negative Affect, Neuroticism, Positive Affect

BIBLIOGRAPHY

Watson, D. (2000). *Mood and temperament.* New York: Guilford.

JATIN G. VAIDYA

Multidimensional Health Locus of Control Scale

The Multidimensional Health Locus of Control (MHLC) Scales are a family of measures developed in the mid-20th century by Ken Wallston and colleagues. These scales are designed to assess a person's beliefs regarding whether his or her health status is determined by the actions of individuals (as opposed to fate, luck, or chance) and, if so, whether the locus of that control is "internal" (i.e., residing in the person's own actions) or "external" (i.e., dependent on the actions of other people).

The predecessor of the MHLC Scales, the 11-item unidimensional Health Locus of Control (HLC) Scale developed in 1976 by Wallston, was a health-specific version of J. Rotter's 1966 I-E Scale, which was used to classify individuals as "internals" or "externals." By the time the HLC Scale was published, however, it became clear that locus of control was multidimensional; internality and externality were basically uncorrelated rather than being opposite ends of the same pole.

The initial version of the MHLC Scales, still very much in use in the early 21st century, consisted of two more or less equivalent forms (A and B), each of which contained three six-item subscales. Modeled after Levenson's (1973) I, P, & C Scales, which separated externality into two dimensions—powerful others and chance—the MHLC Scales soon became the instrument of choice for health researchers wanting to assess perceived control of health. The three MHLC subscales are IHLC (e.g., "The main thing that affects my health is what I myself do"), PHLC (e.g., "My family has a lot to do with my becoming sick or staying healthy"), and CHLC (e.g., "If it is meant to be, I will stay healthy"). In most populations, IHLC and PHLC are uncorrelated with each other, IHLC and CHLC are slightly negatively intercorrelated ($-.10$ to $-.20$), and the two external dimensions, PHLC and CHLC, are somewhat positively intercorrelated ($.20$ to $.30$). The alpha reliabilities of the six-item subscales hover around .70 ($.65–.75$), and the test–retest reliabilities are in the range of $.70–.80$.

Forms A/B of the MHLC Scales have been used in hundreds of studies since the scales were first developed. Sufficient evidence has accumulated to support a claim for the validity of the MHLC Scales, although a stronger case can be made for their association with indicators of health status (self-perceived or objective) than for their ability to predict specific health behaviors. They were never intended to be used by themselves to predict either health behavior or health status; instead, they were intended to moderate or be moderated by other theoretically relevant variables such as health value, other expectancies, or disease severity.

Form C of the MHLC Scales was designed to be a generic, medical-condition-specific assessment of locus of control beliefs. Each item of Form C contains the word "condition," which can be left intact or substituted with the name of an existing condition (e.g., "diabetes"). Form C has the same subscale structure as Forms A/B, except that PHLC consists of two three-item subscales—"doctors" and "other people"—signifying a more complex discrimination of the role that physicians play in determining the health status of those already diagnosed.

Although not formally a part of the MHLC Scales, in 1999 Wallston and colleagues developed a God Locus of Health Control (GLHC) subscale to assess the extent to which people attribute their health status to a supreme being. The GLHC subscale is more internally consistent than the traditional MHLC subscales (alpha greater than .90); however, there is no evidence that scoring high on the GLHC is associated with a better health status.

BIBLIOGRAPHY

Levenson, H. (1973). Multidimensional locus of control in psychiatric patients. *Journal of Consulting and Clinical Psychology, 41,* 397–404.

Rotter, J. B. (1966). Generalized expectancies for interval versus external control of reinforcement. *Psychological Monographs, 80,* 609.

Wallston, K. A., Malcarne, V. L., Flores, L., et al. (1999). Does God determine your health? The God Locus of Health Control scale. *Cognitive Therapy and Research, 23,* 131–142.

Wallston, K. A., & Smith, M. S. (1994). Issues of control and health: The action is the interaction. In N. P. Gillian, P. Bennett, & M. Herbert (Eds.), *Health psychology: A lifespan perspective* (pp. 00–00). Philadelphia: Harwood.

Wallston, K. A., Stein, M. J., & Smith, C. A. (1994). Form C of the MHLC Scales: A condition-specific measure of locus of control. *Journal of Personality Assessment, 63,* 534–553.

Wallston, K. A., & Wallston, B. S. (1981). Health locus of control scales. In Herbert M. Lefcourt (Ed.), *Research with the locus of control construct: Vol. 1. Assessment methods* (pp. 00–00). New York: Academic.

Wallston, K. A., Wallston, B. S., & DeVellis, R. (1978). Development of the multidimensional health locus of control (MHLC) scales. *Health Education Monographs, 6,* 160–170.

Wallston, B. S., Wallston, K. A., Kaplan, G. D., et al. (1976). The development and validation of the health related locus of control (HLC) scale. *Journal of Consulting and Clinical Psychology, 44,* 580–585.

KENNETH A. WALLSTON

Nn

National Institutes of Health

The National Institutes of Health (NIH) is the U.S. federal government's principal agency for the support of medical research. The mission of the NIH is to develop knowledge that will lead to improved human health. With a 2002 budget of about $23.5 billion, the NIH's institutes and centers award 84 percent of their money via grants to investigators in the United States and abroad. A smaller in-house research program operates on the NIH's campus in Bethesda, Maryland, and on ancillary sites.

This current configuration emerged after World War II, but the NIH traces its roots to the 1887 bacteriological laboratory within the Marine Hospital Service. Initially, infectious diseases were the primary concern of the laboratory. Beginning in 1902, research expanded into the areas of pharmacology, chemistry, and zoology, and after 1912, research into noncontagious diseases was also included. Basic research, especially in chemistry, became an interest of laboratory scientists in the 1920s and 1930s. In 1937 the first categorical institute, the National Cancer Institute, was created.

The 1944 reorganization of the Public Health Service introduced features that shaped the subsequent development of the NIH. The NIH was permitted to award grants in aid of research and to conduct clinical research. Following the war, Congress created the National Institute of Mental Health (NIMH) and shortly thereafter institutes for heart disease and dental research.

Subsequently, Congress established institutes to investigate arthritis, eye diseases, deafness, and diabetes, among other diseases. The National Library of Medicine developed bioinformatics, and the Fogarty International Center coordinated international biomedical research activities. In addition to disease-focused components, institutes for research on the broad areas of child health, aging, nursing, and general medical sciences were added. Most recently, components for human genome research, complementary and alternative medicine, biomedical imaging and bioengineering, and minority and health disparities research were established. In 2002, 27 institutes and centers sponsored health-related research initiatives in the biomedical, behavioral, and social sciences.

BEHAVIORAL AND SOCIAL RESEARCH

The NIH has had a long and growing commitment to behavioral and social scientific research relevant to health. Almost all NIH institutes and centers have played a role, but NIMH has been the largest single source of support for behavioral and social science research. Following President Lyndon Johnson's call in the 1960s to apply research to the alleviation of social and public health problems, NIMH established various topic-focused research centers to focus basic and applied research, training, demonstration grants, and technical assistance on issues such as crime and delinquency, suicide, metropolitan problems, mental health and aging, minority group mental health, and substance abuse and alcoholism. During the 1960s and 1970s the National Heart, Lung, and Blood Institute (NHLBI) developed a pioneering extramural program on health and behavior, and the National Institute on Child Health and Human Development (NICHD) and the National Institute on Aging (NIA) both established broad-ranging programs in support of basic and applied behavioral and social research.

In 1979 the Alcoholism, Drug Abuse, and Mental Health Administration (ADAMHA) and NIH jointly commissioned a landmark study by the Institute of Medicine, *Health and Behavior: Frontiers of Research in the Biobehavioral Sciences* (Hamburg et al., 1982), which gave direction to NIH's expanding activities in the behavioral and social sciences. Organizationally, NIH recognized the need to coordinate its activities across the institutes and centers and established in 1982 the NIH Working Group on Health and Behavior (now the NIH Behavioral and Social Sciences Research Coordinating Committee).

In 1993 Congress established the Office of Behavioral and Social Sciences Research (OBSSR) within the NIH Office of the Director, in recognition of the key role that behavioral and social factors often play in illness and health. OBSSR's mission is to stimulate behavioral and social sciences research throughout NIH and to integrate these areas of research more fully into the NIH health research enterprise. For example, OBSSR commissioned the National Research Council to develop a trans-NIH agenda for supporting research and training in the behavioral and social sciences, which is serving as one blueprint for developmental activities and directions at the NIH. (Singer & Ryff, 2001). In fiscal year (FY) 2002 about $2.64 billion (10 percent of the NIH's total budget) was devoted to behavioral and social sciences research and training (Table 1).

Behavioral and social science research funded at the NIH may be described by dividing it into core and adjunct areas of research. The core areas of research may be further categorized into basic or fundamental research and clinical research. Many studies have both basic and clinical components. Moreover, basic and clinical investigations are often complementary. Adjunct areas of behavioral and social sciences research include many types of neurobiological research and some research on pharmacologic interventions—areas that have implications for, and are often influenced by, behavioral research. These are beyond the scope of this entry.

Basic Research

Basic research in the behavioral and social sciences furthers understanding of behavioral and social functioning. As is the case for basic research in the biomedical sciences, basic behavioral and social sciences research does not address disease outcomes per se, but instead provides essential knowledge of fundamental processes and states.

Behavioral and Social Processes

Research on behavioral and social processes involves the study of human or animal functioning at the level of the individual, small group, institution, organization, or community. At the individual level, this research may involve the study of behavioral factors such as cognition, memory, language, perception, personality, emotion, motivation, and others. At higher levels of aggregation, it includes the study of social variables such as the structure and dynamics of small groups (e.g., couples, families, work groups, etc.); institutions and organizations (e.g., schools, religious organizations, etc.); communities (defined by

Table 1. Behavioral and Social Research Budgets for NIH Institutes and Centers

NIH institutes and centers	FY2002 Estimated Budget (million $)
National Cancer Institute	275.3
National Heart, Lung, and Blood Institute	124.8
National Institute of Dental and Craniofacial Research	26.0
National Institute of Diabetes and Digestive and Kidney Disease	42.0
National Institute of Neurological Disorders and Stroke	60.3
National Institute of Allergies and Infectious Diseases	34.6
National Institute of General Medical Sciences	0.0
National Institute of Child Health and Human Development	252.7
National Eye Institute	56.3
National Institute of Environmental Health Sciences	10.6
National Institute on Aging	221.3
National Institute of Arthritis and Musculoskeletal Diseases	19.6
National Institute on Deafness and Other Communication Disorders	80.8
National Institute of Mental Health	406.1
National Institute on Drug Abuse	387.4
National Institute on Alcohol Abuse and Alcoholism	175.9
National Institute of Nursing Research	94.2
National Human Genome Research Institute	9.8
National Institute of Biomedical Imaging and Bioengineering	0.0
National Center for Research Resources	59.6
National Center for Complementary and Alternative Medicine	0.0
National Center on Minority Health and Health Disparities	1.6
John E. Fogarty International Center	5.4
National Library of Medicine	1.6
NIH Office of the Director	18.0
Total	2,364.0

Source: NIH Office of the Budget, February 28, 2002.

geography or common interest); and larger demographic, political, economic, and cultural systems. Research on behavioral and social processes also includes the study of the interactions within and between these two levels of aggregation, such as the influence of sociocultural factors on cognitive processes or emotional responses. Finally, this research also includes the study of environmental factors such as climate, noise, environmental hazards, and residential environments and their effects on behavioral and social functioning.

Biopsychosocial Processes

Biopsychosocial research (also known as biobehavioral or biosocial research) involves the study of the interactions of biological factors with behavioral or social variables and how they affect each other (i.e., the study of bidirectional multilevel relationships).

Development of Procedures for Measurement, Analysis, and Classification

Research on the development of procedures for measurement, analysis, and classification involves the development and refinement of procedures for measuring and analyzing behavior, psychological functioning, or the social environment. This research is designed to develop research tools that could be used in other areas of behavioral and social sciences or in biomedical research.

Clinical Research

Clinical research in the behavioral and social sciences is designed to predict or influence health outcomes, risks, or protective factors. It is also concerned with the impact of illness or risk for illness on behavioral or social functioning. Clinical research may be divided into five categories.

Identification and Understanding of Behavioral and Social Risk and Protective Factors

Research on the identification and understanding of behavioral and social risk and protective factors associated with the onset and course of illness, and with health conditions, examines the association of specific behavioral and social factors with mental and physical health outcomes, and the mechanisms that explain these associations. It is concerned with behavioral and social factors that may be health damaging (risk factors) or health promoting (protective factors).

Effects of Illness or Physical Condition on Behavioral and Social Functioning

Research in this category focuses on the consequences of illness for behavior. Included are such questions as the psychological and social consequences of genetic testing behavioral correlates of head injury across developmental stages, emotional and social consequences of HIV infection or cancer, coping responses associated with chronic pain syndromes, effects of illness on economic status, and coping with loss of function due to disability.

Treatment Outcomes Research

Treatment outcomes research involves the design and evaluation of behavioral and social interventions to treat mental and physical illnesses, or interventions designed to ameliorate the effects of illness on behavioral or social functioning. This area also includes research on behavioral and social rehabilitation procedures.

Related Entries: American Psychological Association, Society of Behavioral Medicine

RONALD P. ABELES*

BIBLIOGRAPHY

Hamburg, D. A., Elliott, G. R., & Parron, D. L. (Eds.). (1982). *Health and behavior: Frontiers of research in the biobehavioral sciences.* Washington, DC: National Academy Press.
Singer, B. H., & Ryff, C. D. (2001). *New horizons in health: An integrative approach.* Washington, DC: National Academy Press.

Negative Affect

The majority of mood experiences can be grouped into two overarching categories: negative and positive affect. Rather than being opposite ends of the same dimension, these factors operate relatively independently of one another. Negative affect is a broad dimension of mood representing the extent to which an individual feels unpleasant arousal. High negative affect is reflected in feelings of distress and dissatisfaction; low negative affect is characterized by feelings of calmness and contentment. Negative affect encompasses a range of aversive feelings, including sadness, anger, disgust, contempt, fear, shame, and guilt. This dimension can be conceptualized as either a state or a trait. State negative affect refers to a transient, short-term feeling, often in response to some specific stimulus. Trait negative affect, in contrast, refers to a more consistent, long-term individual difference in the tendency to experience these negative moods over time and situations, even without a specific source of stress.

Related Entries: Mood: The Relationship Between Mood and Health, Positive Affect

BIBLIOGRAPHY

Watson, D. (2000). *Mood and temperament.* New York: Guilford.

ERICKA NUS SIMMS

* This article was prepared as part of the author's official duties as an employee of the U.S. federal government and is consequently in the public domain. Any opinions expressed herein are those of the author and do not necessarily reflect the position or policies of the NIH or the U.S. federal government.

Nervous System

The nervous system is the organ system responsible for our outward behavior and our internal thoughts. The nervous system allows us to receive information about the world around us and to know what is going on within our bodies. Cells in the nervous system are responsible for creating the most beautiful symphonies as well as the most torturing mental illnesses. Whereas most people equate the nervous system with the brain, it is in fact made up of much more than the brain. This entry reviews the cellular structure and functioning of the nervous system as well as the basic anatomy of the central and peripheral nervous systems.

CELLS OF THE NERVOUS SYSTEM

There are two broad categories of cells in the nervous system: glial cells and neurons. Glial cells mainly play a supportive and protective role providing nutrients, physical support, and protection to neurons. Glial cells are small and very numerous. In fact there are about 10 times more glial cells than neurons. Each type of glial cell serves a very specific function. Some common glial cells are astroglia, radial glia, and oligodendrocytes. Astroglia are star-shaped cells that transfer energy molecules and oxygen from the blood to the neurons and carry waste products from the neuron to the blood stream. As such, they play a critical role in protecting neurons from potentially dangerous substances in the blood stream. Astrocytes also remove waste material and form scar tissue in areas where neurons have died. Radial glia are specialized astroctyes that play a critical role in brain development—they provide a "pathway" for developing neurons to follow on their way to their final destination. Oligodendrocytes produce an important material called myelin, which wraps around the axon of a neuron. Cells that produce myelin outside of the central nervous system are called Schwann cells. The process of myelination takes many years to complete and some brain regions do not become fully myelinated until early adulthood. Because glial cells can replicate, they can be added throughout an individual's life span.

Neurons are differentiated from glial cells by the fact that they can transmit messages to and receive messages from other neurons. Neurons are much larger and less numerous than glial cells. Historically, scientists believed that neurons were not capable of regeneration, that is, when neurons died, they were not replaced. Recent research, however, suggests that some neurons, under some conditions, may be capable of regeneration.

Although neurons come in different shapes and sizes, the typical neuron has a cell body covered by fine, branchlike projections called dendrites. There may be thickenings on the end of dendrites called dendritic spines. A single extension called the axon leaves the cell body at a small bump called the axon hillock. Axon length can vary dramatically, ranging from a few micrometers to more than 1 m in length.

As the axon extends farther and farther from the cell body it branches into finer and finer divisions, finally ending in tiny swellings called terminal boutons. Inside the terminal bouton are small packages of neurotransmitter chemicals. These chemicals are typically produced in the cell body and transported to the terminal bouton by tiny tubes within the axon. Some commonly known neurotransmitters are acetylcholine, serotonin, dopamine, norepinephrine, and glutamate.

The terminal boutons of one neuron are situated next to the dendritic spines or cell bodies of other neurons. While the two cells are in very close proximity to each other a very small space called a synapse exists between them. Synapses are about 20–40 nm (1 billionth of a meter) wide.

Some axons are covered by myelin, a thick, fatty substance that acts as an insulator. The presence of myelin allows electrical messages to travel faster along an axon. For example, the speed of conduction in an unmyelinated axon is approximately 10 m/sec, whereas myelinated axons propagate a message at 120 m/sec, At regular intervals along the length of a myelinated axon are bare patches called the nodes of Ranvier.

All cells are surrounded by the cell membrane, in which there are embedded protein channels. These protein channels can open and close to control the passage of various chemicals into and out of the cell.

CELLULAR COMMUNICATION

Neurons communicate with each other by electrical and chemical means. The dendrites and cell body of a neuron are covered by synapses. A typical neuron has between 5,000 and 10,000 synapses, with some specialized neurons having as many as 100,000. Activity at the synapses causes small changes in the electrical charge of the cell membrane surrounding the synaptic connection. If enough synapses are active at the same time or in rapid succession, the change in electrical charge of the cell membrane may be enough to surpass the "threshold of excitation." If this happens, a large electrical event called an action potential is generated at the axon hillock. This electrical event travels the length of the axon via opening of ion channels. When the action potential reaches the terminal bouton, the packets of neurotransmitter move forward, merge with the membrane, and spill their chemicals into the synaptic space. The neurotransmitter crosses the synapse and binds to a protein on the cell membrane of the next neuron. This causes small changes in the electrical charge of the membrane and the process of producing and propagating an action potential begins again.

CENTRAL NERVOUS SYSTEM

The nervous system can be divided into two components: the central nervous system and the peripheral nervous system. The central nervous system is composed of the brain and the spinal cord. There are many ways of describing the organization and structure of the brain. One of the simplest schemes divides the brain into three components: the hindbrain, the midbrain, and the forebrain. The hindbrain is composed of the medulla oblongata, the pons, and the cerebellum. Cells in the hindbrain are responsible for many vital reflexes such as breathing and heart rate as well as for controlling alertness and sleep. The cerebellum plays a role in balance, control of some types of movement, and some forms of learning. The midbrain contains important motor (movement) and sensory regions. The forebrain is the newest part of the brain from an evolutionary standpoint. It contains regions that control sensory processes, movement, and hormonal systems. The forebrain also includes regions that serve learning, memory, and higher order cognitive processes. The two hemispheres of the brain are connected by a huge band of axons called the corpus callosum. This connection allows neurons in one hemisphere of the brain to communicate with neurons in the other hemisphere.

PERIPHERAL NERVOUS SYSTEM

The peripheral nervous system is made up of the cranial nerves, the spinal nerves, and the autonomic nervous system. The autonomic nervous system can be further divided into the sympathetic and parasympathetic components.

The cranial nerves mainly convey sensory and motor information about the head and neck. There are 31 pairs of spinal nerves, which join the spinal cord at regular intervals. These carry sensory information from the body to the spinal cord and the brain and from the spinal cord to the muscles in the body.

The autonomic nervous system is a collection of ganglia (groups of neurons) located in many regions of the body. Neurons in these ganglia provide input to all major body organs, including the heart, stomach, and lungs. The sympathetic division of the autonomic nervous system consists of neurons found in the thoracic and lumbar region of the spinal cord. They innervate smooth muscles in organs and walls of blood vessels. Activation of these neurons prepares the body for action. For example, sympathetic nervous system arousal leads to increased heart rate, faster rate of breathing, and enlargement of pupils. The parasympathetic nervous system is made up of neurons in ganglia located throughout the body. The parasympathetic nervous system is activated during "resting" states and results in increased activity in digestive organs, reduced heart rate, and

lowered blood pressure. Because the sympathetic and parasympathetic divisions often exert opposite effects on organ systems, we have very accurate modulation over these bodily processes. It is noteworthy that the autonomic nervous system is not under our conscious control. Thus we cannot lower and raise our blood pressure at will.

The nervous system is a complex organ system made up of millions of cells working together to maintain the functioning of our bodies as well as to create the complexities our minds.

Related Entries: Dementia, Mental Status Examination

BIBLIOGRAPHY

Finger, S. (1994). *Origins of neuroscience: A history of explorations into brain function.* New York: Oxford University Press.
Kandel, E. R., Schwartz, J. H., & Jessell, T. M (2000). *Principles of neural science* (4th ed.). New York: McGraw-Hill.

DEBRA L. JOHNSON

Neuropsychology

DEFINITION AND HISTORICAL BACKGROUND

The field of neuropsychology is concerned with the relationship between the brain and behavior. "Behavior" in this definition refers not only to observable actions, but also to internal cognitive processes such as memory, attention, visual functions, decision making, and emotions. The term neuropsychology is most often applied to the study of the relationship between brain and behavior in humans, although clearly it could also be applied to the study of animals. In health psychology, the term clinical neuropsychologist is used to denote a psychologist with expertise in how brain–behavior relationships are relevant to the diagnosis, treatment, and well-being of patients with known or suspected brain disease.

The history of neuropsychology in some senses dates back to the early Greeks. However, the beginning of the modern age is most often linked to the 19th century. In the early 1800s Franz Josef Gall (1758–1828) and Johann Casper Spurzheim (1776–1832) proposed that different areas of the brain are dedicated to different traits or abilities and that differences in the shape of the skull would reflect the strength or weakness of underlying "faculties" (see Figure 1). This localizationist approach, called phrenology, was influential in England and the United States. It

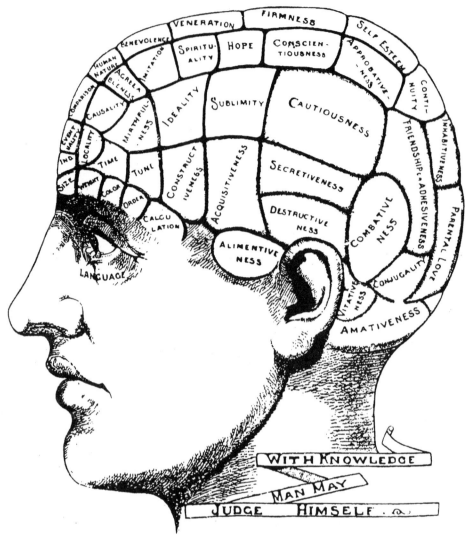

Figure 1.   The areas of the skull presumed to overlie areas of specific personality traits or cognitive abilities according to Spurzheim, based on Gall's original 27 "faculties." From Kolb and Whishaw (1996). Reproduced with permission of Bryan Kolb.

was not long after this that Paul Broca (1824–1880) reported a relationship between language impairments and damage to the left frontal lobe, and Carl Wernicke (1848–1904) subsequently described a different set of language impairments associated with a different part of the left hemisphere. What followed was a series of discoveries by late 19th-century neurologists and psychiatrists concerning some of the fundamental relationships between different areas of the brain and specific behaviors [see Benton (1988) for a review].

By the mid-20th century, psychologists were beginning to investigate how specific tests were performed by patients with brain damage. It was around this time that the term neuropsychology was coined. Early pioneers in this area include Ward Halstead, Arthur Benton, Ralph Reitan, Brenda Milner, and Edith Kaplan. Neuropsychological batteries, or specific collections of mental tests that proved sensitive to brain damage, were

developed by the 1940s and 1950s. Other early neuropsychologists developed formal tests of language, memory, attention, and other cognitive capacities that proved sensitive not only to brain damage generally, but also to specific areas of brain damage.

The advent of neuroimaging techniques such as computerized tomography (CT) in the 1970s and magnetic resonance imaging (MRI) in the 1980s marked the beginning of the most recent major advances in neuropsychology. Until that time, researchers often had to wait until autopsy of the brain to establish a relationship between areas of brain damage and neuropsychological impairment. However, neuroimaging techniques allowed neuropsychologists to examine, in living humans, the relationship between specific areas of brain damage and performance on standardized mental tests. This resulted in an explosion of knowledge in relation to brain function, culminating in the "decade of the brain" of the 1990s. Alongside these neuroimaging techniques, which enable researchers to see the brain in living humans, are newer "functional" neuroimaging techniques such as functional MRI (fMRI) and positron emission tomography (PET), which allow researchers to evaluate areas of the brain that are utilized during different mental tasks.

TRAINING IN NEUROPSYCHOLOGY

Clinical neuropsychology is a practice-oriented subspecialty of clinical psychology that aims to evaluate or treat behavioral deficits produced by brain damage or dysfunction. Clear guidelines for training have been published (Hannay et al., 1998). Training usually begins with an undergraduate degree in psychology. After they obtain a college degree, students typically enroll in a graduate program in clinical psychology that is approved by the American Psychological Association or other appropriate national organization. The end point of such a graduate program is the doctoral (PhD) degree. Attainment of the doctoral degree requires both breadth and depth in the field of psychology, including study in areas such as statistics and methodology, social psychology, and biological bases of behavior, in addition to more clinically oriented areas of training such as psychopathology, interviewing and assessment techniques, and professional ethics. During graduate training, students who want to become clinical neuropsychologists generally also study areas more specific to that specialty, including functional and structural neuroanatomy, neurological and medical disorders related to behavioral or cognitive change, psychopharmacology, and entry-level classes in the practice of neuropsychology. Graduate training usually takes 5–6 years and includes 1 year of full-time supervised clinical internship prior to the granting of the PhD degree. The clinical internship usually includes at least one major rotation in neuropsychology for those students wanting to specialize in the field.

The last stage of training in clinical neuropsychology is the residency. After they obtain the PhD degree, students of neuropsychology complete a 2-year residency aimed at further training in the specialty of clinical neuropsychology. It is at this level that students branch out in the specialty area, principally through supervised training in specific neuropsychological procedures. These specific procedures include all aspects of assessment including knowledge of measures and tests, report writing, and detailed knowledge of medical, psychiatric, and neurological conditions in relation to behavior and cognition change. In recent years, additional training in neuropsychological rehabilitation has been offered with increasing frequency. The residency is a 2-year program, and is viewed as a mandatory part of training in clinical neuropsychology. Research is viewed as a fundamental component of this stage, and most residency programs in clinical neuropsychology provide time for independent and collaborative research. The residency is generally considered to be complete after 2 years, assuming the resident shows evidence of competence in all relevant areas. Board certification can be obtained following residency training through the American Board of Clinical Neuropsychology (ABCN), which is affiliated with the American Board of Professional Psychology (ABPP). The ABCN–ABPP serves to designate individuals who have undergone extensive written and practice examinations of their competence as clinical neuropsychologists.

ACTIVITIES OF A NEUROPSYCHOLOGIST

Clinical

Most neuropsychologists maintain a clinical practice. In a clinical setting, neuropsychologists typically administer and interpret the results of standardized tests of mental and behavioral ability. There can be many reasons for such an assessment. For example, the results of neuropsychological assessments may be used to determine the management of patients with brain disease, such as a person's ability to handle finances, drive, or live independently. Also, such assessments are often used to monitor the recovery of cognitive abilities following certain brain disorders (e.g., stroke) or the rate and nature of cognitive decline in progressive conditions (e.g., Alzheimer's disease). Finally, in some disorders (e.g., mild traumatic brain injury) all other medical tests may be normal and neuropsychological assessment may be the only means by which to establish the diagnosis.

There are many methods and several schools of assessment, but all have in common the fact that tests are standardized and based on published scientific normative data. A neuropsychological assessment typically takes from 2 to 6 hr of patient time, depending on the referral question, the stamina of the patient, and the results of other tests. Screening examinations may last as little as 30 min, and extended examinations may last 8 hr or more. It is common to measure multiple cognitive abilities in the course of a single assessment, including memory and orientation, language, higher visual functions, spatial abilities, decision-making ability, and mood and personality.

Research

Many neuropsychologists conduct research, particularly in academic settings such as university departments of psychology or in medical schools. Usually, the aim of such research is to examine the relationship between the brain and behavior. For example, many neuropsychologists study the relationship between the structure of the brain and a person's ability to produce language, have memory, or have normal vision. Although such studies can be traced to discoveries from the mid-19th century, it is fair to say that most modern knowledge of the relationship between the brain and behavior has been derived from research in the last 30–50 years. Such research has yielded information now considered to be fundamental in the diagnosis of many disorders. For example, neuropsychological research has substantiated the fact that early memory impairments are the hallmark of Alzheimer's disease, which in turn has helped with early diagnosis of the condition. This early diagnosis of Alzheimer's disease has helped clinicians to provide more timely interventions for patients with the disorder, and has thereby improved the quality of life for millions of patients.

More recent neuropsychological research has focused on treatment and rehabilitation of acquired brain problems such as memory disorders (amnesia), language disorders, and vision impairments. For example, recent studies have begun to investigate ways in which patients with amnesia following stroke may benefit most from memory aids, using tools such as notebooks, pagers, handheld computers, and other automatic reminders and mnemonic strategies. This research is in its infancy, but reflects a straightforward application of neuropsychological principles developed in the last 50 years to the direct alleviation of suffering due to acquired cognitive impairments.

Teaching

Many neuropsychologists are in academic settings, and in that context those neuropsychologists typically have responsibilities that include teaching at the college level or in graduate schools or medical schools. Neuropsychologists, given that they are usually trained as clinical psychologists, often have basic teaching responsibilities in departments of psychology. Courses taught might include introductory courses in psychology and clinical psychology, but typically also include advanced courses in assessment, brain function, clinical neuropsychological assessment, and psychopharmacology. Similarly, neuropsychologists employed in medical schools often teach medical students or medical residents about the fundamentals of clinical neuropsychology and brain–behavior relationships. Particularly in departments of neurology and psychiatry, it is a common part of a young physician's training to learn about formal neuropsychological assessment and the ways that such assessment may benefit patients.

Related Entries: Clinical Psychology, Nervous System

BIBLIOGRAPHY

Benton, A. L. (1988) Neuropsychology: Past, present, and future. In F. Boller & J. Grafman (Eds.), *Handbook of neuropsychology* (Vol. 1, pp. 00–00). Amsterdam: Elsevier Science.
Hannay, H. J., Bieliauskas, L. A., Crosson, B. A., Hammeke, T. A., Hamsher, K. deS., & Coffer, S. P. (1998). Proceedings: The Houston conference on specialty education and training in clinical neuropsychology. *Archives of Clinical Neuropsychology, 13*, 157–249.
Kolb, B., & Whishaw, I. Q. (1996). *Fundamental of human neuropsychology* (4th ed.). New York: Freeman.

R. D. JONES

Neuroticism

Neuroticism is one of five major dimensions of normal personality that make up the five-factor model of personality. The central feature of neuroticism is proneness to experience negative emotions. Individuals high in neuroticism also have characteristics that are related to emotional distress such as low self-esteem and self-consciousness. High levels of neuroticism have been related to an increased risk for the development of depression, anxiety disorders, and hypochondriasis. Low neuroticism is characterized by emotional stability.

Neuroticism is of interest to health psychologists because it is related to higher reports of physical symptoms and ratings of poor health. However, some researchers have called into question whether poorer ratings of health among individuals high in neuroticism are related to actual underlying differences in health or simply to differences in illness behavior. Thus, it has been suggested that neurotic individuals are more likely to perceive physical sensations, may misinterpret benign sensations as pathological, or may have a lower threshold for reporting physical symptoms to others. Additionally, the link between neuroticism and negative mood states influences perceptions of health. For example, when individual high in neuroticism who is experiencing depressed mood may interpret changes in his or her physical health more negatively and may be more likely to remember past negative health events.

The effects of the foregoing constellation of illness behaviors and symptom-related emotional distress among highly neurotic individuals on actual health is unclear. Some research suggests that the attention to signs of illness and associated worry may, under some circumstances, lead to better self-care and more-positive health outcomes. However, other studies have found no relationship between neuroticism and physical illness. Still other research has demonstrated that neuroticism and/or components of neuroticism, such as depression and anxiety, are linked to negative health outcomes such as poorer immune functioning, hypertension, coronary heart disease, and premature mortality. Clearly, many questions remain regarding the extent to which neuroticism is related to actual physical health.

Much of the research on mechanisms for the relationship between neuroticism and health has focused on psychological stress. There is substantial evidence that individuals high in neuroticism report more stressors, experience more distress in response to stressors, and have higher levels of some stress hormones, such as cortisol. There is also evidence that individuals high in neuroticism may engage in poorer health behavior (i.e., diet, exercise, sleep), particularly under conditions of high stress. Poorer health practices, in turn, may influence both perceived and actual health.

In summary, the relationship between neuroticism and health is complex. The chronic negative emotional states associated with neuroticism may lead to illness behavior (e.g., reports of symptoms, health care use) in the absence of objective illness and, in some contexts, may lead to better health outcomes if translated into more attentive health self-care. However, in other contexts, chronic negative mood states can clearly have adverse effects on physical health. Future research will need to further explore the mechanisms by which neuroticism affects self-assessed health, health behavior, and disease outcomes.

Related Entry: Five-Factor Model of Personality

BIBLIOGRAPHY

Smith, T. W., & Gallo, L. C. (2001). Personality traits as risk factors for physical illness. In A. Baum, T. A. Revenson, & J. E. Singer (Eds.), *Handbook of health psychology* (pp. 139–173). Mahwah, NJ: Erlbaum.

Suls, J., Green, P., & Hillis, S. (1998). Emotional reactivity to everyday problems, affective inertia, and neuroticism. *Personality and Social Psychology Bulletin, 24,* 127–136.

Watson, D., & Pennebaker, J. (1989). Health complaints, stress, and distress: Exploring the central role of negative affectivity. *Psychological Review, 96,* 234–254.

Williams, P. G., Colder, C. R., Lane, J. D., McCaskill, C. C., Feinglos, M. N., & Surwit, R. S. (2002). Examination of the neuroticism–symptom reporting relationship in individuals with Type 2 diabetes. *Personality and Social Psychology Bulletin, 28,* 1015–1025.

PAULA G. WILLIAMS

NK Cells

Natural killer (NK) cells are large, granulated lymphocytes found in the spleen, lymph nodes, bone marrow, and blood (lymphocytes are a subset of white blood cells including NK, T, and B cells). NK cells destroy tumor cells and cells that have been invaded by viruses or bacteria. Unlike T and B cells, NK cells do not require prior contact with targets for activation and therefore can act instantly against target cells. They are particularly important in defense against development and metastases of tumors, and NK cell activity has been associated with relapse, disease progression, and disease-free survival in cancer patients. NK cells are also important in controlling viral replication following infection. NK cell activity is sensitive to social and psychological factors, possibly via adrenergic and glucocorticoid receptors. Although NK cell activity increases briefly following acute stressors, decrements in NK cell activity are found in chronically stressed individuals. Reduced NK cell activity has also been related to pessimism, depression, and bereavement. In contrast, social support, sense of meaning, and relaxation practice have been associated with greater NK cell activity.

Related Entries: Cancer: Biopsychosocial Aspects, Immune System: Structure and Function, Psychoneuroimmunology

ERIN S. COSTANZO

Nociception

Nociception is the transmission of nerve impulses that signal possible tissue damage. Nociception begins with activation of sensory receptors, called nociceptors, which respond to stimuli that are potentially harmful. Nociceptors can be activated by mechanical (e.g., pinching, crushing), thermal (e.g., hot, cold), chemical, and electrical stimulation. Once stimulated, nociceptors transmit their information to the spinal cord. The degree to which incoming nociceptive signals are forwarded by the spinal cord to the brain is determined by a complex interaction of incoming signals from the peripheral nervous system, local mechanisms within the spinal cord, and descending input from the brain. As a result, the amount of pain we experience is not only related to the amount of tissue damage or nociceptor stimulation. For example, an athlete involved in an intense competition may not notice an injury or experience any pain until after the competition is over.

Related Entries: Gate Theory of Pain, Pain

CHRISTOPHER R. FRANCE

Nutrition

Good nutrition is vital for growth, health, and well-being throughout the life cycle. Nutritional status both preconceptionally and during pregnancy has an impact on pregnancy and infant outcomes. Good nutrition is essential during infancy, childhood, and adolescence, when nutrient needs are high, to ensure optimal growth and development. Nutritional factors are important in the prevention of 4 of the leading 10 causes of death in the United States: coronary heart disease, certain cancers, stroke, and Type II diabetes. Nutrition is also related to other chronic health conditions such as obesity and osteoporosis. Relationships between dietary factors and health are becoming clearer. Thus, increased attention is being placed on the importance of preventive nutrition.

Many dietary components are involved in the link between nutrition and health. For instance, excessive intake of saturated fat is related to heart disease and inadequate intake of fruits and vegetables is associated with an increased risk for certain cancers. The 2000 *Dietary Guidelines for Americans* recommend that to stay healthy, persons aged 2 years and older should aim for a healthy weight, be physically active each day, choose a diet that is low in saturated fat and cholesterol and moderate in total fat, choose beverages and foods to moderate sugar intake, choose and prepare foods with less salt, and, if drinking alcoholic beverages (for adults), do so in moderation. The *Dietary Guidelines for Americans* also recommend selecting foods and portions based on guidelines outlined by the *Food Guide Pyramid*. The *Food Guide Pyramid* suggests consuming grains, fruits, and vegetables as the basis for healthy eating, accompanied by a moderate amount of low-fat foods from the milk and meat/beans groups and limited amounts of foods that are high in fat and sugars (Table 1).

Given the interrelationship between nutrition and health, it is important to review the priority nutrition-related concerns affecting Americans today. *Healthy People 2010* is a National Health Promotion and Disease Prevention Agenda that was established by the U.S. Department of Health and Human Services. Several nutrition-related goals have been established through *Healthy People 2010* to promote health and reduce chronic disease associated with diet and weight. Table 2 reviews the key nutrition-related objectives.

PRIORITY NUTRITION CONCERNS

Overweight and Obesity

Overweight and obesity have reached epidemic proportions in the United States. Currently, approximately two-thirds of U.S. adults are overweight or obese. There are also nearly twice as many overweight children and almost three times as many overweight adolescents as there were in 1980. These startling percentages are continuing to increase. Thus, the prevention and treatment of overweight and obesity is an important public health goal and is considered one of the leading health indicators in *Healthy People 2010*.

Overweight adults are at increased risk for morbidity and mortality from many acute and chronic medical conditions such

as hypertension, coronary heart disease, Type II diabetes, certain cancers, and musculoskeletal disorders such as osteoarthritis. Approximately 300,000 deaths a year in the United States are associated with overweight and obesity. Overweight children are more likely to become overweight adults, and are also at increased risk for morbidity and mortality during adulthood. Overweight and obesity are increasing across all ages, among both genders, and in all population groups. However, they are particularly prevalent among Native Americans, Hispanics, and African-American females.

Overweight and obesity are caused by a complex variety of social, behavioral, cultural, environmental, physiological, and genetic factors. Nonetheless, a healthy diet consistent with guidelines recommended in the *Dietary Guidelines for Americans* and regular physical activity (30 min of moderate activity daily) are both essential for maintaining a healthy weight. Efforts to maintain a healthy weight should begin during childhood and continue throughout adulthood.

INADEQUATE OR EXCESSIVE DIETARY INTAKES

Fruits, Vegetables, and Whole Grains

Dietary patterns characterized by a high intake of fruits, vegetables, and whole grains are associated with a variety of health benefits including a lower risk of developing heart disease, stroke, hypertension, and certain cancers. *The Dietary Guidelines for Americans* recommend consuming 3–5 servings of vegetables daily, 2–4 servings of fruits daily, and 6–11 servings daily of grain products with at least three being whole grains. Most Americans fail to meet these recommendations. Data from national food consumption surveys showed that only 28 percent of Americans consumed at least two servings of fruit daily, 3 percent of Americans consumed three servings of vegetables daily, and 7 percent of Americans consumed six grain servings daily with at least three being whole grains. A national survey found that although knowledge of the recommendation to consume five or more fruits and vegetables daily was associated with higher consumption, only 8 percent of the population was aware of this recommendation. Public health campaigns, such as the Five-A-Day for Better Health Program, to promote awareness and behavior change are underway.

Dietary Fat

The public health recommendation is that all healthy people aged 2 years and older reduce dietary fat intake to less than 30 percent of calories and dietary saturated fat intake to less than 10 percent of calories. However, results from population-based food consumption surveys indicate that consumption of

Table 1. Daily Food Guide

Food Group	Serving Size	Servings/Day
Breads, cereal, rice, pasta (preferably whole grains)	One slice bread	6–11
	One-half cup cooked rice, pasta, or cooked cereal	
	One ounce (3/4–1 cup) dry cereal	
	One-half bun, bagel, or English muffin	
	One 6-in. tortilla	
	Four small, plain crackers	
Vegetables	One cup raw leafy vegetables	3–5
	One-half cup other vegetables, raw or cooked	
	Three-fourths cup vegetable juice	
Fruits	One medium apple, banana, or orange	2–4
	One-half cup chopped fruit	
	Three-fourths cup fruit juice	
Milk, yogurt, cheese (preferably low fat or fat free)	One cup milk or yogurt	3
	One and one-half ounces natural cheese	
	Two ounces processed cheese	
Meat, poultry, fish, dry beans, peas, eggs, and nuts (preferably lean or low fat)	Two to three ounces lean meat, poultry, or fish	2
	One-half cup cooked dry beans or peas	
	One egg, or 2 tbsp. peanut butter = 1 oz. lean meat	
Fats, oils, and sweets	Use sparingly	—

Source: Modified from U.S. Department of Agriculture (1992). *The Food Guide Pyramid* (Home and Garden Bulletin No. 252). Hyattsville, MD: Author.

Table 2. Healthy People 2010: Key Nutrition-Related Objectives

Increase the proportion of adults who are at a healthy weight from 42 percent to 60 percent

Reduce the proportion of adults who are obese from 23 percent to 15 percent

Reduce the proportion of children and adolescents who are overweight or obese from 10–11 percent to 5 percent

Increase the proportion of persons aged 2 years and older who consume at least two daily servings of fruit from 28 percent to 75 percent

Increase the proportion of persons aged 2 years and older who consume at least three daily servings of vegetables, with at least one-third being dark green or deep yellow vegetables, from 3 percent to 50 percent

Increase the proportion of persons aged 2 years and older who consume at least six daily servings of grain products, with at least three being whole grains, from 7 percent to 50 percent

Increase the proportion of persons aged 2 years and older who consume less than 10 percent of calories from saturated fat from 36 percent to 75 percent

Increase the proportion of persons aged 2 years and older who consume no more than 30 percent of calories from fat from 33 percent to 75 percent

Increase the proportion of persons aged 2 years and older who consume 2,400 mg or less of sodium daily from 21 percent to 65 percent

Increase the proportion of persons aged 2 years and older who meet dietary recommendations for calcium from 46 percent to 75 percent

Reduce iron deficiency among young children and females of childbearing age from 9 percent to 5 percent among children aged 1 to 2 years, from 4 percent to 1 percent among children aged 3 to 4 years, and from 11 percent to 7 percent among nonpregnant females aged 12 to 49 years

Reduce anemia among low-income pregnant females in their third trimester from 29 percent to 20 percent

Reduce iron deficiency among pregnant females

Increase the proportion of children and adolescents aged 6–19 years whose intake of meals and snacks at school contributes proportionally to good overall diet quality

Increase the proportion of worksites that offer nutrition or weight management classes or counseling

Increase the proportion of physician office visits made by patients with a diagnosis of cardiovascular disease, diabetes, or hyperlipidemia that include counseling or education related to diet and nutrition

Increase food security among U.S. households and in so doing reduce hunger

Increase the proportion of mothers who breast-feed their babies from 64 percent to 75 percent in the early postpartum period, from 29 percent to 50 percent at 6 months, and from 16 percent to 25 percent at 1 year

Source: U.S. Department of Health and Human Services. (2000). *Healthy People 2010: National health promotion and disease prevention objectives.* Washington, DC: Public Health Service.

total and saturated fat remains above recommended levels for a large proportion of the population. Only 30 percent of Americans consume diets containing no more than 30 percent of calories from total fat, and 36 percent of Americans consume diets containing less than 10 percent of calories from saturated fat. These findings are due in part to an increased reliance by Americans on takeout and restaurant foods, which are typically higher in fat.

Diets that are high in total fat are associated with an increased risk for obesity, certain cancers, and gallbladder disease. Diets high in saturated fat and cholesterol are associated with a greater risk for coronary heart disease. Saturated fatty acids, which are found in meats and dairy products that contain fat, and trans-fatty acids, which are found in hydrogenated margarine and shortening, raise blood low-density-lipoprotein cholesterol levels, thereby increasing the risk for heart disease. Monounsaturated fatty acids, found in olive and canola oil, and polyunsaturated fatty acids, found in corn, sunflower, and safflower oils, do not raise blood cholesterol levels and should replace saturated fats in the diet to lower health risks.

Sodium

Excess sodium and salt intake has been linked to high blood pressure in many people. Food consumption survey data indicate that approximately 80 percent of Americans consume greater than the recommended maximum of 2,400 mg of sodium daily. Most dietary sodium is added to foods during processing. It is also added in the form of condiments such as table salt, soy sauce, ketchup, and mustard. *The Dietary Guidelines for Americans* recommend choosing a diet moderate in salt and sodium by limiting processed foods, added salt, and high-sodium condiments.

Calcium

Calcium is essential for the formation and maintenance of bones and teeth. In fact, the level of bone mass achieved at full growth (peak bone mass) appears to be related to the level of calcium intake during childhood and adolescence. Achieving optimal peak bone mass is thought to protect against fractures and osteoporosis later in life.

The DRI (dietary reference intake) for adequate daily calcium intake is 800 mg for children aged 4–8 years, 1,300 mg for adolescents aged 9–18 years, 1,000 mg for adults aged 19–50 years, and 1,200 mg for adults aged 51 and older. The DRI for pregnant adolescents and women is not increased above prepregnancy levels because calcium absorption increases during pregnancy. Population-based survey data indicate that more than 50 percent of the population consumes less calcium than recommended. These findings are particularly prevalent among adolescents and adult females.

Approximately three-fourths of calcium in the American diet comes from dairy products such as milk, yogurt, and cheeses. Individuals who suffer from lactose intolerance can often tolerate smaller amounts of milk with meals, aged cheeses, yogurt with active cultures, and/or lactose-reduced milk. Other high-calcium food sources include fortified orange juice, cereals, breakfast bars, and breads.

Iron

Iron deficiency is the most prevalent nutritional deficiency disorder in the United States. Iron deficiency can progress to iron deficiency anemia and cause preterm births, low birth weight, and delays in infant and child development. Iron deficiency is most common among minority and low-income children, females of childbearing age due to blood loss during menstruation, and pregnant women due to increased iron requirements during pregnancy. Food consumption data indicate that only 25 percent of women of child-bearing age meet the RDA (recommended dietary allowance) of 15 mg of iron daily. Iron deficiency among women of childbearing age and children can be prevented by consumption of iron-rich foods such as meats, poultry, fish, leafy greens, dried beans, and iron-enriched grains and cereals. Vitamin C-rich foods (orange juice and other citrus foods) should be consumed with iron-rich foods, as they enhance iron absorption. Supplementation with 30 mg of elemental iron is recommended for all pregnant women during the second and third trimesters to prevent iron deficiency anemia during pregnancy. Also, exclusive breast-feeding during the first 4–6 months and the use of iron-fortified formulas for formula-fed infants is recommended to prevent iron deficiency during infancy.

Nutritional factors are important throughout the life span. Nutritional status before and during pregnancy has an impact on maternal and infant outcomes. During childhood, nutritional factors can affect growth and development, resistance to disease, and risk for future chronic diseases. Nutrition is also related to several acute and chronic health conditions such as overweight, hypertension, coronary heart disease, stroke, certain cancers, and Type II diabetes. Behaviors to promote good nutrition should begin during infancy and childhood, and the development of healthy eating habits should continue throughout life.

BIBLIOGRAPHY

Healthy People 2010 & U.S. Department of Health and Human Services. (2000). *Healthy people 2010: Tracking healthy people 2010*. Washington, DC: U.S. Department of Health and Human Services.

Heimendinger, J., and Chapelsky, D. (1996). The National 5-A-Day for Better Health Program. *Advances in Experimental Medicine and Biology, 401*, 199–206.

Institute of Medicine. Standing Committee on the Scientific Evaluation of Dietary Reference Intakes. (1997). *DRI, Dietary reference intakes: For calcium, phosphorus, magnesium, vitamin D, and fluoride*. Washington, DC: National Academy Press.

Institute of Medicine. Subcommittee on Nutritional Status and Weight Gain During Pregnancy & Institute of Medicine. Subcommittee on Dietary Intake and Nutrient Supplements During Pregnancy. (1990). *Nutrition during pregnancy: Part I, Weight gain: Part II, Nutrient supplements*. Washington, DC: National Academy Press.

Lozoff, B., Jimenez, E., & Wolf, A. W. (1991). Long-term developmental outcome of infants with iron deficiency. *New England Journal of Medicine, 325*, 687–694.

National Center for Health Statistics & Centers for Disease Control and Prevention. (1997). *Atlas of United States mortality.* Hyattsville, MD: National Center for Health Statistics.

National Research Council Committee on Diet and Health. (1989). *Diet and health: Implications for reducing chronic disease risk.* Washington, DC: National Academy Press.

Subar, A. F., et al. (1995). Fruit and vegetable intake in the United States: The baseline survey of the Five A Day for Better Health Program. *American Journal of Health Promotion 9*, 352–360.

U.S. Agricultural Research Service. (2000). *1994–96, 1998 Continuing survey of food intakes by individuals (CSFII) and related survey materials, etc., April 2000* [CD-ROM]. Washington, DC: U.S. Department of Agriculture.

U.S. Department of Agriculture. (1992). *The food guide pyramid* (Home and Garden Bulletin No. 252). Washington, DC: Author.

U.S. Department of Agriculture & U.S. Department of Health and Human Services. (1995). *Nutrition and your health: Dietary guidelines for Americans* (4th ed., Home and Garden Bulletin No. 232). Washington, DC: Author.

U.S. Department of Health and Human Services. (2001). *The Surgeon General's call to action to prevent and decrease overweight and obesity.* Rockville, MD: U.S. Department of Health and Human Services, Public Health Service, Office of the Surgeon General.

Van Duyn, M. A., & Pivonka, E. (2000). Overview of the health benefits of fruit and vegetable consumption for the dietetics professional: Selected literature. *Journal of the American Dietetic Association, 100*, 1511–1521.

Yolanda Cartwright
Mary Story

Oo

Operant Conditioning

Operant conditioning is learning that occurs when an action becomes governed by its consequences. Operant conditioning is also referred to as instrumental learning because a certain type of responding is instrumental in leading to a desired consequence. An exemplar of operant conditioning is Edward Thorndike's law of effect, which states that if a response in the presence of a stimulus leads to satisfying effects, the association between the stimulus and the response is strengthened.

The law of effect operates through a mechanism called reinforcement. Reinforcement occurs when an event following a response increases an organism's tendency to make that response. Positive reinforcement occurs when a response is strengthened because it is followed by a reward. Negative reinforcement occurs when a response is strengthened because it is followed by the removal of an unpleasant stimulus. Researchers make a distinction between unlearned (primary) and learned (secondary) reinforcers. Primary reinforcers are rewards that are satisfying because they fulfill a biological need, such as food and water. Secondary reinforcers are rewards that are satisfying because of their relationship with primary reinforcers, such as money and praise.

Punishment is conceptualized as a consequence that weakens responding. Punishment has several drawbacks; for example, punishment can lead to a inhibition of behavior in all domains, not just the domain that is the target of modification. In addition, punishment can trigger a strong emotional response, such as fear, anxiety, anger, and resentment.

The basic processes involved in operant conditioning are acquisition, shaping, generalization, discrimination, and extinction. Acquisition refers to the initial stage of learning a new pattern of responding. Shaping occurs when closer approximations of the desired response are rewarded. Discrimination is the recognition of which specific stimuli (referred to as discriminative stimuli) indicate that a reward will probably follow, and responding only to those stimuli. In contrast, stimulus generalization occurs when the organism responds to stimuli that are similar to the original conditioned stimulus. Extinction refers to the gradual weakening and disappearance of a response tendency because it is no longer reinforced. Some behaviors are particularly resistant to extinction; for example, substance abusers have a hard time resisting substances even when they have ceased to be rewarding.

One of the factors that determines how resistant a behavior is to extinction is the schedule of reinforcement. The schedule of reinforcement describes which occurrences of the desired response get rewarded. When responses are reinforced only part of the time, called intermittent reinforcment, the behavior is more resistant to extinction than when the behavior is reinforced every time it is performed.

Evidence suggests that organisms have a species-specific preparedness to be conditioned to some stimuli and not others. Research has demonstrated that taste aversions can develop from foods that produce nausea despite long periods of time between consuming the food and the onset of the nausea. Additional research has demonstrated that phobic responses are more easily conditioned to stimuli that are more commonly feared (such as spiders and snakes) than those that are rarely feared (such as flowers and houses).

Related Entries: Classical Conditioning, Modeling

BIBLIOGRAPHY

Garcia, J. (1989). Food for Tolman: Cognition and cathexis in concert. In T. Archer & L. G. Nilsson (Eds.), *Aversion, avoidance, and anxiety: Perspective on aversively motivated behavior* (pp. 45–85). Hillsdale, NJ: Erlbaum.

Mineka, S., & Tomarken, A. J. (1989). The role of cognitive biases in the origins and maintenance of fear and anxiety disorders. In T. Archer & L. G. Nilsson (Eds.), *Aversion, avoidance, and anxiety: Perspective on aversively motivated behavior* (pp. 195–221). Hillsdale, NJ: Erlbaum.

Skinner, B. F. (1974). *About behaviorism.* New York: Knopf.

CHRISTINA L. FRANKLIN

Optimism and Health

Optimism is typically defined by psychologists as (1) having a generally positive view of the future, (2) attributing negative life events to factors unlikely to cause problems again, or (3) estimating one's personal chances of experiencing specific negative outcomes to be low (and positive outcomes high). Traits related to optimism include hardiness (the tendency to appraise stresses as challenges), self-efficacy (a belief in one's ability to effect positive outcomes), internal locus of control (feeling in control of what happens to oneself), and hope (a belief in one's ability to achieve goals, combined with planned strategies to achieve those goals). This entry discusses various definitions of optimism, their relation to health, and explanations for this link.

DISPOSITIONAL OPTIMISM

Dispositional optimism is usually measured by the Life Orientation Test (LOT), which includes items such as, "In uncertain times, I usually expect the best." Michael Scheier, Charles Carver, and others have shown that dispositional optimists experience relatively better physical health, report fewer illness symptoms, cope more effectively with stress, recover more quickly from surgery, are better able to deal with illness, are less likely to need rehospitalization, and have better survival rates following serious disease. The association between dispositional optimism and these outcomes holds even when taking into account other related traits such as neuroticism, and holds not only for self-reported outcomes, but also for more objective measures of those outcomes. The link has been demonstrated in a wide variety of different samples, including HIV-infected men, adult-daughter caregivers, and patients with head and neck cancer.

ATTRIBUTIONAL STYLE

Two methods have been used to measure attributional style. In the Attributional Style Questionnaire (ASQ), participants imagine experiencing a negative event and then report what they would consider to be the major cause. Then they evaluate whether this cause has something to do with them (internal vs. external dimension), whether it affects other personal outcomes (specific vs. global dimension), and whether it can be considered to be a temporary aberration (unstable vs. stable dimension). The second method is to subject written essays to a procedure (Content Analysis of Verbatim Explanations, or CAVE) that assesses each of the foregoing dimensions. When responses in either of these methods suggest an external, specific, and unstable attribution, the person is said to have an optimistic explanatory style. On the other hand, individuals who make internal, global, and stable attributions for negative events are said to have a pessimistic explanatory style, and tend to be more prone to depression. Optimism scores based on explanatory style are positively (though moderately) correlated with scores on the LOT.

Christopher Peterson and Lisa Bossio, in their 1991 book on optimism and health, reviewed several studies linking an optimistic explanatory style with positive health outcomes including general health (based on patient ratings or physician ratings), illness symptoms, illness onset, physician visits, illness susceptibility, immune system functioning, survival times following cancer diagnosis, survival times following heart attack, completion of rehabilitation programs, and longevity. Some work suggests that the globality and stability dimensions may be more important than the internality dimension.

EVENT-SPECIFIC OPTIMISM

The third common method of assessing optimism is to ask people to estimate their chances of experiencing one or more outcomes. Estimates of absolute risk are usually made on verbal scales (e.g., "How likely are you to get cancer") or numerical scales (e.g., "What is the percentage chance you will get cancer?"). Paul Windchitl and Gary Wells showed that verbal scales are more reliable because of people's difficulty in working with numbers. Often people are also asked to compare their risk with that of the typical person (comparative risk). Individuals who rate their absolute or comparative risk as low are defined as optimistic.

Nathan Radcliffe and William Klein, among others, found that optimism defined in this way is related to lower actual risk, less anxiety and worry, greater attention to health risk information, higher frequencies of health-promoting behavior, and better coping. Some studies (such as one by Karina Davidson and Kenneth Prkachin) linked such optimism with poorer health practices and less attention to risk information, but often these studies defined optimism based on estimates for a number of different health problems (increasing the chance that some estimates are inaccurate; see next section), or they measured optimism and health at the same time (opening the possibility that optimistic risk estimates reflect rather than cause health behavior). It is possible to be optimistic on one scale and not on another; for example, Isaac Lipkus and his colleagues found that women tend to be pessimistic about their breast cancer risk when measured on an absolute scale, yet optimistic when measured on a comparative scale. Comparative optimism is often not correlated (or only modestly correlated) with dispositional optimism, which may be due to the specificity of comparative optimism to a particular life event.

IMPORTANCE OF ACCURACY

Whether optimism promotes good health may depend on whether the beliefs underlying that optimism are accurate. One cannot easily assess the accuracy of a dispositionally optimistic orientation (because it is not based on specific predictions that can be verified), yet it is possible to verify the accuracy of a person's attribution for a negative event or that person's prediction of whether an event will happen. No research has examined the accuracy of attributions (which is not surprising, given that identifying the multiple causes of an event is a largely subjective exercise), yet much work has looked at the accuracy of predictions. As explained in a paper by Alexander Rothman, William Klein, and Neil Weinstein, this research shows that people often (1) overestimate small numerical risks, such as HIV risk, and underestimate large risks, such as the risk of getting divorced; (2) consider the chances of experiencing both high and low risks to be lower than that of the typical person, meaning that many people are unrealistically optimistic because not everyone can have below-average risk; and (3) overestimate the risk of other people experiencing health problems. Whereas people are unrealistically optimistic about their chances of having a health problem, Hart Blanton and his colleagues showed that people are unrealistically pessimistic about how well they would cope with the problem if they experienced it.

The question of whether biased optimistic beliefs are beneficial to health is a controversial one. Some studies show that even when optimistic beliefs are unrealistic, they may lead to the same positive health consequences noted earlier. For example, in a study by Shelley Taylor and colleagues, HIV-seropositive men considered their risk of getting AIDS to be lower than did HIV-seronegative men, a belief that was clearly biased. Yet the seropositive men also were engaging in more health-promoting behavior. On the other hand, a study by Nathan Radcliffe and William Klein showed that people who are unrealistically optimistic are less likely to be taking measures to reduce their (relatively higher) risk, and are less attentive to new risk information. Based on the evidence so far, unrealistic optimism may be particularly beneficial when it is mild, when it concerns a proximal threat, and when it motivates one to achieve the outcomes about which one is optimistic. David Armor and Shelley Taylor reviewed several studies consistent with such a conclusion.

HOW DOES OPTIMISM PROMOTE HEALTH?

Michael Scheier and Charles Carver found that dispositional optimism helps individuals cope with potential stressors, such as by using problem-focused strategies and by persisting in anxiety-provoking situations, which in turn enhances immune functioning and well-being. The trait is also associated with better health habits such as vitamin intake and exercise and nondefensive responses to health threats. People with an optimistic explanatory style seem to exhibit less negative affect and fewer depressive tendencies, possess better levels of social support, respond better to stress, set realistic and reachable goals, persevere at difficult tasks, bounce back well from setbacks, have immune systems that are more responsive to antigens, and have better health habits. In reviewing these possible reasons for the effect of optimism, Christopher Peterson and Lisa Bossio emphasized that no one mechanism is thought to be more powerful than the others—they seem to act together. It is unclear whether optimism exerts most of its influence on the onset or the course of an illness, or both.

CONCLUSION

The evidence suggests that optimism—defined in various ways—is associated with better physical health, and this link may be attributable to a variety of different factors including better health habits and coping strategies. Despite these findings, optimism still seems to influence health less strongly than family history, past health history, and other traits such as hostility and neuroticism. This is important because anecdotal evidence—such as the story of Norman Cousins, who maintained he cured his cancer by being positive—has a firm place in popular culture. An exaggerated belief in the power of optimism could lead to the blaming of ill people for their condition, and social support centered on "staying positive" might fail to help ill patients cope with their feelings. Nevertheless, the research suggests that programs designed to increase optimism, such as those that help people to attribute negative outcomes to external, specific, and unstable factors, may promote better health. As Christopher Peterson and Lisa Bossio noted, early attempts at this approach have been promising.

Related Entry: Pessimistic Explanatory Style

BIBLIOGRAPHY

Armor, D. A., & Taylor, S. E. (1998). Situated optimism: Specific outcome expectancies and self-regulation. *Advances in Experimental Social Psychology, 30*, 309–379.

Blanton, H., Axsom, D., McClive, K., & Price, S. (2001). Pessimistic bias in comparative evaluations: A case of perceived vulnerability to the effects of negative life events. *Personality and Social Psychology Bulletin, 27*, 1627–1636.

Chang, E. C. (2001). *Optimism and pessimism: Implications for theory, research, and practice.* Washington, DC: American Psychological Association.

Davidson, K., & Prkachin, K. (1997). Optimism and unrealistic optimism have an interacting impact on health-promoting behavior and knowledge changes. *Personality and Social Psychology Bulletin, 23*, 617–625.

Lipkus, I. M., Kuchibhatla, M., McBride, C. M., Bosworth, H. B., Pollak, K. I., Siegler, I. C., & Rimer, B. K. (2000). Relationships among breast cancer perceived absolute risk, comparative risk, and worries. *Cancer Epidemiology, Biomarkers and Prevention, 9*, 973–975.

Peterson, C., & Bossio, L. M. (1991). *Health and optimism.* NY: Free Press.

Radcliffe, N. M., & Klein, W. M. P. (2002). Dispositional, unrealistic, and comparative optimism: Differential relations with knowledge and processing of risk information and beliefs about personal risk. *Personality and Social Psychology Bulletin, 28*, 836–846.

Rothman, A. J., Klein, W. M., & Weinstein, N. D. (1996). Absolute and relative biases in estimations of personal risk. *Journal of Applied Social Psychology, 26*, 1213–1236.

Scheier, M. F., & Carver, C. S. (1992). Effect of optimism on psychological and physical well-being: Theoretical overview and empirical update. *Cognitive Therapy and Research, 16*, 201–228.

Taylor, S. E., Kemeny, M. E., Aspinwall, L. G., Schneider, S. G., Rodriguez, R., & Herbert, M. (1992). Optimism, coping, psychological distress, and high-risk sexual behavior among men at risk for acquired immunodeficiency syndrome (AIDS). *Journal of Personality and Social Psychology, 63*, 460–473.

Windschitl, P. D., & Wells, G. L. (1996). Measuring psychological uncertainty: Verbal vs. numeric methods. *Journal of Experimental Psychology: Applied, 2*, 343–364.

WILLIAM M. P. KLEIN

Organ Transplantation

Transplantation is an accepted therapeutic option for end-stage diseases of the kidneys, heart, liver, and lungs. Other forms of transplantation, including stem cell transplantation for diseases of the blood and intestinal transplantation for severe gastrointestinal disorders, are also becoming viable alternatives for extending and improving the quality of patients' lives. Thousands of persons receive the "gift of life" each year, and the majority are able to resume a lifestyle that was no longer possible with their end-stage disease. The new organs may extend their lives by years or even decades.

As for all medical therapies, there are psychological and health-related costs and benefits associated with transplantation, both for the organ recipients and for their families. Many of these costs and benefits are linked to specific phases of the transplantation process: Organ transplantation is best considered not as a discrete event (i.e., the surgery itself), but as a series of events and time periods that are associated with unique stressors and demand specific coping strategies. Figure 1 illustrates the typical time line for most individuals, whose initial contact and evaluation by the transplant medical team marks the beginning of the process of waiting for an organ, undergoing the surgery and initial postsurgical recovery period, returning home for the first year of rehabilitation after the transplant, and coping with new health challenges during the extended years after the surgery. Although some elements of the process can vary considerably in their duration (e.g., the length of the waiting period before transplant), the basic ordering of events and time periods is similar for all patients and all types of organ transplants. This entry discusses the key issues facing patients and their families during these events and time periods.

THE INITIAL EVALUATION FOR ORGAN TRANSPLANT

The formal medical evaluation for transplant candidacy is usually the first occasion during which patients and their families seriously consider transplantation as a therapeutic option. The evaluation may evoke conflicting feelings, including relief and the hope of having a healthy future, fears about surgical risks and adapting to life with "someone else's" organ, anxiety about whether the patient will be judged to be a suitable candidate, and realistic concerns that an organ will not become available soon enough to save the patient's life. Patients' heightened psychological distress related to these issues and their deteriorating physical health may significantly increase the perceived stressfulness of the medical evaluation.

The evaluation is usually lengthy and complex because it is designed to assess all aspects of patients' clinical and psychosocial status. In addition to biomedical and laboratory tests, mental health and substance use history, cognitive status, history of compliance with medical treatments for the disease, available social supports, and coping styles are routinely assessed because these factors may influence patients' psychological adaptation to waiting for the transplant and to life after the transplant. These psychosocial elements of the medical evaluation often serve as important additional stressors to patients and families because the information obtained may be used to decide whether patients should be immediately listed as transplant candidates or whether they need to undergo additional interventions to improve their health status and adherence to the medical requirements set by the transplant team. For example, they may need to enroll in alcohol or smoking cessation programs before they can be accepted onto the waiting list.

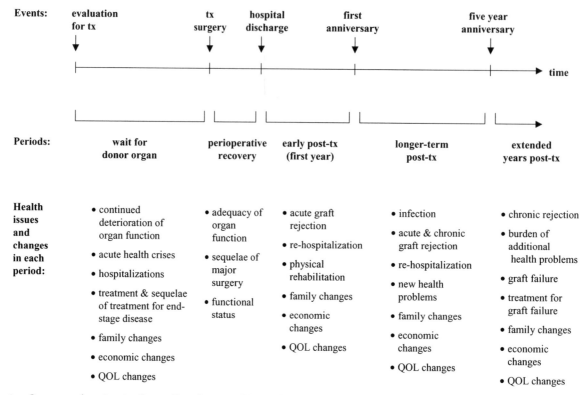

Figure 1. Organ transplantation time line. tx, Transplantation; QOL, quality of life. Reprinted with permission from *Medscape Transplantation* (http://www.medscape.com/viewpublication/704—about). © 2002, WebMD, Inc.

THE WAITING PERIOD

Many patients and their families perceive the waiting period to be the most psychologically stressful part of the transplant experience, due in large part to the patients' continued physical health deterioration and the inherent uncertainties about whether and when a suitable donor organ will become available. Like many chronic disease populations, transplant candidates are at high risk for psychological distress and depressive and anxiety-related disorders. Transplant candidates' cognitive status is often impaired as well. For example, hepatic encephalopathy is common in liver candidates. Heart transplant candidates often show cognitive deficits due to reduced blood flow to the brain. Kidney candidates who are not well dialyzed may have a range of subtle cognitive deficits. Continued elevations in psychological distress and/or mental status changes may lead patients to have difficulty adhering to the healthy lifestyle and medical regimen requirements set by the transplant team. For example, it may become difficult to follow specific diets or refrain from smoking or drinking.

As their organ function declines, patients may require increasingly complicated medical technologies and treatment regimens. These treatments themselves serve as stressors for patients. The strain may extend to the family as well. The patient's

marriage and relationships with primary family caregivers (who are most often spouses of adult patients and parents of pediatric patients) are particularly vulnerable due to role changes within the family and changes in daily living activities and schedules.

THE SURGERY AND THE PERIOPERATIVE RECOVERY PERIOD

This phase of the transplant process is characterized by major, but often positive, physical and emotional transitions. With the surgery completed, a majority of patients and their families are optimistic about prospects for recovery. The central concerns for most patients and families usually involve how well the new organ is functioning and the probable speed of the patient's physical recovery. These concerns are sometimes heightened by knowledge that, due in part to health insurance coverage limitations, hospital stays following the surgery are brief, ranging from 1 week to several weeks in the absence of major complications.

Moreover, the brief posttransplant hospital stay is often perceived as stressful because patients and families typically receive many educational materials about life posttransplant during this time. (This information may have been provided before the transplant as well, but it is likely to have been difficult for patients to absorb due to other stresses and/or cognitive impairment during the waiting period.) The positive feelings and optimism that often dominate after the surgery can interfere with educational efforts during the perioperative period because these feelings may lead patients and their families to be less able to accept and focus on information concerning potential complications, financial issues, and family difficulties that can arise posttransplant.

THE FIRST YEAR AFTER THE TRANSPLANT

For most transplant recipients, the first year after the surgery brings gradual improvements in all domains of quality of life, including physical functional status, emotional well-being, and social functioning. Many important psychosocial issues, however, may slow patients' improvement and may also affect family members' well-being. These issues are related to patients' need to (1) cope with physical and emotional changes induced by the immunosuppressive medications required to prevent organ rejection, (2) alter their self-image beyond that of a critically ill individual and resume a less illness-focused lifestyle, (3) psychologically accept the transplant and the fact that, in cadaver donation, donors lost their lives just when recipients regained theirs, and (4) manage the continuing financial costs associated with the transplant and follow-up care.

A likely result of these concerns is that risks of experiencing emotional distress and clinically significant episodes of depressive and anxiety-related disorders are higher during the first year posttransplant than during later years. Some psychiatric disorders, for example, posttraumatic stress disorder related to the transplant, may be limited almost exclusively to the first year.

An additional area of difficulty for many patients is compliance with their complex posttransplant treatment regimen. Not only must patients take multiple medications, but they have exercise and diet requirements, follow-up medical evaluations and laboratory tests, and restrictions on smoking, alcohol, and other substance use. Compliance in most areas of these areas worsens over the first year after the transplant, just as it does for most patients with complex regimens. Psychosocial and emotional strains during the year exacerbate patients' risk of having difficulty with the medical regimen.

THE EXTENDED YEARS AFTER THE TRANSPLANT

Compared to the other phases of the transplant experience, less is known about psychosocial and adjustment issues that arise in the long term posttransplant. This is due largely to the fact that, with the exception of kidney transplantation, long-term survival in solid organ transplantation (heart, liver, lung) has only become a reality in recent years. Nevertheless, as shown in Figure 1, the years beyond the first anniversary of the transplant can be divided into at least two periods. There is usually a multiyear period following the first anniversary in which patients achieve maximal functioning of the transplanted organ, with a relatively low level and severity of complications and infrequent episodes of acute organ rejection. Patients' physical functional capabilities and quality of life are often high. With time, however, other problems with the organ often develop (e.g., "chronic" rejection), and patients may become more limited functionally due to long-term immunosuppressive medication complications, including diabetes, hypertension, and cancer.

Many of the psychosocial and health-related concerns that emerged during the first year posttransplant carry over into subsequent years. Focal issues for patients in the long term concern maintaining as high a quality of life as possible and postponing the effects of declining organ function and related complications. Financial strains related to continuing medication and health care needs may assume greater prominence. These sources of stress may provoke renewed increases in distress and rates of psychiatric disorders in over the very long term.

CONCLUSION

Each phase of the organ transplant process, from the initial evaluation through the long-term years after the transplant, is associated with unique stressors and psychosocial issues that are of concern to both patients and their families. Patients' physical and mental health at one phase of the process are affected by, and in turn affect, their health in other phases. Moreover, the transplant experience influences the well-being of the patient's family. Identification of the unique difficulties and concerns experienced by patients and families during this process will allow for the development of interventions to reduce the impact of these difficulties on individuals' health.

Related Entries: Body Image, Coping, Posttraumatic Stress Disorder (PTSD), Stressful Life Events

BIBLIOGRAPHY

Cupples, S. A., & Ohler, L. (Eds). (2002). *Solid organ transplantation: A handbook for primary health care providers.* New York: Springer.
Dew, M. A., Manzetti, J., Goycoolea, J. M., Lee, A., Zomak, R., Vensak, J. L., et al. (2002). Psychosocial aspects of transplantation. In S. L. Smith &

Linda Ohler (Eds.), *Organ transplantation: Concepts, issues, practice and outcomes* (Chapter 8). New York: Medscape Transplantation. Available at WebMD, Inc., www.medscape.com/transplantationhome

Trzepacz, P., & DiMartini, A. (2000). *The transplant patient: Biological, psychiatric and ethical issues in organ transplantation.* Cambridge: Cambridge University Press.

United Network for Organ Sharing. Available at www.unos.org

USTransplant.org. *Scientific registry of transplant recipients*, available at www.ustransplant.org

MARY AMANDA DEW
LARISSA MYASKOVSKY
GALEN E. SWITZER
ANDREA F. DIMARTINI

Pp

Pain

Pain is one of the most complex of human experiences. It is the most common reason for which patients seek medical care. More than 80% of all physician visits are due to pain. Pain accounts for over $70 billion annually in health care costs and lost productivity. It is defined by the International Association for the Study of Pain as "an unpleasant sensory and emotional experience associated with actual or potential tissue damage." Accordingly, the perception of pain is not only a sensory experience, but also an emotional experience. It is important to distinguish between acute and chronic pain. The distinction between the two is not simply a matter of duration: (1) Acute pain is biologically useful; it serves as the body's alarm of an underlying medical condition, whereas chronic pain loses this function. (2) The etiology of acute pain is almost always identifiable, whereas the complex interaction of physical and emotional factors in chronic pain make the etiology murky. (3) Cure and relief are almost always attainable in acute pain, but is often not possible with chronic pain; the goal in chronic pain treatment is to improve functionality. (4) Acute pain may lead to anxiety, whereas chronic pain is often associated with depression.

The first psychological model of chronic pain was the psychodynamic approach, which emphasized the psychological etiology of pain. Freud viewed pain as a symptomatic expression of an unconscious conflict seeking awareness. In 1965, Melzack and Wall revolutionized the way we think about pain with their "gate control" theory. For the first time, pain theory incorporated higher brain functions such as cognition and affect. The theory postulated the existence of a "spinal gate" in the dorsal horn of the spinal column, which modulates transmission cells influenced by inhibitory and facilitative fibers. Quite significantly, the theory postulated that cognitive and affective states can help open or close the gate. Although the theory has been revised due to new physiological discoveries, its basic premises remain.

Behavioral models, particularly operant conditioning, proposed by William Fordyce in the 1970s became popular. Fordyce proposed that the behavioral expression of pain, pain behavior, is the result of positive and negative reinforcers from the patient's environment such as social reinforcement from family and friends, medications from physicians, financial incentives, or avoidance of activities. Subsequently, cognitive–behavioral models of pain became more popular, and remain the prevailing theory with regard to the assessment and treatment of chronic pain. The cognitive–behavioral model theorizes that the experience of pain is a reciprocal interaction of thoughts, feelings, physiology, and behavior.

The traditional medical model of chronic pain was that pain had either a physical basis or a psychological one. It is now well accepted that chronic pain is the end product of physiological, psychological, and social processes. These biopsychosocial determinants of chronic pain interact with one another: Neurophysiological responses to noxious stimuli can trigger psychological responses, whereas psychological states such as depression or anxiety can affect the neurophysiological system by enhancing or inhibiting the transmission of noxious signals. Social factors such as stress, environmental reinforcers of pain (such as an overly attentive spouse), or financial compensation (such as through disability or litigation) can significantly influence a patient's perception of pain. Many patients with chronic pain, particularly if pain resulted from an accident at work, will go on disability because they cannot or will not return to work. The disability system, however, often works against the best interests of the patient and the goals of pain management by offering compensation comparable to work, by promoting activity restrictiveness, by leading to extensive delays in medical and psychological authorizations, and by the not offering light duty work or trial return-to-work periods.

The most prevalent psychological characteristic of chronic pain patients is depression. Depression and chronic pain occur together so frequently that it is often difficult to determine whether the depression is a precipitant of the pain or a consequence of living with intractable pain. Levels of depression can range from minor mood state disturbances to major clinical depressions with active suicidal ideation. Other characteristics of patients with "chronic pain syndrome" include increased dependency on others, increased illness behaviors (such as grimacing), overreliance on medications, increased health care utilization, and family dysfunction (spouses may display clinically significant levels of emotional distress).

The multidisciplinary evaluation and treatment approach to the patient suffering with chronic pain is widely practiced and considered to be the standard of care. The psychological evaluation and assessment of chronic pain patients has evolved from unidimensional to multidimensional models. Since the formation of the first multidisciplinary pain center in 1961 by John Bonica at the University of Washington, there are over 350 such centers. A multidisciplinary pain center is a facility in which comprehensive treatment is provided by a team of health care professionals including physicians, psychologists, physical therapists, occupational therapists, and nurses. A major advantage of the team approach is that a broad base of knowledge and expertise is available, which can facilitate a team analysis of the etiology of pain and the appropriate treatment approach.

Despite the increasing recognition of the importance of appropriate pain control, as evidenced by the formation of national professional societies such as the American Pain Society and the recently revised accreditation criteria of the Joint Commission on Accreditation of Hospitals mandating pain evaluations of every hospitalized patient, pain is often undertreated. Lack of knowledge on the part of health care professionals regarding the appropriate evaluation and treatment of pain, as well as poor attitudes, particularly the unwarranted fear of addiction on the part of both patient and provider, hamper proper pain control efforts. Appropriate pain control therefore continues to be a significant challenge for the patient, the patient's family, and health care providers.

Although the treatment of a patient with chronic pain mandates a comprehensive evaluation of the medical as well as psychological contributors to the etiology, maintenance, and exacerbation of pain, evaluating and treating chronic pain patients with a unimodal, strictly medical approach still occurs. Relying solely on radiographic results of the spine, which have been shown to be unreliable indices of pain, to explain a patient's pain can lead to failed surgical interventions. Additionally, significant spinal abnormalities are found in patients who are not experiencing back pain. Other detrimental effects of a strictly medical approach to chronic pain include not evaluating

chronic pain patients for maladaptive behaviors, such as drug-seeking behaviors or addictive personality traits, which can lead to inappropriate pharmacologic management. Another example of psychological issues that can be overlooked without a comprehensive psychological evaluation are patterns of somatization, which can lead to repeated medical interventions by all-too-willing pain specialists, and further contribute to medical and psychological morbidity. Therefore, the Commission on Accreditation of Rehabilitation Facilities (CARF) only accredits chronic pain programs that are interdisciplinary in both their evaluation and treatment of patients and require as part of the core pain team a psychologist or psychiatrist.

PSYCHOLOGICAL ASSESSMENT OF THE CHRONIC PAIN PATIENT

The objectives of the psychological evaluation of the patient with chronic pain are as follows: (1) To determine the degree of psychological adaptation to chronic pain, including mood state, coping skills, effect on family, and level of physical functioning. (2) To evaluate the patient's psychological state before his or her pain began, which would include personality factors that may influence pain etiology. (3) To determine the role of psychological factors in terms of the etiology, maintenance, and exacerbation of pain. (4) To identify environmental reinforcers of chronic pain and illness behaviors such as family, litigation status, and disability insurance status. (5) To evaluate the likelihood of the development of a chronic pain-related disability. (6) To predict outcome of invasive procedures such as surgical implantation of spinal cord stimulators or continuous infusion pumps.

The standard pain center evaluation protocol utilizes a pain questionnaire, a structured clinical interview, pain assessment measures (including pain intensity rating scales and the McGill Pain Questionnaire), and a psychological evaluation of the patient.

The pain questionnaire should be designed to yield objective clinical outcome measures, and include information such as demographic characteristics, pain descriptors such as throbbing or gnawing, what makes the pain better and worse, whether there is interference with sleep, and circumstances related to the onset of pain. Also included typically are a review of prior nonpharmacologic interventions and their efficacy, specific current and past medication use to treat symptoms, litigation and compensation status, job status, job satisfaction, and specific occasions when pain interferes with quality of life.

The clinical interview should review the patient's pain complaints, onset of pain and relationship to trauma, prior medical and psychiatric history, prior alcohol and drug usage, current marital and family environment, current functional level, utilization of coping skills, disability status, motivational level to return to work, the possibility of secondary gain issues, ability to experience restful sleep at night, and beliefs and cognitions about his or her pain.

Measures of psychological status typically include a measure of mood state such as the Beck Depression Inventory (BDI). The BDI, a 20-item test using a 0–3 rating scale for each item, is one of the most widely used tests with chronic pain patients because it is a relatively quick measure of depression, a mood state closely linked with chronic pain. The Minnesota Multiphasic Personality Inventory (MMPI, MMPI-2), one of the most widely used and researched tests, is used quite extensively with chronic pain patients. The MMPI is a 566-question true–false test that evaluates the presence of psychopathology through three validity scales (the degree to which respondents may be trying to distort their true persona), and 10 clinical scales: Hypochondriasis, Depression, Hysteria, Psychopathic Deviance (history of antisocial behavior and nonconformance), Paranoia, Psychasthenia (obsessive–compulsive tendencies and other expressions of anxiety), Schizophrenia, Hypomania, Masculinity–Femininity, and Social Introversion. Other measures include the Symptom Checklist 90–Revised (SCL–90R), a commonly used assessment of psychological symptom patterns, which evaluates nine symptom dimensions: somatization, obsessive–compulsive, interpersonal sensitivity, depression, anxiety, hostility, phobic anxiety, paranoid ideation, and psychoticism.

The Coping Strategies Questionnaire, a 48-item questionnaire using a 7-point Likert-type scale, assesses six cognitive coping responses and two behavioral responses to pain: catastrophizing, ignoring sensations, reinterpreting pain sensations, coping self-statements, diverting attention, praying and hoping, increasing behavioral activity, and increasing pain behaviors. It is an extensively used measure designed to evaluate how pain patients cope with their pain. Coping techniques have been well researched and found to be important mediators of pain perception and functionality. Active coping strategies such as staying busy, ignoring pain, and distraction have been associated with less pain, whereas passive coping strategies such as restricting activities, wishful thinking, and depending on others tend to lead to more pain. Specific coping strategies such as "catastrophizing" correlate strongly in a negative manner with a pain patient's prognosis.

As pain management has become more technologically sophisticated and aggressive in its approach, one of the more common uses of the psychological evaluation has been to determine the appropriateness of a potential candidate for an interventional technique. A meta-analysis of the literature on this topic concluded that patients should be excluded from implantable spinal cord stimulators if they have active psychosis, suicidality, untreated major depression, somatization disorder, alcohol or drug dependency, compensation/litigation disincentive to recovery, lack of social supports, or cognitive deficits (severity and type unspecified). Additional considerations for exclusion include unusual pain ratings, significant personality disorders, physical incongruence, a high elevation on the Depression scale of the MMPI, or elevations on four or more MMPI scales.

The clinician needs to take the results from the pain questionnaire, clinical interview, and psychological assessment measures, and with sound clinical judgment formulate a diagnosis and treatment plan that is individually geared to each patient. To paraphrase Sir William Osler, "It is not the type of disease that a patient has that is as important as the type of patient that has the disease."

PSYCHOLOGICAL MANAGEMENT OF PAIN

The psychological intervention with the patient who has chronic pain is an integral part of a multidisciplinary approach to pain management. The overall goal of pain management centers is to return the patient to a more optimal level of functioning. Improved functionality rather than cure of pain is often the focus of pain management. The most commonly utilized psychological approach is the cognitive–behavioral modality. The general objective of cognitive–behavioral treatment strategies is to assist the patient in reconceptualizing his or her belief about pain as an uncontrollable medical symptom to a belief that the patient's response to pain can be under his or her control. The initial step is educating the patient about the mind–body relationship. The effectiveness of this step depends on the patient's defensiveness, level of knowledge about the mechanism of pain, and attitudes about the mind–body relationship. The mainstay of this approach is relaxation training, which helps patients to redirect their focus away from pain, reduce autonomic reactivity, and enhance a sense of self-control. Relaxation training can be accomplished through guided imagery, progressive muscular relaxation, biofeedback, and hypnosis. Relaxation seems to work through reduction of muscle tension, distraction of the patient from his or her pain and body, and a feeling of enhanced control over the body.

Guided imagery has the patient focus on a multisensory imaginary scene. Typically, the image is elicited from the patient, and the psychotherapist guides the patient through the image, substituting sensations such as warmth or numbness for pain. Diaphragmatic breathing is an important part of the relaxation experience, distracting the patient even further.

In progressive muscular relaxation, patients are taught to alternately tense and relax individual muscle groups throughout the body. Only nonpainful muscle groups and body locations are used. Patients learn to recognize and differentiate feelings of tension and relaxation.

Biofeedback is a particularly effective modality for teaching chronic pain patients relaxation as well as self-regulation of physiological processes. Biofeedback monitors ongoing physiological processes such as muscle tension, heart rate, temperature, and even brain waves (called electroencephalographic neurofeedback) and provides the patient with visual and auditory feedback. Body sensors attached to a computer enables the patient to achieve relaxation, which can increase pain tolerance, decrease emotional distress, and even relax specific muscle spasms. Physiological self-control leads to a sense of control, better coping skills, and hopefulness. Pain syndromes with which biofeedback is most effective include headaches, transmandibular joint dysfunction, myofascial pain syndrome, fibromyalgia, and pain exacerbated by stress or anxiety.

Hypnosis is another particularly effective therapeutic technique with pain patients. It not only teaches patients relaxation, but also enables them to experience an analgesic reinterpretation of their pain, experiencing numbness, for example, instead of pain. In one study, women with metastatic breast carcinoma pain undergoing weekly group therapy with self-hypnosis had significantly lower pain ratings over 1 year than a control group.

In addition to education and relaxation training, an essential part of the cognitive–behavioral approach is cognitive restructuring. With this technique, patients are taught to identify maladaptive negative thoughts that pervade their thinking and to replace them with more constructive and adaptive positive thoughts. The maladaptive thoughts often take the form of statements about oneself or one's illness that are negative, and can include overgeneralizing or catastrophizing. Maladaptive thoughts patients with chronic pain typically have include "Pain signifies something is terribly wrong," "Pain means I need more surgery," and "No one can help me, it's hopeless."

A National Institutes of Health technology assessment conference on the efficacy of mind–body approaches for the treatment of chronic pain and insomnia found "strong" to "moderate" evidence to support the use of relaxation techniques, hypnosis, cognitive–behavioral therapy, and biofeedback in reducing chronic pain. The American Psychological Association has specified that the psychological treatment of chronic pain is one of 25 areas for which there is empirical validation for psychological intervention.

Psychotherapy also plays an essential role in the psychological intervention with pain patients. This can include supportive psychotherapy, group therapy, psychoanalytic (dynamic) psychotherapy, and/or family therapeutic interventions.

Nevertheless, there are barriers to the integration of these psychological therapies into chronic pain management practice. These barriers include a continued overemphasis on the biomedical model, a lack of standardization of psychological techniques, physician reluctance to refer to psychologists (due to lack of awareness of benefits, and concern regarding patient feeling that the physician perceives their pain as imaginary or "in their head"), and poor insurance reimbursement.

In conclusion, the psychological evaluation of patients suffering with chronic pain is based on a comprehensive evaluation of them and their pain. The evaluation protocol typically uses a pain questionnaire, a structured clinical interview, pain assessment measures, and psychological testing of the patient. The psychological treatment of the patient with pain is most often a cognitive–behavioral approach, with relaxation training as the mainstay. The assessment and management of the patient with chronic pain underscore the important role of mental health care providers in their care.

Related Entries: Gate Theory of Pain, McGill Pain Inventory, Placebo Effects

BIBLIOGRAPHY

Beck, A. T., Rush, A. J., Shaw, B. F., & Emery, G. (1979). *Cognitive therapy of depression.* New York: Guilford.

Block, A. R., Kremer, E. F., & Fernandez, E. (Eds.). (1999). *Handbook of pain syndromes—Biopsychosocial perspectives.* Mahwah, NJ: Erlbaum.

Bradley, L. A. (1996). Cognitive–behavioral therapy for chronic pain. In R. Gatchel & D. Turk (Eds.), *Psychological approaches to pain management* (pp. 00–00). New York: Guilford.

Butcher, N. B., Dahlstrom, W. G., Graham, J. R., et al. (1989). *MMPI–2, manual for administration and scoring.* Minneapolis: University of Minnesota Press.

Derogatis, L. R. (1977). *The SCL–90R: Administration scoring and procedures manual I.* Baltimore: Clinical Psychometrics Research.

Flor, H., & Birbaumer, N. (1993). Comparison of the efficacy of EMG biofeedback, cognitive–behavior therapy, and conservative medical interventions on the treatment of chronic musculoskeletal pain. *Journal of Consulting and Clinical Psychology, 61,* 653–658.

Fordyce, W. E. (1976). *Behavioral methods in chronic pain and illness.* St. Louis, MO: Mosby.

Gatchel, R., & Turk, D. C. (Eds.) (1996). *Psychological approaches to pain management—A practitioner's handbook.* New York: Guilford.

Holzman, A. D., & Turk, D. C. (Eds.). (1986). *Pain management—A handbook of psychological treatment approaches.* New York: Pergamon.

Keller, L. S., & Butcher, J. N. (Eds.). (1991). *Assessment of chronic pain patients with the MMPI–2.* Minneapolis: University of Minnesota Press.

Lefkowitz, M., Lebovits, A. H., Wlody, D., & Rubin, S. (Eds.). *A practical approach to pain management.* Boston: Little Brown.

Melzack, R. (1975). The McGill Pain Questionnaire: Major properties and scoring methods. *Pain, 1,* 277–299.

Nelson, D. V., Kennington, M., & Novy, D. M. (1996). Psychological selection criteria for implantable spinal cord stimulators. *Pain Forum, 5,* 93–103.

Romano, J. M., & Turner, J. A. (1985). Chronic pain and depression: Does the evidence support a relationship? *Psychological Bulletin, 97,* 18–34.

Rosenstiel, A. K., & Keefe, F. J. (1983). The use of coping strategies in chronic low back pain patients: Relationship to patient characteristics and current adjustment. *Pain, 17,* 33–44.

Spiegel, D., & Bloom, J. (1983). Group therapy and hypnosis reduce metastatic breast carcinoma pain. *Psychosomatic Medicine, 45,* 333–339.

Turk, D. C., & Melzack, R. (2001). *Handbook of pain assessment* (2nd ed.). New York: Guilford.

ALLEN LEBOVITS

Panic Disorder

Panic disorder is one of the most widely recognized, publicized, and investigated anxiety disorders. Individuals diagnosed with panic disorder experience discrete, recurrent, unexpected episodes of fear or discomfort that develop abruptly and reach a peak within 10 min. These episodes of fear are accompanied by four or more symptoms such as racing heart, chest pain, shortness of breath, dizziness, sweating, numbness, chills, shaking, fear of dying, fear of losing control, and/or fear of going crazy. Individuals with panic disorder experience persistent concern about experiencing future panic attacks, and worry about the consequences of the panic attacks and/or a change in behavior because of them (e.g., reducing time spent at work or cutting back on social activities). As with the other anxiety disorders, these symptoms cannot be directly caused by a substance, such as caffeine, or by a general medical condition, such as an overactive thyroid.

PANIC DISORDER WITH AGORAPHOBIA

Panic disorder may occur with or without agoraphobia. Individuals with panic disorder with agoraphobia (PDA) avoid situations that might be difficult to leave or escape from, or avoid situations in which help would be unavailable should a panic attack occur. For individuals with PDA, situations that are commonly avoided include being in grocery stores, shopping malls, restaurants, movie theaters, and churches or temples, driving far from home, traveling over bridges, being in crowds, and using public transportation. Agoraphobic avoidance typically develops as a coping strategy for trying to avoid having another panic attack. Individuals with PDA avoid going places or being in situations where panic attacks may occur or have occurred in the past. It seems that secondary gain in the form of negative reinforcement (anxiety diminishing when the person leaves a situation) and/or positive reinforcement (extra attention or help from other people) may also contribute to the development of agoraphobia. Agoraphobic avoidance may interfere mildly (e.g., grocery shopping during a time of day when lines are minimal) or severely, to the point that an individual may be entirely housebound or only venture outside with a specific "safe" person.

Individuals with PDA may also try to avoid physical symptoms that resemble panic attacks. They may avoid physical activities such as exercise (which may cause racing heart or chest tightness), being in hot, stuffy rooms (which may cause sweating or shortness of breath), or alcohol (which may cause dizziness). White and Barlow refer to this cluster of responses as "interoceptive avoidance," and hold that it is just as important as the situational avoidance just described.

Epidemiologic studies worldwide indicate that between 1.5% and 3.5% of people have panic disorder at some point during their lifetime. Between 1% and 2% of the population is affected with panic disorder during any 1-year period. Additionally, about 33%–50% of individuals with panic disorder also have agoraphobia. Panic disorder is typically a disorder of adults, beginning at a median age of 24 years. The average age for seeking treatment is 34 years. Twice as many women experience panic disorder as men, and increasing severity of agoraphobia is associated with a higher proportion of women. The most common explanation for this marked difference in rate of occurrence among men and women involves cultural factors, in that it is generally more acceptable for women to report fear and to avoid various situations due to fear.

PDA tends to be chronic and result in high levels of occupational, social, and physical disability according to several important studies that followed individuals over time. Antony and colleagues found that people with panic disorder reported *more* impairment than people with chronic medical conditions such as end-state renal disease or multiple sclerosis.

ETIOLOGY

Most individuals with panic disorder (more than 70%) can clearly remember a stressful situation (e.g., either interpersonal difficulties, concern about their physical well being, or having a frightening experience with drugs such as anesthetics or marijuana) that was going on when their panic attacks began. Barlow's model of the etiology of panic disorder posits a nonspecific biological predisposition to react to negative events with emotionality, anxiety, and possibly panic attacks. This biological predisposition, combined with a psychological predisposition to focus anxiety on somatic events that are perceived to be uncontrollable and potentially threatening or dangerous, creates a diathesis. This focus on somatic events or life stress then triggers an unexpected panic attack. Among those with the specific biological and psychological vulnerabilities (the diathesis), anxiety becomes focused on experiencing future panic attacks and worry about the consequences of the attacks, and panic disorder subsequently develops.

FREQUENT HEALTH CARE SEEKING

Because panic attack symptoms mimic a variety of cardiac, respiratory, neurological, and gastrointestinal symptoms, a key component of a diagnostic assessment of panic disorder includes ruling out potential medical causes for the panic symptoms through a medical evaluation. Most patients with panic disorder (80%–89%) initially seek treatment in general medical and not mental health settings. This is somewhat problematic, given that panic disorder is not typically recognized in medical settings. Seventy percent of patients with panic disorder see an average of 10 physicians before being correctly diagnosed. Of patients with panic disorder, 61%–80% are not recognized as having panic disorder in the primary care setting and 98% are not correctly identified in emergency departments. When compared to people with other psychological disorders (such as depression), those with panic disorder use medical services far more frequently, and are among the highest utilizers of medical services, especially emergency departments.

Why is panic disorder so rarely diagnosed in medical settings? Roy-Byrne and Katon suggest that patient barriers (e.g., the stigma of mental illness, lack of knowledge of the mind–body connection), physician barriers (e.g., the tendency to look for physical causes of somatic symptoms, overemphasis on not missing a medical disorder due to our litigious society), and system and process of medical care barriers (e.g., lack of adequate time for primary care physician diagnosis, an overwhelmed medical system) all contribute to the problem of panic disorder not being recognized.

In primary care settings, physicians may rule out an organic etiology for a patient's physical symptoms, but offer no additional treatment or explanation beyond the feedback that there is nothing physically wrong with him or her. Although the medical community may assume that informing patients they do not have a medical problem is reassuring, for patients with panic disorder this can be frustrating because they still do not have an explanation for their intense and frightening physical symptoms.

TREATMENT

Psychological Approaches

Recent studies have suggested that in general, patients with anxiety disorders are seldom treated, and those who are treated often receive ineffective treatments. The psychological treatment for panic disorder that has received indisputable empirical support is cognitive–behavioral therapy (CBT). More than 25 independently conducted, controlled clinical trials have demonstrated the effectiveness of CBT. Craske and Barlow recently summarized statistics from all randomized controlled trials and concluded that 76% of treatment completers are free of panic at the end of treatment, and 78% are still panic free 2 years later. Importantly, 66% of patients maintained or improved on the gains made in treatment even after treatment ended. In addition to eliminating panic attacks, researchers found that CBT improves quality of life.

The CBT approach to treating panic disorder is based on cognitive and learning theory principles of fear acquisi-

tion and reduction. The goal is to reduce patients' fear and avoidance of internal and external cues associated with panic attacks. CBT is directed at correcting patients' maladaptive thoughts and behaviors that initiate, sustain, or exacerbate panic symptoms. CBT targets fears of bodily sensations as well as anxious apprehension over the recurrence of panic. CBT is typically conducted in a structured, short-term modality of 10–15 sessions, and may be done in an individual or group format.

There are several key components of CBT for panic disorder. These include use of daily monitoring forms and homework, psychoeducation to correct misappraisals of bodily sensations, cognitive restructuring to challenge fearful thoughts regarding the meaning of bodily sensations, diaphragmatic breathing retraining to achieve somatic control, interoceptive exposure to reduce the fear of bodily sensations, and (if indicated) *in vivo* exposure to reduce the fear of agoraphobic situations. Some experts argue that the interoceptive exposure component of treatment is the most important. Interoceptive exposure involves deliberately provoking feared physical sensations like breathlessness, dizziness, and accelerated heart rate by means of exercises such as forced hyperventilation, spinning, and running in place, with the goal of reducing the fear of bodily sensations through habituation.

Additionally, the CBT approach to treating panic disorder discourages avoidance of activities that may produce physical sensations (e.g., ingesting caffeine, exercise, hot conditions). Moreover, any activity that is done to keep the person's mind off feelings of anxiety (distraction) is also discouraged. This includes counting, reading coping statements, playing loud music, drinking water, and so on. These activities are discouraged because they are not helpful in the long run and do not alter the underlying processes that lead to panic attacks, and thus prevent corrective learning from occurring. More recently, the argument has been made that diaphragmatic breathing is a form of distraction, and therefore should not be taught as a coping skill. For individuals with agoraphobic avoidance, situational *in vivo* exposure treatment typically begins by creating a hierarchy of feared situations or activities that have been regularly avoided such as grocery stores, driving, malls, crowds, and so on. Patients are then encouraged to repeatedly enter and remain in these feared situations, utilizing therapeutic coping skills until their anxiety diminishes.

Pharmacologic Approaches

In general, pharmacotherapy for panic disorder is concerned primarily with the elimination of panic and limited symptom attacks, with the expectation that when those are controlled, reductions in anticipatory anxiety and agoraphobic avoidance will follow. The three major classes of medications used to treat panic disorder are benzodiazepines, tricyclic antidepressants (TCAs), and selective serotonin reuptake inhibitors (SSRIs).

The efficacy of benzodiazepines, such as alprazolam (Xanax), diazepam (Valium), clonazepam (Klonopin), and lorazepam (Ativan), in the acute treatment of panic disorder has been demonstrated in several trials. In most studies, 50%–75% of patients were panic free by the end of treatment. With aggressive treatment, panic attacks can be reduced within a few days, and global improvement commonly appears within a few weeks. Unfortunately, approximately 50% of patients relapse when the drug is discontinued. There is some risk of drug tolerance, abuse, and dependence, although this appears to be a problem principally among individuals with a personal or family history of drug abuse or dependence. Nonetheless, physiological dependence develops in most patients with prolonged benzodiazepine use, as indicated by the appearance of withdrawal symptoms during drug discontinuation.

Since the 1960s, over 15 controlled clinical trials have demonstrated the efficacy of tricyclic antidepressants with panic disorder, and have demonstrated both short-term and long-term effectiveness. Imipramine (Tofranil), and less studied clomipramine (Anafranil), desipramine (Norpramin), and nortriptyline (Pamelor), are thought to selectively suppress uncued panic attacks. Despite their empirical effectiveness, clinically, the TCAs are often accompanied by troublesome side effects that are difficult to tolerate, such as weight gain, constipation, and blurred vision. The termination of TCA use is also linked with high relapse rates.

The selective (SSRIs) are considered by many to be the state-of-the-art treatment for panic disorder. Numerous studies have demonstrated the efficacy of SSRIs including paroxetine (Paxil), fluoxetine (Prozac), and sertraline (Zoloft). SSRIs are often preferred to other medications because they are considered to be safer, have fewer side effects, and are easier to dose than the TCAs, and lack the abuse and dependence potentials of the benzodiazepines. Additionally, the SSRIs are also effective in the treatment of depression and other comorbid disorders.

In many clinical settings as well as research studies, patients with panic disorder receive combined (psychological and pharmacological) treatment for panic disorder. In the largest combined treatment study to date, by Barlow and colleagues, five treatment groups were compared: CBT alone, imipramine alone, placebo, CBT plus imipramine, and CBT plus placebo. The authors concluded that although both CBT alone and imipramine alone are clearly effective, there does not seem to be an advantage to combining the treatments. However, after treatment was stopped, CBT had better effects in follow-up, whereas people on medication typically lost the gains they made after they stopped treatment.

Although CBT is an effective psychological treatment for panic disorder, disseminating effective psychological treatments to those who need them remains one of the major obstacles facing mental health practitioners. There has been a trend toward making treatments briefer, more intense, and more self-directed. There is wide agreement that primary care settings will become an increasingly important arena for the delivery of behavioral health care in general. Because so many patients with panic disorder present for treatment initially in medical settings, including primary care and emergency departments, innovative treatments that are adapted to be suitable in these settings are important. Studies of treating panic attack patients in the emergency department with exposure-based principles have been effective. Additionally, treatments for noncardiac chest pain using cognitive–behavioral techniques delivered in emergency department and cardiology settings have also showed promise. Because we have effective psychological and pharmacologic treatments for panic disorder, efforts focused on improving recognition and treatment of panic disorder patients in medical settings has recently attracted much attention and is becoming an important focus for future research and changes in clinical practice settings.

BIBLIOGRAPHY

American Psychiatric Association. (1994). *Diagnostic and statistical manual of mental disorders* (4th ed.). Washington, DC: Author.

Antony, M. M., Roth, D., Swinson, R. P., Huta, V., & Devins, G. M. (1998). Illness intrusiveness in individuals with panic disorder, obsessive compulsive disorder, or social phobia. *Journal of Nervous and Mental Disease, 186,* 311–315.

Barlow, D. H., Gorman, J. M., Shear, M. K., & Woods, S. W. (2000). Cognitive–behavioral therapy, imipramine or their combination for panic disorder: A randomized control trial. *Journal of the American Medical Association, 283,* 2529–2536.

Craske, M. G., & Barlow, D. H. (2001). Panic disorder and agoraphobia. In D. H. Barlow (Ed.), *Clinical handbook of psychological disorders: A step-by-step treatment manual* (3rd ed., pp. 1–59). New York: Guilford.

Craske, M. G., Miller, P. P., Rotunda, R., & Barlow, D. H. (1990). A descriptive report of features of initial unexpected panic attacks in minimal and extensive avoiders. *Behaviour Research and Therapy, 28,* 395–400.

Esler, J. L., Barlow, D. H., Woolard, R. H., Nicholson, R. A. Nash, J. M., & Erogul, M. H. (2003). A brief cognitive–behavioral intervention for patients with noncardiac chest pain. *Behavior Therapy, 34,* 129–148.

Fleet, R. P., Dupuis, G., Marchand, A., Burelle, D., Arsenault, A., & Beitman, B. D. (1996). Panic disorder in emergency department chest pain patients: Prevalence, comorbidity, suicidal ideation, and physician recognition. *American Journal of Medicine, 101,* 371–378.

Roy-Byrne, P. P., & Katon, W. (2000). Anxiety management in the medical setting: Rationale, barriers to diagnosis and treatment, and proposed solutions. In D. I. Mostofsky and D. H. Barlow (Eds.), *The management of stress and anxiety in medical disorders* (pp. 1–14). Boston: Allyn & Bacon.

Spitzer, R. L., Williams, J. B. W., Kroenke, K. Linzer, M., deGruy, F. V., Hahn, S. R., Brody, D., & Johnson, J. G. (1994). Utility of a new procedure for diagnosing mental disorders in primary care: The PRIME-MD 1000 study. *Journal of the American Medical Association, 272,* 1749–1756.

Swinson, R. P., Soulis, C., Cox, B. J., & Kuch, K. (1992). Brief treatment of emergency room patients with panic attacks. *American Journal of Psychiatry, 149,* 944–946.

White, K. S., & Barlow, D. H. (2001). Panic disorder and agoraphobia. In D. H. Barlow (Ed.), *Anxiety and its disorders: The nature and treatment of anxiety and panic* (2nd ed., pp. 00–00). New York: Guilford.

JEANNE L. ESLER

Passive Smoking

Passive smoking refers to the involuntary exposure of nonsmokers to the cigarette smoke of smokers. This smoke is commonly referred to as environmental tobacco smoke (ETS) and consists of mainstream smoke, which is inhaled and then exhaled by the smoker, and sidestream smoke, which is produced at the smoldering end of a cigarette when the smoker is not puffing. ETS is made up of numerous harmful chemicals including over 50 compounds identified as carcinogens. ETS is recognized as having harmful effects on children including impaired fetal growth, sudden infant death syndrome, lower respiratory tract infections (e.g., bronchitis and pneumonia), asthma, middle ear infections, and chronic respiratory symptoms. In adults ETS is thought to be responsible for eye and nasal irritation, lung and sinus cancer, and heart disease. The California Environmental Protection Agency estimates that in the United States passive smoking causes approximately 3,000 lung cancer deaths per year and 35,000–62,000 deaths due to heart disease.

Related Entries: Cancer: Biopsychosocial Aspects, Coronary Heart Disease, Respiratory System, Smoking Cessation, Smoking Prevention

BIBLIOGRAPHY

California Environmental Protection Agency. *Health effects of exposure to environmental tobacco smoke: the report of the California Environmental Protection Agency.* Available at www.oehha.ca.gov

Samet, J. M., & Yang, G. (2001). Passive smoking, women and children. In J. M. Samet & S.-Y. Yoon (Eds.), *Women and the tobacco epidemic: Challenges for the 21st century* (pp. 00–00). Geneva: World Health Organization. Available at www.who.int

DELWYN CATLEY
JAMES BUTLER

Patient Adherence

Adherence is a term used to describe the extent to which an individual's behavior corresponds to the health-related recommendations of that individual's health care provider. The term has been used broadly, in reference to medication regimens, dietary restrictions, exercise recommendations, smoking cessation, screening participation, and other health-protective behaviors. Although similar in meaning to "compliance," the word "adherence" is preferred by many providers because it emphasizes the collaborative nature of treatment and prevention, rather than implying a passive and perfunctory approach on the part of the patient.

Several emerging trends have amplified the importance of adherence over the last century. With advances in modern medical treatment and prevention research, providers are increasingly able to offer helpful behavioral recommendations to their patients. Also, with the growing significance of chronic illnesses rather than acute conditions as major health threats (as reported by the National Center for Chronic Disease Prevention and Health Promotion), patients have been obligated to assume a more active role in their own health care. Especially when treating conditions that require lifestyle changes and self-care on the part of the patient, health care providers often find the efficacy of their interventions limited by the extent to which patients are willing and able to adhere to their recommendations.

This entry summarizes the extent and significance of nonadherence. It also describes the different ways in which adherence is assessed, focusing on the strengths and weaknesses of each method. Finally, it reviews research on the prediction of adherence using information about patients, providers, and regimens, and discusses intervention strategies used to promote adherence.

EXTENT AND IMPLICATIONS OF NONADHERENCE

The problem of nonadherence has been well documented for many years. Though prevalence estimates vary depending on the type of behavior, the length and complexity of the regimen, and the assessment method employed, estimates indicate that overall, patients follow provider recommendations only about half of the time. In the first comprehensive review of the literature in 1976, David Sackett and Brian Haynes reported that adherence to chronic medication regimens averaged about 54%. They found that adherence to short-term regimens was highly variable, but tended to decrease sharply with time. They also reported prevalence of nonadherence for other health behaviors, finding, for example, that attendance at scheduled appointments was only about 47% for asymptomatic patients, but that it jumped to 81% for patients actively seeking care for a medical condition. More recent work has generally supported these results, suggesting that nonadherence is frequent enough to seriously limit the efficacy of therapeutic interventions.

The overall impact of poor adherence is difficult to estimate. Not only may it render treatments ineffective, making more intensive intervention necessary, but inconsistent medication adherence has been identified as a key factor in the development of new, treatment-resistant strains of some infectious diseases. A review by Irina Cleemput and her colleagues in 2002 reported on 18 economic impact studies with widely variable results, pointing out that differences in the definition of adherence and inconsistencies in assessment methods make estimates problematic. However, from lost productivity to increased hospitalization and premature death, there is general agreement that the cost is in the billions of dollars each year, and estimates have ranged to more than 100 billion dollars per year in costs associated with medication nonadherence in the United States alone.

ASSESSMENT OF ADHERENCE

Adherence has been measured, both directly and indirectly, using a multitude of methods for both clinical and research purposes. Perhaps the most simple and widely used method of assessment involves asking patients to report their own behavior. Self-report strategies can vary from single questions asked by clinicians to gauge their patients' adherence to detailed retrospective accounts of adherence over periods of several days or weeks. Patients may be asked to monitor their own behavior as it occurs for a period of time, and keep a written record that may be examined by a clinician or researcher. Although most adherence assessment methods are targeted at medication usage, an advantage of self-report methods is that they are flexible enough to use with any type of behavior, including exercise, diet, and substance use. They are also inexpensive to implement, and are unlikely to underestimate actual adherence behavior. However, they are plagued by potential reporting biases. Patients may say what they think the provider wants to hear in an attempt to form a positive impression, or they may have inaccurate memory for their behavior, especially if they are not asked in advance to keep a record. Finally, if patients are informed in advance that they will be asked to report on their adherence, that knowledge alone may cause a difference in the extent to which they adhere.

Noting the difficulties inherent in self-report measures, some researchers have asked health care professionals to provide estimates of their patients' adherence, a method with clear and immediate clinical implications. However, research has consistently demonstrated that providers perform poorly when estimating patient behavior, tending to overestimate adherence. This tendency does not appear to decrease with experience or training. In fact, as early as 1966, Milton Davis found that senior physicians tend to overestimate adherence more dramatically than their junior counterparts. A study by John Steiner and his colleagues determined that even nurse practitioners, who may interact extensively with their patients, have difficulty accurately estimating patient behavior.

In an attempt to counter some of the problems associated with such subjective report measures, some researchers have turned to counting pills and weighing or measuring liquid medications to estimate adherence to medication regimens. In each of these strategies, patients are asked to bring their medications with them to medical appointments, and the difference between the amount of medication dispensed and the amount remaining is compared to the amount that the patients were instructed to ingest. Because patients may not always bring their medications with them for appointments, some providers use a variation on the pill count method, involving the examination of pharmacy refill records. These methods, while objective and reliable, are limited in that they do not provide information about how or when medication is taken. In fact, if patients are aware that their medication usage is to be assessed, they may simply dump large quantities of pills prior to an appointment to convey the appearance of adherent behavior.

In recent years, the evolution of microelectronics has permitted the development of electronic monitoring devices that may be used to record events related to adherence. For instance, Joyce Cramer and her colleagues were among the first researchers to use specially designed medication bottle caps to record the date and time on each occasion the bottles were opened. The advantages of such a method are clear: The results are objective and easily retrieved, and a single device can record thousands of medication-related events. However, there are significant logistical obstacles to using monitoring devices: the devices can be quite expensive, they may be impractical for use with multiple-drug regimens or large pills that must be taken frequently, there are often legal limitations associated with repackaging of prescription medications, and patients may neglect to return their medication bottles for monitoring. In addition, data may be misleading if patients leave a bottle open between doses, open the bottle without ingesting medication, or transfer their pills to pill boxes or organizers. Similar monitoring devices that are somewhat easier to apply are those that record the amount of time patients use respiratory therapy equipment for such conditions as sleep apnea or asthma.

Finally, biochemical assays or other laboratory tests may be used to estimate adherence. These tests may measure either the actual amount of a drug or drug tracer in a patient's blood or urine, or the outcome of a treatment, assuming a close link between adherence and outcome. Biochemical markers can be helpful, objective indices of adherence to the extent that they are available and affordable. However, some drugs are broken down and cleared from the body rapidly, causing unreliability in such tests. Aside from funded research studies and applications of medicines with high potential toxicity, the cost of these assays may preclude their use as a part of regular clinical care. Clinical outcome measures are often only indirectly related to adherence. For example, hemoglobin A_1C is frequently used as an index of adherence in diabetic patients, reflecting glycemic control over extended periods of time. Whereas its association with adherence to multiple regimen components (e.g., insulin injection, dietary restriction, exercise) may make it an attractive measure, glycemic control is also affected by other factors, such as psychological stress. If factors beyond the patient's control have a significant impact on the measure, or if a regimen is not well tailored to a patient or has limited efficacy, adherence may have very little association with clinical outcome.

There is no single gold standard in the measurement of patient adherence. Whereas the selection of an assessment method might depend on its intended purpose, the strengths and weaknesses of different methods illustrate the importance of obtaining multiple indices of adherence in research, and even clinical, settings. The factors that cause the results of different measures to vary from one another are not well understood. Further research may more clearly document in specific populations why self-report and laboratory measures are so often poorly correlated, or why providers' estimates differ from more objective behavioral indices.

PREDICTION OF ADHERENCE

By far, the area of adherence prediction that has received the least attention is the study of characteristics of the health care provider. Not only is such research logistically difficult to accomplish, but, since Davis's early study, the literature has shown that physicians are more likely to attribute nonadherence to patient factors rather than to factors within their own control. Those studies that have examined provider characteristics have shown significant effects of the use of clear communication and the provision of support by the provider. For example, a meta-analysis of process studies by Judith Hall and her colleagues found greater adherence among patients when providers provided more information, asked questions specifically about adherence, and engaged in positive communication, avoiding negative conversational content.

Several characteristics of the medical regimen itself have been associated with adherence. Chief among these is the complexity of the regimen. For instance, Cramer and her colleagues found that as the number of pills patients were asked to take each day increased from one to four, adherence dropped sharply, from 87% to 39%. In addition to regimen complexity, the length of the regimen can negatively impact adherence. Adherence tends to erode with time not only for acute regimens, as noted earlier, but also for longer-term regimens. Thus, adherence to lifestyle change recommendations is especially challenging for patients.

A great deal of research has examined individual differences among patients and how they are related to adherence, with mixed results. Studies of demographic characteristics, such as age, gender, and race have generally shown little direct and consistent association with adherence. Perhaps surprisingly, there has also been little evidence for a link between patient knowledge and adherence. Although knowledge of an illness and its treatment is clearly necessary for adherence to occur, it is usually not sufficient to induce change in behavior. Some personality constructs have been found to predict adherence to a modest extent. In their extensive review of the early literature, Sackett and Haynes reported that such characteristics as cooperativeness, high frustration tolerance, a futuristic orientation, low authoritarianism, and low demandingness were associated with good adherence. Other researchers have found similar effects for variables such as conscientiousness and low neuroticism. However, most studies attempting to link personality characteristics to adherence have had little or inconsistent success.

The difficulty in reliable prediction of adherence using any single variable, or even combinations of variables related to the patient, the provider, or the treatment context, has caused some researchers to look to the interaction of these variables. A review by John Wiebe and Alan Christensen cited a number of studies that have been successful in predicting adherence by considering the interaction of patient factors and characteristics of the treatment context. For instance, patients who tend to become highly involved in their care tend to adhere and adapt best in a disease or treatment context that allows greater patient control. However, if the disease or treatment context offers the patient little control, a less active coping style may be associated with better adherence. Although there is relatively little research on such interaction, it remains a promising area for further work.

INTERVENTION TO INCREASE ADHERENCE

Interventions to simplify regimens have often been quite successful in increasing patient adherence. Data showing increased adherence with reduced dosing frequency has led to the marketing of sustained-release drugs with longer half-lives that may be taken less frequently, from antibiotics to antiretroviral medications for HIV infection, as reported by the Body Health Resources Corporation. Other work has pursued more convenient treatment modalities. For example, James Burris and his colleagues showed that patient adherence with a transdermal patch used to treat hypertension was nearly double the rate for even a sustained-release oral medication taken once per day.

Interventions directed toward the health care system have seldom been conducted in isolation. However, when combined with individual-level strategies in comprehensive disease management programs, they have had some success, especially with chronic illnesses. For instance, Neil Grey and his colleagues reported on a multidisciplinary hospital-based disease management program for diabetic patients. They constructed a team including a primary care physician, an advanced practice nurse, and a registered dietician, focused heavily on patient education, and scheduled frequent follow-up appointments. With this approach they observed a 22% improvement in glycemic control, sustained and increased over a 6-month follow-up period, which they attributed largely to increased adherence.

Overall, the majority of work has been targeted directly at patients. The approaches used with patients have been primarily either educational or behavioral in focus. Patient education programs, whether delivered individually, in groups, or via lectures, have had mixed results in targeting nonadherent behavior. As Donald Meichenbaum and Dennis Turk pointed out in their review of the subject, education tends to be most effective when it involves explicit recommendations about how to implement newly acquired knowledge into the treatment regimen, when it avoids unnecessary jargon and reiterates key points, and when it does not make excessive use of fear appeals to change behavior. However, even when education is appropriately delivered, a multitude of barriers may prevent the increase in knowledge from being translated into behavior change. For example, Sackett and Haynes found that only 8 of the 14 educational-only interventions they studied led to significant increases in adherence.

Behavioral interventions have had slightly better success. Although they may include educational aspects, these programs have focused on such techniques as providing reminder cues and organization strategies, teaching patients to monitor their own behavior and set adherence goals, and delivering feedback and reinforcement for adherent behavior. In comparing the results of educational and behavioral intervention studies, a review by Leonard Epstein and Patricia Cluss found that behavioral approaches had a greater effect on adherence, especially when they included feedback and reinforcement components. However, because few studies have been conducted with long-term follow-up assessments, it remains unclear whether the effects of these behavior modification techniques endure after the intervention is terminated. Some researchers have attempted to maximize the long-term efficacy of behavioral intervention efforts by teaching patients to monitor, evaluate, and reinforce themselves for adherent behavior, rather than having a therapist administer reinforcement. For example, Christensen and his colleagues reported a controlled study of a self-management

intervention with hemodialysis patients in which effects on adherence were actually greater at an 8-week follow-up assessment than at the conclusion of therapy. However, this intervention, like most behavioral strategies, included not only the use of standard behavior modification principles, but also education regarding the effects of nonadherence. In fact, research has generally supported the use of integrated educational and behavioral programs as most effective in increasing adherence.

Perhaps the most extreme form of intervention to promote adherence is directly observed therapy (DOT). In this approach, patients take their medications in the presence of a health worker. Generally reserved for communicable diseases that pose a significant public health threat, DOT has been most frequently applied in the treatment of tuberculosis, where the treatment regimen is of limited duration. The strategy is quite cost effective when compared to inpatient hospitalization, but its clinical efficacy remains unclear. A review by Jimmy Volmink and his colleagues in 2000 found significant improvements in adherence associated with the use of DOT, but pointed out that the strategy is applied inconsistently across studies and often combined with other interventions, making it difficult to isolate its effect.

CONCLUSIONS

Patient adherence constitutes a vital link between provider recommendations and health outcomes, and it is becoming more important in modern health care as patients assume greater self-care responsibilities. However, nonadherence is commonplace, with significant public health and economic implications. Multiple measures of adherence are available, each with its own limitations. Results using different measures are not necessarily highly correlated with one another, and accurate assessment can be a challenging and expensive task. Although there has been a tendency on the part of health care providers to attribute nonadherence to patient characteristics, the literature has not supported this assertion well. Researchers are beginning to examine the interaction between patient characteristics and the treatment context in an attempt to better predict adherence. In efforts to improve adherence, progress has been made toward the simplification of treatment regimens and the development of systemic approaches to disease state management. Behavioral interventions directed toward increasing patient adherence have shown slightly better results than patient education in isolation, but it is likely that integrated approaches are most effective. Finally, in cases where nonadherence may have extreme consequences, directly observed therapy may be instrumental in achieving desired clinical outcomes.

Related Entries: Chronic Illness, Health Promotion, Treatment Delay

BIBLIOGRAPHY

Body Health Resources Corporation. Once a day treatment. Available at www.thebody.com/treat/onceaday.html

Burris, J. F., Papademetriou, V., Wallin, J. D., Cook, M. E., & Weidler, D. J. (1991). Therapeutic adherence in the elderly: Transdermal clonidine compared to oral verapamil for hypertension. *American Journal of Medicine, 91* (Supplement), 22–28.

Christensen, A. J., Moran, P. J., Wiebe, J. S., Ehlers, S. L., & Lawton, W. J. (2002). Effect of a behavioral self-regulation intervention on patient adherence in hemodialysis. *Health Psychology, 21,* 393–397.

Cleemput, I., Kesteloot, K., & DeGeest, S. (2002). A review of the literature on the economics of noncompliance: Room for methodological improvement. *Health Policy, 59,* 65–94.

Cramer, J. A., Mattson, R. H., Prevey, M. L., Scheyer, R. D., & Ouellette, V. L. (1989). How often is medication taken as prescribed? A novel assessment technique. *Journal of the American Medical Association, 261,* 3273–3277.

Davis, M. S. (1966). Variations in patients' compliance with doctors' orders: Analysis of congruence between survey responses and results of empirical investigations. *Journal of Medical Education, 41,* 1037–1048.

Epstein, L. H., & Cluss, P. A. (1982). A behavioral medicine perspective on adherence to long-term medical regimens. *Journal of Consulting and Clinical Psychology, 50,* 950–975.

Grey, N., Maljanian, R., Staff, I., & Cruzmarino de Aponte, M. (2002). Improving care of diabetic patients through a collaborative care model. *Connecticut Medicine, 66,* 7–11.

Hall, J. A., Roter, D. L., & Katz, N. R. (1988). Meta-analysis of correlates of provider behavior in medical encounters. *Medical Care, 26,* 657–675.

Meichenbaum, D., & Turk, D. C. (1987). *Facilitating treatment adherence: A practitioner's guidebook.* New York: Plenum.

National Center for Chronic Disease Prevention and Health Promotion. *Chronic disease overview.* Available at www.cdc.gov/nccdphp/overview.htm

Sackett, D. L., & Haynes, R. B. (1976). *Compliance with therapeutic regimens.* Baltimore: Johns Hopkins University Press.

Steiner, J. F., Fihn, S. D., Blair, B., & Inui, T. S. (1991). Appropriate reductions in compliance among well-controlled hypertensive patients. *Journal of Clinical Epidemiology, 44,* 1361–1371.

Volmink, J., Matchaba, P., & Garner, P. (2000). Directly observed therapy and treatment adherence. *Lancet, 355,* 664–669.

Wiebe, J. S., and Christensen, A. J. (1996). Patient adherence in chronic illness: Personality and coping in context. *Journal of Personality, 64,* 815–835.

JOHN S. WIEBE

Patient–Provider Communication

For the process of health care to be successful, patients and their providers must be able to communicate with one another clearly and efficiently. Interpersonal communication involves an exchange of messages or meanings between people, in this case between patient and provider. Communication can have many differing kinds of content and can take several forms. Whereas many people associate communication messages in medical practice with an exchange of thoughts or information, communication can also involve an exchange of feelings or emotions. In addition to verbal communication, the content of what patients and practitioners say to one another, communication can also be nonverbal. Touch, facial expressions, body position, and the use of space communicate important messages, and sometimes the way in which things are said (paralinguistic cues such as tone, speed, and inflection) can be as important as content. Although patient–provider communication is typically face to face, communication may also take place across media such as e-mail and the Internet.

It is not difficult to see how failures of communication can create problems. Patients who are told to take two pills a day for 4 weeks are not likely to do well if they understand the instructions as four pills a day for 2 weeks. Yet the nature of patient–practitioner communication can be considerably more subtle than this. How much each party communicates and what is communicated provide evidence of the very nature of the patient–provider relationship.

COMMUNICATION AND THE PATIENT–PROVIDER RELATIONSHIP

Although others have updated and elaborated their classic description, Szasz and Hollender described three models of the patient–provider relationship that are characterized by different styles of communication. The activity–passivity model is one in which the pattern of communication is highly asymmetrical. The physician is the expert, the patient is treated much like a work object, and little communication is necessary because it is assumed that the patient has little to contribute. Although this might be appropriate clinically in the cause of acute trauma or coma, when a provider takes this sort of attitude toward the treatment of patients in general, the provider's communications are often in the form of *orders*.

The guidance–cooperation model involves more of a give and take between patient and provider, but the exchange is still far from symmetrical. Providers ask for input from the patient, the patient is valued for being able to add relevant information, but decision making is still in the hands of the provider. Rather than giving orders, communication from provider to patient takes the form of *recommendations*. Third, the model of mutual participation involves a pattern of communication in which patient and provider are seen as relative equals. The patient's input is openly invited and valued, and the provider offers patients *alternatives* or *options* from which to choose. The kind of communication pattern found here is more like that between two adults than between adult and adolescent, or adult and child, as in the previous two models.

PATIENT-CENTERED CARE

The most typical way in which patient–practitioner communication has been described is from the perspective of patient-centered care. Patient-centeredness has been studied from two closely related perspectives. Contrasting the patient-centered style with one that is doctor-centered, Byrne and Long distinguished the two in terms of authority and power. Providers who are doctor-centered set the agenda for communication, monopolize the discussion, and offer relatively little information to patients. Those who are patient-centered allow their patients to help set the agenda for the visit, invite their patients' participation, offer information, and ask for feedback to be sure that the transfer of information has been successful.

Contrasting patient-centeredness with a style that is disease-centered, others such as Moira Stewart have suggested that the purpose of patient-centered communication is to allow the provider to see the problem through the patient's eyes, to understand the patient's ideas, expectations, and feelings. This approach focuses on the concept of "illness," the problem as subjectively interpreted by the patient, rather than "disease," the problem as objectively defined from a biomedical perspective. According to this approach, patient-centered providers communicate with their patients about the their lifestyles and other relevant psychosocial issues with the goal of satisfying the needs and meeting the expectations of the patient for treatment. Although the term patient-centered care has been one of the most widely used in the field of medical communication, some researchers have proposed the term relationship-centered care as preferable because it places the emphasis on neither the provider nor the patient alone, but on the two-person unit as the focus of greatest interest.

EMPIRICAL FINDINGS

Studies of patient–provider communication have found that the communication process leaves considerable room for improvement. The average length of a visit with a physician is in the range of 16 to 26 min, although, surprisingly, the quantity of time for patient and practitioner to communicate has not decreased in spite of the movement toward managed care. At the beginning of the visit, patients typically get about 18 to 24 sec to speak before they are interrupted, which is usually while explaining their first concern (which is not necessarily their most important one). Interruptions during the patients' exposition of problems can result in the raising of hidden agendas at the end of the visit, or the possibility that the concern is never raised at all. In a recent study by Robert Bell and his colleagues, almost 10% of the patients studied had at least one unvoiced desire. In other studies, patients and their physicians were found not to agree on the main presenting problem in 50% of their visits;

half of the psychosocial and psychiatric problems that patients had were missed by their physicians.

Differences in the communication styles of male and female practitioners are considerable. On the average, female physicians who practice primary care have visits that are 10% longer than those of their male counterparts. They engage in more talk that is positive, involve their patients more often as partners, and focus more on emotions. Male and female physicians do not differ in the amount they talk about biomedical issues; however, female physicians ask their patients more questions about psychosocial issues and offer more counseling in this arena.

COMMUNICATION AND OUTCOMES

The quality of patient–provider communication can affect many significant outcomes. Good communication is associated with greater satisfaction on the part of both the patient and the practitioner and with higher levels of adherence to medical recommendations. When providers want to change their patients' behavior (such as getting them to stop smoking or to drink more responsibly), the style of communication can make a significant difference. When patients are counseled in a way that is argumentative and controlling (e.g., "You must . . . "; You should . . . "), they are not likely to adhere to recommended changes, but when their autonomy is supported and providers acknowledge the resistance or ambivalence of their patients, patients are more likely to accept their providers' recommendations and change their behavior. Other outcomes associated with good communication include improvement in patients' emotional health and better physical functioning and symptom resolution.

A finding of considerable interest is that patient–provider communication is closely associated with malpractice claims. Among the most significant reasons sighted in malpractice suits are that patients feel deserted by their doctors, their views have been devalued, and they have received poor information, and that the doctor failed to take into account their perspective. In a comparison of the behavior of a sample of internists who had been sued twice or more to those who had never been sued, nonsued physicians more often told their patients what was going to happen during a visit, encouraged their patients to talk, solicited their opinions, checked to see if patients understood what they were told, and used more humor.

ASSESSING AND IMPROVING COMMUNICATION

Given the importance of good communication skills, increasing attention has been directed to assessing competence in communications among practitioners, and using this information for important decisions. The accreditation status of residency programs in the United States will soon be determined by the achievement of educational outcomes in six areas, one of which is communications. In addition, the American Board of Medical Specialties has agreed to base the certification and recertification of specialists according to their ability to demonstrate competence in communications in addition to other biomedically related skills. Finally, because not all practitioners are born with good communications skills, training programs for medical students and other clinicians-in-training as well as practicing medical providers have grown in number. A review of these indicates that communications skills can be learned, and that education and training in communications skills result in changed provider behavior and greater patient satisfaction.

Debra Roter and Judith Hall asserted that "talk is the main ingredient of medical care . . . it is the fundamental instrument by which the doctor–patient relationship is crafted and by which therapeutic goals are achieved." In recent years, a growing body of research has documented this, showing that patient–provider communication can be measured and that it affects important outcomes. Future research is likely to identify those elements of the communication that are most critical, thereby enabling providers to further master the art of medicine.

Related Entry: Patient Adherence

BIBLIOGRAPHY

Beckman, H. B., & Frankel, R. M. (1984). The effect of physician behavior on the collection of data. *Annals of Internal Medicine, 101,* 692–696.

Beckman, B. B., Markakis, K. M., Suchman, A. L., & Frankel, R. M. (1994). The doctor–patient relationship and malpractice: Lessons from plaintiff depositions. *Archives of Internal Medicine, 54,* 1365–1370.

Bell, R. A., Kravitz, R. L., Thom, D., Krupat, E., & Azari, R. (2001). Unsaid but not forgotten: Patients' unvoiced desires in office visits. *Archives of Internal Medicine, 161,* 1977–1984.

Bertakis, K. D., Roter, D. L., & Putnam S. (1991). The relationship of physician medical interview style to patient satisfaction. *Journal of Family Practice, 32,* 175–181.

Byrne, P. S., & Long, B. E. L. (1976). *Doctors talking to patients.* London: Her Majesty's Stationary Office.

Davenport, S., Goldberg, D., & Millar, T. (1987). How psychiatric disorders are missed during medical consultations. *Lancet, 2,* 439–440.

DiMatteo, M. R., Reiter, R. C., & Gambone, J. C. (1994). Enhancing medication adherence through communication and informed collaborative choice. *Health Communication, 6,* 253–265.

Emmanuel, E. J., & Emmanuel, L. L. (1992). Four models of the physician–patient realtionship. *Journal of the American Medical Association, 267,* 2221–2226.

Levenstein, J. H., Brown, J. B., Weston, W. W., Stewart, M., McCracken, M. C., & McWhinney, I. (1989). Patient centered clinical interviewing. In M. Stewart, & D. Roter (Eds.), *Communicating with medical patients* (pp. 107–120). Newbury, CA: Sage.

Levinson, W., Roter, D. L., Mullooly, J. P., Dull, V. T., & Frankel, R. M. (1997). Physician–patient communication: The relationship with malpractice claims among primary care physicians and surgeons. *Journal of the American Medical Association, 277,* 553–559.

Lewin, S. A., Skea, Z. C., Entwhistle, V., Zwarenstin, M., & Dick, J. (2001). Intervention for providers to promote a patient-centered approach in clinical consultations. *Cochrane Database of Systematic Reviews, 4.*

Mechanic, D., McAlpine, D. D., & Rosenthal, M. (2001). Are patients' office visits with physicians getting shorter? *New England Journal of Medicine, 344,* 198–204.

Miller, M. R., Benefield, G., & Tonigan, J. S. (1993). Enhancing motivation for change in problem drinking: A controlled comparison two therapist styles. *Journal of Consulting and Clinical Psychology, 61,* 455–461.

Robbins, J. A., Bertakis, K. D., Helms, L. J., Azari, R., Callahan, E. J., & Creten, D. A. (1993). The influence of physician practice behaviors on patient satisfaction. *Family Medicine, 25,* 17–20.

Rost, K., & Frankel, R. M. (1993). The introduction of the older patient's problems in the medical visit. *Journal of Aging and Health, 5,* 397–401.

Roter, D. L., & Hall, J. A (1992). *Doctors talking with patients/patients talking with doctors.* Westport, CN: Auburn House.

Roter, D. L, Hall, J. A., & Aoki, Y. (2002). Physician gender effects in medical communication: A meta-analytic review. *Journal of the American Medical Association, 288,* 756–764.

Starfield, B., Wray, C., Hess, K., Gross, R., Birk, P. S., & D'Lugoff, B. C. (1981) The influence of patient–practitioner agreement on outcome of care. *American Journal of Public Health, 71,* 127–131.

Stewart, M. A. (1995) Effective physician–patient communication and health outcomes: A review. *Canadian Medical Association Journal, 152,* 1423–1433.

Stewart, M. A., Brown, J. B., Donner, A., McWhinney, I. R., Oates, J., Weston, W. W., et al. (2000) The impact of patient-centered care on outcomes. *Journal of Family Practice, 49,* 796–804.

Suchman, A. L., Roter, D., Green, M., & Lipkin, M., Jr. (1993). Physician satisfaction with primary care office visits. *Medical Care, 31,* 1083–1092.

Szasz, P. S., & Hollender, M. H. (1965). A contribution to the philosophy of medicine: the basic model of the doctor–patient relationship. *Archives of Internal Medicine, 97,* 585–592.

Tresolini, C. P., and the Pew-Fetzer Task Force. (1994). *Health professions education and relationship-centered care.* San Francisco: Pew Health Professions Commission.

Williams, G. C., & Deci, E. L. (2001). Activating patients for smoking cessation through physician autonomy support. *Medical Care, 39,* 813–823.

EDWARD KRUPAT

Pediatric Psychology

Pediatric psychology, the interface of health psychology and clinical child psychology, has grown over the past 35 years to become an independently recognized field. Pediatric psychology explores the interrelationship between the psychological and physical well-being of children, adolescents, and families, attending to developmental processes and physical, cognitive, social, and emotional functioning as they relate to health and illness. Specific topics of importance to this field include how psychosocial and developmental factors contribute to the etiology, course, treatment, and outcome of pediatric conditions; assessment and treatment of behavioral and emotional concomitants of disease, illness, and developmental disorders; and the promotion of health and health-related behaviors and prevention of illness and injury among youth. Entire volumes have been devoted to describing and summarizing the field of pediatric psychology. This entry discusses some of the tenets of pediatric psychology, followed by an overview of four topic areas of concern to the field and a succinct discussion of two ethical issues confronted by pediatric psychologists.

BASIC TENETS OF PEDIATRIC PSYCHOLOGY

To understand pediatric psychology, it is important to explore the basic assumptions that underlie and guide the field. The biopsychosocial model, the systems approach, a developmental perspective, and an emphasis on prevention reflect the basic assumptions of the field.

Biopsychosocial Model

As in health psychology, pediatric psychology recognizes that multiple factors converge and interact to influence the etiology, course, and outcome of mental and physical conditions. More specifically, biological, emotional, behavioral, interpersonal, and cultural factors are accepted as influencing health and illness.

Systems Approach

Pediatric psychologists generally accept that children are embedded within and reciprocally interact with various social systems. The social–ecological model provides a framework for understanding these various systems, which range from the child's immediate family, to peers, to social institutions such as schools, hospitals, and religious organizations, to the broadest influences of the legal system, societal values, technology, and culture. Each of these systems influences and is influenced by childhood medical conditions.

Developmental Perspective

Childhood is a time in which many dramatic changes occur in biological, cognitive, emotional, and social abilities. Thus, pediatric psychologists espouse a developmental perspective, accepting that individuals of different ages have different abilities (e.g., physical, cognitive), needs (e.g., caretaking), goals (e.g., autonomy, intimacy), and social environments (e.g., home, school). Families, as systems, are also accepted to have developmental trajectories. The way in which health and illness issues are addressed by children and families is influenced by developmental stage.

Focus on Prevention

Much like pediatric medicine, pediatric psychology aims to promote healthy behaviors and prevent adverse health conditions. This tenet of pediatric psychology is evident in efforts to identify and intervene with families at risk for adjustment difficulties in response to chronic illness, promote adherence to medical regimens, educate children and parents regarding the development and sustenance of healthy lifestyle behaviors (i.e., exercise, proper diet/nutrition), and prevent drug and alcohol abuse, accidents, and injuries.

TOPICS OF INTEREST IN PEDIATRIC PSYCHOLOGY

Pediatric psychology is a broad field. Four topic areas are presented to provide an overview of the types of issues important to this field: adaptation to chronic illness, adherence, management of pain and distress, and developmental disabilities.

Adaptation to Chronic Illness

Because of advances in medicine, previously fatal childhood conditions can now be treated with consistently applied, often long-term, medical regimens. Thus, the number of children living with chronic medical conditions such as asthma, cancer, cardiovascular disease, cerebral palsy, cystic fibrosis, diabetes, muscular dystrophy, renal disease, rheumatoid arthritis, sickle cell disease, and spina bifida has risen. Pediatric psychology is concerned with the emotional and behavioral adaptation of children and families to such chronic medical conditions.

Research has demonstrated that there is no simple or direct universal relationship between chronic physical conditions and psychological adjustment. Most children and families facing chronic medical conditions adjust well; however, these families are at increased risk for adjustment difficulties. To aid clinical remediation and preventative efforts, research within pediatric psychology has attempted to identify correlates and predictors of adjustment to chronic conditions. These research efforts suggest that children and families are at higher risk for difficulties when the child's disorder impairs brain functioning, when the child reports high levels of stress and low levels of self-esteem, when the child's mother is highly distressed, and when the child's family is characterized by low levels of cohesion and supportiveness.

Adherence

Rates of nonadherence (i.e., failure to adopt and/or maintain prescribed medical regimens) among pediatric samples have been estimated to range from 50% to 89%. Given these alarming numbers, a major effort within pediatric psychology has been the identification of factors contributing to treatment adherence and methods for improving adherence. Although this area of investigation faces methodological challenges, such as how to accurately measure this construct, certain factors have been identified across studies as contributing to adherence. These factors include characteristics of the child's disease, the child's developmental level, individual psychological characteristics of the child (e.g., emotional and behavioral problems), the functioning of the family, and the interface between the family and the health care team.

Research has suggested that adherence is more difficult to maintain when a disease is chronic and the treatment regimen complex. Furthermore, adolescents, compared to younger children, and youngsters with emotional and behavioral problems, contrasted with those who are functioning within normal limits, have more difficultly with adherence. The family plays an important role in medical regimen adherence. Generally, parents who are knowledgeable and skilled with the treatment regimen and who are supportive have youngsters who are more adherent. Finally, adherence is more common when there is a positive relationship between the medical team and the family. Successful interventions to improve adherence involve simplifying the medical regimen, educating the child and family about the treatment, ensuring parental involvement or oversight, encouraging developmentally appropriate self-monitoring of behaviors, and reinforcing desired behaviors.

Management of Pain and Distress

Managing pain and distress is one of the most difficult, yet common, problems for pediatric psychology. Because of this, research on assessment and management of pediatric pain has grown dramatically over the last 10 years. Experts generally agree that pediatric pain experiences can be classified into one of four categories: pain associated with chronic disease (e.g., arthritis, sickle cell), pain associated with injuries or traumas (e.g., burns), pain associated with nonobservable events (e.g., headache, abdominal pain) and pain associated with medical procedures (e.g., lumbar punctures).

By definition, pain is a subjective experience. As such, assessment of pediatric pain is complex, and often involves a combination of child report, parent report, and independent observation depending on the type of pain and the child's developmental level. The majority of treatments for pediatric pain involve cognitive–behavioral techniques, including positive reinforcement, imagery/distraction, relaxation, modeling, role playing, and coaching by the therapist, medical personnel, or parents. Such techniques have been demonstrated to be effective in reducing pain and distress and improving cooperativeness of children during procedures and may be most effective

when used in combination with pharmacologic strategies (e.g., numbing creams).

Developmental Problems

Pediatric psychology emphasizes developmental issues and therefore is also concerned with the assessment of and intervention for developmental problems. There is a wide range of developmental problems addressed by pediatric psychologists, including high-risk infancy, feeding disorders, failure to thrive, elimination disorders, habit disorders (e.g., tics), sleep disturbances, attention-deficit/hyperactivity disorder, autism and mental retardation, anorexia nervosa, bulimia, and obesity, and neglect, physical abuse, and sexual abuse. The majority of these issues overlap with the interests of clinical child psychology, but some have specific medically related aspects, and thus frequently come to the attention of pediatric psychologists. To illustrate the role of pediatric psychology in regard to a developmental problem, high-risk infancy will be discussed.

High-risk infancy may arise due to prematurity, congenital anomalies, prenatal exposure to substances or infections, or difficulties during labor and delivery. Pediatric psychologists serve high-risk infants and their families through assessing and fostering the infant's health, the adjustment of the parent(s), the infant–parent relationship, and collaboration between the family and the neonatal intensive care unit team. The pediatric psychologist may also continue to assess the physical, cognitive, emotional, behavioral, and social development of high-risk infants as they age, to determine whether there are emerging difficulties to be addressed.

ETHICAL ISSUES RELATED TO PEDIATRIC PSYCHOLOGY

Ethical decisions in pediatric psychology are complicated because this field must attend to and balance the needs of the children, their families, the health care system, and society at large. Ethical decisions are further complicated by variations in laws across local jurisdictions (e.g., age of consent). Two particularly salient issues are informed consent and confidentiality.

Because children lack the necessary cognitive capacity to fully comprehend the gravity and nature of their treatment, they are not legally able to give informed consent for their treatment. Instead, parents give consent. Still, it is important to protect the child's right to be an informed participant in his or her care. Therefore, children should have information presented in a way understandable to them and should be given the opportunity to assent voluntarily to treatment without coercion.

Similarly, pediatric psychologists must address issues of confidentiality. Children are not accorded the same right to confidentiality as adults due to their minor status, yet it is important to establish a trusting environment in which the child feels able to disclose sensitive information. Thus, pediatric psychologists must discuss and establish confidentiality guidelines in conjunction with the parent(s) and child, specifying the types of information that will be shared with the parent. Of course, the legal limits of confidentially (mandatory reporting of abuse and intention to harm oneself or others) must be upheld and explained to children in terms they can comprehend.

To summarize, pediatric psychology is a multidisciplinary field that has grown out of clinical child and health psychology. Pediatric psychology incorporates the biopsychosocial model, the systems approach, a developmental perspective, and an emphasis on prevention. Areas of interest to pediatric psychologists include adaptation of children and families to chronic disease, adherence, management of pain and distress, and developmental disorders. Informed consent and confidentiality are important ethical issues for this field.

Related Entries: Patient–Provider Communication, Stressful Life Events

BIBLIOGRAPHY

Brown, R. T. (2002). Society of Pediatric Psychology presidential address: Toward a social ecology of pediatric psychology. *Journal of Pediatric Psychology*, *27*, 191–201.

Harper, D. C. (1997). Pediatric psychology: Child psychological health in the next century. *Journal of Clinical Psychology in Medical Settings, 4*, 180–192.

Holmbeck, G. N. (2002). A developmental perspective on adolescent health and illness: An introduction to the special issues. *Journal of Pediatric Psychology*, 27, 409–416.

Kazak, A. E. (1997). A contextual family/systems approach to pediatric psychology: Introduction to the special issue. *Journal of Pediatric Psychology*, *22*, 141–148.

Mullins, L. L., & Chaney, J. M. (2001). Pediatric psychology: Contemporary issues. In C. E. Walker & M. C. Roberts (Eds.), *Handbook of clinical child psychology* (3rd ed., pp. 910–927). New York: Wiley.

Olsen, R. A., Mullins, L. L., Gillman, J. B., & Chaney, J. M. (1994). *Sourcebook of pediatric psychology*. Needham Heights, MA: Allyn & Bacon.

Roberts, M. C. (Ed.). (1995). *Handbook of pediatric psychology* (2nd ed.). New York: Guilford.

MELISSA A. ALDERFER

Pennebaker, James W. (1950–)

James Whiting Pennebaker was born March 2, 1950, in Midland, Texas. He is professor of psychology at the University of Texas in Austin. Between his birth and his current position, several things happened. He grew up in the oil-rich, but scenery-

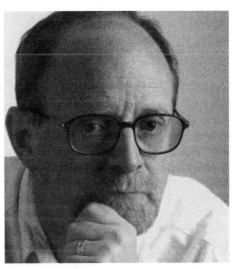

Pennebaker, James W.

challenged flatlands of West Texas in a middle-class home with a younger brother and sister. He attended the University of Arizona on a music scholarship and later transferred to and graduated from Eckerd College in St. Petersburg, Florida, in 1972. After college, Pennebaker married Ruth Burney, who had also spent most of her life in West Texas. After 1 year working as a research assistant and janitor at Eckerd, Pennebaker started graduate school at the University of Texas, where he graduated in 1977. His academic positions include being an assistant professor at the University of Virginia (1977–1983), and an associate and full professor at Southern Methodist University (1983–1997, including 2 years as departmental chair). He finally returned to the University of Texas in 1997 with two well-adjusted children, two seriously disturbed cats, and a truckful of books.

Pennebaker's research falls into three broad domains. His early work focused on how people perceive physical symptoms and sensations. Physical symptoms, he discovered, are the results of normal perceptual processes and distortions. His studies revealed that the correspondence between actual and perceived biological activity is often very poor. Further, various personality dimensions (e.g., negative affectivity), gender, early childhood experiences, and peoples' ongoing social concerns can influence the symptom perception process.

Beginning in the mid-1980s, Pennebaker began exploring the links between traumatic experience, emotional disclosure, and physical health. With a number of colleagues, he found that traumatic experiences that were kept secret resulted in far worse health problems than similar traumas that were openly discussed. This led to his developing a writing paradigm wherein individuals were encouraged to write about their traumas for only 20 min a day for 4 days. Compared to controls, the writing technique yielded striking improvements in physical health. This phenomenon was later extended to major and minor physical and mental diseases among widely diverse samples in labs around the world.

Most recently, Pennebaker has delved into the world of words in an attempt to explain why the act of putting emotional problems into language is beneficial. With the aid of a text analysis program, he is finding that the words people use in daily life, as well as in emotional writing, can reflect their personalities, physical health, and other aspects about them.

BIBLIOGRAPHY

Pennebaker, J. W. (1982). *The psychology of physical symptoms.* New York: Springer-Verlag.

Pennebaker, J. W. (1997). *Opening up: The healing power of expressing emotions.* New York: Guilford.

Pennebaker, J. W., Mehl, M. R., & Niederhoffer, K. (*in press*). Psychological aspects of natural language use: Our words, our selves. *Annual Review of Psychology.*

Pennebaker, J. W., Paez, D., & Rimé, B. (Eds.). (1997). *Collective memories of political events: Social psychological perspectives.* Mahwah, NJ: Erlbaum.

JAMES W. PENNEBAKER

Pessimistic Explanatory Style

The concept of explanatory style originates from the work of social psychologists on how causal attributions for events are made. However, the idea that there are stable differences between people in the ways that they attribute causation across situations came to prominence with research on cognitive theories of depression. These individual differences in explaining the causes of events have been dubbed "explanatory style" by Martin Seligman and his colleagues. Researchers examining explanatory style have focused on three dimensions of the concept: internality, the tendency to attribute the causes of events to one's own actions rather than the actions of others; stability, the tendency to attribute events to temporally constant rather than transient causes; and globality, the tendency to attribute events to factors with far-reaching consequences, rather than those with more limited focus. A pessimistic explanatory style, then, is characterized by a tendency toward internal, stable, and global attributions for negative events.

Explanatory style has been assessed most commonly with questionnaires, although methods have been developed to analyze the content of speeches, therapy sessions, media interviews, and other sources for patterns of causal attribution. Early problems with the reliability of questionnaire measures caused some researchers, such as Carolyn Cutrona and her colleagues, to question whether attributions were really the function of a "style"—an enduring individual difference—or whether they might be largely dictated by situational factors. However, refinements to questionnaire measures and the introduction of alternative assessment methods have demonstrated that individuals do appear to show consistency in the types of attributions they make for different events.

Initial applied work on pessimistic explanatory style centered on its impact on psychological, rather than physical, health. Researchers found that a pessimistic explanatory style served to predispose individuals to depression in the presence of negative events. Specifically, the tendency toward stable and global explanations for negative events (termed "negative generality" by Gerald Metalsky and his colleagues) was shown to predict severity of depression. The tendency toward internal explanations for negative events has been found to have somewhat different effects. For instance, David Pillow and his colleagues found that internality predicts depression indirectly, through its association with low self-esteem. As the role of explanatory style in psychological health has become clear, researchers have turned to study its role in physical health as well. Pessimistic explanatory style has been associated with reduced immune functioning, self-reported increases in poor health habits, physician visits, and sick days.

Finally, although theoretical and empirical work suggest that explanatory style is a relatively stable characteristic, initial efforts have shown that it may be altered through intensive cognitive therapy. For instance, a study by Seligman and colleagues found sustained reduction in pessimistic explanatory style associated with cognitive therapy for depression in a small group of patients. However, further research is necessary to determine whether changes in explanatory style are responsible for corresponding changes in psychological and physical health outcomes.

Related Entries: Depression, Optimism and Health

BIBLIOGRAPHY

Buchanan, G. M., & Seligman, M. E. P. (1995). *Explanatory style.* Hillsdale, NJ: Erlbaum.

Cutrona, C. E., Russell, D., & Jones, R. D. (1985). Cross-situational consistency in causal attributions: Does attributional style exist? *Journal of Personality and Social Psychology, 47,* 1043–1058.

Kamen-Siegel, L., Rodin, J., Seligman, M. E. P., & Dwyer, J. (1991). Explanatory style and cell-mediated immunity in elderly men and women. *Health Psychology, 10,* 229–235.

Kelley, H. H. (1973). The process of causal attribution. *American Psychologist, 28,* 107–128.

Metalsky, G. I., & Joiner, T. E. (1992). Vulnerability to depressive symptomatology: A prospective test of the diathesis–stress and causal mediation components of the hopelessness theory of depression. *Journal of Personality and Social Psychology, 4,* 667–675.

Pillow, D. R., West, S. G., & Reich, J. W. (1991). Attributional style in relation to self-esteem and depression: Mediational and interactive models. *Journal of Research in Personality, 25,* 57–69.

Seligman, M. E. P., Castellon, C., Cacciola, J., Schulman, P., Luborsky, L., Ollove, M., et al. (1988). Explanatory style change during cognitive therapy for unipolar depression. *Journal of Abnormal Psychology, 97,* 1–6.

JOHN S. WIEBE

Placebo Effects

DEFINITION

The word placebo derives from the Latin *placere,* meaning "to please." Placebo literally means "I shall please." In medicine, a placebo is a therapeutic intervention that is used intentionally or unintentionally for its nonspecific psychological or psychophysiological effects. Placebos may be used under a variety of circumstances, such as when the patient demands medication that the physician feels is unjustified, or when the physician wishes to provide hope and an expectation of improvement even though medication is unlikely to have any physical effect. The physician is, in effect, enacting the phrase "I shall please." Patients receiving placebos do improve and this improvement is referred to as a placebo effect.

THE ROLE OF PLACEBOS IN MEDICAL RESEARCH

Placebos play an important role in medical research. In evaluating a new medication, the standard research design is to randomly assign participants to receive either the medication or an identical-looking, placebo pill. In these studies, all who are directly involved should be "blind," that is, unaware of whether a particular participant is receiving the pill or a placebo. The patient, clinician, and outcome evaluator all need to be blind so that they are not influenced by their various expectations for medication or placebo effects.

Unfortunately, in medication trials, the blinding procedures may not work perfectly. Many medications have side effects, and patients who experience side effects may be more convinced that they are receiving active medication, and patients who do not experience side effects may suspect that they are on a placebo. The clinician and independent evaluator may also be influenced by the report of side effects and may also guess the medication status of the patient. This problem has been the focus of a recent article criticizing the effectiveness of antidepressant medication by Kirsch and colleagues. They argued that most of the effect we see in research trials of antidepressant medication may be due to placebo effects heightened by positive expectations for patients with side effects.

There are research strategies to improve the maintenance of the blinding in research trials. Active placebos are medications that produce side effects similar to those of the medication under investigation, but without the active ingredient. For example, in studies assessing antidepressant medication, antihistamines are sometimes used as the placebo because they may cause dry mouth and blurred vision, which are side effects of certain antidepressants. Because participants receiving placebo may also experience side effects, all still remain blind.

Placebo conditions in medical research may go beyond pill placebos. For example, Moseley and colleagues studied the effectiveness of a particular form of knee surgery for arthritis. Two different forms of surgery were compared to placebo surgery in which an incision was made, but no further surgical work was done. In this study neither form of actual surgery did better than the placebo in reducing pain or in increasing knee functioning.

THE ROLE OF PLACEBOS IN PSYCHOTHERAPY RESEARCH

Psychotherapy research has adopted the research design used for evaluating new medications. In analogous fashion, a new form of psychotherapy is generally compared to a placebo psychotherapy. Placebo psychotherapy usually consists in seeing a therapist for the same number and length of sessions, but the therapist in the placebo condition refrains from using what are thought to be the active ingredients in the new therapy. The placebo therapy controls for those components that are common to all therapies: a relationship with a caring therapist, a chance to examine closely the problems bothering the person, and so on. Often placebo therapies involve a specific intervention that is thought to be of minimal benefit. For example, in a study of a new therapy for phobias, the placebo condition might consist of relaxation training. Relaxations may be helpful, but alone are not as likely to be as effective as an active treatment that involves exposure to the feared object.

Blinding is quite different in psychotherapy research. Obviously clinicians administering the therapy cannot be blind as to what they are doing. Patients cannot be blind in that they are exposed to different rationales for the experimental and the placebo therapies, either explicitly or implicitly. Only evaluators can be blind, but they must be careful to ask the participant being interviewed to say nothing about the therapy itself that might let the interviewer know which condition they were in.

To be effective, a placebo should produce the same positive expectations of help as the experimental therapy. Borkovec and Nau had people rate the potential effectiveness of therapies from their rationales. They concluded that the results of actual outcome studies were entirely predictable from the rationale ratings. The weaker rationales of placebo conditions corresponded to weaker effects in published papers.

Morris Parloff discussed the various problems associated with placebo psychotherapy conditions and the various ways in which they fail to function in a way analogous to the placebo pill in medical research. He concluded that the psychotherapy placebo condition in psychotherapy research was an inadequate control and he told psychotherapy researchers to "go forth and sine qua non no more."

A number of alternative research designs are available in the psychotherapy literature. One is to compare a new psychotherapy to the best-established therapy in common use. Another is to compare a standard therapy to a new therapy that improves on the standard with some additions. Disassembly designs compare the full treatment to therapy with one or another element removed (disassembled). This design allows for the evaluation of the components of a complex therapy program. Because medications for psychological disorders have been much more extensively studied than psychotherapies, some studies compare psychotherapies to a known effective medication and a placebo drug. The difference between the placebo and the active drug is used as the scale against which to evaluate the psychotherapy.

FACTORS ENHANCING PLACEBO EFFECTS

The expectations of both the clinician and the patient are critical determinants of the placebo effect. Thus, therapist and patient belief that a powerful drug is being used enhances the placebo effect. When patients or clinicians "break the blind" by correctly guessing that a placebo treatment has been administered, expectancy for improvement may result in a diminished placebo effect. Guessing may be based on lack of improvement, lack of side effects, or higher dosage in comparison to medicated patients.

In addition to expectancy effects, various characteristics of the treatment have been found to enhance the placebo effect. Literature reviews report the following general findings: (1) injections are more powerful than pills, (2) capsules are perceived as stronger than tablets, (3) size is positively correlated with perceived strength, and (4) pill color is related to perceived effect. These results underscore the importance of matching the placebo treatment to the active treatment as closely as possible.

Finally, according to Shapiro and Shapiro, greater placebo effects are observed "in pleasant, non-threatening, efficient clinical settings with doctors who are perceived by patients as warm, likable, and interested in them." From a therapeutic perspective, the placebo effect is enhanced by a clinician who allays anxiety and provides a meaning to the illness.

POSSIBLE MECHANISMS OF PLACEBO EFFECTS

Some common psychological and physiological mechanisms that have been proposed to explain the placebo effect include classical conditioning, response expectancy, anxiety reduction, and an opioid-mediated pathway.

According to the classical conditioning model, the placebo response can be conceptualized as a conditioned response. The drug or treatment is the unconditioned stimulus, and its physiological or pharmacologic effects are the unconditioned response. Over the course of one's lifetime, neutral behavioral and environmental stimuli (i.e., clinical setting, doctor, pills, injections, etc.) act as conditioned stimuli, which through repeated pairing with the unconditioned stimulus (i.e., receipt of drug) eventually produce a conditioned response—the placebo response. Experimental animal data, including results that show a conditioned immunosuppressive response can be elicited in rats, provide some support for the conditioning model of the placebo response. Limitations of the classical conditioning theory include the finding that some conditioned responses to drugs occur in the opposite direction of the placebo and drug responses. Thus, the classical conditioning model cannot account for the placebo phenomenon in its entirety.

More contemporary theories of learning, such as Kirsch, suggest that the placebo effect is explained by expectations such as "the anticipation of the occurrence of non-volitional responses, such as pain, sadness, joy, intoxication, vomiting, and alertness." In this framework, although various modes of learning, including conditioning, reading, and observation, can shape expectancies, the expectancies themselves are considered the key mediating mechanism of the placebo response. Placebo effects do not always mimic drug effects, but may elicit responses that are consistent with cultural expectancies. Positive expectancies may be engendered not only in the patient, but in the patient's family and friends. These expectancies may lead to activation of efforts to solve problems and improve the patient's life circumstances, making the patient feel generally better.

The hypothesis that anxiety reduction is a mechanism for the placebo effect is supported by reports that increased pain tolerance is associated with lower situational anxiety following placebo administration. However, findings that placebo effects can be highly specific (e.g., local to a specific part of the body) imply that global changes, such as anxiety reduction, are not satisfactory explanations.

Opioid pathways likely are responsible for at least some instances of the placebo response, namely placebo pain relief. Evidence from animal and human studies supports the idea that an opioid-mediated neural circuit is related placebo pain relief. Specifically, medications that block opioids reduce the pain relief of placebo responders.

BIBLIOGRAPHY

Borkovec, T. D., & Nau, S. D. (1972). Credibility of analogue therapy rationales. *Journal of Behavior Therapy and Experimental Psychiatry, 3,* 257–260.

Evans, F. J. (1985). Expectancy, therapeutic instructions, and the placebo response. In L. White, B. Tursky, & G. E. Schwartz (Eds.), *Placebo: Theory, research and mechanisms* (pp. 215–228). New York: Guilford.

Fields, H. L., and Price, D. D. (1997). Toward a neurobiology of placebo analgesia. In A. Harrington (Ed.), *The placebo effect: An interdisciplinary exploration* (pp. 93–116). Cambridge, MA: Harvard University Press.

Kirsch, I. (1997). Specifying nonspecifics: Psychological mechanisms of placebo effects. In A. Harrington (Ed.), *The placebo effect: An interdisciplinary exploration* (pp. 166–186). Cambridge, MA: Harvard University Press.

Kirsch, I., Moore, T. J., Scoboria, A., & Nicholls, S. S. (2002). The emperor's new drugs: An analysis of antidepressant medication data submitted to the U.S. Food and Drug Administration. *Prevention and Treatment, 5,* Article 23. Retrieved from http://journals.apa.org/prevention/volume5/pre0050023a.html

Moseley, J. B., O'Malley, K., Petersen, N. J., Menke, T. J., Brody, B. A., Kuykendall, D. H., et al. (2002). A controlled trial of arthroscopic surgery for osteoarthritis of the knee. *Journal of Family Practice, 51,* 813.

Parloff, M. B. (1986). Placebo controls in psychotherapy research: A sine qua non or a placebo for research problems? *Journal of Consulting and Clinical Psychology, 54,* 79–87.

Ross, S., & Buckalew, L. W. (1985). Placebo agentry: Assessment of drug and placebo effects. In L. White, B. Tursky, & G. E. Schwartz (Eds.), *Placebo: Theory, research and mechanisms* (pp. 67–82). New York: Guilford.

Shapiro, A. K., and Shapiro, E. (1997). Is it much ado about nothing? In A. Harrington (Ed.), *The placebo effect: An interdisciplinary exploration* (pp. 12–36). Cambridge, MA: Harvard University Press.

Thompson, W. G. (2000). Placebos: A review of the placebo response. *American Journal of Gastroenterology, 95,* 1637–1643.

LYNN P. REHM
NISHA NAYAK

Positive Affect

Affect is a general psychological construct that refers to mental states involving evaluative moods and emotions. Affect, therefore, can be studied as a temporary, transient state or as a long-term, stable trait. Empirical evidence suggests that affect can be characterized by two largely independent, broad, hierarchical dimensions: positive and negative affect. Generally, measures of positive and negative affect are weakly correlated with one another, and in empirical studies show largely different associations with personality and real-world outcomes. The broad dimension of positive affect comprises positively valenced mood and emotion states including enthusiasm, energy, engagement, pleasure, confidence, and affiliative feelings. Trait positive affectivity reflects an individual's stable level of pleasurable engagement with the environment. State positive affect reflects an individual's short-term, often context-specific experience of positive emotions such as confidence or joy. Both state and trait positive affect are strongly and reliably correlated with personality measures of extraversion.

Related Entries: Mood: The Relationship Between Mood and Health, Negative Affect

BIBLIOGRAPHY

D., Ed, & Emmons, R. A. (1985). The independence of positive and negative affect. *Journal of Personality and Social Psychology, 47,* 1105–1117.

Watson, D., & Clark, L. A. (1992). On traits and temperament: General and specific factors of emotional experience and their relation to the five-factor model. *Journal of Personality, 60,* 441–476.

ELIZABETH K. GRAY

Postpartum Depression

Postpartum depression refers to a nonpsychotic mood disorder that meets diagnostic criteria for major or minor depression. There is no specific diagnosis of "postpartum depression" listed in the *Diagnostic and Statistical Manual of Mental Disorders,* 4th ed. (DSM-IV), although there is a "postpartum onset specifier." According to the *DSM-IV* specifier, an episode may only be termed postpartum onset if it occurs within the first 4 weeks after delivery; however, the term postpartum depression is often used to describe women who experience a depressive episode up to 1 year after delivery. There is no particular time during the first year postpartum when depressive episodes are most likely to occur. Depressive episodes occurring in the postpartum period can be quite persistent, and can last 6–9 months. Furthermore, women experiencing postpartum depressive episodes are at increased risks for future depressions both associated with and independent of childbirth.

Although there is much debate surrounding the issue, postpartum depression does not appear to differ significantly from depressions occurring at other times in a woman's life. However, a fluctuating course and mood lability may be more commonly found in postpartum episodes. Symptoms can include the full range of symptomatology experienced with major depression (e.g., depressed mood, loss of interest in usual activities, irritability, fatigue, difficulty making decisions, sleep and appetite disturbances, and suicidal ideation). The prevalence of postpartum depression is estimated in the range of 10%–15% if both minor and major depressions are included and 5%–8% if only episodes meeting criteria for major depression are included.

Women commonly experience mild dysphoria during the first week postpartum; however, such mild mood disturbance may be suggestive of "postpartum blues" rather than the more severe and chronic diagnosis of postpartum depression. Prevalence estimates for postpartum blues range from 26% to 85%. Symptoms of postpartum blues begin within a few days of delivery and may last from a few hours to several days. Women with postpartum blues may be more likely to experience the following symptoms: dysphoric mood, mood lability, crying, anxiety, insomnia, lack of appetite, and irritability. Women experiencing the blues are at increased risk for postpartum depression, but there no other negative sequelae.

A more severe postpartum disorder than the blues or depression is postpartum psychosis. Psychosis is marked by gross impairment in the ability to function, usually due to hallucinations and/or delusions, although severely depressed mood or profound confusion may instead be responsible for the impairment. The general consensus in the literature is that postpartum psychoses are no different from psychoses occurring at other times in a woman's life and that they often take the form of bipolar disorder. Postpartum psychotic episodes typically occur within the first 2–4 weeks after delivery. The first month postpartum has been shown to be a time of elevated risk for a psychotic episode (perhaps a 13-fold increase); however, postpartum psychosis is extremely rare, with prevalence estimated between 1 and 4 in 1,000 deliveries.

The predominant biological explanation for postpartum blues and depression is that levels of specific reproductive hormones and steroids (e.g., estrogen, progesterone, prolactin, cortisol) are either too high or low after delivery or that the rate of change in levels of these hormones after delivery is too rapid. For example, some researchers believe that the large increase in levels of estrogen and progesterone during pregnancy, followed by the abrupt decrease after delivery, may be responsible for postpartum depression. Despite the intuitive attraction of these theories, there is very little evidence to support them. Neurotransmitter abnormalities are central to many theories of psychiatric disturbance, and postpartum depression is no exception. There is currently little information on the possible impact of neurotransmitters (e.g., norepinephrine, epinephrine, monoamine oxidase, α_2-adrenoceptors) on postpartum depression, and findings are mixed. Stronger evidence supports the notion that thyroid dysfunction during pregnancy or after delivery is related to

postpartum depression. It is estimated that a small percentage (i.e., between 1% and 4%) of postpartum depression cases may be specifically due to thyroid dysfunction. It is important to note that hormonal factors may only be important for women who are otherwise vulnerable to mood disorders due to biological/genetic, psychological, or social/environmental factors.

Postpartum depression is also associated with numerous psychosocial risk factors. Women at risk for postpartum depression are more likely to have a poor marital relationship and to believe that they are not receiving adequate social support from others. Those who experience postpartum depression are more likely to have lower incomes and to come from lower social classes. In addition, high-risk women commonly experience significant life stressors during pregnancy and have more difficult pregnancies and deliveries than low-risk women. Finally, women who have experienced prior depressive episodes and showed evidence of at least mild mood disturbances during pregnancy are more likely to experience a postpartum depressive episode.

Psychological characteristics have also been examined for their possible relationships with postpartum depression. Some researchers have reported that higher levels of "neurotic" personality characteristics in depressed versus nondepressed mothers, although others have contradicted this finding. Several studies have found a significant relationship between levels of depression/emotional distress during pregnancy and levels postdelivery. Attributional style (the types of causes women identify for life events) has been found to predict postpartum depression in some, but not all studies. Attitudes regarding self-control, measured during pregnancy, may be a significant predictor of women's level of postpartum depression. Finally, family history of psychopathology has also inconsistently been found to be a predictor of postpartum depression.

Several long-term follow-up studies of women with postpartum depression have reported on the consequences of the disorder for the woman's children. Postpartum depression has been shown to affect the interactions between a mother and her infant. Depressed mothers exhibit fewer positive facial expressions and less animated verbalizations. In turn, infants of depressed mothers exhibit less interest in interactions and show a preference for sad faces and vocalizations. Infants of depressed mothers have been characterized as less securely attached and as showing fewer exploratory behaviors. A number of studies have found that during the preschool years, mothers who experienced postpartum depression rate their children as having more behavioral problems. Additionally, a large body of research suggests that children of women who experienced a postpartum depression perform significantly worse on tests of cognitive abilities than children of mothers who were nondepressed postpartum. Findings suggest that children of postpartum depressed mothers may show deficits in their social and emotional development relative to their peers born to nondepressed mothers.

Postpartum depression has also been shown to negatively affect the spousal relationship. Postpartum depressed women report receiving less support than postpartum nondepressed women in close relationships; however, this perceived lack of social support is most striking within the spousal relationship. Husbands typically disagree with their wives' perceptions, often leading to marital dissatisfaction, a risk factor for depression in both women and men. In addition, depressed women perceive their overall family life to be more negative than nondepressed women. In addition to marital dissatisfaction, living with a depressed spouse is also a risk factor for depression, so that spouses of postpartum depressed women themselves experience more depressed mood than spouses of nondepressed women.

Antidepressant medications are commonly prescribed for postpartum depression; however, there are almost no controlled studies of the efficacy of psychotropic medications with postpartum women. The literature does support the use of nortriptyline, fluoxetine, and sertraline as medical treatments for postpartum depression. Because there are no data from controlled studies regarding the safety of antidepressant medication with breastfeeding women, the use of these medications with breastfeeding women is controversial. Transdermal estrogen, which is a hormonal treatment, has been tested as a treatment for postpartum depression with some success. Pregnant women with a history of postpartum depression have also been treated preventatively with antidepressants. In general, the few studies conducted suggest the efficacy of preventative pharmacologic treatment for women at risk for postpartum depression.

The efficacy of psychotherapeutic approaches to acute treatment of postpartum depression is strongly supported in the literature. Given the paucity of pharmacologic research with postpartum women and the lack of risks to the infant associated with counseling, psychotherapy could be considered a first-line approach to treatment. Interpersonal psychotherapy, client-centered therapy, nondirective therapies, and cognitive–behavioral therapy have all been shown to be superior to no treatment or waiting-list control conditions. A number of studies have also assessed the efficacy of preventative psychological treatments for postpartum depression. Prevention efforts have largely focused on antenatal relaxation training and/or group psychoeducation sessions regarding expectations for the postpartum period. In general, the prevention efforts resulted in a decrease in postpartum emotional distress. The literature suggests that outcome for preventive efforts may be improved by selecting patients who are at high risk for depression and by using aggressive measures to encourage patient retention in treatment.

Related Entries: Depression, Pregnancy

BIBLIOGRAPHY

American Psychiatric Association. (1994). *Diagnostic and statistical manual of mental disorders* (4th ed.). Washington, DC: Author.

Benazon, N. R., & Coyne, J. C. (2000). Living with a depressed spouse. *Journal of Family Psychology, 14,* 71–79.

Goodman, S. H., & Gotlib, I. H. (1999). Risk for psychopathology in the children of depressed mothers: A developmental model for understanding mechanisms of transmission. *Psychological Review, 106,* 458–490.

O'Hara, M. W. (1999). Postpartum mental disorders. In J. J. Sciarra (Ed.), *Gynecology and obstetrics* (Vol. 6, pp. 1–19). Philadelphia: Lippincott Williams & Wilkins.

O'Hara, M. W., & Stuart, S. (1999). Pregnancy and postpartum. In R. G. Robinson & W. R. Yates (Eds.), *Psychiatric treatment of the medically ill* (pp. 253–277). New York: Dekker.

O'Hara, M. W., Stuart, S., Gorman, L. L., & Wenzel, A. (2000). Efficacy of interpersonal psychotherapy for postpartum depression. *Archives of General Psychiatry, 57,* 1039–1045.

Wisner, K. L., Parry, B. L., & Piontek, C. M. Postpartum depression. *New England Journal of Medicine, 347,* 194–199.

MICHAEL W. O'HARA
TRACY E. MORAN

Posttraumatic Stress Disorder (PTSD)

Postraumatic stress disorder (PTSD) is an anxiety disorder characterized by the development of a constellation of cognitive, behavioral, emotional, and physiological difficulties following exposure to a traumatic event or experience. PTSD is a relatively common, recurrent, and debilitating disorder and is the focus of considerable ongoing clinical and research attention. This entry reviews the signs and symptoms, epidemiology, impact, risk factors, etiology, and treatment of this important public health problem.

SIGNS AND SYMPTOMS

The symptoms of PTSD develop following exposure to a trauma. According to the *Diagnostic and Statistical Manual of Mental Disorders*, 4th edition (*DSM-IV*), a trauma is defined as an experience in which (1) there is actual or threatened death or injury of self or others, and (2) the person's response involves intense fear, helplessness, or horror (American Psychiatric Association, 1994). Although there is no discrete list of events that can precipitate PTSD, such experiences may include war or combat, terrorist attacks, natural or human-caused disasters, torture, being held as a prisoner of war or in a concentration camp, severe motor vehicle or other accidents, criminal/physical assault, rape, childhood physical or sexual abuse or severe neglect, diagnosis with a life-threatening illness, seeing someone killed or severely injured, seeing or handling human remains, and learning of a loved one's severe injury, accident, or sudden, unexpected death.

PTSD involves three kinds of trauma-related symptoms: reexperiencing the trauma, avoiding reminders of the trauma or feeling emotionally numb, and hyperarousal. A person may reexperience the trauma by having repeated, distressing memories or thoughts of the experience, having nightmares, having flashbacks when he or she feels as though reliving the trauma, being emotionally upset when reminded of the trauma, and having physical reactions (e.g., racing heart, sweating) when exposed to trauma reminders. Symptoms of avoidance and numbing include avoiding thoughts, feelings, conversations, or activities that remind the person of the trauma, inability to remember important parts of the traumatic experience, loss of interest in previously enjoyable or important activities, feeling distant or detached from others, feeling emotionally numb, and having a sense of a foreshortened future (e.g., not expecting to have a normal life span). Hyperarousal symptoms include sleep difficulty, irritability, concentration problems, hypervigilance, and an exaggerated startle response. In children, PTSD symptoms may be reflected in disorganized or agitated behavior, generally frightening dreams that may not be directly linked to the trauma, and repetitive play in which aspects of the trauma are acted out.

Although many of these symptoms are common as part of the natural adjustment process following a traumatic experience, PTSD is distinguished from a normal response by the duration and impact of these symptoms. If difficulties persist for more than 1 month following the end of the traumatic experience and cause significant distress or impairment in relationships, social interactions, work or school performance, or other important areas of functioning, then a diagnosis of PTSD is likely.

A related disorder, acute stress disorder (ASD), may be diagnosed within the first month following the trauma and is viewed as a precursor to PTSD. ASD is characterized by the development of dissociative symptoms (e.g., feeling numb or detached, being in a daze, derealization, depersonalization, or amnesia), in addition to the reexperiencing, avoidance, and arousal symptoms described earlier. Again, although many of these symptoms are part of the normal trauma response, they are viewed as a disorder if they are persistent in the first month following the trauma and if they cause distress or impairment.

EPIDEMIOLOGY

Almost two-thirds of adult men and half of adult women have had at least one traumatic experience in their lifetime,

although some studies suggest that as many as 9 in 10 adults have experienced a trauma. Of those, roughly 15% to 24% develop PTSD. The lifetime prevalence of PTSD ranges from 1% to 14%, but is twice as high in women as it is in men (10.4% vs. 5%). In addition, a significant percentage of people experience subthreshold or partial PTSD, symptoms that are distressing and impairing, but do not meet the formal diagnostic criteria for PTSD. The incidence of PTSD is higher for those who are younger and for those with fewer resources (e.g., lower socioeconomic status). The traumas most commonly associated with PTSD are combat exposure and witnessing of violence in men, and rape and sexual molestation among women. The incidence of PTSD varies widely by trauma type. For example, the lifetime prevalence of PTSD in Vietnam combat veterans is estimated to be 25% to 30%, with at least an additional 20% suffering from partial PTSD. Approximately 47% of rape victims, 21% of nonsexual assault victims, 14% of those experiencing sudden bereavement, and 9% of motor vehicle accident survivors develop chronic PTSD. Of children exposed to severe traumatic experiences, such as parental homicide or sexual assault, sexual abuse, or community/school violence, 35% to 90% may develop PTSD.

IMPACT

PTSD can have a devastating impact on victims and their families. PTSD is closely associated with other emotional and behavioral difficulties. Many with PTSD also have comorbid problems with depression, anxiety, guilt (e.g., at surviving a trauma when others did not, at not doing more to prevent the trauma), anger, low self-esteem, and chemical (alcohol and/or drug) abuse and dependence. By definition, those with PTSD have trouble in multiple life domains, including social and family relationships, work, school, and ability to participate in daily activities. Not surprisingly, those with PTSD may feel hopeless, often to the point of contemplating or attempting suicide. Importantly, those with PTSD may be more likely to experience a range of physical symptoms and medical problems (e.g., headaches, gastrointestinal distress, hypertension, asthma, pain, immune system problems), to engage in high-risk health behaviors, and to overutilize health care resources. Those with chronic PTSD show changes in central and autonomic nervous system functioning, including altered brain-wave activity, dysregulation of stress hormones (e.g., cortisol, norepinephrine), and alteration of brain structure and functioning (e.g., amygdala, hippocampus).

RISK FACTORS

Risk factors for the development of PTSD include pre-, peri-, and postevent characteristics. Demographic (being younger, female, less educated, of lower socioeconomic status, of minority ethnicity, of lower intelligence) and historical (personal or family history of psychiatric problems, previous exposure to trauma or adverse childhood events such as abuse) have been found to predict development of PTSD in some studies. In addition, there are thought to be biological/genetic vulnerabilities to developing PTSD. Although they account for only a small amount of the variance in symptoms, greater trauma severity and exposure are associated with greater risk of PTSD. Some kinds of events—those that are unpredictable and uncontrollable, involve sexual victimization, are associated with feelings of guilt or self-blame, are felt by the victim to be extremely threatening or dangerous, or are responded to with intense fear, helplessness, or horror or with dissociation—are associated with greater risk of PTSD. Following a traumatic experience, other life stressors, loss of financial, material, or social resources, and limited or aversive social support are also associated with increased likelihood of developing PTSD.

ETIOLOGY

Many theories exist regarding the etiology of PTSD. Learning theories propose that a combination of classical and operant conditioning accounts for the development of PTSD, such that trauma-related stimuli take on an anxiety-provoking quality and that withdrawal from trauma reminders is reinforced, maintaining a cycle of fear and avoidance. Cognitive theories of PTSD focus on dysfunctional thought patterns that develop following a trauma, including overestimation of negative outcomes, misattributions regarding control and blame, and appraisal of benign situations as dangerous. Psychodynamic explanations point to inconsistencies between the individual's view of self/the world and the meaning attributed to the traumatic event—the cycle of intrusion and avoidance is thought to reflect the struggle to reconcile these discrepancies. Biological explanations of the development of PTSD emphasize genetic/neurobiological vulnerabilities and a dysregulated physiological stress response, which result in chronic biological and neuroanatomic alterations.

TREATMENT

Although PTSD symptoms often improve over the first weeks and months following traumatization, the symptoms of approximately one-third of those with PTSD will fail to remit, and become chronic. If PTSD is still present at 3 months posttrauma, it becomes less likely that symptoms will improve without treatment. Recent evidence suggests that for some individuals diagnosed with acute stress disorder, brief cognitive–behavioral intervention initiated at 2 weeks posttrauma may prevent development of PTSD. A variety of treatment approaches have been advocated for use with PTSD. Cognitive–behavioral treatments, particularly trauma-specific exposure and cognitive therapies, have received the strongest empirical support in terms of their impact on PTSD symptoms. Exposure therapy involves systematic repetitive exposure to trauma reminders and memories, most typically via the survivor being encouraged to recount in detail the experience and his or her reactions to it, and to develop and repeat the account until emotional reactions become less intense. Cognitive therapy involves a systematic therapist-facilitated approach to identifying, challenging, and restructuring negative trauma-related beliefs (e.g., guilt). These treatments are usually delivered in 9–16 individual sessions, with additional help provided as necessary. In children with PTSD, play therapy may use games, drawings, and other techniques to help the children process their traumatic memories. Medications are often used to manage sleep difficulties, hyperarousal, and intrusive thoughts. The selective serotonin reuptake inhibitors (SSRIs) have received the most research support in terms of their impact on PTSD symptoms. In addition to cognitive–behavioral and SSRI treatments, other interventions that have received empirical support include eye movement desensitization and reprocessing and stress inoculation training. Because PTSD is associated with a variety of interpersonal difficulties and problems in functioning, group psychotherapy, marital and family therapy, parenting coaching, and social and occupational rehabilitation therapies may also be helpful.

In conclusion, PTSD is a common and potentially incapacitating disorder, which can negatively affect all life domains. Based on empirical studies, important advances are being made in prevention, detection, and treatment of this significant disorder.

Related Entries: Psychotherapy, Stressful Life Events

BIBLIOGRAPHY

American Psychiatric Association. (1994). *Diagnostic and statistical manual of mental disorders* (4th ed.). Washington, DC: Author.

Blanchard, E. B., & Hickling, E. J. (1997). *After the crash: Assessment and treatment of motor vehicle accident survivors*. Washington, DC: American Psychological Association.

Brewin, C. R., Andrews, B., & Valentine, J. D. (2000). Meta-analysis of risk factors for posttraumatic stress disorder in trauma-exposed adults. *Journal of Consulting and Clinical Psychology, 68*, 748–766.

Bryant, R. A., & Harvey, A. G. (2000). *Acute stress disorder: A handbook of theory, assessment, and treatment*. Washington, DC: American Psychological Association.

Foa, E. B., Keane, T. M., & Friedman, M. J. (Eds.). (2000). *Effective treatments for PTSD: Practice guidelines from the International Society of Traumatic Stress Studies*. New York: Guilford.

Foa, E. B., & Rothbaum, B. O. (1998). *Treating the trauma of rape: Cognitive–behavioral therapy for PTSD*. New York: Guilford.

Foy, D. W. (Ed.). (1992). *Treating PTSD: Cognitive–behavioral strategies*. New York: Guilford.

Follette, V. M., Ruzek, J. I., & Abueg, F. R. (Eds.). (1998). *Cognitive–behavioral therapies for trauma*. New York: Guilford.

Friedman, M. J. (2000). A guide to the literature on pharmacotherapy for PTSD. *PTSD Research Quarterly, 11*(1), 1–7. Available at http://ncptsd.org/research

Halligan, S. L., & Yehuda, R. (2000). Risk factors for PTSD. *PTSD Research Quarterly, 11*(3), 1–7. Available at http://ncptsd.org/research

Horowitz, M. (1997). *Stress response syndromes* (3rd ed.). New York: Aronson.

Kessler, R. C., Sonnega, A., Bromet, E., Hughes, M., & Nelson, C. B. (1995). Posttraumatic stress disorder in the National Comorbidity Survey. *Archives of General Psychiatry, 52*, 1048–1060.

Kulka, R. A., Fairbank, J. A., Jordan, B. K., Weiss, D., & Cranston, A. (1990). *Trauma and the Vietnam War generation: Report of findings from the National Vientam Veterans Readjustment Study*. New York: Brunner/Mazel.

Yehuda, R. (2002). Posttraumatic stress disorder. *New England Journal of Medicine, 346*, 108–114.

Wilson, J. P., & Keane, T. M. (Eds.). (1997). *Assessing psychological trauma and PTSD*. New York: Guilford.

Matthew J. Cordova
Josef I. Ruzek

Pregnancy

Pregnancy is the period of embryonic and fetal development, or gestation. In humans, a normal pregnancy lasts 40 weeks from conception to birth. Delivery before 37 weeks of gestation, known as preterm delivery, is associated with greater risk for a number of adverse conditions in the newborn including low birth weight (less than 2,500 g). Low-birth-weight babies are at substantially increased likelihood of dying during their first year of life; many survivors experience long-term physical health and developmental problems.

Pregnancy is a common experience for women. In the United States, more than 4 million births occur each year. The number of pregnancies is higher, however, because not all pregnancies result in a birth. Some women elect to terminate their pregnancies, a procedure known as therapeutic abortion, and approximately 15%–20% of pregnancies end by spontaneous abortion (miscarriage). There is research on psychological aspects of therapeutic and spontaneous abortion, such as how women adapt afterward, but that research is not discussed in this entry. The focus here is on pregnancies that result in a birth.

Studies find that pregnancy is a momentous experience, with women retaining clear memories of their pregnancy and birthing and strong feelings about them as much as 20 years later. A woman's age, health status, reproductive history, education, marital or relationship status, and other important characteristics have been shown to influence her experience of pregnancy. However, researchers find that some aspects of pregnancy are typical of the experience of most women. The most common physical symptoms include nausea and vomiting, fatigue, indigestion or heartburn, swollen feet and hands, difficulty breathing or sleeping, leg cramps, breast tenderness, headaches, hemorrhoids, and frequent urination. Psychological or lifestyle adjustments may be necessary to adapt to these physical discomforts.

Also common in pregnancy are the changes in appearance that women experience. Studies find that some pregnant women feel unattractive, whereas others welcome their body's changes as confirmation of their child's growth. Women view their appearance differently as pregnancy progresses, and these views are affected by how their friends, family, and even strangers treat them. Pregnant women are sometimes subjected to unkind comments about their size, unsolicited advice, touch, and staring.

Pregnancy is an important topic of study for health psychologists because it is both a biomedical and a psychosocial event. In addition to the physiological processes that occur, pregnancy can influence women's emotions, actions, thoughts, and social relationships. Furthermore, a number of interactions occur between pregnant women's physical and psychosocial states. Three topics that comprise most psychological research on pregnancy illustrate the reciprocal effects of biomedical and psychosocial factors. First, how does advancing pregnancy affect women's emotional state? Second, how do women cope with the strains and challenges that they experience during pregnancy? Third, how do psychosocial factors such as stress affect the health of pregnant women and their fetuses? The following sections address each of these questions.

PREGNANCY AND EMOTIONAL STATE

Most studies of women's emotional state in pregnancy have examined levels of anxiety and depression. Well-conducted studies find that most women do not experience fluctuations in anxiety during pregnancy, and most are within normal levels throughout this 9-month period. However, there is evidence that a portion of women experience changes in anxiety across pregnancy, with some experiencing increases, some decreases, and others a combination. Patterns of anxiety in pregnancy are not related to a woman's age, level of education, ethnic background, marital status, or other individual characteristics. Thus, there is no way to identify beforehand the women most likely to become highly anxious during pregnancy.

In comparison to the studies of prenatal anxiety, studies of prenatal depression are less well conducted and their findings are more contradictory. However, most of these studies suggest that for women who do experience depression during pregnancy, the symptoms (such as feeling hopeless or sad) are usually within normal ranges and do not warrant treatment. Of course, some women may desire and need help to overcome depressive symptoms. Women who experience depression prior to pregnancy are more likely to become depressed during their pregnancy, particularly if the pregnancy adds to their preexisting levels of stress.

Taken together, studies of prenatal anxiety and depression illustrate that there is no single, universal emotional response to pregnancy. This is because anxiety and depression are emotional responses to life conditions that vary from woman to woman. Most women experience normal, stable levels of negative emotion during this period of time.

COPING IN PREGNANCY

Coping includes anything people do to manage problems or their emotional responses, whether successful or not. Four types of coping have received most attention in research on pregnancy: avoidance, problem solving, positive appraisal, and prayer. Avoidant coping, by which people remove themselves physically or psychologically from problems, is associated with greater emotional distress in pregnant women, and in other people who cope this way. Avoidant coping may also have harmful nonemotional consequences in pregnancy, such as neglecting to get assistance or medical attention when it is needed.

A second type of coping, called problem solving, active coping, or approach-oriented coping, tends to be effective in other people, but the evidence in pregnancy is mixed. One reason is that these ways of coping may lead to an increased focus on problems that cannot be remedied in pregnancy. For example, in a recent study of pregnant women with medical conditions that put them at high risk for having a miscarriage or a preterm delivery, women were worse off emotionally if they coped by preparing for the baby's arrival, such as acquiring furniture, baby clothes, or supplies. The researchers reason that this type of coping focuses attention on the baby, which is distressing among women whose pregnancy may not result in a healthy child. Although problem-focused coping strategies such as preparation are associated with positive outcomes in some stressful situations, there is evidence that this type of coping is less effective for people facing severe threats.

A third type of coping that has been examined in pregnant women is prayer. A few recent studies find that prayer is the most frequently reported type of coping used by pregnant women. However, in one of these studies, use of prayer was associated with increased emotional distress. The study's authors explained that the type of prayer used by women in their study may have been a form of worrying, or rumination, which typically produces unfavorable emotional consequences.

Positive appraisal is the only type of coping that has consistently been associated with lower distress in pregnant women. This way of coping involves viewing a stressful situation positively, emphasizing what can be gained or what benefits might accrue from it. Positive appraisal has been shown to be an adaptive form of coping in many types of people undergoing stressful events.

What leads pregnant women to use particular ways of coping? There is recent evidence that women who are optimistic and those who view their pregnancy as controllable select more effective ways of coping, and, as a result, they experience lower emotional distress during pregnancy.

EFFECTS OF STRESS IN PREGNANCY

Pregnancy is a stressful event for some women because they are coping with physical strains and psychological challenges while carrying out demanding family, work, and other roles. Research shows that high levels of stress can have a deleterious effect on pregnancy, increasing the likelihood of adverse birth outcomes such as low birth weight and preterm delivery. Studies have examined stress in a variety of ways. Some measure the number of stressful life events that occur during pregnancy, such as whether a close friend or family member dies, or the loss of a home. Other studies examine how women perceive the life events that they experience—specifically, how stressful or disturbing they are. Still other studies measure levels of anxiety in pregnant women. In scientific studies published during the last several decades, a consistent association has emerged between the number of stressful life events experienced in pregnancy and low birth weight, and somewhat less consistent associations with preterm delivery. Anxiety and women's perceptions of life event stress have been linked to serious labor and delivery complications. Additional studies have measured stress by examining the combination of stressful life events, anxiety, and other stress factors such as financial or family strains. These studies provide some of the scientifically strongest evidence documenting the deleterious effects of stress in pregnancy.

What accounts for the impact of stress on birth outcomes? Both physiological and behavioral processes are affected by stress. There is some evidence that stress causes the release of hormones and other chemicals in the nervous system that trigger early delivery. Stress reduces the flow of blood and oxygen to the fetus, which can result in fetal growth problems. In addition, stress may disrupt the immune system, making women more susceptible to infections, which can bring on early delivery or otherwise affect the fetus. Behaviorally, studies find that pregnant women who experience high stress have poorer nutrition and physical activity, and they are more likely to smoke cigarettes, to consume alcohol, and to use other substances that have severe effects on birth weight and newborn health.

CONCLUSIONS

Pregnancy is an important life event that is experienced by most women. It entails physical and psychosocial changes that are stressful for some. Nevertheless, the majority of women cope successfully with the strains and challenges of pregnancy. Those who do experience high levels of stress and resultant emotional distress during pregnancy face increased risk of adverse birth outcomes including low birth weight and preterm delivery.

Related Entries: Postpartum Depression, Reproductive System, Women's Health

BIBLIOGRAPHY

Dunkel-Schetter, C., Gurung, R. A. R., Lobel, M., & Wadhwa, P. D. (2001). Stress processes in pregnancy and birth: Psychological, biological, and sociocultural influences. In A. Baum, T. A. Revenson, & J. E. Singer (Eds.), *Handbook of health psychology* (pp. 495–518). Hillsdale, NJ: Erlbaum.

Dunkel-Schetter, C., & Lobel, M. (1998). Pregnancy and childbirth. In E. A. Blechman & K. D. Brownell (Eds.), *Behavioral medicine and women: A comprehensive handbook* (pp. 475–482). New York: Guilford.

Hoffman, S., & Hatch, M. C. (1996). Stress, social support and pregnancy outcome: A reassessment based on recent research. *Pediatric and Perinatal Epidemiology, 10,* 380–405.

Lazarus, R. S., & Folkman, S. (1984). *Stress, appraisal, and coping.* New York: Springer.

Lederman, R. P. (1995). Relationship of anxiety, stress, and psychosocial development to reproductive health. *Behavioral Medicine, 21,* 101–112.

Lobel, M. (1994). Conceptualizations, measurement, and effects of prenatal maternal stress on birth outcomes. *Journal of Behavioral Medicine, 17,* 225–272.

Lobel, M., Yali, A. M., Zhu, W., DeVincent, C. J., & Meyer, B. A. (2002). Beneficial associations between optimistic disposition and emotional distress in high-risk pregnancy. *Psychology and Health, 17,* 77–95.

Stanton, A. L., & Gallant, S. J. (Eds.). (1995). *The psychology of women's health: Progress and challenges in research and application.* Washington, DC: American Psychological Association.

Stanton, A. L., Lobel, M., Sears, S., & DeLuca, R. S. (2002). Psychosocial aspects of selected issues in women's reproductive health: Current status and future directions. *Journal of Consulting and Clinical Psychology, 70,* 751–770.

Yali, A. M., & Lobel, M. (1999). Coping and distress in pregnancy: An investigation of medically high risk women. *Journal of Psychosomatic Obstetrics and Gynecology, 20,* 39–52.

Marci Lobel

Prevalence

Prevalence is defined as the total number of cases of a disease or disorder reported for a particular population or subpopulation. In epidemiologic research, this number is an indication of the percentage of individuals in a given population who are afflicted with the particular disease. This allows researchers to compare levels of disease or disorder across populations. For example, according to the U.S. Renal Data System, the year 2000 prevalence rates of end-stage renal disease (ESRD), or loss of kidney function, in the United States for Whites was approximately 223,800, for African-Americans it was approximately 121,000, and for Asians was approximately 14,500. Additionally, the 2000 prevalence rates for ESRD for women were 165,800 and 199,500 for men. Using census information, these data suggest that end-stage renal disease is more prevalent among men than women. Prevalence, the total number of cases of a disorder in a particular population, can be compared to incidence, the number of new cases of a disorder in a given population.

Related Entries: Epidemiology, Incidence

Jamie A. Cvengros

Prevention

Prevention is a commonsense concept that has roots in the discipline of public health and in the mental hygiene movement of the early 20th century. It derives from Latin words meaning "to anticipate" or "before something to come." Psychiatrist Gerald Caplan's (1964) conceptualization of primary, secondary, and tertiary types or levels of prevention has been particularly influential in the development of the field.

Interventions for primary prevention are applied to entire populations with no identified distress in order to prevent the occurrence of problems. These interventions target potentially harmful circumstances to proactively reduce or eliminate their effect. Examples of primary prevention include vaccinations, water fluoridation, and social skills programs for preschoolers.

Secondary prevention interventions are directed toward populations showing early signs of problems in order to prevent a full-blown occurrence. Persons targeted are considered at risk of developing a disorder (e.g., shy or withdrawn children, children having academic difficulty, teens with alcoholic parents). The necessity of identifying persons at risk can be a thorny issue because individuals who might never develop a disorder may be stigmatized.

Tertiary prevention includes interventions given to populations who have a disorder in order to limit its impact, prevent its worsening, and reduce its reoccurrence. The similarities between tertiary prevention and treatment are striking and intentional. Caplan's aim was to introduce a new paradigm to his treatment-oriented contemporaries in the mental health fields by emphasizing its similarities to their existing approach. Although current practices attest to his success, the overlap in these concepts has fueled a continuing debate over whether specific interventions should be termed prevention or treatment.

The Institute of Medicine (IOM) report *Reducing Risks for Mental Disorders* (Mrazek & Haggerty, 1994) introduced a conceptual model that has achieved prominence and influences current thinking about prevention. Central to the IOM report are the concepts of risk, protection, and resilience. Risk processes are features of individuals and environments that reduce a person's capacity to maintain well-being and adaptive functioning. Protective processes enhance the functional capacities of individuals. Resilience is a special case of protective processes involving a combination of individual and environmental attributes that enable an individual to better withstand life's stressors.

The IOM report groups prevention measures into categories that roughly parallel Caplan's three prevention types. Universal preventive measures are considered appropriate for everyone in a given population group, typically a population not currently in distress. Selective prevention measures are administered to persons at above-average risk for developing disorders. The source of that risk may be environmental (e.g., low income, high family conflict) or personal factors (e.g., low self-esteem, difficulties in school). These factors are associated with the development of particular disorders, but are not symptoms of those disorders. Indicated prevention measures are applied to individuals at high risk for developing a disorder. Those targeted may be showing early symptoms, but do not meet full criteria for the diagnosis of a disorder.

Two viewpoints that have emerged in the field of prevention distinguish prevention of disorder and promotion of wellness. Wellness promotion aims at the strengthening of overall health and social competence. Prevention of disorder is a construct most popular with those following a medical model. The IOM report locates health promotion in a category distinct from prevention. The field of community psychology favors a wellness promotion paradigm, regarding prevention as a transactional construct that encompasses both the people involved and the contexts within which they live. This entry is based on the discussion of prevention by Dalton and colleagues (2001).

Related Entries: Health Promotion, Public Health

BIBLIOGRAPHY

Caplan, G. (1964). *Principles of preventive psychiatry.* New York: Basic Books. Cowen, E. L. (1991). In pursuit of wellness. *American Psychologist, 46,* 404–408.
Dalton, J. H., Elias, M. J., & Wandersman, A. (2001). *Community psychology: Linking individuals and communities.* Belmont, CA: Wadsworth/ Thomson.
Mrazek, P., & Haggerty, R. (1994). *Reducing risks for mental disorders: Frontiers for preventive intervention research.* Washington, DC: National Academy Press.

ELISE J. HERNDON
ABRAHAM WANDERSMAN

Psychogenic Illness

The term psychogenic is used in contrast to organic, physical, biogenic, or physiological. By definition, psychogenic illnesses have no known organic or physical (physiological, anatomic) basis. Conversion hysteria is one example. Any bodily system can become involved, including gait and voice. Sociocultural processes (imitation, social contagion) could drive symptom expression. The prevalence and symptom profile of psychogenic disorders vary across cultures, birth cohorts, and historical eras.

The boundary between psychogenic and biogenic is often fuzzy. Multiple chemical sensitivities and chronic fatigue syndrome are two poorly understood disorders that some authorities consider psychogenic and others believe to be biogenic. Some illnesses may have both psychogenic and biogenic components.

Mass psychogenic disorders are particularly intriguing. A group of people may fall ill all at once following exposure to an ecological trigger such as a foul odor or chemical spill. Sometimes symptoms develop following other environmental changes, such as the beginning of a new construction site. Media coverage can exacerbate the symptoms.

Related Entries: Conversion Hysteria, Somatization

PAUL R. DUBERSTEIN

Psychoneuroimmunology

INTRODUCTION

Health psychologists are concerned with the effects that psychological states and processes have on health and disease. Credible scientific enquiry into these connections began with Dunbar and Alexander, both of whom proposed that specific psychological factors caused or predisposed individuals to specific diseases, giving rise to the theory of specificity. Engel subsequently described the multifactorial approach, in which diseases have multiple determinants, including psychological factors. Finding correlational evidence that disease and health states are affected by psychological factors necessitates the investigation of processes mediating such links. Psychoneuroimmunology (PNI) is concerned with these processes, examining in particular the bidirectional relationships between the mind and the immune system, through nervous system and endocrine system pathways.

This entry provides a basic introduction to the field of PNI. This includes a brief overview of the immune system followed by a description of nervous and endocrine systems, which provide the channels of communication between the mind and the immune system. Some of the most commonly used methods that have been used to assess these interactions are examined. Conditioning of immunity and the effects of stress on the immune system are then discussed, and finally the clinical applications of PNI are considered, including the importance of PNI for understanding the course of immune-mediated disorders.

The Immune System

The immune system is a highly complex system whose intricate workings are described elsewhere in this text. This section seeks only to set out the basic principles of the system in order to familiarize the reader with key terms and processes.

Self Versus Nonself

The immune system has one basic function: to seek and destroy foreign agents (pathogens). To achieve this, the body must first discriminate between itself and the pathogen. This recognition is achieved first by phagocytes recognizing patterns on the surface of the cell in question. This is termed innate recognition.

Once an agent is recognized as nonself, the system begins a process in which there is a cascade of cells to attack and destroy the specific pathogen. Such defenses are brought about through monocytes and lymphocytes: T cells and B cells. B cells are principally responsible for the production of antibody, which binds to the pathogen to aid in its destruction. There are several types of T cells, including cytotoxic T cells, T suppressor cells, and T helper cells, all of which have specific roles in immune function. The cascade of cells and their functioning is mediated by the presence of certain chemicals, called cytokines, including the interleukins, interferons, and colony–stimulating factors. Alterations in their concentrations regulate immune functioning.

Channels of Communication Between Brain and Immune System

The physiological processes that form the pathway between the brain and the immune system are the nervous and the endocrine systems, both of which are controlled by an area of the brain called the hypothalamus. These are briefly introduced in turn.

The Nervous System

The nervous system consists of two branches: the central nervous system (CNS), which comprises the brain and the spinal cord, and the peripheral nervous system (PNS), which comprises the remainder of the nerves. The PNS is further divided into the autonomous and somatic nervous systems. The somatic system is connected to voluntary muscles, whereas the autonomic system is the one of interest in PNI because it is connected to the involuntary muscles, such as lungs, stomach, and liver, regulating the processes essential for survival. The somatic system is subdivided into the sympathetic and parasympathetic systems. Both systems innervate the same organs, but they have different, but not mutually exclusive, actions. The sympathetic nervous system is concerned with arousal of systems, increasing blood supply to facilitate the activation of a system or organ, and as such is associated with increased heart rate and blood pressure. The parasympathetic nervous system reduces arousal and activation and as such slows down heart rate and reduces blood pressure.

The Endocrine System

The action of the endocrine system is complementary to that of the nervous system and acts through the release of hormones into the bloodstream through a series of glands. The most widely investigated of these are the adrenal glands, which consist of the adrenal medulla and the adrenal cortex. Following stimulation of the sympathetic nervous system, the adrenal medulla secretes epinephrine and norepinephrine (also known as adrenaline and noradrenaline, respectively). Norepinephrine functions like the sympathetic nervous system by extending arousal. Epinephrine has similar effects and is particularly effective in stimulating the heart. The adrenal cortex is stimulated through the release of adrenocorticotropic hormone (ADTH) from the pituitary, which in turn has been stimulated through the release of corticotropin-releasing factor (CRF) by the hypothalamus. When stimulated, the adrenal cortex secretes corticosteroid hormones. There are two basic forms of corticosteroids; mineral corticoids, which affect the utilization of minerals and electrolyte regulation in the blood, and glucocorticoids, which aid in regulation of glucose in the blood. In humans, the main glucocorticoid is cortisol.

Mind–Body Connections

The first experiments linking psychological events with physiological responses were conducted by Selye in 1946 and gave rise to the theory of the general adaptation syndrome

(GAS). In basic terms, GAS proposes that exposure to a stressor elicits a nonspecific adrenocortical response in three stages: alarm reaction, resistance, and exhaustion. Alarm reaction occurs as an animal recognizes a stimulus as a stressor; resistance occurs as an animal attempts to cope with the stressor, and is characterized by increased adrenocorticol activity; and exhaustion occurs when the stress caused by the stressor is not alleviated, and leads to adrenocortical exhaustion and disease or death. Although simplistic (it is clear that the adrenal cortex is not the only mechanism between stress and health), this research demonstrated that external events could influence physiological processes, that the effect was hormonally related, and that this had direct consequences for immune functioning.

These experiments led to the understanding of two important systems responsible for coping with stressors: the active (fight/flight) system and the passive (conservation/withdrawal) system. The pathways for these systems will be set out in turn. They are important in understanding health and disease because they both culminate in the release of hormones that can and do influence immune functioning.

The Sympathoadrenomedullary (SAM) Pathway

The SAM pathway is the pathway for the active system, and involves activation of the sympathetic nervous system and then the adrenal medulla. As previously discussed, this results in the release of epinephrine and norepinephrine.

The Hypothalamic–Pituitary–Adrenocorticol (HPA) Pathway

The HPA corresponds to the passive system, where stress activates the hypothalamus, which secretes CRF, stimulating the pituitary. This activates the adrenal cortex, and culminates in the release of cortisol.

Hormones involved in both of these pathways affect the immune system and therefore influence the body's ability to respond to disease. Some of the evidence linking the SAM, HPA, and immune system is summarized as follows:

SAM and the Immune System

In general, activation of the SAM axis has been associated with an upregulation of the immune system. For example, an early study involving injections of norepinephrine found that this hormone results in the redistribution of lymphocytes from storage into circulation while reducing the efficacy of the cells (Crary et al.) Norepinephrine has also been associated with increased natual killer (NK) cell activity (Locke et al.) and a decrease in gamma interferon (Malarkey et al.). Indeed, Cohen and Kinney, in a recent review of the interactions between the nervous and immune systems, state that there is compelling evidence to support a bidirectional relationship between these systems. This includes evidence that the nervous system is connected to parts of the immune system by nerve fibers and that components of the immune system, in turn, have receptors specific for norepinephrine that respond to norepinephrine released by the sympathetic nervous system.

HPA and the Immune System

In general, the activation of the HPA axis has been associated with a downregulation of the immune system. Most HPA studies have examined the effects of cortisol on immunity and have found that cortisol can kill lymphocytes (Borysenko & Borysenko) and can affect the ability of NK cells and lymphocytes to respond to pathogens (Strausbaugh & Irwin). In a more recent study, Gruzelier and colleagues showed, by using hypnosis to reduce stress in students during examination periods, that changes in cortisol correlate positively with changes in NK cells.

Further description of the relationships among the nervous, endocrine, and immune systems are explored in details in other texts (e.g., Ader et al.).

Before examining the evidence linking psychological processes with immune function, we consider how these relationships are typically measured. This includes an overview of approaches to measuring the immune system and stress.

MEASUREMENT ISSUES IN PSYCHONEUROIMMUNOLOGY

Measuring Immunocompetence

The dramatic increase in PNI research has resulted in a plethora of techniques to measure the effects that psychological states might have on immunity. The breadth of techniques leads to difficulty in interpreting PNI data because direct comparisons among studies can not easily be drawn. This section presents some of the most commonly used techniques and briefly discuss their pros and cons. Vedhara and colleagues provide a more in-depth review of available measures and their relative usefulness.

Immunocompetence can be measured *in vivo* and *in vitro*. *In vitro* assessment is the most common and tends to focus on the presence, quantity, and function of individual parts of the immune system. *In vivo* assessment is much less common and focuses on how the system works as a whole when presented with a specific immune challenge. Both types of technique have advantages and disadvantages. *In vivo* techniques tell us much about the outcome of the immune response, but little about the underlying processes, whereas *in vitro* techniques tell us about the minutiae of processes within the system, but a limited amount about what impact those processes will have on the functioning of the host. Both approaches involve enumerative and dynamic or functional measures.

Common Enumerative Measures

Enumerative measures involve measuring the amount of a chosen immune substance, for example, total lymphocyte numbers, or numbers of T cells. Adequate functioning of the immune system might depend on adequate numbers of cells. However, it should be noted that cell numbers do not always correspond to cell function. Anesi and colleagues, for example, in a study with people with depression, found that although T cell numbers were not altered, T cell responses were reduced. Additional difficulties arise from variations in cell numbers brought about through physiological events, other than stress or psychological changes, such as circadian rhythms.

Other enumerative measures include the measurement of cytokine and antibody levels. Cytokines up- and downregulate the immune system, and therefore measurement of cytokine levels can be useful in understanding underlying mechanisms for immune dysfunction. Kiecolt-Glaser and colleagues reported that stress in caregivers was associated with poor antibody response to influenza vaccine. Through measurement of several cytokine levels, they were able to speculate on the possible mechanisms underlying this poor response.

Measurement of antibody levels is popular in PNI research, with investigators assessing both total antibody levels or levels of specific types of antibody. Of these, the measurement of total antibody levels is the perhaps the most limited because only a proportion of any circulating antibody will respond to any pathogen, and thus total levels are imprecise in determining functional immunocompetence. Responses to specific pathogens are favored, but even these have difficulties, in particular the fact that antibody levels decrease quickly once the pathogen is removed. Many researchers have circumvented this through focusing on latent viruses (i.e., viruses that are always present in the body).

Common Functional Measures

Functional measures typically involve assessing the immune system in action. One of the most common techniques involves measuring the extent of proliferation in immune cells in response to a pathogen. Despite the widespread use of these proliferation assessments, there is no proof of a linear relationship between proliferation and efficacy of the immune response, and it is not always clear which lymphocytes are responding to the pathogen.

Measurement of the ability to kill pathogens (cytotoxicity) also provides a measure of immune system efficacy. Active killing or cytotoxicity can be carried out by T cells and NK cells. The assays for measuring this inform us about the T or NK cells potential for killing. However, cytotoxicity assays only inform us about the endpoint—that cytotoxicity is affected. Such an end result could be the result of many different changes, such as decreased proliferation.

Integrated inVivo Measures

The foregoing methods of measuring immunocompetence provide indications of how specific parts of the immune system are functioning. However, there is little empirical evidence associating such methods with clinical outcomes. Methods of measuring immunocompetence *in vivo* offer outcomes of the greatest clinical significance because evidence concerning how the system works as a whole offers the most accurate way to judge the efficacy of the system. As previously mentioned, there are very few *in vivo* methods that have been used in this field, largely due to the ethical difficulties in exposing human participants to immune challenges. Those that have been used include delayed hypersensitivity tests and responses to live or attenuated virus preparations. These are briefly discussed here.

Delayed Hypersensitivity Test. Hypersensitivity is an exaggerated immune response leading to tissue damage. There are four types, but only type IV or delayed hypersensitivity has been adopted as an index of immunity in PNI. In this response, lymphokine release following T cell–pathogen interaction causes inflammation. In humans this test is often used to determine whether previous exposure to a particular pathogen has occurred. Although this method provides an indication of a system working in context, it does not illustrate where the immune impairment has taken place or provide an easily quantifiable immune response.

Response to Live or Attenuated Virus Preparations. This method involves healthy individuals being given a vaccine and different responses, most commonly the antibody response, being examined. This has clear advantages because the pathogen is naturalistic and the ethical difficulties of introducing a pathogen into a participant are removed. The only caveat with such methods is that previous exposure to pathogen can have a profound effect on immune response to current assault, and therefore any results from such studies should be interpreted with this in mind. Vaccination studies tend to use populations who would be receiving vaccinations without involvement in a study; for example, influenza viruses are commonly examined in older adults, who receive the vaccination in winter, and hepatitis B vaccinations are often examined in medical students, who receive this vaccination before beginning clinical work involving potential exposure to blood.

PNI AND PSYCHOLOGICAL APPLICATIONS

Conditioning of Immunity

Ader and Cohen in the 1970s conducted a revolutionary experiment in which they paired a saccharin solution (the conditioned stimulus) with an immunosupressant drug (the nonconditioned stimulus) in a classical conditioning paradigm. In classical conditioning a stimulus that will naturally affect a specific response (the nonconditioned stimulus) is given at the same time as a stimulus that by itself would produce no response (the conditioned stimulus). Conditioning occurs when the stimulus that would typically produce no response begins to produce the response that is associated with the other stimulus. Ader and Cohen were able to show that immunosuppression could be conditioned because the saccharin solution given without the immunosupressant drug began to produce immunosupressant effects. These findings have been replicated many times using various paradigms, and it is now widely accepted that the immune system can be conditioned, although robust findings have only been shown in T cell conditioning, not B cell conditioning.

Exton and colleagues showed that immunosuppression could be conditioned in rats that had undergone heart grafts to prevent rejection of the graft and prolong survival. They proposed that this occurred by inhibiting the release of cytokines in the spleen, imitating and supplementing the action of the standard drug treatment, which also works in this way.

Most studies have used pharmacologic agents to elicit immunosupression, but perhaps of even more interest to health psychologists are experiments using nonpharmacologic stimuli to elicit a conditioned immune response. Sato and colleagues, for example, found that if mice were stressed using electric shock, a conditioned immunosupression related to the stress of the shock could be elicited.

The conditioning of immunoenhancement has also been the subject of only limited research. Most studies have used conditioning of enhancement of NK cell activity, and most have been carried out using animals. One exception to this is the work of Ikemi and Nakagawa, who elicited a conditioned skin inflammatory response in a sample of four participants. Although not being beneficial in itself, this work showed that the immune system could be upregulated as well as downregulated by conditioning.

Stress and Immune Functioning

The relationship between stress and immunity is perhaps the most researched area of PNI within health psychology. Experiments have considered the effects of both acute and chronic stress in animals and humans and in healthy and diseased populations, including people with HIV, cancer, rheumatoid arthri-

tis, and multiple sclerosis. These studies have employed many paradigms to assess the efficacy of the immune response, including response to vaccine, wound healing, and progression of disease.

With regard to experimental acute stress, Bachen and colleagues found that experimentally induced acute stress, caused by a 21-min Stroop test, was associated with a reduction in lymphocyte numbers and their proliferation in response to pathogen. Illustrating the importance of appraisal of stress, Sieber and colleagues found that participants who reported a noise stressor as less controllable had a higher reduction in NK cell activity than those who perceived they did have control over the noise, and were therefore probably less stressed.

Examination stress is the most widely used naturalistic acute stress paradigm. For example, Glaser and colleagues found that students had a lower percentage of CD4+ cells and reported more infectious illnesses during exam periods. More recently, Marucha and colleagues used a within-subject design to compare wound healing in students during examination and vacation periods. They found that each individual student healed more slowly during their examination period and that the time to heal was an average of around 40% longer during this time.

In terms of chronic stress, evidence for downregulation of immunity due to chronic stress has been found in hospitalized groups, people with clinical depression, people who have been bereaved, and caregivers. These studies have shown reductions in NK cell activity and T cell percentages and increased antibody levels (indicating increased viral activity) and increased plasma cortisol, indicating activation of the HPA system. Kiecolt-Glaser and colleagues (1987) examined the immune function of the caregivers of people with Alzheimer's disease. They noted a decline in T cell percentages, a decline in the number of T helper cells, and an increase in antibody levels to Epstein–Barr virus (the virus responsible for glandular fever). In a more recent study with caregivers, Kiecolt-Glaser and colleagues (1995) gave caregivers punch biopsy wounds, and observed that healing times were approximately 25% longer than those of controls.

There is now a large body of literature on the effects of stress on the progression of disorders such as HIV infection. Whether stress can mediate the course of a disease is a difficult question to answer, given the multifactorial nature of disease aetiology. However, investigations using a wide range of research designs appear to suggest that stress may indeed be a significant cofactor in the progression of such illnesses.

Cross-Sectional, Longitudinal, and Long-Term Survivor Studies: HIV Infection, an Example

In a cross-sectional study of HIV-positive men, Goodkin and colleagues found greater NK cell cytotoxicity in participants with an active coping style. Longitudinally, Weiss found that greater anger and less suppression of anger in HIV-positive men was associated with more rapid disease progression as evidenced by CD4+ decline over a 5- to 6-year follow-up. In a key study in the area of HIV infection, Soloman and colleagues retrospectively compared people who had died with AIDS-related pneumocystis corinic pneumonia and those still alive. Survivors were found to have made more use of problem-solving social support and had significantly higher scores on the control dimension of Kobasa's hardiness measure. Interviews with long-term survivors revealed the presence of active coping associated with realistic acceptance and adjustment to their diagnosis. These studies suggest that psychological variables, in particular coping styles, might influence the course of immune-mediated diseases such as HIV infection.

Intervention Studies

Despite the fact that the field of PNI is in its infancy, it has been possible to give persuasive evidence that conditioning, stress, and other psychological factors can influence immune function. However, researchers have also examined how such immune changes can be used in clinical applications to improve health.

In a study of hypnosis and relaxation in a healthy student population, Kiecolt-Glaser and colleagues (1987) found that during examination periods, those in the intervention group had an increase in the number of T helper cells. More recently, Petrie and colleagues examined the effect of emotional disclosure on medical students. Emotional disclosure is a technique in which people are encouraged to write about traumatic or upsetting experiences usually for around 20 min a day on four consecutive days. Petrie found that the disclosure group had significantly increased antibody levels in response to hepatitis B vaccine, indicating enhanced immune functioning.

A classic study investigating interventions in a clinical population was that of Spiegel and colleagues, who examined the effect of 1 year of weekly group therapy sessions and self-hypnosis in a group of women with breast cancer. The women involved in the groups lived an average of 18 months longer than women not in the groups. Similarly, Stanton and colleagues investigated the effect of emotional disclosure on a group of women with breast cancer. They found that the participants in the emotional disclosure group attended clinics for illnesses related to their cancer, and self-reported symptoms at 3-month follow-up significantly less than the control group. However, Rosenberg and colleagues in a pilot study with 30 men with prostate cancer found that although emotional disclosure was linked to improved psychological outcomes, there was no evidence that immunity was affected.

CONCLUSIONS

PNI is a burgeoning area of research. The research endeavor has provided compelling evidence of a potent bidirectional relationship between psychological factors and physiological and immunological functioning. The challenges that lie ahead include gaining a greater understanding of the mechanisms underlying these relationships, exploring the clinical relevance of the observed effects on immunity, and developing interventions to harness the effects of the mind on the body.

Related Entries: Cancer: Biopsychosocial Aspects, Immune System: Structure and Function

BIBLIOGRAPHY

Ader, R., & Cohen, N. (1975). Behaviourally conditioned immunosupression. *Psychosomatic Medicine, 37,* 333–340.

Alexander, F. (1950). *Psychosomatic medicine.* New York: Norton.

Anesi, A., Franciotta, D., Di Paolo, E., Zardini, E., Melzi, D., Eril, G., et al. (1994). PHA-stimulated cellular immune function and T-lymphocyte subsets in major depressive disorders. *Functional Neurology, 9,* 17–22.

Bachen, E. A., Manuck, S. B., Marsland, A. L., Cohen, S., Malkoff, S. B., Muldoon, M. F., et al. (1992). Lymphocyte subset and cellular immune responses to a brief experimental stressor. *Psychosomatic Medicine, 54,* 673–679.

Borysenko, M., & Borysenko, J. (1982). Stress, behaviour and immunity: Animal models and mediating mechanisms. *General Hospital Psychiatry, 4,* 59–67.

Cohen, N., & Kinney, K. S. (2001). Exploring the phylogenetic history of neural–immune system interactions. In R. Ader, D. L. Felten, & N. Cohen (Eds.), *Psychoneuroimmunology* (3rd ed., Vol. I, pp. 21–54). New York: Academic.

Cohen, S., Kamarck, T., & Mermelstein, R. (1983). A global measure of perceived stress. *Journal of Health and Social Behavior, 24,* 385–396.

Crary, B., Hauser, S. L., Borysenko, M., Kutz, I., Hoban, C., Ault, K. A., et al. (1983). Epinepherine induced changes in the distribution of lymphocyte subsets in the peripheral blood of humans. *Journal of Immunology, 131,* 1178–1181.

Delongis, A., Folkman, S., & Lazarus, R. S. (1988). The impact of daily stress on health and mood: Psychological and social resources as mediators. *Journal of Personality and Social Psychology, 54,* 486–496.

Dunbar, H. F. (1943). *Psychosomatic diagnosis.* New York: Harper.

Engel, G. L. (1954). Selection of clinical material in psychosomatic medicine. *Psychosomatic Medicine, 16,* 368–378.

Exton, M. S., Schult, M., Donath, S., Strubel, T., Nagel, E., Westermann, J., et al. (1998). Behavioral conditioning prolongs heart allograft survival in rats. *Transplantation Proceedings, 30,* 2033.

Glaser, R., Rice, J., Sheridan, J., Fertel, R., Stout, J., Speicher, C., et al. (1987). Stress-related immune suppression: Health implications. *Brain Behaviour and Immunity, 1,* 7–20.

Goodkin, K., Blaney, N., Feaster, D., Fletcher, M. A., Baum, M. K., MenteroAtineza, E., et al. (1992). Active coping style is associated with natural killer cell cytotoxicity in asymptomatic HIV-1 seropositive homosexual men. *Journal of Psychosomatic Research, 36,* 635–650.

Gruzelier, J., Smith, F., Nagy, A., & Henderson, D. (2001). Cellular and humoral immunity, mood and exam stress: The influences of self-hypnosis and personality predictors. *International Journal of Psychophysiology, 42,* 55–71.

Holmes, T., & Rahe, R. (1967). Holmes–Rahe Life Changes Scale. *Journal of Psychosomatic Research, 11,* 213–218.

Ikemi, Y., & Nakagawa, S. (1962). A psychosomatic study of contagious dermatitis. *Kyushu Journal of Medical Science, 13,* 335–350.

Kanner, A. D., Coyne, J. C., Schaefer, C., & Lazarus, R. S. (1981). Comparison of two models of stress management: Daily hassles and uplifts versus major life events. *Journal of Behavioural Medicine, 4,* 1–37.

Kiecolt-Glaser, J. K, Glaser, R., Shuttleworth, E. C., et al. (1987). Chronic stress and immunity in family caregivers of Alzheimer's-disease victims. *Psychosomatic Medicine, 49,* 523–535.

Kiecolt-Glaser, J. K., Marucha, P. T, Malarkey, W. B., et al. (1995). Slowing of wound-healing by psychological stress. *Lancet, 346,* 1194–1196.

Kirschbaum, C., Pirke, K.-M., & Hellhammer, D. H. (1993). The Trier Social Stress Test—A tool for investigating psychobiological stress responses in a laboratory setting. *Neuropsychobiology, 28,* 76–81.

Kobasa, S. C. (1979) Stressful life events, personality, and health: An inquiry into hardiness. *Journal of Personality and Social Psychology, 37,* 1–11.

Lazarus, R. S., & Folkman, S. (1987). Transactional theory and research on emotions and coping. *European Journal of Personality, 1,* 141–170.

Locke, S., Krause, L., Kutz, I., Edbril, S., Phillips, K., & Benson, H. (1984). Altered natural killer cell activity during norepinephrine infusion in humans. In *Proceedings of the 1st International Workshop on Neuroimmunomodulation* (pp. 00–00). New York: Gordon & Breach.

Malarkey, W. B., Wang, J., Cheney, C., Glaser, R., & Nagaraja, H, (2002). Human lymphocyte growth hormone stimulates interferon gamma production and is inhibited by cortisol and norepinephrine. *Journal of Neuroimmunology, 123,* 180–187.

Marucha, P. T., Kiecolt-Glaser, J. K., & Favagehi, M. (1998). Mucosal wound healing is impaired by examination stress. *Psychosomatic Medicine, 60,* 362–365.

Petrie, K. J, Booth, R. J., Pennebaker, J. W., Davison, K. P., & Thomas, M. G. (1995). Disclosure of trauma and immune response to a hepatitis B vaccination program. *Journal of Consulting and Clinical Psychology, 63,* 787–792.

Rosenberg, H. J., Rosenberg, S. D., Ernstoff, M. S., Wolford, G. L., Amdur, R. J., Elshamy, M. R., et al. (2002). Expressive disclosure and health outcomes in prostate cancer population. *International Journal of Psychiatry and Medicine, 32,* 37–53.

Sato, K., Flood, J. F., & Makinodan, T. (1984). Influence of conditioned psychological stress on immunological recovery in mice exposed to low-dose x-irradiation. *Radiation Research, 98,* 381–388.

Selye, H. (1946). The general adaptation syndrome and the diseases of adaption. *Journal of Clinical Endocrinology, 6,* 117.

Sieber, W. J., Rodin, J., Larson, L., Ortega, S., Cummings, N., Levy, S., et al. (1992). Modulation of human natural killer cell activity by exposure to uncontrollable stress. *Brain Behaviour and Immunity, 6,* 141–156.

Soloman, G. F., Temoshok, L., O'Leary, A., & Zich, J (1987). An intensive psychoimmunological study of long term surviving persons with AIDS. *Annals of the New York Academy of Sciences, 496,* 647–655.

Spiegel, D., Bloom, J. R., Kraemer, H. C., & Gottheil, E. (1989). Effects of psychosocial treatment on survival of patients with metastatic breast cancer. *Lancet, 2,* 886–901.

Stanton, A. L., Danoff-Burg, S., Sworowski, L. A., Collins, C. A., Branstetter, A., Rodriguez-Hanley, A., et al. (2002). Randomized, controlled trial of written emotional expression and benefit finding in breast cancer patients. *Journal of Clinical Oncology, 20,* 4160–4168.

Strausbaugh, H., & Irwin, M. (1992). Central corticotrophin-releasing hormone reduces cellular immunity. *Brain, Behaviour and Immunity, 6,* 11–17.

Vedhara, K., Fox, J. D., & Wang, E. C. Y. (1999). The measurement of stress-related immune dysfunction in psychoneuroimmunology. *Neuroscience and Biobehavioural Reviews, 23,* 699–715.

Lucie M. T. Byrne-Davis
K. Vedhara

Psychophysiology

Psychophysiology, a discipline that traces its roots back to ancient Greek society, is one of several scientific disciplines that examine relations between mind and body. Psychophysiology has traditionally been defined as any research in which the dependent variable is a physiological measure and the independent (or predictor) variable is a behavioral one. Studies examining how different stimuli (e.g., nude photos and accident victims) affect physiological parameters (e.g., heart rate and palmar sweating) accurately reflect the discipline of psychophysiology. Psychophysiology differs from related disciplines such as physiological psychology mainly in that psychophysiological research tends to be conducted on humans and is noninvasive, whereas physiological psychology tends to be conducted on animals and is more likely to use invasive procedures.

Recent decades have witnessed a dramatic increase in psychophysiological research. New technology, user-friendly equipment, and increasing expertise of researchers have aided this trend. More importantly, however, psychophysiological measures have allowed researchers to assess theoretical constructs that hitherto had remained hypothetical. In doing so, psychophysiological methods have facilitated theoretical advances. Classic areas of psychophysiology include study of orienting, attentional activity, and defensive reflexes; cognitive processing; anxiety, stress, and, emotion; and personality.

Although all are interested in central nervous system processing, most psychophysiologists are either "neck up" or "neck down," a distinction that reflects the measures they use and more specifically the placement of their sensors. Neck-up psychophysiologists tend to study brain electrical activity and potentials, whereas neck-down psychophysiologists tend to study the endpoints of autonomic nervous system activity (e.g., heart rate and blood pressure) or musculoskeletal activity.

Perhaps no area exemplifies psychophysiology better than the study of stress, a phenomenon uniquely suited to psychophysiological investigation because of its familiar association with bodily responses. Rare is the individual who has never felt his or her heart leap with excitement or his or her blood boil with anger. For good and bad, stress is part of being alive. Moreover, stress has been related to a host of diseases including hypertension, cardiovascular disease, and stroke. As such, stress-related psychophysiology has a long and distinguished history, as well as a bright future.

Stress-related psychophysiology has focused on the activity of the autonomic nervous system (ANS) in general and the cardiovascular system in particular. Indeed this area is often called the study of cardiovascular reactivity to stress (CVR). Researchers in this area typically assess ongoing cardiovascular activity during a rest or baseline period and then during a stress period in which where participants are required to perform mental arithmetic, solve complicated problems, present a short speech, or similar task. Cardiovascular reactivity refers to the change in physiological activity from resting levels to task levels. The general hypothesis guiding this research is that exaggerated, repeated, or prolonged cardiovascular reactivity to stress indicates enhanced risk for cardiovascular diseases and/or hypertension. The autonomic reaction responsible for cardiovascular changes is also responsible for other physiological sequella, including changes in neuroendocrine and immune system activity. The health-damaging effects of stress have been attributed to the activity of the sympathetic nervous system (SNS), the system historically associated with the fight-or-flight response.

The simplest and most widely used measures of CVR are heart rate and blood pressure (i.e., systolic and diastolic). Researchers can assess these measures with minimal equipment and training. Unfortunately, measures such as heart rate and blood pressure lack sufficient specificity in terms of their autonomic origin because they have multiple ANS determinants. Take heart rate, for example, which is dually controlled by the SNS and parasympathetic (PNS) branches of the ANS. Because of tonic PNS suppression of heart rate under normal circumstances, increases in heart rate from baseline to stress may be caused by (1) release of normal parasympathetic restraint, (2) increased sympathetic activation, or (3) some combination of the two. As such, increased heart rate does not necessarily indicate SNS activity. Moreover, what may appear to be no change in heart rate may reflect countervailing parasympathetic and sympathetic influences, which effectively cancel each other out. A similar conundrum exists for blood pressure changes, which may reflect (1) increased cardiac output, (2) increased peripheral resistance, (3) a synergistic combination of the two, or (4) a countervailing combination of the two.

The inability of these measures to provide unambiguous information about SNS activity has prompted the search for measures that can provide such information. One notable development in this regard is a technique called impedance cardiography.

Impedance cardiography (ZCG) is a noninvasive technique that allows researchers to assess cardiac stroke volume on an ongoing, beat-by-beat, basis. In addition, the waveform resultant from ZCG can be used in combination with other waveforms, such as the electrocardiogram (ECG), to derive a wealth of information about ongoing cardiac performance and to better specify the ANS origins of such activity.

Briefly, impedance cardiography works by sending a high-frequency (alternating current or radio) current across the thoracic cavity and assessing the electrical impedance of the thorax. Small variations in this activity, magnified mathematically and electronically, indicate discrete cardiac events including the onset of left ventricular ejection, the peak ejection velocity, and the closing of the aortic valve, the latter signaling the end of systole. Using specialized equations, one can score the ZCG waveform to estimate cardiac stroke volume (SV). Stroke volume estimates, in turn, can be combined with heart rate estimates to derive cardiac output (CO = HR × SV).

In addition to stroke volume and cardiac output, the ZCG and ECG waveforms can be used to assess several systolic time intervals (STIs), expressed in milliseconds. STIs describe various aspects of the heart's performance during the contraction process. Systole consists of two phases, the preejection period (PEP) and the left ventricular ejection time (LVET). PEP reflects the time from depolarization of the ventricular nerve fibers and muscle tissue to the onset of ventricular ejection and reflects how long it takes the contracting heart to generate sufficient force to eject blood into the atrial system. A heart that is beating hard (i.e., with great contractile force) will have a relatively short PEP, whereas a heart that is beating less hard will have a relatively long PEP. As such, PEP directly reflects changes in cardiac contractile force. Because anatomic studies have shown that cardiac contractile force is almost exclusively under control of the SNS, with little or no countervailing PNS influence, PEP provides a relatively unambiguous measure of sympathetic influence on the heart. PEP's counterpart, LVET, reflects the time in milliseconds from onset of ventricular ejection to closing of the aortic valve. Although important in the calculation of SV, LVET alone does not convey unique information on ANS function.

Impedance cardiography also allows derivation of other useful measures, most notably, total peripheral resistance (TPR), which reflects the overall state of arterial vasoconstriction and/or vasodilation. TPR is estimated by taking mean arterial pressure (MAP) and factoring out changes in cardiac output (TPR = MAP/CO * 80). Theoretically, after factoring out the effect of cardiac output on blood pressure change, what remains must reflect changes in total peripheral resistance.

Total peripheral resistance is important to psychophysiologists because they can use it along with CO to explore the underlying hemodynamics of blood pressure. For example, increases in systolic blood pressure and diastolic blood pressure might reflect a change in cardiac output, a change in peripheral vascular resistance, or both. Perhaps more importantly, what appears as no change in blood pressure might reflect reflect increasing CO combined with decreasing TPR, influences that can cancel each other out in terms of overall blood pressure.

Measures derived from impedance cardiography can shed considerable light on this issue. Moreover, disorders such as cardiac arrest and hypertension may differentially relate to cardiac versus vascular reactions.

Total peripheral resistance is also important as an indicator of sympathetic nervous system activity. This is because processes of vasoconstriction and vasodilation—the origins of TPR—are controlled exclusively by the SNS, with no countervailing PNS influence. Therefore, an increase in TPR can indicate increased SNS activity in terms of vasoconstriction. Unfortunately, the global assessment of TPR, as is done in most psychophysiological research, can reflect countervailing vasoconstrictive and vasodilatory influences, the former caused by SNS neural stimulation, the latter by circulating epinephrine primarily at the heart, lungs, and large muscles. Thus, no change in TPR may reflect no measurable autonomic activity, or may reflect countervailing vasoconstriction and vasodilatory effects.

How does stress affect these parameters? There is no straightforward answer to this question, primarily because the construct of stress is not singular. Despite prevailing belief to the contrary, psychophysiologists have known for some time that there is no single form of stress, but that stress takes several forms. These forms are distinguished by different combinations of parasympathetic and sympathetic activity and patterns of activity within the SNS (e.g., vasoconstriction vs. vasodilation, increased cardiac output vs. increased peripheral resistance, presence or absence of epinephrine and cortisol). Complicating matters, researchers do not agree regarding the form or utility of specific types of stress, nor do they agree regarding the psychological significance of each. Nonetheless, several good candidates exist in this regard. For example, although they use different nomenclature, researchers have identified an energy mobilization response that consists of large increases in cardiac performance, increased vasodilation and receptivity of the arteries to blood flow, and the release of epinephrine. Moreover, this cardiovascular pattern has been associated with both appetitive (e.g., challenge) and aversive affective reactions (e.g., fear, anger). A second good candidate reflects a more restrained form of stress, and consists of strong increases in peripheral vascular resistance and low or reduced cardiac output. This form has been associated more uniformly with negative affective states such as threat and vigilance.

Although more work is needed to delineate the various types of stress reaction, the important lesson here is that no single physiological measure can suffice as an indicator of "stress." Instead, researchers taking a psychophysiological approach should employ as many measures of autonomic function as they can, and use these measures to look for patterns of physiological response. In addition, researchers should also take care to supplement their physiological measures with measures of behavioral activity or performance and affective reaction to

further delineate the type or types of stress being evidenced by participants in their studies.

BIBLIOGRAPHY

Blascovich, J., & Katkin, E. S. (Eds.). (1993). *Cardiovascular reactivity to psychological stress and cardiovascular disease: An examination of the evidence.* Washington, DC: American Psychological Association.

Cacioppo, J. T., Tassinary, L. G., & Berntson, G. G. (Eds.). (2000). *Handbook of psychophysiology.* New York: Cambridge University Press.

Tomaka, J., Blascovich, J., Kelsey, R. M., & Leitten, C. L. (1993). Subjective, physiological, and behavioral effects of threat and challenge appraisal. *Journal of Personality and Social Psychology, 65,* 248–260.

JOE TOMAKA

Psychosomatic Medicine

The term psychosomatic is derived by combining two Greek roots, *psyche* ("mind") and *soma* ("body"). Psychosomatic medicine refers both to a scientific paradigm and medical institutions (journals, textbooks, learned societies, medical schools) that are premised on the inextricable physiological relationship between mind and body. The psychosomatic approach to research, education, and treatment acknowledges the potential contributions of emotions and psychological states to the onset, exacerbation, course, and recurrence of disease. Psychosomatic medicine can be contrasted to health psychology or medical sociology in its relative emphasis on physiological processes as opposed to psychological (social–cognitive, behavioral) processes or socioeconomic conditions.

HISTORY

Psychosomatic concepts have been discussed for millennia. The term psychosomatic medicine was used more frequently after the 1935 publication of Helen Flanders Dunbar's *Emotions and Bodily Changes.* The formation of the American Psychosomatic Society and the creation of its influential flagship journal *Psychosomatic Medicine* in 1939 were other defining events.

Psychosomatic medicine insinuated itself into American culture by the late 1940s. Popular magazines such as *Reader's Digest* featured articles on psychosomatic topics. Not coincidentally, psychoanalysis also gained popularity at that time. In 1950, Franz Alexander likened psychosomatic specificity to microbial specificity in his attempt to reconcile psychoanalytic theory with mainstream medicine. His approach provided a stark contrast to the psychoanalysis of the 1920s, when Georg Groddeck, a self-proclaimed "wild" analyst, maintained that all physical conditions, including myopia, represented unconscious conflicts. (After hearing Groddeck deliver a presentation, Sigmund Freud asked him whether he meant to be taken seriously; Freud supported him nonetheless.)

From Alexander's perspective, diseases such as asthma or ulcers resulted from unresolved needs and intrapsychic conflicts. Alexander's bold but unsuccessful attempt to appeal to his physician colleagues may have contributed to the marginalization of psychosomatics within internal medicine. Still, psychosomatics gained momentum in psychiatry. The Academy of Psychosomatic Medicine, an organization of psychiatrists, was founded in 1954. Its official journal, *Psychosomatics*, was launched in 1960.

While Alexander and other psychoanalytic investigators pursued creative if occasionally strange ideas with dubious validity, the 1950s and 1960s saw a dramatic increase in research on the health consequences of stress. Devoid of psychoanalytic content, these studies ushered in a new era in psychosomatics. The endocrinologist Hans Selye examined the deleterious effects of an overactive hypothalamic–pituitary–adrenal axis, Hinkle and Wolff conducted groundbreaking research in social epidemiology, and experiments demonstrated that animals subjected to stress show greater susceptibility to infection. A multidisciplinary, empirically driven psychosomatic medicine emerged from the shadow of psychoanalysis. Stress, not intrapsychic conflict or unconscious motivation, took center stage in this new paradigm.

IS PSYCHOSOMATIC MEDICINE MERELY A HISTORICAL NOVELTY?

The *institution* of psychosomatic medicine has not been particularly successful. Witness its peripheral role in the curriculum of most medical schools, the long-term trend toward reductionism in internal medicine and even in psychiatry, and the failure of the label "psychosomatic medicine" to appear anywhere on the organizational chart of the National Institutes of Health. Still, the ascendancy of new journals, societies, and textbooks in the 1980s and 1990s devoted to psychyoneuroimmunology and psychoneuroendocrinology testifies to the power, validity, and heuristic value of the fundamental premise of the psychosomatic paradigm, the inextricable physiological relationship between mind and body.

Related Entries: American Psychosomatic Society, Society of Behavioral Medicine, Somatization

BIBLIOGRAPHY

Ader, R., Felten, D. L., & Cohen, N. (Eds.). (2001). *Psychoneuroimmunology.* (3rd ed.). San Diego; CA: Academic.

Brown, T. M. (2000). *The rise and fall of psychosomatic medicine.* Available at www.human-nature.com/free-associations/riseandfall.html

National Library of Medicine, History of Medicine Division, Emotions and Disease. Available at www.nlm.nih.gov/hmd/emotions/ emotionshome.html

Weiner, H. (1999). Praise be to *Psychosomatic Medicine. Psychosomatic Medicine, 61,* 259–262.

PAUL R. DUBERSTEIN

Psychotherapy

The term psychotherapy refers to the use of psychological (as opposed to physical) treatments to improve physical and mental health by relieving symptoms, helping patients manage or adjust to stressors, decreasing distress, and enhancing well-being. To some practitioners psychotherapy is a science; to others it is more of an art form. An abiding belief in the value of talking about one's concerns is a key premise shared by the thousands of psychotherapies and nearly as many theoretical perspectives.

Psychotherapy is typically conducted on a one-to-one basis, with an individual. Treatments for couples, families, and groups are also available. Psychotherapy is practiced throughout the world, with different types gaining popularity in different parts of the world.

HISTORICAL OVERVIEW

In Western cultures, at least four prominent schools of individual psychotherapy can be identified: psychoanalytic, behavioral, cognitive, and humanistic/existential. Psychoanalysis is the original "talking cure." Joseph Breuer and Sigmund Freud developed it in 19th-century Vienna when they discovered that uncovering and talking about repressed intrapsychic conflict led to the removal of symptoms in hysterical patients. Psychoanalysis posits that human behavior is in part driven by unconscious wishes and conflicts often originating in early childhood, and that the work of therapy is to uncover and analyze patients' intrapsychic conflicts. Freud refined the techniques of classical psychoanalysis in the early 20th century, and charismatic leaders such as Harry Stack Sullivan, Otto Kernberg, and Heinz Kohut subsequently developed numerous forms of psychodynamically oriented treatments. Because many of these leaders shared Freud's disdain for empirical scrutiny, psychodynamically oriented clinicians were unprepared to respond to the demand for greater economic and scientific accountability in the 1980s.

The same was not true of behavior therapy. Derived from scientific research by I. Pavlov and B. F. Skinner on conditioning and how people learn, behavior therapy was developed and disseminated in the middle of the 20th century, most notably by Joseph Wolpe. Unlike their psychodynamically oriented colleagues, behavior therapists were interested in demonstrating scientifically the effectiveness of the treatment. Behavior therapists explain pathological behaviors as consequences of maladaptive learning and reinforcement systems, rather than unconscious dynamic conflicts. In psychotherapy, behaviorists work with patients to identify new behaviors to replace problematic ones, and to substitute new reinforcement systems that will maintain the new behaviors. So, for example, a behavior therapist might determine that a child who resisted going to school was having this behavior reinforced by parents giving the child more attention. Treatment would involve restructuring the reinforcement system to have parents give greater attention and other rewards to the child when he or she attends school.

Due largely to the pioneering work of Aaron Beck, cognitive therapy rose to prominence in the 1960s and preeminence in the mid-1970s. By the early 1980s cognitive–behavioral therapies, integrating behavioral and cognitive approaches, became influential. Solid empirical research documenting their effectiveness is perhaps the main reason why the number of clinical psychologists whose primary theoretical orientation is psychodynamic fell from 35% in 1960 to half that in 1995. Cognitive and cognitive–behavioral therapies are concerned with the impact of patients' thoughts and beliefs on their moods and behaviors. Cognitivists identify the automatic, negative thoughts and beliefs that patients have about themselves and others, and work to restructure thinking patterns in more appropriate and adaptive ways. A cognitive–behavioral therapist could, for example, assist a male patient who was depressed after not receiving a job promotion by identifying the negative thought patterns underlying the depression ("If I'm not promoted, I'm no good; I'll never succeed at work") with more adaptive ones ("I am a worthwhile person whether or not I have a job promotion; just because I wasn't promoted doesn't mean I'll never have job success again").

Carl Rogers and Victor Frankl, among others, propounded humanistic and existential therapies. In contrast to the relatively more disorder-focused approaches of psychoanalysis and behaviorism, proponents of humanistic and existential approaches strive to understand the whole person and to assist patients' in their search for personal meaning, identity, or self-actualization. Therapists do not view themselves as authority figures; instead, the relationship with the *client* (not *patient*) is meant to be more egalitarian.

CONCEPTUAL OVERVIEW

Given the plethora of psychotherapies and theoretical perspectives, it is useful to think about psychotherapists as varying along three related dimensions: their conceptualization of the patient's problem, psychological focus, and behavior in the session.

Perhaps the most salient conceptual dimension that distinguishes therapists is the extent to which they view the patient's current presenting problem as emanating from earlier (often childhood) experiences. Another distinction concerns how literally the presenting symptom is conceptualized. Psychodynamic therapists may view a symptom such as anxiety as a symbolic expression of repressed emotional conflict, and they will attempt to uncover and help the patient work through the conflict. Cognitive therapists will conceptualize anxiety as fueled by maladaptive thinking, and they will help patients think about themselves as effective and powerful in a relatively benign world.

With respect to psychological focus, therapists differ in the relative emphasis placed on the patient's thoughts, use of language, emotions, interpersonal relationships, behaviors, motives, and goals. The name of the psychotherapy often is derived from the psychological focus. For example, cognitive therapists focus on thoughts, behavior therapists concentrate on behavior, cognitive–behavior therapists attend to the thoughts that accompany particular behaviors, and psychodynamic therapists analyze the driving (or dynamic) unconscious wishes and conflicts behind behaviors and emotions.

Turning to in-session behavior, we can say that therapists differ in their level of activity, warmth, and attention to how they are perceived or treated by their patients. Active therapists dispense advice, reveal much of themselves, prescribe behavioral regimens, or assign homework, such as asking patients to maintain diaries or journals. Passive therapists say very little, never talk about themselves, and do not assign homework. That does not mean that they are less intellectually or emotionally engaged in the treatment.

Another in-session dimension concerns the therapist's level of warmth or empathy. At one end of this spectrum, some therapists exude warmth and approach the patients with unconditional positive regard. At the other end, therapists could be confrontational or critical in an effort to help patients take a closer look at themselves. That does not mean that they like the patient less than therapists who display unconditional positive regard.

A third dimension concerns the extent to which the relationship between therapist and patient is analyzed or even discussed. Psychodynamic therapists pay very close attention to their patients' emotional responses to them because those responses are thought to derive from deep-seated and often unconscious feelings about early caregivers in patients' lives.

Other therapies do not make the therapeutic relationship a central concern.

PRAGMATIC CONSIDERATIONS

Therapies need to be tailored to the age, educational level, and cognitive status of the patient. Many psychotherapies require reasonably intact, adult-level cognition and are therefore not appropriate for children or for patients with cognitive impairment. The patient's socioeconomic circumstance, notably his or her insurance coverage, is another important pragmatic consideration. In response to increasing economic constraints and calls for scientific accountability, there has been movement toward scientific study of briefer treatments (defined in terms of weeks or months) as opposed to longer-term therapies. Structured, or manualized, brief treatments for disorders such as acute depression and panic disorder have proven successful. However, as evidence mounts that therapy's beneficial effects are often not sustained, longer-term maintenance therapies are now being used to maintain good mental health outcomes.

WHO PRACTICES PSYCHOTHERAPY AND WHERE?

Psychotherapy is practiced by individuals trained in a number of professional disciplines, including psychology, psychiatry, family medicine, nursing, education, social work, and theology. It is practiced in diverse settings, including schools and universities, places of worship, the workplace, primary care clinics, community mental health centers, psychiatric inpatient units of hospitals, and private offices.

PSYCHOTHERAPY IN THE CONTEXT OF MEDICAL TREATMENT

Practitioners in virtually every medical specialty are potentially positioned to make referrals for psychotherapy. Primary care physicians often see patients with depression, anxiety, or multiple unexplained physical symptoms. Many will make a referral to a mental health professional only after conducting a course of psychotherapy themselves. Panic disorder patients will often present to a primary care physician or cardiologist before seeking help from a mental health professional. Surgeons may refer patients with posttraumatic stress disorder following a motor vehicle accident or other accidental injury. Many skin conditions, such as eczema or dermatitis, are stress responsive and may abate in response to stressreducing treatments. Depression is not uncommon following myocardial infarction, coronary artery bypass graft surgery, or the diagnosis and treatment of many forms of cancer. These patients (and their spouses) may often benefit from psychotherapy. The advent of genetic testing may have solved a number of problems, but it has created others, some of which may be amenable to psychotherapy.

EFFECTIVE TREATMENTS

As noted by Peter Nathan and Jack Gorman, research has identified a number of effective therapies for particular symptoms or disorders For example, cognitive–behavioral interventions can be used effectively in the treatment of ritualistic behaviors and thoughts associated with obsessive–compulsive disorder. Cognitive–behavioral interventions are also effective at improving body image in patients with body dysmorphic disorder, and decreasing the frequency of binge and purge behavior in patients with bulimia nervosa. Behavior therapies have proven effectiveness in treating several disorders commonly seen in medical settings, especially panic disorder with agoraphobia and sleep disorders. Cognitive–behavior therapy, psychodynamic therapy and interpersonal therapy have all been shown to be effective in treating some forms of depression.

Most of the rigorous studies and subsequent meta-analyses on treatments for mental disorders have been conducted on patients seen in the context of mental health care delivery settings, not medical settings. Research on the effectiveness of psychotherapeutic treatments for medical patients seen in medical settings will help advance the science and art of psychotherapy.

Related Entries: Coping, Cognitive–Behavioral Therapy, Disclosure and Health, Stress Management

BIBLIOGRAPHY

Beck, A. T. (1976). *Cognitive therapy and the emotional disorders.* New York: International Universities Press.

Brenner, C. (1982). *An elementary textbook of psychoanalysis.* New York: International Universities Press.

Frank, J. D. (1961). *Persuasion and healing: A comparative study of psychotherapy.* New York: Shocken.

Frankl, V. E. (1959). *Man's search for meaning: An introduction to logotherapy.* New York: Simon & Schuster.

Meichenbaum, D. H. (1977). *Cognitive behavior modification: An integrative approach.* New York: Plenum.

Nathan, P. E., & Gorman, J. M. (1998). (Eds.). *A guide to treatments that work.* New York: Oxford University Press.

Rogers, C. R. (1949). *Client-centered therapy: Its current practice, implications and theory.* Boston: Houghton Mifflin.

Wolpe, J. (1973). *The practice of behavior therapy.* New York: Pergamon.

PAUL R. DUBERSTEIN
NANCY L. TALBOT

Public Health

Public health refers to those activities by which a society attempts to increase life expectancy, decrease morbidity, and help improve health-related quality of life. A distinction is sometimes made between clinical or high-risk approaches to disease treatment and prevention versus population-based strategies. Although there is some utility in distinguishing between these approaches, they should be seen as complementary because neither strategy is effective for all behaviors or all target groups. Thus, an important public health task is to identify which risk behaviors are amenable to individual-based versus population-based interventions and how to make these interventions synergistic with one another.

Application of the social and behavioral sciences to improve health and combat disease occurs at multiple levels and requires implementation of different skills both within and across levels. Genetic counseling for those at familial risk of disease, family counseling to reduce substance abuse or interfamilial violence and group counseling to help those living with HIV/AIDS are examples of interpersonal interventions at the individual level. At the organizational level, interpersonal intervention such as blood pressure screenings and smoking cessation programs, the provision of physical fitness facilities, and media communication have been used in schools, work sites, and community centers. Finally, societal-type interventions involving media and policy actions can occur at the community, state, or federal level. Seat-belt laws, public service announcements about drunk driving, and taxation of cigarettes are examples of interventions at this level.

To achieve public health objectives, it is sometimes useful to deal with intransigent problems at multiple levels. Although behavioral interventions administered at the individual level tend to produce successful weight loss in the short term, few people maintain their weight loss over the long term. In order for individual-based interventions to succeed on a population basis, such interventions should take place in a sociocultural environment that is conducive to healthful eating and exercise. Improving the availability of healthy food choices, providing economic incentives for healthy eating by selective taxation, ensuring through the schools that children and adolescents get adequate exercise, enhancing accessibility of physical activity for the general public by providing bicycle paths and highway lanes, and initiating mass media campaigns supporting a healthy lifestyle could be useful for maintaining weight loss.

The relatively recent successes in tobacco control in the United States provide a heartening example of how multilevel approaches to a major public health problem can lead to a decline in disease. In this case the improvements have occurred in coronary heart disease (CHD), some cancers including lung cancer, and respiratory diseases. At the interpersonal level, smoking cessation interventions, sometimes in conjunction with pharmacologic treatment, have been effective. At the organizational level, smoking cessation support groups, school campaigns against smoking, restrictions on smoking in restaurants and work sites, and reductions in health insurance premiums for nonsmokers have been instituted. Finally, at the societal level, laws against juvenile smoking, taxation of cigarettes, governmental restrictions on tobacco advertising, and government-sponsored antismoking campaigns have all been implemented. These measures have led to a marked reduction in cigarette smoking and a concomitant improvement in the nation's health. Unfortunately, the export of tobacco products to other countries remains a threat to improvements in global public health.

An important cornerstone of public health is prevention. Primary prevention refers to measures taken to reduce the incidence of disease. In the case of CHD, for example, people may be encouraged to quit smoking, decrease intake of dietary fat, and increase physical activity before diseases become evident. In contrast, secondary prevention involves reducing the prevalence of disease by shortening its duration and limiting adverse physiological and psychological effects. Screening programs are examples of secondary prevention strategies. Breast cancer and prostate cancer mortality are decreased by early detection of cancers when they are still treatable. Still another form of prevention is tertiary prevention. This involves reducing the complications associated with chronic diseases and minimizing disability and suffering. Medication adherence training in HIV/AIDS patients is a form of tertiary prevention.

The first half of the 20th century witnessed an unprecedented increase in longevity primarily in economically advanced countries. This decrease in mortality rate was largely due to a decline in infectious diseases related to vaccination, decreased exposure to infection because of improved hygiene, improved nutrition, and the development of antibiotics to cope with bacterial infections. As infectious diseases declined as the leading cause of mortality in economically advanced countries, they were eclipsed by chronic diseases. By the middle of the 20th century, CHD, cancer and stroke accounted for more than 60% of the death rate in the United States.

As scientists attempted to find specific causal agents in the pathogenesis of cancer and CHD throughout most of the 20th century, they became increasingly frustrated. Unable to find single causes of diseases, attention shifted to the role of environment and host in the pathogenesis of chronic diseases. Whereas single cause-and-effect models proved successful in studying the genesis of infectious diseases, an understanding of the basis of chronic diseases turned to probabilistic models based on the presence of risk factors. The identification of risk factors makes prediction of chronic diseases more likely, but individual risk factors cannot be identified as necessary and sufficient causes for many diseases. In this respect, interactions among agent, host, and the environment have now taken center stage.

At the beginning of the risk-factor revolution, it was widely believed that the causes of chronic diseases such as CHD could be explained in terms of a few biological (e.g., high cholesterol, high blood pressure) and lifestyle (e.g., smoking) risk factors. This turned out not to be the case. Other variables contributing to CHD turned out to include physical inactivity, excess consumption of alcohol, and obesity. Still other factors under investigation include individual difference variables such as depression and hostility and sociocultural variables including low socioeconomic status, ethnic minority status, lack of social support, and occupational stress.

At the turn of the 21st century the major causes of death in the United States included (1) heart disease (2) cancer (3) stroke (4) unintentional injuries (5) chronic obstructive pulmonary disorder (6) pneumonia and influenza (7) diabetes (8) suicide (9) liver disease (10) HIV/AIDS and (11) homicide. Behavioral, psychosocial, and sociocultural factors associated with lifestyle contribute to virtually all of these causes of mortality. Even in the case of an infectious disease such as pneumonia, risk factors can be related to disruptions of natural pulmonary host mechanisms related to lifestyle factors such as smoking and alcohol abuse. Similarly, infection from HIV is primarily spread through high-risk sexual practices and the sharing of contaminated drug paraphernalia.

In conclusion, public health efforts to eradicate infectious diseases led to an unprecedented increase in longevity in economically developed and even many less developed countries during the first half of the 20th century. Similarly, improvements in healthy lifestyle led to decreases in morbidity and increases in longevity in these countries during the second half of the 20th century. In contrast, the dissolution of the Soviet Union toward the end of the 20th century led to a precipitous drop of life expectancy in Russia and several other Eastern European countries. This has been related to increases in poverty, social disintegration, and environmental pollution superimposed on high rates of alcoholism and tobacco use. At the same time, the HIV/AIDS pandemic in sub-Saharan Africa has led to an even steeper decline in life expectancy. The growing spread of HIV/AIDS across the Asian continent is ominous. Widespread social disorganization and the growing disparity in income within and between nations also pose a global threat to public health. Because public health is a global matter that is closely tied to international policies, hope for future improvements in public health will largely depend on global improvements in public policy.

Related Entry: Prevention

BIBLIOGRAPHY

Centers for Disease Control and Prevention. (1999). Achievements in public health, 1900–1999; Changes in the public health system. *Morbidity and Mortality Weekly Report, 48,* 1141–1147.

Institute of Medicine. (2001). *Health and behavior: The interplay of biological, behavioral and societal influences.* Washington, DC: National Academy Press.

Institute of Medicine. (2001). *New horizons in health: An integrative approach.* Washington, DC: National Academy Press.

Ironson, G., Balbin, E., & Schneiderman, N. (2002). Health psychology and infectious diseases. In S. B. Johnson, N. W. Perry, Jr., and R. H. Rozensky (Eds.), *Handbook of clinical health psychology* (pp. 5–36). Washington, DC: American Psychological Association.

Kawachi, I. (1999). Social capital and community effects on population and individual health. *Annals of the New York Academy of Sciences, 896,* 120–130.

McKinlay, J. B., and McKinlay, S. M. (1977). The questionable contribution of medical measures to the decline of mortality in the United States in the twentieth century. *Milbank Memorial Fund Quarterly, 55,* 405–428.

Orth-Gomér, K., & Schneiderman, N. (Eds.). (1996). *Behavioral medicine approaches to cardiovascular disease prevention.* Mahwah, NJ: Erlbaum.

Smedley, B. D., and Syme, S. L. (Eds.). (2000). *Promoting health: Intervention strategies from social and behavioral research.* Washington, DC: National Academy Press.

World Health Organization. (2000). *The world health report 2000: Executive summary.* Geneva: Author.

NEIL SCHNEIDERMAN
MARC GELLMAN

Qq

Quality of Life

Health is probably the most valued human asset. In fact, studies on the preference for different states of being show that virtually everyone rates health as most important. Despite the perceived importance of health, health status has remained difficult to define. There are two common themes in definitions of health. First, premature death is undesirable, so one aspect of health is the avoidance of mortality. The health status of nations is often evaluated in terms of mortality rates or infant mortality rates (infant mortality is the number of children who die before 1 year of age per 1,000 live births).

Second, quality of life is also very important. Disease and disability are of concern because they affect either life expectancy or life quality. For example, cancer and heart disease are the two major causes of premature death in the United States. In addition, disease or disability can make life less desirable. A person with heart disease may face restrictions in daily living activities and may be unable to work or participate in social activities. Even relatively minor diseases and disabilities affect quality of life. A cold, for example, may interfere with the ability to concentrate, work, or attend school. A cold, however, lasts only a short time. A chronic disease, such as arthritis, may affect the quality of life for a long time

Within the recent years, medical scientists have come to realize the importance of quality-of-life measurement. Many major diseases, including arthritis, heart disease, and diabetes, and digestive problems are evaluated in terms of the degree to which they affect life quality and life expectancy. One can also evaluate treatments for these conditions by the amount of improvement they produce in quality of life. The Food and Drug Administration now considers quality-of-life data in their evaluations of new products, and nearly all major clinical trials in

medicine use quality-of-life assessment measures. Several approaches to quality-of-life measurement are reviewed in the following sections.

WHAT IS HEALTH-RELATED QUALITY OF LIFE?

There are numerous methods for the assessment of health-related quality of life. There is now an entire journal devoted to quality-of-life measurement, and several professional societies focus on the topic. Methods of assessment of health-related quality of life represent at least two different conceptual traditions. One grows out of the tradition of health status measurement. Several efforts to develop measures of health status were launched in the late 1960s and early 1970s. All the projects were guided by the World Health Organization's (WHO) definition of health status as a "complete state of physical, mental, and social well-being and not merely absence of disease" (WHO, 1948). The projects resulted in a variety of assessment tools, including the Sickness Impact Profile, the Quality of Well-Being Scale, the SF-36, and the Nottingham Health Profile. Many of the measures examine the effect of disease or disability on performance of social role, ability to interact in the community, and physical functioning. Some of the systems have separate components for the measurement of physical, social, and mental health. The measures also differ in the extent to which they consider subjective aspects of life quality.

Perhaps the most important distinction among methods used to assess quality of life is the contrast between psychometric and decision-theoretic approaches. The psychometric approach attempts to provide separate measures for the many different dimensions of quality of life. Perhaps the best-known example of the psychometric tradition is the Sickness Impact Profile (SIP). The SIP is a 136-item measure, and yields 12 different scores displayed in a format similar to a Minnesota Multiphasic Personality Inventory profile.

The decision-theoretic approach attempts to weight the different dimensions of health to provide a single expression of health status. Supporters of this approach argue that psychometric methods fail to consider that different health problems are not of equal concern. A runny nose is not the same as severe chest pain. In an experimental trial using the psychometric approach, one will often find that some aspects of quality of life improve while others get worse. For example, a medication might reduce high blood pressure but also produce headaches and impotence. Many argue that the quality-of-life notion is the subjective evaluation of observable or objective health states. The decision-theoretic approach attempts to provide an overall measure of quality of life that integrates subjective function states, preferences for these states, morbidity, and mortality.

COMMON METHODS FOR THE MEASUREMENT OF QUALITY OF LIFE

Various methods have been proposed to measure quality of life, but rather than attempt to review and critique them all here, this section presents some of the most widely used psychometric and decision-theory-based methods. Readers interested in more detailed reviews should consult Walker and Rosser (1993) and McDowell and Newell (1996).

Psychometric Methods
SF-36

Perhaps the most commonly used outcome measure is the Medical Outcome Study Short Form-36 (SF-36). The SF-36 grew out of work by the RAND Corporation and the Medical Outcomes Study (MOS). Originally, it was based on the measurement strategy from the RAND Health Insurance Study. The MOS attempted to develop a very short, 20-item instrument known as the Short Form-20, or SF-20. However, the SF-20 did not have appropriate reliability for some dimensions. The SF-36 includes eight health concepts: physical functioning, role-physical, bodily pain, general health perceptions, vitality, social functioning, role-emotional, and mental health The SF-36 can be either administered by a trained interviewer or self-administered. It has many advantages. For example, it is brief, and there is substantial evidence for its reliability and validity. The SF-36 can be machine scored and has been evaluated in large population studies.

Despite its many advantages, the SF-36 also presents some disadvantages. For example, it does not have age-specific questions, and one cannot clearly determine whether it is equally appropriate at each level of the age continuum. The items for older, retired individuals are the same as those for children. Nevertheless, the SF-36 has become the most commonly used behavioral measure in contemporary medicine.

Nottingham Health Profile

The Nottingham Health Profile (NHP) is another profile approach, and has been used widely in Europe. One of the important features of the NHP is that the items were originally generated on the basis of extensive discussions with patients. The NHP has two parts. The first includes 38 items divided into six categories: sleep, physical mobility, energy, pain, emotional reactions, and social isolation. Items within each of these sections are rated in terms of relative importance. Items are rescaled to allow them to vary between 0 and 100 within each section. The second part of the NHP includes seven statements related to the areas of life most affected by health: employment, household activities, social life, home life, sex life, hobbies and interests, and holidays. The respondent indicates whether a health condition has affected his or her life in these areas. Used in a substantial number of studies, the NHP has considerable evidence for its reliability and validity.

An important strength of the NHP is that it is based on consumer definitions of health derived from individuals in the community. The language in the NHP is simple, and the scale requires only a low level of reading ability. Psychometric properties of the NHP have been evaluated in a substantial number of studies. However, the NHP, like most profile measures, does not provide relative-importance weightings across dimensions. As a result, it is difficult to compare the dimensions directly with one another.

Decision-Theoretic Approaches

Within recent years, interest has grown in using quality-of-life data to help evaluate the cost/utility or cost-effectiveness of health-care programs. Cost studies have gained in popularity because health care costs have grown so rapidly in recent years. Not all health care interventions equally return benefit for the expended dollar. Objective cost studies might guide policymakers toward an optimal and equitable distribution of scarce resources. Cost-effectiveness analysis typically quantifies the benefits of a health care intervention in terms of years of life, or quality-adjusted life-years (QALYs). Cost/utility analysis is a special case of cost-effectiveness analysis, which weights observable health states by preferences or utility judgments of quality. In cost/utility analysis, the benefits of medical care, behavioral interventions, and preventive programs are expressed in terms years of life adjusted for reduced quality of life, or QALYs.

If a man dies of heart disease at age 50 years and he was expected to live to age 75 years, we might conclude that the disease was responsible for 25 lost life-years. If 100 men died at age 50 years, each of whom had a life expectancy of 75 years, we might conclude that 2,500 (100 men × 25 years) life-years had been lost. Yet death is not the only relevant outcome of heart disease. Many adults suffer myocardial infarctions, which can leave them somewhat disabled for a long time. Although they are still alive, they suffer diminished quality of life. The QALY measure takes into consideration such consequences. For example, a disease that reduces quality of life by one-half will take away 0.5 QALY over the course of each year. If the disease affects two people, it will take away 1 life-year (2 × 0.5) over each year. A medical treatment that improves quality of life by 0.2 for each of five individuals will result in the equivalent of 1 QALY if the benefit persists for 1 year. This system has the advantage of considering both benefits and side effects of programs in terms of common QALY units.

The need to integrate mortality and quality-of-life information is clearly apparent in studies of heart disease. Consider hypertension. People with high blood pressure may live shorter lives if untreated, and longer lives if treated. Thus, one benefit of treatment is to add years to life. However, for most patients, high blood pressure does not produce symptoms for many years. Conversely, the treatment for high blood pressure may cause negative side effects. If one evaluates a treatment only in terms of changes in life expectancy, the benefits of the program will be overestimated because one has not taken side effects into consideration. On the other hand, considering only current quality of life will underestimate the treatment benefits because information on mortality (death) is excluded. In fact, considering only current function might make the treatment look harmful because the side effects of the treatment might be worse than the symptoms of hypertension. A comprehensive measurement system takes into consideration side effects and benefits and provides an overall estimate of the benefit of treatment (Russell, 1986).

Most of the several different approaches for obtaining quality-adjusted life years are similar. The three most commonly used methods are the EQ-5D, the Health Utilities Index (HUI), and the Quality of Well-being Scale (QWB).

EQ-5D

The approach most commonly used in the European community is the EQ-5D. This method, developed by Paul Kind and associates, has been developed by a collaborative group from Western Europe known as the EuroQol group The intention of this effort was to develop a generic currency for health that could be used commonly across Europe. The concept of a common EuroQol was stimulated by the desire for a common European currency—the Eurodollar. The original version of the EuroQol had 14 health states in six different domains. Respondent health was placed on a continuum ranging from death (0.0) to perfect health (1.0). The method was validated in postal surveys in England, Sweden, and the Netherlands. More recent versions of the EuroQol, known as the EQ-5D, are now in use in a substantial number of clinical and population studies Although the EQ-5D is easy to use and comprehensive, there have been some problems with ceiling effects. Substantial numbers of people obtain the highest possible score.

Health Utilities Index

Another approach has been developed in Canada by Torrance, Feeny, Furlong, and associates. This method, known as the Health Utilities Index (HUI), is derived from microeconomic theory. There have been several versions of the measure, typically identified by "Mark" designations. The HUI Mark I was developed for studies in the neonatal intensive care unit. The measure had 960 unique health states. In 1992, the HUI Mark II was developed, and included 24,000 unique health states. The HUI Mark III, released in 1995, had 972,000 health states. The eight components of the HUI Mark III include vision (six levels), hearing (six levels), speech (five levels), ambulation (six levels), dexterity (six levels), emotion (five levels), cognition (six levels), and pain (five levels). Multiplying the number of levels across the eight dimensions gives the 972,000 states. Using multiattribute utility scaling methods, judges evaluate levels of wellness associated with each level of each domain. A multiattribute model is used to map preference for the 972,000 possible states onto the 0.0–1.0 continuum. The HUI has been used in many population and clinical studies. Figure 1 shows estimates of the HUI for men and women in the U.S. population. For overall health status, men obtain higher scores early in the life cycle. However, after about age 45 years, women obtain higher scores, and this difference grows systematically through the remainder of the life span.

Quality of Well-being Scale (QWB)

A third method, known as the Quality of Well-being Scale, integrates several components into a single score. First, patients are classified according to objective levels of functioning. These levels are represented by the scales of mobility, physical activity, and social activity. Once observable behavioral levels of functioning have been classified, each individual is placed on the 0–1.0 scale of wellness, which describes where a person lies on the continuum between optimum function and death.

Most traditional measures used in medicine and public health consider only whether a person is dead or alive. In other words, all living people get the same score. We know, however, that there are different levels of wellness, and there is a need to quantify these levels of wellness. To accomplish this, the observable health states are weighted by quality ratings for

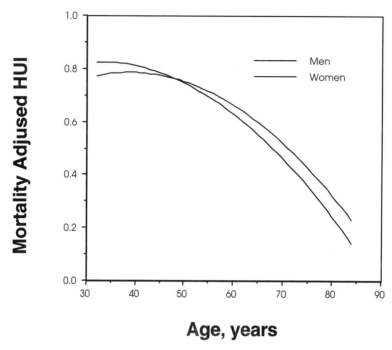

Figure 1. Difference between men and women for fitted Health Utilities Index (HUI).

the desirability of these conditions. Human value studies have been conducted to place the observable states onto a preference continuum, with an anchor of 0 for death and 1.0 for completely well. Studies have shown that the weights are highly stable over a 1-year period and that they are consistent across diverse groups of raters. Finally, one must consider the duration of stay in various health states. Having a cough or a headache for 1 day is not the same as having the problem for 1 year. A health measure must take these durations into consideration. Using this information, one can describe health-related quality of life in terms similar to years of life. For example, one year in a state assigned the weight of 0.5 is equivalent to 0.5 of a QALY.

The QWB combines preference-weighted values for symptoms and functioning. The preference weights were obtained by ratings of 856 people from the general population. These judges rated the desirability of health conditions in order to place each on the continuum between death (0.00) and optimum health (1.00). Symptoms are assessed by questions that ask about the presence or absence of different symptoms complexes. Functioning is assessed by a series of questions designed to record functional limitations over the previous 6 days, within three separate domains (mobility, physical activity, and social activity). The three domain scores are combined into a total score that provides a numerical point-in-time expression of well-being that ranges from zero (0) for death to one (1.0) for asymptomatic optimum functioning.

Disease-Specific Measures

This entry has focused on generic quality-of-life scales. However, there are a significantly larger number of disease-specific measures. Validated measures of health-related quality of life are available for illnesses such as arthritis, diabetes, heart disease, and kidney failure, and virtually every other major health condition. Two examples are the Arthritis Impact Measurement Scale and the UCSD Shortness of Breath Questionnaire, which is used in studies of patients with emphysema.

The Arthritis Impact Measurement Scales (AIMS) is a health index designed at the Multi-purpose Arthritis Center at Boston University. It is intended to measure physical health and social well-being for patients with rheumatoid arthritis. The resultant scale includes 67 items, with questions about functioning, health perceptions, morbidity, and demographics. The AIMS contains scales for mobility, physical activity, social activity, activities of daily living, depression and anxiety, and arthritis-related symptoms. In effect, it is an adaptation of an early version of the QWB with a series of items designed to tap more specifically the effect of arthritis on functioning and the quality of life. Factor analysis of the AIMS has produced three subscales: physical function, psychological function, and pain. Most current applications of the AIMS use composite scores for these three areas.

The University of California, San Diego Shortness of Breath Questionnaire (SOBQ) includes 25 items, which evaluate self-reported shortness of breath during the performance of various activities of daily living. Evaluations of the measure show it to be highly correlated with other quality-of-life measures such as the Quality of Well-Being Scale and the Center for Epidemiologic Studies Depression Scale. The measure has high internal consistency (alpha = 0.96) and is significantly correlated with performance measures such as the amount of distance that can be walked in 6 minutes.

SUMMARY

Assessment of health-related quality of life has become a standard component of health outcome evaluation. There are several important distinctions among commonly used approaches. Generic measures are used to evaluate health outcome for any illness or disease state. Generic measures can typically be classified as derived from psychometric or decision theory. Psychometric approaches include the Sickness Impact Profile, the SF-36, and the Nottingham Health Profile. Decision-theoretic approaches are used to estimate outcomes in terms of quality-adjusted life years. Methods used for this purpose include the EQ-5D, the HUI, and the QWB. Disease-specific measures are available for a wide variety of health conditions. Although disease-specific measures may be more sensitive for outcomes of a particular condition, they cannot be used for cross-illness comparisons or for cost-effectiveness analysis. Assessment of health-related quality of life is a rapidly developing field, and major new developments can be anticipated over the next decade.

BIBLIOGRAPHY

Bergner, M., Bobbitt, R. A., Carter, W. B., & Gilson, B. S. (1981). The Sickness Impact Profile: Development and final revision of the health status measure. *Medical Care, 19*, 787–805.

Brown, M., Gordon, W. A., & Haddad, L. (2000). Models for predicting subjective quality of life in individuals with traumatic brain injury. *Brain Injury, 14*, 5–19.

Feeny, D., Furlong, W., Mulhern, R. K., Barr, R. D., & Hudson, M. (1999). A framework for assessing health-related quality of life among children with cancer. *International Journal of Cancer, 12* (9 Supplement), 2–9.

Kaplan, R. M. (1996). Measuring health outcomes for resource allocation. In R. L. Glueckauf, R. G. Frank, et al. (Eds.), *Psychological practice in a changing healthcare system: Issues and new directions* (pp. 101–133). New York: Springer.

Kind, P. (1997). The performance characteristics of EQ-5D, a measure of health related quality of life for use in technology assessment [Abstract]. In *Annual meeting of International Society of Technology Assessment in Health Care* (Vol. 13, p. 81).

Koloski, N. A., Talley, N. J., & Boyce, P. M. (2000). The impact of functional gastrointestinal disorders on quality of life. *American Journal of Gastroenterology, 95*, 67–71.

Lowe, D., O'Grady, J. G., McEwen, J., & Williams, R. (1990). Comparisons of five health status instruments for orthopedic evaluation. *Medical Care, 28*, 632–642.

McDowell, I., & Newell, C. (1996). *Measuring health: A guide to rating scales and questionnaires* (2nd ed.), New York: Oxford University Press.

Walker, S. R., & Rosser, R. (1993). *Quality of life assessment: Key issues in the 1990s.* Dordrecht: Kluwer.

Ware, J. E., Jr., & Gandeck, B. (1998). Overview of the SF-36 Health Survey and the International Quality of Life Assessment (IQOLA) Project. *Journal of Clinical Epidemiology, 51*, 903–912.

World Health Organization. (1948). *Constitution of the World Health Organization.* Basic documents. Geneva: Author.

ROBERT M. KAPLAN

Rr

Reactance Theory

The theory of psychological reactance assumes that people believe themselves to have specific behavioral freedoms. For example, having beef for dinner, taking photos of one's child, and riding a bicycle to school or work could all be behavioral freedoms. The theory specifies that each behavioral freedom has a certain amount of importance to the individual, largely depending on what needs are satisfied by the particular freedom. The freedom to be a vegetarian, for example, could be much more important to a given person than the freedom to chew gum. These freedoms can be threatened or eliminated in many ways, and when they are, the theory asserts that psychological reactance will occur. Reactance is defined as an urge (motivation) to restore any freedom that has been threatened or taken away. In addition to this urge, reactance theory says that the behavior that is threatened or taken away will become more attractive to the individual. Thus, a threat to the freedom to engage in a particular behavior will result in attempts to engage in the threatened behavior as well as increased attractiveness of the behavior.

The magnitude of reactance increases as (1) the number of current freedoms threatened increases, (2) the proportion of current freedoms threatened increases, and (3) other freedoms are threatened by implication. The most likely implication is that the same freedom will be threatened on future occasions, but threat by implication also occurs when, for example, a person is advised to stop getting exposure to the sun without sunscreen, which carries the implication that one may also have to stop sunbathing even with sunscreen.

When a person must decide between important alternatives such as when making a career decision, recommendations from others can threaten or eliminate that person's freedom of choice. For example, even unsolicited advice from a person of equal status such as one's friend can easily create reactance and result in a tendency to reject the advice, no matter how good it is.

Specifically in the health arena, advice or even orders from a physician can threaten free behaviors having to do with health and thereby create resistance and motivation to preserve personal freedoms. Even relatively simple instructions, such as those to take specific medications daily, to exercise, or to avoid unhealthy foods, can create reactance, especially when they interfere with long-term habits. Reactance to advice from a physician or a therapist may take different forms, from verbal opposition to recommendations, to disengagement and premature termination of the treatment.

In addition to the investigation of situational factors that may create reactance in medical settings, research has also examined medical noncompliance as a function of individual differences in client reactance, and scales have been developed to assist in identifying appropriate treatments. Research has revealed that directive interventions worked best among patients with low levels of trait-like reactance, whereas nondirective and paradoxical interventions were found to work best with highly reactant patients.

BIBLIOGRAPHY

Beutler, L. E., Moleiro, C., & Talebi, H. (2002). Resistance to psychotherapy: What conclusions are supported by research. *Journal of Clinical Psychology, 58*, 207–217.

Brehm, J. W. (1966). *A theory of psychological reactance.* New York: Academic.

Brehm, S. S., & Brehm, J. W. (1981). *Psychological reactance: A theory of freedom and control.* New York: Academic.

Buboltz, W. C, Thomas, A., & Donnell, A. (2002). Evaluating the factor structure and internal reliability of the Therapeutic Reactance Scale. *Journal of Counseling and Development, 80*, 120–125.

Dowd, E. T., Milne, C. R., & Wise, S. L. (1991). The therapeutic reactance scale: A measure of psychological reactance. *Journal of Counseling and Development, 69,* 541–545.

Fogarty, J. S. (1997). Reactance theory and patient noncompliance. *Social Science and Medicine, 45,* 1277–1288.

Graybar, S. R., Antonuccion, D. O., Boutilier, L. R., & Varble, D. L. (1989). Psychological reactance as a factor affecting patient compliance to physician advice. *Scandinavian Journal of Behavior Therapy, 18,* 43–51.

Hong, S. M., & Page, S. (1989). A psychological reactance scale: Development, factor structure and reliability, *Psychological Reports, 64,* 1323–1326.

Horvath, A. V., & Goheen, M. D. (1990). Factors mediating the success of defiance- and compliance-based interventions. *Journal of Counseling Psychology, 37,* 363–371.

Seibel, C. A., & Dowd, E. T. (1999). Reactance and therapeutic noncompliance. *Cognitive Therapy and Research, 23,* 373–379.

Tennen, H., Press, S., Rohrbaugh, M., & White, L. (1981). Reactance theory and therapeutic paradox: A compliance–defiance model. *Psychotherapy, 18,* 14–22.

JACK W. BREHM
ANCA MIRON

Reactivity Hypothesis

CARDIOVASCULAR REACTIVITY TO LABORATORY AND REAL-LIFE CHALLENGES

Although homeostasis is a common characteristic of the underlying physiology of humans and most other life forms, our regulatory systems possess the adaptive capacity to mount relatively dramatic temporary changes to respond to and even anticipate challenges. For the cardiovascular system, some challenges are as simple and routine as changing from supine to standing posture. Others involve dealing with complex interpersonal interactions based on prior learning and experience, like job interviews or driving a car in heavy traffic. The regulatory systems that allow transitory increases in blood pressure, heart rate, cardiac output, and/or vasoconstriction include efferent activity via sympathetic and parasympathetic nerves to the heart and blood vessels; adrenocortical and adrenomedullary hormones such as epinephrine, norepinephrine, and cortisol; neuropeptides such as oxytocin, vasopressin, and atrial natriuretic peptide; and other substances with endocrine activity. The hypothalamus plays a major role in the integration of cardiovascular responses and thus is always part of the initiation, maintenance, and posttask recovery of cardiovascular responses to behavioral events.

Historically, the best-recognized pattern of cardiovascular responses has been labeled the defense reaction, an increase in heart rate and blood pressure and a decrease in vasoconstriction seen in cats during hypothalamic stimulation that also engaged motor responses mimicking those occurring when the animal was faced with a predator. Also described as the fight-or-flight

response, the hemodynamic adjustments were adaptively designed to mobilize the cardiovascular system to provide extra oxygenated blood flow to working muscles before and during vigorous activity. In modern industrialized societies, however, the remnants of this response pattern (minus much of the dilation of blood vessels) are frequently evoked during cognitive and emotional stressors where physical activity does not increase. Then the mobilization increases cardiac work and stresses the vasculature with no apparent benefit.

The primary interest in human research on cardiovascular reactivity is actually on the study of individual differences. Who is a high reactor to this challenge and who is a low reactor? Can we use the magnitude of reactivity or change in physiological response to reveal an underlying response that is excessively great or small, and therefore indicates dysregulation in a key physiological system? Can we show that someone who is a high reactor to one challenge will be a high reactor to others, and will high or low responses to laboratory stressors reflect the relative responses to natural life demands?

The classic reactivity hypothesis in its most general form posits that individuals who are high reactors to behavioral challenges or stressors will over time be more likely to develop elevated blood pressure and hypertensive heart disease (characterized by left ventricular remodeling and hypertrophy) and/or coronary heart disease (characterized by stenosis in coronary vessels, which can lead to myocardial infarction). High stress response may be simply a marker of increased cardiovascular risk, or it may play a more direct role. In the latter case, it is suggested that transitory episodes of elevated adrenergic and cardiovascular activity, if evoked on a frequent basis by stressors in an individual's environment at home or work, may eventually induce secondary changes leading to resetting of homeostatic mechanisms to a higher level of blood pressure (BP) maintained even in the resting state, and to structural changes in the heart and vessels.

The reactivity hypothesis has generated considerable research and much debate since the 1970s. High heart rate, blood pressure, cardiac output, and vascular resistance responses to stressors have been shown to be relatively stable characteristics of certain individual across challenges and over time intervals from a few months to as long as 10 years. Several longitudinal studies have confirmed the expected association between high cardiovascular response to stressors and higher incidence of hypertension, but others have found this relationship to be modest or absent after partialing out higher resting BP, which is associated with both high stress response and later hypertension. In two recent prospective studies, high pressor response to active coping tasks predicted increased BP after 5 and 6.5 years of follow-up in men but not women, and showed stronger relationships in persons of lower than of higher socioeconomic status (SES). This may be related to the fact that women have a low incidence of hypertension prior to the age of menopause, perhaps due to protective effects of reproductive hormones, and to the likelihood that lower-SES persons are exposed to greater economic and social stress.

Updated variations of the reactivity hypothesis differ from the original in several respects, but are likely to yield stronger predictive relationships to cardiovascular disease outcomes. First, using BP reactivity scores in a simple linear regression model to predict subsequent BP or hypertension seems much less powerful than comparing individuals in the highest quartile (top 25%) versus the lower three quartiles of reactivity. That is, there appears to be a threshold effect rather than a continuous increment of risk. Second, one recent 10-year follow-up study demonstrated that high stress responses were much more predictive of later hypertension among those with genetic susceptibility, defined as one or more hypertensive parents, and risk was further enhanced in those reporting greater daily life stress exposure. Thus, it is recommended that future tests of the reactivity hypothesis should be specifically designed to examine interactions between extreme versus lesser cardiovascular responsivity and family history of hypertension or other indexes of enhanced genetic or environmental susceptibility.

Related Entry: Coronary Heart Disease

BIBLIOGRAPHY

Carroll, D., Smith, G. D., Shipley, M. J., Steptoe, A., Brunner, E. J., & Marmot, M. G. (2001). Blood pressure reactions to acute psychological stress and future blood pressure status. *Psychosomatic Medicine, 63*, 737–743.

Everson, S. A., Kaplan, G. A., Goldberg, D. A., & Salonnen, J. T. (1996). Anticipatory blood pressure response to exercise predicts future high blood pressure status. *Hypertension, 27*, 1059–1064.

Kasagi, F., Akahoshi, M., & Shimaoki, K. (1995). Relation between cold pressor test and development of hypertension based on 28-year follow-up. *Hypertension, 25*, 71–76.

Light, K. C. (2001). Hypertension and the reactivity hypothesis: The next generation. *Psychosomatic Medicine, 63*, 744–746.

Light, K. C., Girdler, S. S., Sherwood, A., Bragdon, E. E., Brownley, K. A., West, S. G., et al. (1999). High stress responsivity predicts later blood pressure only in combination with positive family history and high life stress. *Hypertension, 33*, 1458–1464.

Markovitz, J. H., Raczynski, J. M., Wallace, D., Chettur, V., & Chesney, M. A. (1998). Cardiovascular reactivity to video game predicts subsequent blood pressure increases in young men: The CARDIA Study. *Psychosomatic Medicine, 60*, 186–191.

Matthews, K. A., Woodall, K. L., & Allen, M. T. (1993). Cardiovascular reactivity to stress predicts future blood pressure status. *Hypertension, 22*, 479–485.

Menkes, M. S., Matthews, K. A., Krantz, D. D., Lundberg, V., Mead, L. A., Qaqish, B., et al. (1989). Cardiovascular reactivity to the cold pressor as a predictor of hypertension. *Hypertension, 14*, 524–530.

Sherwood, A., Girdler S. S., Bragdon, E. E., West, S. G., Brownley, K. A., Hinderliter, A. L., et al. (1997). Ten-year stability of cardiovascular responses to laboratory stressors. *Psychophysiology, 34*, 185–191.

KATHLEEN C. LIGHT

Rehabilitation Psychology

Due to the increased awareness of the important influences of emotional and behavioral factors on health and illness, the last two decades have seen a substantial increase in the number of psychologists working in medical settings. Although most are employed in departments of psychiatry, psychologists have also become valuable members of other medical specialties including pediatrics, geriatrics, primary care, family medicine, anesthesiology/pain, and rehabilitation. In fact, over the last decade, the field of rehabilitation has been hailed as perhaps the greatest opportunity for psychologists to make unique contributions in the lives of health care patients (Frank, Gluck, & Buckelew, 1990). Rehabilitation psychology is a specialized discipline within the broad domain of clinical health psychology, and focuses on researching and providing clinical services to a broad group of health care patients to facilitate their adjustment to, coping with, and recovering from illness or injury. The American Medical Association (2002) generally defines impairment as the loss of, or loss of use of, a body part or system due to an injury or illness. Whereas impairment is solely a medical description of loss, disability is defined as a limitation or loss of one's ability to meet personal, social, or occupational demands due to one's illness or injury. Thus, disability is defined in terms of the functional impact of one's impairment, and a person may have a physical impairment, but no corresponding functional disability. Finally, the AMA defines an individual as having a handicap if their impairment substantially limits their involvement with work, social, or leisure activities. As such, a handicap is generally interpreted as a barrier or obstacle to certain functional activities. The goal of rehabilitation psychology is to assist individuals in increasing their ability to function independently and to minimize any disability or handicap associated with a medical impairment. Rehabilitation psychology services may address issues in any or all of the physical, cognitive/affective, and social domains to improve quality of life.

TRAINING

Rehabilitation psychologists typically complete doctoral-level training in clinical psychology programs that offer specialized coursework, practica, and predoctoral internships in health care facilities. After graduation, postdoctoral fellowship programs can provide additional specialized training, often directly in a rehabilitation environment. For practicing professionals, a variety of professional organizations, conferences, journals, books, and websites offer access to rehabilitation information and continuing educational training. The American Board of Professional Psychology (ABPP) recognizes rehabilitation psychology as a specialized area of psychological practice for certification. The American Psychological Association (APA) contains a specialized division for rehabilitation psychology, and this division's website provides an important resource for information sharing and professional interaction among rehabilitation psychologists.

SCOPE OF PRACTICE

Rehabilitation psychologists are employed in a variety of work settings including university medical schools, public and private hospitals, community-based rehabilitation centers that specialize in treatment for a specific rehabilitation population (e.g., brain injury or spinal cord injury), nursing homes, assisted-living facilities, and specialized private practices. Fewer than 5% of psychologists working in U.S. medical schools are specifically employed in rehabilitation medicine departments (APA, 1998), but instead provide services in the variety of work settings listed.

The process of rehabilitation is widely referred to as multidisciplinary in nature, and interventions are most often team based rather than being provided by a single person. Persons served are empowered to actively contribute to treatment goal setting and ongoing care decisions with their health care providers, and many professional specialties contribute their expertise toward achieving these goals. Rehabilitation psychologists are members of treatment teams that include physicians, nurses, physical and occupational therapists, speech language pathologists, and recreational therapists. Additionally, other mental health professionals including psychiatrists, social workers, neuropsychologists, specialized clinical health psychologists (i.e., pain management, biofeedback), and school psychologists may also contribute to the assessments, goal setting, and treatments of rehabilitation patients. Outside of the immediate medical environment, rehabilitation psychologist's work may have far-reaching impact as they interact with schools, employers, state/federal agencies, correctional facilities, or courts regarding the various aspects of physical and emotional rehabilitation.

Surveys of practicing rehabilitation psychologists suggest that they spend the majority of their professional time providing clinical care or conducting research on health, cognitive, or emotion issues. Other duties include consulting with health or community services, teaching psychologists and physicians in training, contributing to program development, or consulting on the development of public policies addressing rehabilitation and public reintegration of people with certain disabilities or handicaps.

CLINICAL CHALLENGES

As the field of rehabilitation medicine provides treatment to people with specialized injuries or illnesses, rehabilitation psychologists provide clinical services to individuals coping with limb loss, brain injury, spinal cord injury, burn injuries, neurological diseases (e.g., multiple sclerosis), sports medicine or athletic injuries, persistent pain problems, and mobility challenges (e.g., those using wheel chairs, walkers, or artificial limbs for movement). Rehabilitation psychologists serve people of all ages, ethnicities, and cultures, and interventions commonly involve both the patient and family members. In certain instances, members of the treatment team may be trained in specific behavioral or psychosocial interventions to promote improved patient functioning, and specific family members may receive training to provide care at home. The wide-ranging clinical assessment and treatment challenges addressed by rehabilitation psychologists are well described in several recently published books (Cushman & Scherer, 1995; Frank & Elliott, 2000; Radnitz, 2000).

DESIRABLE SKILLS FOR REHABILITATION PSYCHOLOGISTS

Whereas rehabilitation psychologists need to be competent in the professional skills of most practicing psychologists (i.e., psychological interviewing, testing, and psychotherapy), it is the specialized application of these skills to the unique rehabilitation populations that demands enhanced skill training for these practitioners. Rehabilitation psychologists rarely work in isolation from other multidisciplinary team members, and must be skilled in medical team consultation regarding cognitive or emotional issues, and capable of coordinating psychosocial assessment and treatment schemes within the context of a broad-based rehabilitative plan.

Rehabilitation psychologists employ psychological testing in several areas to assess patient's cognitive functioning (e.g., mental status, intelligence, memory, learning, problem solving), emotional functioning (e.g., depression, anxiety, anger, personality issues, readiness for change, locus of control, self-efficacy, motivation, health-related beliefs and attitudes), and ability to cope with illness or injury (e.g., cognitive coping skills, active or passive coping, perceived control, confidence in one's coping ability, social support). The typical goal of psychological testing in rehabilitation is to determine the extent to which emotional, behavioral, cognitive, or attitudinal factors may influence or interfere with an individual's recovery from illness or injury. For example, results of cognitive testing (typically conducted by a neuropsychologist) can be used to estimate or predict a person's ability to independently and safely perform activities in his or her home environment including self-care, child care, driving, managing money, self-administering medications, performing wound care, or understanding and consistently following health recommendations.

Rehabilitation psychology therapy is intended to enhance a person's understanding of his or her illness or injury, and to determine the individual and family's readiness to begin making adjustments to any physical, cognitive, behavioral, or emotional changes they have encountered. Rehabilitation therapy must be individualized in all cases because people adjust to, cope with, and accept change in many different ways and at different paces. For some, psychological adjustment may be rapid and there may be few struggles after weeks. However for others, it may take months or years of psychological assistance to gain even partial acceptance of changes brought about by illness or injury. Instructing patients and family members in any of several behavioral or cognitive coping skills, and allowing them to gain confidence in their ability to perform these skills, can facilitate personal adjustment. Specific skills taught in rehabilitative therapy might include ways to manage emotional extremes (e.g., depression, anxiety, or anger) or other important psychosocial issues such as self-esteem, body image, grief and loss, or pain and stress management exercises. Furthermore, assisting individuals and families in making cognitive changes, forming realistic expectations for recovery, or challenging unhealthy beliefs and attitudes about the patient after injury may aid recovery.

Rehabilitation psychologists are often involved in preparing people to undergo invasive medical tests or procedures (e.g., magnetic resonance imaging, injections, surgeries) by providing information and instructing in relaxation, imagery, and cognitive distraction skills (Deardorff & Reeves, 1997). Rehabilitation psychologists encourage patients to adopt healthy lifestyle practices including following healthy diets, increasing exercise, improving sleep patterns, consistently following treatment recommendations, and decreasing tobacco, alcohol, or drug use. The ultimate evaluation of the benefit of rehabilitation psychology therapies may include improved emotional functioning and either independent or modified reintegration of the person into his or her pre-injury or illness family roles and work, school, and leisure activities. All efforts in rehabilitation are aimed at improved quality of life for the person with illness or injury-related impairment. The value of providing psychological support to patients with physical and emotional disorders has been well established from both treatment efficacy and cost-saving perspectives (Friedman et al., 1995).

In summary, the impact of emotional, cognitive, and behavioral influences on recovery from illness or injury is being increasingly recognized in medical care. Rehabilitation psychologists play an important role in assisting persons with illness or injury to successfully return to their home, work, family, and leisure environments. The activities of rehabilitation psychologists encompass many settings, populations, and multidisciplinary treatment partners, and may have far-reaching effects in clinical, teaching, research, and program and public policy development areas.

Related Entries: Clinical Psychology, Neuropsychology

BIBLIOGRAPHY

American Medical Association. (2002). *Guides to the evaluation of permanent impairment* (5th ed.). Chicago: AMA Press.

American Psychological Association. (1998). *1997 Employment characteristics and salaries of medical school psychologists.* Washington, DC: Author.

American Psychological Association, Division 22, Rehabilitation Psychology. Available at www.apa.org/divisions/div22

Cushman, L. A., & Scherer, M. J. (Eds.). (1995). *Psychological assessment in medical rehabilitation.* Washington, DC: American Psychological Association.

Deardorff, W. W., & Reeves, J. L. (1997). *Preparing for surgery: A mind–body approach to enhance healing and recovery.* Oakland, CA: New Harbinger.

Frank, R. G., & Elliott, T. R. (Eds.). (2000). *Handbook of rehabilitation psychology.* Washington, DC: American Psychological Association.

Frank, R. G., Gluck, J. P., & Buckelew, S. P. (1990). Rehabilitation: Psychology's greatest opportunity? *American Psychologist, 45,* 757–761.

Friedman, R., Sobel, D., Myers, P., Caudill, M., & Benson, H. (1995). Behavioral medicine, clinical health psychology, and cost offset. *Health Psychology, 14,* 509–518.

Radnitz, C. L. (Ed.). (2000). *Cognitive–behavioral therapy for persons with disabilities.* Northvale, NJ: Aronson.

BRENT VAN DORSTEN

Relapse

Relapse is the lack of maintenance of behavior change. In relation to drug use, the term refers to a return to drug-using behaviors after a period of nonuse or harm-reduced use. Because addiction to drugs is a chronic disease, there is a tendency toward relapse. The binary model of relapse posits that one instance of nonadherence to behavior change results in relapse. The process model of relapse posits that lapses in behavior change are a part of the essential components of recovery. Biological (e.g., hereditary influences), behavioral (e.g., learned behavior), personality (e.g., personality traits), cognitive (e.g., cognition), and environmental factors (e.g., family and social networks) have been shown to relate to relapse. One illustration of relapse can be grounded using the relapse component of the transtheoretical model, also known as stages of change, which posits that individuals may spiral back in their behavior change as they attempt to modulate drug-using behaviors. In this view, persons experience or return to previous affect, behavior, and cognition as related to their initial phase of the behavior. For example, a person who relapses into drinking behavior after having terminated the behavior for a period of time may be viewed as spiraling back along the continuum of change, which may lead to the ultimate termination of the drinking behavior.

Related Entry: Relapse Prevention

BIBLIOGRAPHY

National Institute on Drug Abuse. (1999). *Principles of drug addiction treatment.* Bethesda, MD: Author.

National Institute on Drug Abuse. (2000). *Approaches to drug abuse counseling.* Bethesda, MD: Author.

Prochaska, J. O., & DiClemente, C. C. (1984). *Transtheoretical approach: Crossing traditional boundaries.* Homewood, IL: Dow Jones–Irwin.

Tims, F. M., Leukefeld, C. G., & Platt, J. J. (Eds.). (2002). *Relapse and recovery in addictions.* New Haven, CT: Yale University Press.

Perry N. Halkitis
Leo Wilton

Relapse Prevention

Mark Twain has been quoted as saying, "Quitting smoking is easy. I've done it hundreds of times." This quote provides an illustrative example of the common outcome of attempts at behavior change: People tend to be unsuccessful. The phenomenon of relapse, or the return to previous maladaptive behaviors after a period of positive behavior change, is the most common outcome for individuals attempting to modify health habits, including dieting, smoking, drinking, and drug use. For the last 30 years researchers and clinicians have attempted to describe, predict, and prevent relapse, with limited success.

The most successful model of the relapse process is based on cognitive–behavioral theory. It is believed that health habits are learned behaviors and changing a health habit requires a relearning process, in which initial setbacks (or lapses) should be expected. Marlatt and colleagues have developed a cognitive behavioral model, which emphasizes the importance of an individual's response during high-risk situations. A high-risk situation is defined as any situation that poses a threat to an individual's ability to maintain the positive behavior change. To provide an analogy, consider the process of learning to ride a bicycle. Initially, riding a bicycle is difficult, and imbalance is common. A small rock in the road or a distracting sound will often cause the novice bicyclist to lose balance and fall from the bicycle. The small rock or distracting sound could be defined as a high-risk situation. In the area of substance abuse, drug cues, social pressure to use, and stressful life events are examples of common high-risk situations.

Relapse prevention (RP) is a psychological treatment designed to identify a client's unique profile of high-risk situations for relapse. Once problematic situations are identified, RP teaches clients coping strategies to recognize warning signs and then plan for more effective responses to high-risk situations. In addition to teaching effective coping responses, a major component of RP is the enhancement of self-efficacy. Self-efficacy is defined as the extent to which an individual feels capable of performing a specific task. Higher levels of self-efficacy are predictive of improved ability to maintain positive behavior change in the face of high-risk situations. One should encourage clients to remember the words of the little engine that could, "I think I can, I think I can..."

As in most cognitive–behavioral treatments, RP incorporates psychoeducation techniques to correct misperceptions, such as myths related to positive outcome expectancies. A positive outcome expectancy is the glorification of previous health habits, such as drug use, by focusing on positive consequences of use (e.g., euphoria and relaxation), while ignoring the more negative consequences of the experience (e.g., legal and health problems).

The experience of a relapse is often an inevitable problem encountered during the change process. Using RP skills, clients are encouraged to use relapses as learning experiences to get back on track toward positive behavior change. RP has been shown to be an effective adjunct to psychological treatment for a variety of psychological disorders and as a stand-alone treatment for substance use disorders.

Related Entries: Addiction, Alcoholism, Smoking Cessation, Transtheoretical Model

G. Alan Marlatt
Katie Witkiewitz

Relaxation Response

Despite inconsistencies and ambiguities associated with the concepts of stress and coping, the popular press regularly discusses the ill effects of stress on physical and psychological well-being and a variety of behavioral antidotes, including aroma therapy, biofeedback, and meditation. Although the possible adverse effects of stress have been noted for thousands of years, the scientific study of stress and coping did not burgeon until after World War II. Indeed, a body of research suggests that the technological developments of our modern life are a double-edged sword. One one hand, technological and industrial advances (e.g., improved sanitation, housing, and medical care) reduced infectious diseases and trauma, the chief causes of death prior to 1900; on the other hand, other developments fostered diseases of lifestyle (e.g., heart disease, high blood pressure, diabetes, and some cancers) associated with the transition from a hunter–gatherer society to our modern Western age of industrialization and technology. Unhealthy aspects of the Western lifestyle include poor nutrition, pollution, lack of exercise, increased substance abuse, loss of social support from an extended family and community, and a chronic sense of "hurry–worry" triggered by the demands of a fast-paced society. That is, the disease-producing features of our modern ways appear linked to behavioral and psychological processes that are discordant with the Stone Age biology we inherited during the evolution of our species.

In the 1970s, a cardiologist affiliated with Harvard Medical School, Dr. Herbert Benson, synthesized scientific evidence with ancient Eastern and Western writings in the formulation of an innate human ability he termed the relaxation response. The relaxation response is innate in that it is grounded in our evolution. Since this time, Benson has published research and written extensively on the daily use of the relaxation response as a component of a lifestyle designed to counter the unhealthy aspects of modern life.

Following a brief introduction to the structure of the nervous system, this entry discusses the fight-or-flight response and the relaxation response, and compares the two. The elicitation the relaxation response is then described, including a simple method to use. Other methods that can elicit the relaxation response and evidence of their salubrious effects are also presented. The entry closes with future directions and implications.

STRESS, RESTORATION, AND THE NERVOUS SYSTEM

The central nervous system (CNS) is composed of the brain and the spinal cord, both encased in bone. Many unconscious and voluntary bodily responses are regulated by the CNS; this regulation is based on information, emanating from both inside and outside the body, transmitted to and from the CNS via peripheral nerves not encased in bone (namely, the peripheral nervous system, PNS). A subdivision of the PNS, namely, the autonomic nervous system (ANS), contains nerve fibers designed to regulate internal organs and glands for the purpose of homeostasis, an internal physiological balance conducive to the maintenance of life. Hence, the ANS is constantly working at striking a balance between energy conservation (rest and restoration) and energy expenditure (physiological adaptations for exercise, and attack or defensive maneuvers). Rest and restoration are the domain of the parasympathetic nervous system (PSNS) and are linked to the relaxation response, whereas adaptation to states of physical exertion, threat, and emergency are the domain of the sympathetic nervous system (SNS), which is linked to the fight-or-flight response. The brain's registering of threatening or crisis situations triggers the SNS and reduces PSNS activity, and sets in motion a cascade of events inducing the release of stress hormones (bodily created substances released into the bloodstream for regulation of the body's responses).

Table 1. Comparison of the Relaxation Response with the Fight-or-Flight Response

Response	Relaxation response	Fight-or-flight response
Felt distress and arousal	Decreased	Increased
Felt calmness and relaxation	Increased	Decreased
Muscle tension	Decreased	Increased
Metabolism	Decreased	Increased
Blood flow to large muscles of upper and lower body	Stable	Increased
Heart rate and blood pressure	Decreased	Increased
Respiration rate	Decreased	Increased
Slow brain waves (alpha)	Increased	Decreased

A COMPARISON OF TWO INNATE RESPONSES

Table 1, based on Benson's conceptualization, shows the physiological differences between the fight-or-flight response and the relaxation response. Because the fight-or-flight response is for adaptation to threat, blood flow is channeled to the brain, heart, and muscles of the legs and arms and away from the viscera and skin (hence, one has cold hands when stressed). Activation of the SNS, release of stress hormones, and increased respiration and cardiovascular system activity move oxygen and nutrients liberated from bodily stores to large muscles and the brain; this response is quickly activated for a vigilant mental state and the behavioral and affective responses of fighting or fleeing. These physiological reactions mark an increase in metabolism induced by environmental exigencies (e.g., jogging or being attacked by a bear); metabolism basically is the process whereby oxygen is consumed or burned for the generation of energy necessary for the body's functioning. Although this Stone Age response system is metabolically appropriate for running from or fighting a bear, it represents a set of responses in excess of metabolic demand for many modern stressors (i.e., events or objects, whether actual or imagined, that trigger stress). In contrast to the stressors of hunting or defending against attacking animals, our modern stressors are mostly symbolic in nature (e.g., reacting to a playful joke as an injurious insult). It is thought that a frequent or chronic triggering of the fight-or-flight response across life can contribute to bodily changes that pose a risk for such diseases as coronary heart disease, high blood pressure, diabetes, and some cancers. As indicated, diseases involving psychosocial stress appear to result, in part, from the mismatch between the modern way of life and our primordial stress reactivity.

As shown in Table 1, Benson characterizes the relaxation response, with its decreased respiration, muscle tension, and cardiovascular activation, as a hypometabolic state characterized by a quieting and calming of both the mind and the body. It is linked to the PSNS and, thus, rest and restoration.

According to Benson, regular use of the relaxation response helps to counter negative mental states (e.g., anxiety, tension, irritability, and depression) and the damaging aspects of the fight-or-flight response. That is, excessive use of the quick-acting, SNS-driven fight-or-flight response is counterbalanced by the less quickly elicited relaxation response of the PSNS. In essence, regular elicitation of this hypometabolic state of relaxation is thought to aid in tuning out daily worries, stresses, and strains while contributing to the body's needed rest and restoration by augmenting PSNS activation and diminishing SNS activation.

ELICITATION OF THE RELAXATION RESPONSE

In the course of his systematic and extensive study of Eastern and Western forms of meditation, Benson formulated four components related to bringing forth the relaxation response.

First, a quiet place without distractions is necessary. This place can be a room in one's home, a place of worship, or even a distraction-free area at work. Again, the key feature of a good relaxation context is a quiet place where one feels safe, calm, and free from distracting sights and sounds. Distracting sights and sounds can evoke negative affective states (e.g., irritation and frustration) and vigilance, both of which are associated with SNS activation. In essence, the place must be conducive to an effortless or easy direction of awareness to events or stimuli generated within oneself.

Second, a "mental device" or ongoing stimulus is used to orient the individual inwardly and away from logical and vigilant thought. This device can be a sound, a phrase, or a word repeatedly silently or aloud with eyes closed; it also can be a passive fixing of one's eyes on an object, a slow, repetitive series of movements as in Tai Chi Chuan, or pondering a Zen koan (unsolvable riddle). A passive attending to one's breathing can aid in use of the mental device and turning one's attention inward. Some examples of mental devices are presented in Table 2.

Third, cultivation of a passive or nonjudgmental attitude is crucial to elicitation of the relaxation response. Distracting thoughts and feelings will occur. One should easily favor the sound (e.g., repetition of a Sanskrit word or mantra), phrase, awareness of breathing, gazing at an object, or whatever is chosen as the mental device. One should simply notice the distracting thoughts, feelings, or both, and then easily restart the mental device without judging the distractions, the momentary disruption of the use of the mental device, or the level of relaxation. The elicitation of the relaxation response is designed to give a break from the stress of comparisons and judgments imposed by oneself and others. It is important not to judge one's relaxation!

Table 2. A Partial List of Mental Devices for Eliciting the Relaxation Response

Secular words or phrases	Religious phrases	Mantras
One	Christianity:	Transcendental
Love	Our father who art in	Meditation
Tranquil	heaven	Eng
Calm	The Lord is my	Enga
Peace	shepherd	Shirim
Relax	Hail Mary, full of grace	Hirim
I am relaxed (or	Judaism	Yoga
tranquil, calm, etc.)	Shalom	Aham Braham Asmi
Inhale relaxation	Echod	Aham-sah
Exhale tension (stress,	S'hma Yisroel	Sohang
worry, etc.)	Islam	Hansa
	Insha' allah	
	Hinduism:	
	Om	

Rather, it should simply be experienced for what it is, whether it be deep or light, or a letting go of many or few mental and affective states. Depth of relaxation will vary within and across periods of elicitation of the relaxation response, which is alright. Relaxation cannot be willed, only permitted to happen in a permissive, passive state of awareness.

Finally, a comfortable position is important as a means of avoiding undue muscular tension, which can serve as a distracter or contribute to SNS activity. Some people sit with legs crossed (e.g., using the lotus position of a yogi); cross-legged or kneeling positions are designed to keep the practitioner from falling asleep. Hence, lying down, although comfortable, is not suggested due to the tendency to fall asleep rather than to bring forth a wakeful hypometabolic state.

The following is a procedural outline for eliciting the relaxation response:

1. Sit comfortably in a quiet place. You may place your hands in your lap.
2. Close your eyes and simply notice your inhalations and exhalations.
3. Relax muscles, starting with the feet and moving up to the head. Sink or settle into the furniture or floor.
4. As you slowly breath in and out of your nose, think the word "one" during exhalation (i.e., breath in . . . breath out, think "one"). As stated before, phrases can be used. For example, think "I am" as you slowly inhale, and then think "relaxed" as you slowly exhale.
5. Continue the process for 10–20 min. Feel free to shift your body for comfort, look at your watch to check on time, scratch, and so forth. Once the relaxation period

is over, sit quietly for several minutes, at first with eyes closed, prior to standing up.

6. As discussed earlier, maintain a passive attitude toward your experience.

OTHER METHODS DEPLOYING THE RELAXATION RESPONSE

Progressive muscle relaxation (PMR), guided imagery, autogenic training, and hypnosis have been deployed to manage stress. During the initial stages of learning, a therapist teaches the client the procedures, which are followed by practice outside the treatment context. All of these techniques share the features necessary to induce the relaxation response. PMR involves closing the eyes, passively attending to verbal instructions to tense and relax large muscle groups (e.g., lower leg, upper leg, forearms, biceps, torso, and shoulders), to feelings characteristic of relaxation (warmth, heaviness, and tingling sensations), to suggestions of letting go of tension, and, in many instances, to imaging of serene contexts. An extension of PMR, cue-controlled relaxation, involves associating a word cue (e.g., "calm" or "relaxed") as one exhales while in a deep state of PMR-induced relaxation. The objective is to condition the cue word to elicit relaxation before, during, and after states of stress. For decades, PMR has been integrated into the behavior therapy of phobias, fear, and generalized anxiety. Over the years, stress management procedures using PMR have been reported to be effective in the behavioral treatment of a number of health-related conditions (e.g., hypertension, coronary disease-prone behavior, reduction of the side effects of chemotherapy in cancer patients, pain, and insomnia).

It is typical for a technique to share a number of features with other techniques. Like PMR, hypnosis, guided imagery, and autogenic training all involve therapist verbalization of suggestions/instructions as the client is in a comfortable position (e.g., recumbent in recliner) with eyes closed. A comparison of these techniques reveals that all share the components necessary for elicitation of the relaxation response. First, all involve a quiet, safe environment. Second, all involve a mental device as a means of orienting away from active perceptions and transactions with ongoing environmental changes: Guided imagery can involve the mental revivification of a tranquil place (e.g., sitting in a forest looking at the sun streaming through the trees); hypnosis can start with fixation on an object (e.g., a watch) until the eyes close, followed by attending to internal physical sensations, images, and thoughts suggested by the hypnotist; autogenic training typically involves covert repetition of phrases (e.g., "My right arm is warm and heavy"); therapists using PMR will suggest sensations connected to relaxation as clients attend inwardly to the tensing and relaxing of muscle groups. Finally, these techniques usually encourage a nonjudgmental/passive at-titude to foster relaxation and receptiveness to suggestion while clients are comfortably positioned.

RESEARCH EVIDENCE

For quite some time, the effects of interventions containing a relaxation component or focusing just on relaxation have been investigated in relation to high blood pressure, rehabilitation following a heart attack, insomnia, anxiety disorders, reduction of the side effects of chemotherapy for cancer, tension headaches, and pain. Although salubrious effects have been reported for this partial list of disorders, there are a number of unanswered questions. The results of meta-analytic reviews will now be reviewed. In meta-analysis, statistics used to test differences between groups (e.g., persons taught relaxation vs. those who were not taught) are combined across research studies to yield an average statistic showing the strength or magnitude of the treatment effect.

In the treatment of panic disorder (intense, disabling states of anxiety, as in fear of open spaces), treatment packages focusing on coping strategies, relaxation training, cognitive restructuring (changing ones view and interpretation of things), and exposure (use of imagery and actual behavior to approach the feared context) provided the most consistent positive results. Behavioral assessment showed less of an effect than other assessments (e.g., physiological and self-report), and the biggest effects were obtained for comparisons of treatment with a drug placebo. All in all, meta-analyses show that exposure is required to effectively treat panic and agoraphobia (fear of open spaces). Trait anxiety, or the general tendency to experience signs of anxiety (e.g., physical symptoms such as rapid heart rate and sweaty hands, as well as such mental states as worry, tension, and low self-worth) across situations, also has been examined. Interestingly, Transcendental Meditation, which utilizes repetition of a Sanskrit mantra, displayed the strongest effect of all the relaxation techniques. Moreover, concentration meditation (i.e., focusing on an external object like a vase) showed the weakest effect in the treatment of trait anxiety.

Chronic sleep disturbance, or insomnia, is a frequent health complaint. Relaxation techniques targeting cognitive arousal (intrusive thoughts, racing mind) were slightly superior to those focusing of physiological arousal (muscle tension); attention-focusing techniques like meditation and imagery training were categorized as targeting cognitive arousal, whereas biofeedback, PMR, and autogenic training were categorized as focusing on somatic arousal. Relaxation training also has been deployed as a component of rehabilitation programs for people with heart disease and high blood pressure. Regarding rehabilitation programs for heart disease, the total package appears to have a favorable impact on mortality and factors, such as decreased blood pressure, decreased smoking, and increased exercise, linked to increased risk of death. However, it is unclear whether relaxation training contributes to treatment effectiveness above that obtained from interventions designed to increase awareness of risk factor modification and deployment of behavioral strategies for risk factor modification. High blood pressure, a disease thought to be stress related in some cases, has been treated with interventions by meditation, PMR, and stress management packages using relaxation and interventions designed to alter the way people think about stressful circumstances. In general, relaxation has been associated with reduction of high blood pressure. However, the best results are linked to tailoring the stress management to the stresses and strains of the individual. For example, some people may deploy relaxation to help manage frequent daily bouts of anger, whereas others may deploy relaxation to aid in the management of daily bouts of social anxiety.

CONCLUSIONS

The hypometabolic relaxation response is thought to counter the deleterious effects of the stress of modern times, and a large body of research supports use of relaxation in a variety of treatment contexts, including cardiac rehabilitation, high blood pressure, insomnia, and anxiety disorders. A daily elicitation of the rest and restoration of the PSNS is believed to be the mechanism underlying the health-fostering effects of the relaxation response.

For quite some time, it has been thought and shown that people vary in the triggers, mechanisms, and physical and psychological expressions of the SNS-linked fight-or-flight response. Likewise, evidence is arising suggesting variability among people regarding the ability of the PSNS to counter excessive SNS activity; that is, some people may experience frequent anxiety and stress attacks due to a decreased capacity of the PSNS to keep excessive and unwarranted SNS activation in check. Interestingly, some people experience high anxiety while practicing relaxation, which is termed relaxation-induced anxiety (RIA). Effective stress management deploying relaxation tailors the treatment to the individual, and it is possible that RIA could be avoided in some cases by using a relaxation technique (e.g., PMR with its focus on muscle tension vs. relaxation) that does not focus on mental activity (e.g., mantra meditation), and thereby reduces the likelihood of ruminations evoking anxiety.

Despite positive advances in understanding the relaxation response, much work is necessary to fully comprehend its role in the treatment of stress-related problems. More component analyses, or isolation of the effects of individual aspects of a stress management package, are required to assess the treatment efficacy of the relaxation response relative to other factors (e.g., alteration of thinking). The relaxation response is associated with multiple factors connected to physiological, mental, and contextual (e.g., familial support for relaxation practice) dimensions that are conducive to a positive outcome. In other words, more fine-tuned research is required to understand why the relaxation response works in some cases but not in others. Does the state of the ANS (e.g., an impaired capacity for the PSNS to counter the SNS) affect relaxation induction? Can such ANS imbalance be adjusted with a relaxation intervention? Are cognitive changes (e.g., generalizing to daily living the ability to let go of stressful thoughts while meditating) necessary to maximize generalization of relaxation training to everyday stress management? Are certain people best suited for certain techniques? These and related questions await further inquiry.

Related Entries: Coping, Fight-or-Flight Response, Meditation, Nervous System, Stress Management, Stressful Life Events

BIBLIOGRAPHY

Benson, H. (1976). *The relaxation response*. New York: Avon.

Benson, H. (1996). *Timeless healing*. New York: Scribner.

Clum, G. A., Clum, G. A., & Surls, R. (1993). A meta-analysis of treatments for panic disorder. *Journal of Consulting and Clinical Psychology, 61*, 317–326.

Dusseldorp, E., van Dlderen, T., Maes, S., Meulman, J., & Kraaij, V. (1999). A meta-analysis of psychoeducational programs for coronary heart disease patients. *Health Psychology, 18*, 506–519.

Eaton, S. B., Konner, M., & Shostak, M. (1988). Stone Agers in the fast lane: Chronic degenerative diseases in evolutionary perspective. *American Journal of Medicine, 84*, 739–749.

Eppley, K. R., Abrams, A. I., & Shear, J. (1989). *Journal of Clinical Psychology, 45*, 957–974.

Jones, F., & Bright, J. (2001). *Stress: Myth, theory and research*. London: Pearson Educational.

Lichstein, K. L. (1988). *Clinical relaxation strategies*. New York: Wiley.

Mattick, R. P., Andrews, G., Hadzi-Pavlovic, D., & Christensen, H. (1990). Treatment of panic and agoraphobia: An integrative review. *Journal of Nervous and Mental Disease, 178*, 567–576.

Morin, C. M., Culbert, J. P., & Schwartz, S. (1994). Nonpharmacological interventions for insomnia: A meta-analysis of treatment efficacy. *American Journal of Psychiatry, 151*, 1172–1180.

Rice, P. L. *Stress and health* (3rd ed.). Pacific Grove, CA: Brooks/Cole.

Thayer, J. R., & Lane, R. D. (2000). A model of neurovisceral integration in emotion regulation and dysregulation. *Journal of Affective Disorders, 61*, 201–216.

RANDALL S. JORGENSEN

Religion and Health

Religion and health have always been, and continue to be, important aspects of human existence. Throughout history, civilizations believed that health and disease were related to particular religious beliefs or practices. For example, some Christians believed that good health was the result of proper Christian living and poor health was a punishment for sin. Though the relation between religious or spiritual dimensions of life and health has been a significant concern, it was not until the 20th century that notable scientific evidence addressed this topic. In fact, the number of scientific studies devoted to religion/spirituality and its relation to health remained at a relatively low annual level until the mid-1990s. Since then the topic has gained significant attention from scientists in many different fields including psychology, sociology, anthropology, epidemiology, medicine, nursing, and public health.

This increased scientific interest was due to many factors. First, Western society became more interested in multicultural understanding of human behavior and health. Religious groups and their customs, beliefs, behaviors, and health became a focus of increased study as a result of this renewed emphasis on the diversity of human societies. Second, many patients became unsatisfied with modern medicine, believing that it had become too technology driven, specialized, and impersonal, and had consequently sacrificed uniquely individual aspects and treatment of the whole person. This led to burgeoning emphasis on alternative medical treatments, some rooted in religious traditions. Finally, interest in spirituality may be the result of other factors in modern society such as a sense of social disconnection or alienation, lack of formative religious experiences during youth for many adults, and the fact that life expectancy is longer and therefore people live with chronic diseases for significant lengths of time. Whatever the reasons, the trend toward increased scientific study of the relation between religion and health continues.

SPIRITUALITY VERSUS RELIGIOUSNESS

A compelling problem for scholars is determining what is meant by the words religion, religiousness, and spirituality. Although the terms are commonly used, their precise definitions are elusive. Nevertheless, it is important for scientific investigators to carefully define what they are examining.

Religion is often viewed in terms of an institutional basis, that is, religions are associated with organized societal groups, which have members who believe in certain rules, rituals, or formal procedures that address what they believe to be transcendent or ultimate reality and are carried out in the context of their gathering or worship. Religiousness is the term used to convey an individual's personal experience of his or her religion. This carries with it the important implication that two individuals may be members of the same religious organization, yet have a very different religiousness. Spirituality is similarly used to describe the individual, rather than the group, experience,

and to some authors it is synonymous with religiousness. Many, however, distinguish spirituality from religiousness on the basis of whether a societal institution (e.g., a church) is involved. They view the individual's experience in the context of a defined religion as religiousness. Spirituality, from this perspective, has more to do with the individual's experience of the important subjective features of life (such as meaning and purpose, hope, and compassion for others) apart from a religious context.

It is important to note that almost all of the scientific research has concerned religiousness and not spirituality per se. Research on spirituality is underway and more will be known in the near future. Consequently, what follows is best described as a review pertaining to religiousness and health.

SCIENTIFIC EVIDENCE REGARDING THE RELATION BETWEEN RELIGIOUSNESS AND HEALTH

The best conclusion based on the scientific evidence is that religiousness or religious involvement appears to be related to better health and greater length of life. Some specific findings from particular studies indicate that religious involvement is related to lower rates of many diseases including heart disease and heart attacks, high blood pressure, emphysema, cirrhosis of the liver, lung cancer, and suicide. Other studies note many mental health benefits of religious involvement such as reduced rates of depression and anxiety and greater quality of life. Some investigators have found that religiousness helps individuals cope better when they have a chronic ailment or disease. Religiousness has also been related to longer life in numerous studies. Thus, although for some specific diseases there are few published scientific investigations, overall there is a large collection of research that, when viewed together, supports the conclusion that religiousness is related to good health.

Despite these conclusions, there is room for skepticism. For example, although some of the studies are of high scientific quality and were designed to look directly at the topic of religiousness and health, most studied religiousness as an afterthought. Consequently, these studies were not designed to rule out other possible causes for their findings. In addition, whereas many of the studies produced results suggesting that religiousness is related to better health, the strength of this finding was often weak. One could question whether a weak finding, though observed with the use of precise scientific instruments and statistical analyses, is of practical meaningfulness. By way of illustration, a person with very high blood pressure may reduce it by two points. This may be observable in a scientific study, yet have no beneficial effect for the person's health. Some of the studies of religiousness have similarly produced insubstantial findings. Finally, not all studies have found the beneficial effects of religion for health, and some of those that have found these effects have only found them on a portion of the characteristics of health studied. Thus, although the best evidence suggests a beneficial effect of religiousness on health, there is room for further investigation of this topic and for healthy skepticism about how strong this effect may be.

POSSIBLE WAYS THAT RELIGIOUSNESS MAY INFLUENCE HEALTH

If religiousness has a beneficial influence on health, how does it achieve this effect? In other words, what mechanisms may account for the relationship between religiousness and health? Several have been proposed. First, one way that religion affects health is by enforcing adherence to certain behavioral patterns based on religious beliefs. For example, many religious groups teach abstinence or moderation of alcohol use, abstinence from tobacco, or consumption of a vegetarian diet. These behaviors have known health effects. To the extent that engagement in these behaviors is motivated by religious beliefs, one can claim that religion has an impact on health.

Another way that religiousness may affect health is through social support. Religious groups provide their members with contact with others who believe in many of the same principles and are often concerned about the welfare of other members of the group. This amount and quality of social support are related to better health because it alleviates stress, provides for coping resources, and in some cases helps meet important material and physical needs. Religious individuals who are connected with organized local bodies of like-minded believers may have an advantage in terms of their social support.

The familiarity and ritual of religious services may also provide a source of support or comfort to individuals who engage in religious activity. These ceremonies carry with them meaning regarding purpose in life and even comfort in the afterlife. The predictability of the services along with their comforting message is likely to reduce distress for some.

Life presents many trials. The uncertainty of day-to-day interactions along with the precarious nature of life and the knowledge of one's own mortality pose significant challenges to people as they adapt and cope with their circumstances. The belief systems found in religious codes may provide a buffer for these challenging and potentially stressful aspects of human existence. Religions provide answers to many of life's biggest questions, such as why am I here, where am I going, what will happen to me when I die, how should I treat other people, and does my life really have meaning? To the extent that religions provide comforting answers to these questions, they may help

individuals live lives that are relatively free of depression, anxiety, and worry. It is well known that these negative emotional states influence health in a detrimental manner.

Finally, some religious persons believe that their health benefits from direct intervention from God or a supernatural power. From a research perspective, studies of intercessory prayer have been cited to potentially support this position. These studies involve having patients with a given health condition being prayed for by other people. In the best of these studies from a scientific point of view, neither the patient nor the patient's doctor knows that the patient is being prayed for. Thus, it is believed that any beneficial differences found for those in the prayer group versus a control group that was not prayed for would be due to the prayer and, by implication, some higher power. There are a number of studies that report such differences. It is important to note that these effects are small and are often found for only a few of many health variables studied. Thus, it is possible, indeed likely, that these results will not stand the test of time nor be consistently found when the studies are repeated.

CONCLUSIONS

The best evidence suggests a beneficial relationship between religiousness and health, but the strength and causes of this relationship remain areas for further study. More precise measurement of the dimensions of religiousness and spirituality and stronger scientific studies will facilitate better understanding of which aspects have prohealth impacts and which may have detrimental effects.

BIBLIOGRAPHY

Koenig, H. G. (1997) *Is religion good for your health? Effects of religion on mental and physical health.* New York: Haworth.

Larson, D. B., Swyers, J. P., & McCullough, M. E. (Eds.). (1998). *Scientific research on spirituality and health: A consensus report.* Rockville, MD: National Institute for Healthcare Research.

Levin, J. S. (1994). Religion and health: Is there an association, is it valid, and is it causal? *Social Science and Medicine, 38,* 1475–1484.

McCullough, M. E., Hoyt, W. T., Larson, D. B., Koenig, H. G., & Thoresen, Carl. (2000). Religious involvement and mortality: A meta-analytic review. *Health Psychology, 19,* 211–222.

Pargament, K. I. (1997). *The psychology of religion and coping.* New York: Guilford.

Sloan, R. P. & Bagiella, E. (2002). Claims about religious involvement and health outcomes. *Annals of Behavioral Medicine, 24,* 14–21.

Thoresen, C. E. (1999). Spirituality and health: Is there a relationship? *Journal of Health Psychology, 4,* 291–300.

Thoresen, C. E. & Harris, A. H. S. (2002). Spirituality and health: What's the evidence and what's needed? *Annals of Behavioral Medicine, 24,* 3–13.

KEVIN S. MASTERS

Renal System

COMPONENTS OF THE RENAL SYSTEM

The renal system consists of two kidneys, two ureters draining urine from each kidney into one bladder, and the urethra, which drains urine. Each kidney, about the size of a fist, has a renal artery, which carries blood from the heart into the kidney; the renal vein drains the blood. The kidneys are located on either side of the vertebra (back bone) above the waist. Under the microscope, the renal arteries divide several times, eventually forming little globes of one-cell-thick vessels (specialized capillaries) called glomeruli. The glomeruli are filters for the blood, and the filtered fluid is the beginning of urine. The blood cells remain within the capillary tubes and eventually return via the renal veins to the heart. Once this beginning urine is formed, it travels down renal tubules, which are highly specialized in their function.

Physiology

Even though each kidney only weighs 1/3 lb and represents less than 1/200 of the body weight, the kidneys receive 20% of the output of the heart, or about 1 quart (1 L) per minute. The kidneys contain approximately 2.5 million glomeruli and tubules. The glomeruli filter about 100 times the final volume of urine produced in 24 hr, and thus the tubules are extremely active in their function to retain and regulate water, minerals, and waste products.

Function of the Renal System

There is a "sea" within us, which the kidneys very precisely regulate to provide the optimal environment for cell function. The careful maintenance of the various salts, minerals, chemicals, and water help maintain normal blood pressure. In addition, the kidneys remove waste products from the body, which are generated from the normal turnover or metabolism of cells and tissues throughout the body. The kidneys, in conjunction with the lungs, cooperate to maintain the normal acid–base condition of the body. In addition, the kidneys have a major function in handling and degrading (metabolizing) naturally occurring compounds such as insulin. They also clear and metabolize many drugs, including certain antibiotics. Another large area of kidney function involves its endocrine function and its role as a chemical factory. The kidneys produced certain chemicals that are used within the kidney and throughout the body to regulate the blood pressure and flow to vital organs (renin–angiotensin system). They also send a chemical to the bone marrow to stimulate the production of red blood cells (erythropoietin). In addition, the kidney completes the formation of vitamin D, which is needed in regulating calcium.

COMMON DISORDERS

Blood Vessels

Each of the parts of the kidneys can be affected. The major blood vessels leading into the kidneys can be affected by hardening of the arteries (atherosclerosis), leading to narrowing of the renal arteries and reduction to the blood supply to the kidneys. This usually occurs in older age and may lead to high blood pressure or reduction in kidney function.

Glomeruli

The filters (glomeruli) may become involved as an innocent bystander when the body is fighting certain infections, such as streptococcus. This leads to inflammation with increased accumulation of white blood cells in these glomeruli, which reduce their function. This type of problem is usually temporary. On the other hand, the glomeruli can become replaced with certain types of foreign material and also become scarred. This happens with diabetes mellitus, which leads to eventual loss of kidney function. Scarring can also be seen in patients with long-standing hypertension, and less severe scarring is also a part of the natural aging process.

Tubules

These may be involved in infections of the kidney and many medications. The kidney itself can also be affected by cancer.

Ureters and Bladder

The tubes that drain urine from the kidney, the ureters, are thin and delicate and can be affected by kidney stones, which might obstruct the drainage from the kidneys. In addition, tumors in the abdomen can compress the ureters and also cause blockage of urine flow. The bladder can develop cancer, which can lead to bleeding. Kidney stones and renal cancers may produce pain. In addition, enlargement of the prostate, located at the outlet of the bladder, can produce narrowing of the drainage passage from the bladder (the urethra) and cause blockage of urine.

Normal Changes with Aging

A slow but natural decline of the filtering capacity of the kidney occurs with age. This begins after age 40 years, and by age 80 years, the filtering ability (glomerular filtration rate) is about half of that of a younger person. The remaining renal function in the elderly is sufficient to keep an individual feeling healthy and produces no symptoms. However, it does affect the ability of the body to handle certain medications, and thus certain drugs need to be given in a reduced dose in the elderly.

End-Stage Renal Disease

If the disorders of the kidney, some of which were listed in the foregoing, progress and cannot be reversed, kidney function declines. Generally, a person may have minimal or almost no symptoms until kidney function declines to less than 25% of normal. Once kidney function is reduced to less than 15% of normal, a person becomes ill. Kidney function less than 10% of normal may produce certain life-threatening conditions and eventually is incompatible with life. Some of the symptoms and signs are apparent from an understanding of normal kidney function. For example, some of the harmful effects include the retention of fluid, the development of swelling in the feet and legs and elsewhere, and the development of high blood pressure (hypertension). In addition, the build-up of waste products in the blood may lead to nausea, vomiting, chest pain, cognitive decline, confusion, somnolence, and anemia. Until two generations ago, severe chronic kidney failure was uniformly fatal. End-stage renal disease is a term applied to kidney function that will no longer sustain life.

Two categories of treatment are available for end-stage renal disease. The first is dialysis. There are two types of dialysis. One is hemodialysis, a process in which the blood is transported outside the body through tubing to a filter or artificial kidney connected to a dialysis machine. The most common artificial kidneys consist of a series of hollow straws or fibers. The blood runs through the center of the hollow fibers. A clean, physiological bathing fluid (called dialysate) flows around the blood-containing fibers, removing waste products and adjusting various minerals and chemicals within the blood, as well as removing fluid. This process requires 3–5 hr three times per week. During this time, the patient is connected generally through two needles and tubing to the dialysis machine. Approximately one cup of blood is outside of the body at any given moment. Complications of hemodialysis include low blood pressure, blood loss, and infection.

Another type of dialysis involves the placement of clean physiological fluid inside the abdomen by means of a tube or catheter. The peritoneal dialysis fluid remains inside the abdominal cavity, removing waste products and again adjusting minerals, chemicals, and volume. After a certain period of time, the fluid from within the abdominal cavity is drained and a new clean solution is placed. Peritoneal dialysis is less efficient than hemodialysis and is performed each day, several times during the day, or at night. Complications of peritoneal dialysis include infection (peritonitis).

The other major treatment for end-stage renal disease is kidney transplantation. This involves the placement of a healthy kidney from another person by a surgeon. The new kidney is placed inside the lower abdomen and does not go in the location of the person's native kidneys. An individual may receive a kidney from a family member (a living, related donor) or from a person who has recently died (cadaveric donor). In recent years, a spouse or very close friend (living, unrelated donor) has been able to be a donor. If an individual does not have a living donor, he or she is placed on a waiting list, and may wait for several years. Complications from kidney transplantation include the risks from surgery and an increased risk of infection and certain cancers due to the antirejection medicine (immunosuppression).

Dialysis and kidney transplantation undoubtedly are life saving. Each has pros and cons. An option for some individuals, especially those with other severely debilitating or serious life-shortening illnesses, may be to not undergo dialysis or transplantation at all. No matter which form of treatment for end-stage renal disease is chosen, there are obviously major changes in a person's lifestyle, with major changes in diet, activities, and medications. These adjustments produce major psychosocial and family stresses and require the integrated input of the health care team including the physician (kidney specialist, or nephrologist), nurses, dietitian, social worker, and often psychologists, psychiatrists, and clergy.

Related Entry: End-Stage Renal Disease

WILLIAM J. LAWTON
MARY LEE NEUBERGER

Reproductive System

The human reproductive system is highly complex and comprises features unique to each sex. Unlike the basic similarities between most male and female anatomic structures and physiological processes, the anatomy and functioning of the human reproductive system is drastically different in males and females. For males, the primary reproductive structures include the testes, vas deferens, penis, and scrotum. In females, the ovaries fallopian tubes, uterus, cervix, and vagina are the major reproductive structures.

Of the reproductive structures, the testes and ovaries are the actual reproductive organs or so-called gonads. The testes and ovaries are regulated by the hypothalamus and pituitary gland. The regulatory process involves a synchronized series of negative and positive feedback signals, which begin with the release of gonadotropin-releasing hormone (GnRH) by the hypothalamus. GnRh then stimulates the pituitary gland to release the gonadotopins follicle-stimulating hormone (FSH) and luteinizing hormone (LH). In males, FSH facilitates the production of sperm in the testes and LH stimulates the production of the male sex hormone, testosterone. In females, FSH signals follicle and egg maturation in the ovaries. Also in females, FSH and LH together stimulate the production of the two female sex hormones in the ovary, estrogen and progesterone, as well as the male hormone, testosterone.

Reproductive capacities vary between the sexes. In males, mature sperm are produced continually throughout life. However, the number and quality (e.g., motility, shape) of sperm decline with increasing age. By contrast, the reproductive capacity of females is limited in years, beginning with a girl's first menstrual period or menarche in puberty (~age 12–13 years) and ending with menopause, the cessation of menstrual cycles (~age 50 years).

The average length of a woman's menstrual cycles is 28 days. On about day 14, ovulation takes place. During ovulation, the mature egg is released from the ovary into the fallopian tube. From there, the egg travels through the fallopian tube, and if sperm are present, may be fertilized. If fertilization takes place, the egg implants itself in the uterine wall and begins its development into a human fetus.

The human reproductive system is intricate, and the process of becoming pregnant can be hindered or obstructed by several factors. Although the majority of couples become pregnant within 1 year, between 10% and 15% of couples experience infertility problems. Infertility is typically diagnosed if a couple is unable to become pregnant during 1 year of unprotected intercourse. A variety of psychosocial and biological factors can lead to infertility. Psychosocial factors include increased age, obesity, exposure to toxins or chemicals, and unhealthy lifestyles, which include smoking, substance/alcohol use, and sexual practices that increase the risk of sexually transmitted diseases. Biological factors that may lead to infertility include hormone irregularities, ovarian cysts, and structural anomalies of reproductive structures. Forty percent of infertility problems in couples is the result of male infertility, another 40% is associated with female infertility, and the remaining 20% is the result of infertility in both members of the couple or is unexplained.

Diagnostic evaluation is the first step in treating infertile couples. Depending on the determined or undetermined cause of infertility, treatment interventions are varied and may include modifying unhealthy lifestyles, using fertility drugs such as clomiphene (Clomid), undergoing surgery (to unblock fallopian tubes), using artificial insemination, or using assisted reproductive technologies (ARTs) such as *in vitro* fertilization, gamete intrafallopian transfer, and zygote intrafallopian transfer. Whereas artificial insemination involves the collection of sperm, which is then placed directly into the woman's uterus or cervix, current ARTs involve retrieval of eggs from the ovary, followed by fertilization with sperm either under laboratory conditions or in the uterus. The success rates of ARTs, reported as live births per egg retrieval, was 27% in 1997.

Advances in medical technology have greatly affected human reproduction. Although the processes and physiology of human reproduction are highly biological, or in the case of ARTs involve advanced medical procedures, psychosocial and psychological factors play major roles.

Related Entries: Genetics and Health, Human Sexuality, Pregnancy, STD Prevention

BIBLIOGRAPHY

Infertility in Women. (2003). MDConsult. Available at http://mdconsult.com/
Infertility in Men. (2003). MDConsult. Available at http:/mdconsult.com/

LAURA GORMAN

Respiratory System

The main function of the respiratory system is gas exchange. During respiration, oxygen is exchanged for carbon dioxide, which is eliminated from the body. This process requires the coordinated interaction of the conduction and respiratory passages. The conduction portion of the respiratory system consists of the nasal cavity, pharynx, larynx, trachea, and bronchi. The larynx leads into the trachea, which branches into the left and right bronchi. The bronchi continue to divide, and finally terminate in the alveolar ducts. The conducting airways are designed to warm, humidify, and filter the air. They are lined by pseudostratified ciliated columnar epithelium and mucus-secreting goblet cells. The mucus traps particulate matter, and the beating action of the cilia removes this material from the body. Paralysis of ciliary action can arise from congenital structural defects in the ciliated cells or from acquired defects caused by products of cigarette smoke. These defects can result in the familiar smoker's cough, pulmonary infection, and chronic lung disease.

Distal to the bronchi and bronchioles are the respiratory passages, which include the respiratory bronchioles, alveolar ducts, alveolar sacs, and alveoli. The alveolar wall is lined by a squamous epithelium composed of Type I cells. Type II cells produce pulmonary surfactant, which coats the alveolar walls and reduces the surface tension between opposing alveolar surfaces. A deficiency in the production of surfactant in newborns is known as respiratory distress syndrome. Alveolar macrophages defend the alveoli against foreign materials that escaped the conducting airways.

Gas exchange occurs via diffusion across the thin walls of the alveoli. The pulmonary capillaries, which are distributed throughout the alveoli, allow oxygen to move from the air into the blood and carbon dioxide to exit the pulmonary circulation.

Oxygenated blood leaves the lungs through the pulmonary veins and enters the left atrium of the heart. Oxygen binds to hemoglobin in red blood cells and is transported throughout the body. Hemoglobin also returns carbon dioxide to the lungs to be expired. Deoxygenated blood returns to the lungs via the pulmonary arteries, which exit the right ventricle of the heart. The central nervous system contains special control centers in the brainstem, which regulate the rhythm and depth of breathing. The vagus nerve also interacts with the circulatory system, the diaphragm, and the chest wall musculature to control breathing.

The lungs are constantly exposed to the environment, which makes them vulnerable to many biological and physical agents. Asthma is an allergic disease that affects millions of individuals. It is characterized by intermittent airway constriction, due to the contraction of smooth muscle in response to specific allergens (e.g., pollen). When the diameter of the airways becomes reduced, individuals experience shortness of breath, wheezing, and coughing. An obstructive respiratory disease that is associated with smoking and air pollution is emphysema. In emphysema, the normal elasticity of the airways and alveolar sacs is destroyed, and the lungs become damaged. The result of emphysema is poor gas exchange, shortness of breath, and advanced difficulty breathing.

Respiratory infections vary in severity and treatment. Pneumonia is a severe respiratory infection, which can be caused by viruses, bacteria, or fungi. In pneumonia, the lungs become inflamed and congested with fluid. The symptoms include a cough, fever, chills, and loss of appetite. Pneumonia was once the leading cause of death in the United States, but antibiotic therapy has largely brought it under control. Another illness that invades the respiratory tract is influenza, also known as the flu. The symptoms of influenza appear suddenly and may include fever, headache, dry cough, and nasal congestion. Influenza is transmitted as a virus, so it cannot be treated with antibiotics. However, the administration of a yearly influenza vaccine can prevent the flu and its most severe complications.

Related Entries: Asthma, Chronic Obstructive Pulmonary Disease

HEATHER WADE

Risk Factor Screening

As research findings accumulate, health professionals are becoming better and better at identifying people who are at risk of developing a variety of health problems. Moreover, knowledge is accumulating at a rapidly escalating pace, especially since

Table 1. Screening Methods and Examples of Risk Factors

Screening method	Example risk factor	Disease risk
Background and behavior	Age	As a woman gets older, her risk of breast cancer increases
Personality	Type A personality	People with Type A personalities characterized by hostility are more likely to have a heart attack
Medical testing	Cholesterol level	High levels of some types of cholesterol increase risk of a heart attack
Genetic testing	Gene for Huntington's disease	Children with the affected gene will eventually develop Huntington's disease

the human genome has been specified. The idea that one can identify at birth whether an infant is more or less likely to suffer from diseases later in life is no longer the stuff of science fiction. This entry describes what is known about how to screen for risk and some of the factors that elevate risk, who gets screened, and the consequences of risk factor screening.

SCREENING FOR RISK

Four general methods are available to identify people who are at risk of developing different diseases (see Table 1). Perhaps the oldest, simplest, and least expensive approach is to ask people to report information about their background and behavior. Background characteristics can be important predictors of risk for disease. For example, Black men are more at risk of prostate cancer than White men, and Black men and women in the United States face a higher risk than Whites for the sickle cell trait. White women, on the other hand, are more likely to suffer from osteoporosis than Black women. Other important background characteristics besides race and gender are family history, income, and education. Family history is an especially important variable, in part because a strong family history of disease suggests that a person is more likely to have a genetic predisposition for the disorder.

In addition to background characteristics, risk factor screening often includes the identification of current behaviors or behavior patterns (i.e., personality) related to disease. A person who smokes cigarettes, for example, is at great risk of numerous diseases, including a variety of different cancers and heart disease, the two biggest causes of early death in the United States. Overweight individuals are also at higher risk of disease, especially coronary heart disease, and individuals who are inactive also place themselves at higher risk for illness. Persons who combine these types of risk factors are at the greatest risk: Type II diabetes, for example, is typically associated with a family history of diabetes, being overweight, and inactivity. Finally, one can also assess personality dimensions. Perhaps the best known of these is the Type A personality. Psychologist Tim Smith has shown that the hostility component of this personality type is a good predictor of later heart disease.

A third means of identifying people at risk is to conduct some type of medical screening that can alert a health professional about the probability of disease. Such screenings are becoming available for more and more diseases, but it is important to recognize that these tests are imperfect: They can produce correct identification, but also false positives (indicating risk when there is actually none) and false negatives (indicating no risk when risk actually exists). Examples of this type of screening include mammography (for breast cancer), cholesterol levels (for heart disease), prostate-specific antigen tests (for prostate cancer), and blood pressure measurement (for stroke).

The final way to identify people at risk is to determine whether they have a gene associated with the disease. In the past, genetic screening was accomplished by constructing extensive family histories of persons with the disease. More recently, health professionals can collect genetic material (typically from blood) and identify whether the genes are predictive of the disease. Such tests will be more available in the future, but it is important to recognize that genes are not necessarily destiny. For breast cancer, as an example, estimates are that a young woman with the BRCA1 gene has greater than a 50/50 chance of developing breast cancer in her lifetime. The vast majority of breast cancers, perhaps as many as 90%, are not associated with any particular genetic abnormality.

WHO GETS SCREENED?

The most powerful predictor of whether a person will get screened is probably a physician's recommendation. Indeed, some risk factor screening is done almost automatically at a physician visit, including recording weight and blood pressure. A recommendation for more invasive screening by a physician is likely to be based on the doctor's knowledge of a patient's personal characteristics, such as a family history of the disease. People also can get screened for some risks in the community. For example, some employers might screen everyone at their worksite. It is also the case that people who feel at risk—who feel vulnerable and worry about contracting disease—are likely to seek out screening. In this case, objective risk factors may be less important than the person's beliefs about his or her susceptibility to disease. It is worth noting that disparities in screening rates

exist among different groups. Persons of lower socioeconomic status are less likely to have been screened for a variety of diseases. Less frequent or delayed screenings can have important negative consequences in that some diseases may be detected later after the illness has progressed further and is more difficult to treat successfully.

A number of barriers have also been indicated as inhibitors of screening. These include such factors as the costs of screening, difficulties obtaining a screening (e.g., transportation problems, lack of time), and concerns about the screening test itself (e.g., fear of radiation, worry about pain).

CONSEQUENCES OF SCREENING

The purpose of screening is to identify risks that, if addressed, may allow people to minimize or avoid disease. How people react to learning that they are at risk depends on the answer they receive. When people receive a negative message (e.g., "Your cholesterol is 250, which is higher than we would like"), they usually respond defensively, trying to minimize the threat inherent in the information. A person might, for example, deemphasize the seriousness of the disease (e.g., "People recover from heart attacks"), question the reliability of the screening test (e.g., "You can't trust these cholesterol readings anyway"), or think about alternative ways to reduce the severity of the threat (e.g., "My high score doesn't matter, because I exercise three times a week and exercise lowers blood pressure"). In summary, when a person receives a threatening message about elevated risk of health problems, he or she is motivated to reduce the negative implications of that information.

People are much more likely to eagerly accept information that they are not at risk. Even here, though, evidence suggests that people will sometimes reject information that they are less at risk than they had believed before testing. For example, researchers have provided risk counseling to women who overestimate their risk of breast cancer. These women learn that their risk is lower than they had thought, but many of them fail to adopt the new risk level: To some extent, they continue to maintain their original belief. People may retain their old beliefs because they wish to hedge their bets, and thus they may note that the new risk information fails to take into account special circumstances. It may also be the case that women avoid new risk information because it interferes with a consistent view of the self, even if this view is somewhat negative.

It is probably possible to communicate risk so that defensive reactions are lessened, but much needs to be learned about the risk communication process. It has been learned that it is possible in some circumstances to change inaccurate perceptions. In a large study of more than 1,000 patients waiting for medical care, Matthew W. Kreuter and Victor J. Strecher measured risk perceptions and provided individualized risk feedback about stroke, cancer, heart attack, and car crashes. The feedback increased stroke risk for those who were underestimating and reduced cancer risk for those who were overestimating. The feedback had no effect, however, on perceived risks of heart attack or car crashes. Not only is it possible to change some risk perceptions, the evidence is also solid that risk information can prompt people to protect their health. Smokers, for example, are more likely to quit when their physician reminds them about their increased health risk and advises them to quit. People with a family history of disease are much more likely to seek out screening, and to adopt behaviors that might lower their chances of contracting the health problem. Although we may not yet know the best ways to communicate risk information so as to persuade people to change their risk perceptions, we do know that the provision of such information can have positive benefits in motivating behavior change among those at greater risk of disease.

BIBLIOGRAPHY

Croyle, R. T., Sun, Y., & Hart, M. (1997). Processing risk factor information: Defensive biases in health-related judgments and memory. In K. J. Petrie and J. A. Weinman (Eds.), *Perceptions of health and illness: Current research and applications.* (pp. 267–290). Amsterdam: Harwood.

Kreuter, M. W., & Strecher, V. J. (1995). Changing inaccurate perceptions of health risk: Results from a randomized trial. *Health Psychology, 14,* 56–63.

Lerman, C., Croyle, R. T., Tercyak, K. P., & Hamann, H. (2002). Genetic testing: Psychological aspects and implications. *Journal of Consulting and Clinical Psychology, 70,* 784–797.

McCaul, K. D., and Tulloch, H. E. (1999). Cancer screening decisions. *Journal of the National Cancer Institute Monographs, No. 25, Cancer Risk Communication: What We Know and What We Need to Learn, 1999,* 52–58.

National Cancer Institute. *Risk communication bibliography.* Available at http://dccps.nci.nih.gov/DECC/riskcommbib/

National Research Council. (1989). *Improving risk communication.* Washington, DC: National Academy Press.

Smith, T. W., & Gallo, L. C. (2001). Personality traits as risk factors for physical illness. In A. Baum, T. A. Revenson, & J. E. Singer (Eds.), *Handbook of health psychology* (pp. 139–174). Mahway, NJ: Erlbaum.

KEVIN D. MCCAUL
AMANDA J. DILLARD

Ss

Schneiderman, Neil (1937–)

Neil Schneiderman, PhD, was born February 24, 1937. He is James L. Knight Professor of Health Psychology, Medicine, Psychiatry and Behavioral Sciences, and Biomedical Engineering at the University of Miami. Schneiderman is also director of the university-wide Behavioral Medicine Research Center. He received his PhD in psychology at Indiana University and postdoctoral training at the University of Basle, Switzerland, in neurophysiology, before joining the faculty of the University of Miami in 1965. He is director of program projects and research training grants in cardiovascular behavioral medicine from the National Heart, Lung, and Blood Institute and in the behavioral management of HIV/AIDS from the National Institute of Mental Health, both institutes in the National Institutes of Health (NIH).

Schneiderman's research has ranged from the neurophysiology of Pavlovian conditions, through the study of stress–endocrine immune interactions in HIV/AIDS and the central nervous system control of the circulation, to the behavioral management and stress research in HIV/AIDS, cardiovascular disease, and cancer. He has served as editor-in-chief of *Health Psychology* and of the *International Journal of Behavioral Medicine.* He is a fellow of Divisions 3, 6, and 38 of the American Psychological Association (APA) as well as the Academy of Behavioral Medicine Research, Society of Behavioral Medicine, and the American College of Clinical Pharmacology. He has served as president of the Division of Health Psychology (APA), Academy of Behavioral Medicine Research, and the International Society of Behavioral Medicine. He is a recipient of the Distinguished Scientist Award from APA and from the Society of Behavioral Medicine. He has served on multiple review

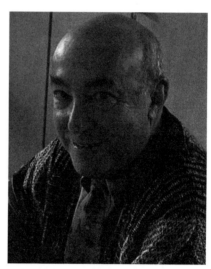

Schneiderman, Neil

committees at the NIH and as advisor to several offices and institutes at the NIH.

NEIL SCHNEIDERMAN

Schwartz, Gary E.

Gary E. Schwartz received his BA in psychology, with an emphasis in pre-medicine, from Cornell University. He received his MA in clinical psychology, and his PhD in personality psychology and psychophysiology, from Harvard University. From 1971 to 1976 he taught at Harvard. He moved to Yale

258

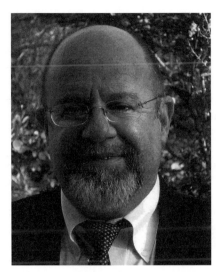

Schwartz, Gary E.

served as its third president. In his presidential address, he illustrated how concepts and findings in contemporary physics addressed challenging and controversial questions in health and illness.

With a distinguished group of students and colleagues, he has conducted research on transcendental and mindfulness meditation, emotion and repression, electroencephalograph registration of subliminal odors, and parental love as a predictor of long-term health. His latest research integrates body–mind–spirit, including controversial research on the possibility of survival of consciousness after death and spirit-assisted healing.

Schwartz is a fellow of the American Psychological Association, the American Psychological Society, the Academy of Behavioral Medicine Research, and the Society of Behavioral Medicine. He has received a Young Psychologist Award and an Early Career Award for distinguished research from the American Psychological Association.

University, where he was a professor of psychology and psychiatry, director of the Yale Psychophysiology Center, and codirector of the Yale Behavioral Medicine clinic until 1988, when he moved to the University of Arizona. He is professor of psychology, medicine, surgery, neurology and psychiatry; director of the Center for Frontier Medicine in Biofield Science; and director of the Human Energy Systems Laboratory at the University of Arizona.

Schwartz began his undergraduate studies in electrical engineering, and seriously considered becoming a philosophy major. His career has emphasized interdisciplinary and integrative science, working at the leading edges of psychology, psychophysiology, and medicine. This has led to his current National Institutes of Health-funded research on the human biofield, energy medicine, and spiritual healing, and his teaching in integrative health psychology.

Schwartz's early research was on biofeedback and the self-regulation of psychophysiological processes. With David Shapiro and Bernard Tursky at Harvard, he conducted pioneering studies demonstrating voluntary control of patterns of blood pressure and heart rate through feedback and reward in college students and hypertension patients. From 1971 to 1976 he authored or coauthored six papers in the journal *Science* on biofeedback and related topics in human psychophysiology and emotion.

While at Yale University, he played a central role in the birth and evolution of the interdisciplinary fields of behavioral medicine and health psychology. With Steven Weiss of the National Heart, Lung, and Blood Institute, he sponsored the Yale Conference on Behavioral Medicine, which helped define the field. He also helped establish the Health Psychology Division of the American Psychological Association, and

BIBLIOGRAPHY

Schwartz, G. E. (1973). Biofeedback as therapy: Some theoretical and clinical issues. *American Psychologist, 29*, 666–673.

Schwartz, G. E. (1984). Psychobiology of health: A new synthesis. In C. J. Scheirer & B. L. Hammonds (Eds.), *Psychology in health: Master lecture series volume III*. Washington, DC: APA.

Schwartz, G. E., & Russek, L. G. (1999). The living energy universe: A fundamental discovery that transforms science and medicine. Charlottesville, VA: Hampton Roads Press.

Schwartz, G. E., & Simon, W. L. (2002). *The afterlife experiments: Breakthrough scientific evidence for life after death*. New York: Pocket Books/Simon & Schuster.

GARY E. SCHWARTZ

Secondary Gain

The concept of secondary gain is based on the learning principle of reinforcement. In the context of health psychology, a secondary gain is a desired response, or elimination of an unwanted consequence, that is the result of an illness, circumstance, or particular behavior. This may be illustrated by the proclivity of a patient to continue to engage in illness behavior (e.g., disengaging from rehabilitation) because the consequence of doing so results in continued time away from an undesirable job. Time off from work is a gain that is secondary to the illness being maintained. Another example of secondary gain may be understood in the context of injury. An injured patient who is not ambulatory may receive benefits that are secondary to the disability, such as having meals prepared and served. Although this may not always be the case, secondary gains can serve as reinforcements to maintain illness behavior or thwart recovery.

Related Entry: Illness Stereotypes

KATHERINE RAICHLE

Self-Efficacy

Self-efficacy is the centerpiece of a theory of human agency developed by psychologist Albert Bandura of Stanford University. In his 1997 book, *Self-Efficacy: The Exercise of Control*, Bandura defined self-efficacy as consisting of "beliefs in one's capabilities to organize and execute the courses of action required to produce given attainments" (p. 3). Very simply, self-efficacy is the belief that one is able to perform a specified action. Bandura argued that, by developing ways to identify, measure, and alter self-efficacy beliefs, behavioral scientists can devise effective methods to help people control their behavior and influence events that shape their lives and societies.

A large body of research supports this. Beliefs about self-efficacy affect personal decisions about what courses of action to pursue, how much effort to invest in a goal, how long to persevere when the going gets tough, how to cope with adversity, how much stress one experiences, and the amount of success achieved. The evidence supports Bandura's (1997) claim that "beliefs of personal efficacy constitute the key factor of human agency" (p. 3). Self-efficacy, however, is not the only factor. Bandura argued that people also must believe that their actions will produce a desired result or outcome. Personal beliefs about the potential consequences of acting, or "outcome expectancies," work together in concert with self-efficacy beliefs to shape human actions.

This may sound straightforward. Understanding self-efficacy, however, is not as simple as it might appear. For one thing, self-efficacy involves more than believing that one can perform the specific behaviors needed to complete a given task, such as preparing a healthy low-fat meal. One must be able to do more than read food labels, measure ingredients, adjust cooking temperatures, and peel, slice, and dice vegetables. All of these behaviors must be timed and coordinated in the right way. Two would-be chefs may be equally skilled at reading, measuring, slicing, and dicing. Yet the two may have very different self-efficacy beliefs about being able to orchestrate everything into a delicious meal. If advised to alter their diets, these two individuals might react in different ways because their levels of self-efficacy are not the same.

SOURCES OF CONFUSION

It is very easy to confuse self-efficacy with several concepts that seem similar. Here are some common examples and distinctions.

Self-confidence. This familiar term is more general, and far less precise, than self-efficacy. A patient's self-confidence when facing an illness may involve a variety of considerations, some related to self-efficacy beliefs and some not. Whereas self-confidence may involve believing that one can perform actions needed to recover (self-efficacy), it also may include feeling loved and supported by one's family or trusting one's health care team.

Self-concept. People have many beliefs about themselves; the composite blend of these beliefs is called the self-concept. Unlike self-efficacy, the self-concept usually is defined as a global self-image. Bandura (1997) argued that this fails to do justice to the complexity of efficacy beliefs, which "vary across different domains of activities, within the same activity domain, at different levels of difficulty, and under different circumstances" (p. 11). Research shows that people's self-efficacy beliefs predict their behavior more reliably than do their self-concepts.

Self-esteem. Self-efficacy refers to beliefs about one's capabilities; self-esteem, on the other hand, refers to judgments about one's worth or value as a person. These are very different things. Doubting one's ability to sing a Verdi aria, for example, may not damage the self-esteem of those who lack operatic pretensions.

Locus of control. Health researchers have considered that motivation to adopt health behaviors may depend on believing that one's actions will generate desired results; people who believe that they can greatly improve their health by dieting would be said to have a strong internal health locus of control. Self-efficacy, however, refers to the belief that one is capable of performing a specified action quite apart from considering its outcome. For example, an overweight person may strongly believe that he or she can lose 10 lb, yet not believe that dieting will affect his or her health. This individual would exhibit strong dieting self-efficacy, but weak internal health locus of control.

General self-efficacy. It would be very convenient if we could measure a person's general or overall self-efficacy with a single scale. Bandura cautioned against this. Research indicates that beliefs about personal efficacy are not general across all activity domains and situations, but vary according to the type of performance and the setting. The term general self-efficacy thus should be considered an oxymoron.

SELF-EFFICACY IN SOCIAL COGNITIVE THEORY

It is misguided to focus on self-efficacy beliefs in isolation, for they are part of a larger explanatory framework, social cognitive theory (SCT), which Bandura developed from earlier social learning theory. According to SCT, human agency involves the interplay of three major factors that influence each other through a process of "triadic reciprocal causation" (Bandura, 1997, p. 7). This triad consists of *personal* factors (cognitive, affective, and biological events), *behavior* factors (what one says or does), and the *environment* (including one's social milieu). As a belief, self-efficacy is considered a personal factor in this scheme. As part of the causal triad, however, self-efficacy shapes, and is shaped by, behavior and the environment. Self-efficacy shapes behavior by influencing what one chooses to do; it shapes one's environment by influencing the types of social situations to which one gravitates. The causal process also works the other way around: A performance success or failure (behavior), or a change in one's social setting (environment), may cause self-efficacy to rise or fall. Environmental changes can have powerful effects on self-efficacy; for example, dieters often find it easier to control calorie consumption in some settings than in others (e.g., lunching alone at work vs. dining with friends at a restaurant).

MEASURING SELF-EFFICACY

Self-efficacy is measured by asking people whether they can perform a specified behavior or task. Many researchers have used a measurement model developed originally by Ewart and his associates at Stanford in their research with cardiac patients. A questionnaire lists performances of increasing difficulty (e.g., walk, run, or climb various distances). For each item, patients are asked, "How confident are you that you could do this activity now?" They are told to indicate their level of certainty on a scale that ranges from "0 = Definitely *cannot* do it" to "100 = Definitely *can* do it" (for some populations, an 11-point scale from 0 to 10 is used). Other questions ask about self-efficacy for dietary changes to lower fat intake (e.g., limit myself to two or fewer egg yolks per week, switch from whole milk to nonfat or 1% fat milk), controlling eating (e.g., when anxious, when watching TV, when it is impolite to refuse), and refraining from smoking (e.g., when bored, after a meal, when offered a cigarette). It is important for the behavior to be specific (e.g., walk 2 miles) and to ask whether the person can do it *now* or within a specified time period (e.g., lose 1 lb per week for 10 weeks). Critical measurement issues must be considered when constructing self-efficacy scales (see sources in the Bibliography).

STRENGTHENING SELF-EFFICACY

What is the best way to increase self-efficacy? According to Bandura, personal beliefs are altered by new information,

and the information we gain directly from our experience has the greatest impact on our self-efficacy. Thus the best way to increase self-efficacy for a particular activity is to perform the activity in gradually increasing amounts. For example, heart patients who doubt their ability to jog 1 mile would be encouraged to start with much shorter distances and gradually increase the distance as their efficacy grows. Next to direct experience, observing someone very much like oneself perform the activity can have a powerful influence. It is important, however, that this person be someone like oneself who appears to have similar ability. A somewhat less powerful but still helpful source of efficacy information consists of feedback from a person one judges to be highly credible, as when a cardiologist explains to a patient, "Your treadmill test performance shows that you can jog a mile." Other sources of efficacy information come from one's internal physical states and moods. Discomfort after exercising may undermine self-efficacy if the sensations are interpreted as indicating injury. A negative mood can bias memory, making it easier to recall past failures, which undermines a sense of efficacy, whereas a positive mood can make it easier to recall past efficacy-boosting successes. Training people how to respond to internal cues and manage mood states may help.

SELF-EFFICACY AND HEALTH PROMOTION

Self-efficacy's most important contribution to health is in suggesting practical methods for changing health behaviors. Programs derived from SCT have been developed to help people recover from heart disease, manage arthritis, cope with pain, curb addictions, and develop healthy eating and exercise habits. Efforts to apply SCT and self-efficacy to public health problems have led to the development of social action theory, an expanded conceptual framework that integrates self-efficacy with other behavior change mechanisms that must be coordinated when implementing health promotion on a wide scale.

CONCLUSION

Self-efficacy and SCT offer powerful evidence-based principles for understanding, measuring, predicting, and altering patterns of health behavior. The Bibliography is an introduction to the extensive literature on self-efficacy, scale construction, and applications to health.

Related Entry: Bandura, Albert

BIBLIOGRAPHY

Bandura, A. (1997). *Self-Efficacy: The exercise of control*. New York: Freeman.

DeVellis, B. M., & DeVellis, R. F. (2001). Self-efficacy and health. In A. Baum & T. Revenson & J. Singer (Eds.), *Handbook of health psychology* (pp. 235–247). Mahwah, NJ: Erlbaum.

DiClemente, C. C., Fairhurst, S. K., & Piotrowski, N. A. (1995). Self-efficacy and addictive behaviors. In J. E. Maddux (Ed.), *Self-efficacy, adaptation and adjustment: Theory, research and application* (pp. 109–141). New York: Plenum.

Ewart, C. K. (1991). Social action theory for a public health psychology. *American Psychologist, 46,* 931–946.

Ewart, C. K. (1995). Self-efficacy and recovery from heart attack: Implications for a social cognitive analysis of exercise and emotion. In J. E. Maddux (Ed.), *Self-efficacy, adaptation, and adjustment: Theory, research and application* (pp. 203–226). New York: Plenum.

Ewart, C. K. (2003). How integrative theory building can improve health promotion and disease prevention. In R. G. Frank, J. Wallander, & A. Baum (Eds.), *Models and perspectives in health psychology* (in press). Washington, DC: American Psychological Association.

Lorig, K., & Gonzalez, V. (1992). The integration of theory with practice: A 12-year case study. *Health Education Quarterly, 19,* 355–368.

Maddux, J. E., Brawley, L., & Boykin, A. (1995). Self-efficacy and healthy behavior: Prevention, promotion, and detection. In J. E. Maddux (Ed.), *Self-efficacy, adaptation, and adjustment: Theory, research, and application* (pp. 173–202). New York: Plenum.

Maibach, E., & Murphy, D. A. (1995). Self-efficacy in health promotion research and practice: Conceptualization and measurement. *Health Education Research, 10,* 37–50.

McAuley, E., & Mihalko, S. L. (1990). Measuring exercise-related self-efficacy. In J. L. Duda (Ed.), *Advances in sport and exercise psychology measurement* (pp. 371–381). Morgantown, WV: Fitness Information.

Schwarzer, R., & Fuchs, R. (1995). Changing risk behaviors and adopting health behaviors. In A. Bandura (Ed.), *Self-efficacy in changing societies* (pp. 00–00). Cambridge: Cambridge University Press.

CRAIG K. EWART

Self-Esteem

Self-esteem, often referred to as self-regard or self-worth, refers to one's perception of the self. A high regard for the self is considered to be indicative of high self-esteem. Self-esteem is typically considered to reflect a trait-like characteristic of a person and has implications for health and well-being. People with high self-esteem are less likely to become depressed, more likely to persist in tasks, and more likely to practice better health behavior. Some people contend that high self-esteem may be based partly on illusion because people with high self-esteem engage in a number of self-serving biases. That is, they take credit for their successes and blame others for failure, they perceive their failures as common and successes as unique, and they tend to see themselves as "better than average" in almost any domain. Each of these self-serving biases also has been linked to psychological well-being.

Global self-esteem can be distinguished from domain-specific self-esteem. Some people have a positive view of themselves in some areas but not necessarily others. Common domains of self-esteem that have been examined among children, adolescents, and adults include physical self-esteem (regard for one's body or athletic skills), social self-esteem (ability to get along with others and maintain relationships), and academic self-esteem (intellectual abilities). Not surprisingly, high self-esteem in one domain is likely to be related to high self-esteem in another domain, and each is related to global self-esteem. One theory is that global self-esteem is really based on one's feelings of acceptance or rejection from others.

Level of self-esteem has been distinguished from variability in self-esteem. Many people have a stable high or low self-esteem, which means that their feelings of self-worth are consistent across time and place. Other people have unstable self-esteem, which means that their feelings about themselves fluctuate on a daily or momentary basis. An unstable self-esteem may be based on a poorly developed self-concept or on becoming overly invested in day-to-day activities. Stability of self-esteem may be more important than level of self-esteem, or may interact with level of self-esteem, in predicting depression. Instability among high–self-esteem individuals may be associated with more depression, whereas instability among low–self-esteem individuals may be associated with less depression.

Self-esteem has implications for how one adjusts to illness. Some illnesses, such as HIV disease and cancer, are associated with a stigma, which may affect one's self-image. In those cases, the illness may negatively affect self-esteem. Even if there is not a stigma associated with an illness, self-esteem is challenged because the previously healthy self must now incorporate illness into the self-concept. There is evidence that more severe disability from disease is associated with lower self-esteem. Successful adjustment to illnesses, such as heart disease and cancer, often include restoring one's positive self-image. There are a number of ways in which self-esteem can be restored. One way is by downward comparison, that is, comparing oneself favorably to worse-off others (i.e., "At least I am not as bad off as the other guy"). There is some evidence that people with high self-esteem are more likely to make these self-enhancing comparisons in the face of illness. In general, high self-esteem has been linked with less distress and better adjustment to illnesses such as cancer and heart disease. Self-esteem is one component of the cognitive adaptation index, which has been linked to good adjustment to heart disease, cancer, and AIDS, and also has predicted less relapse among people with heart disease.

BIBLIOGRAPHY

Baumeister, R. F. (Ed.). (1993). *Self-esteem: The puzzle of low self-regard.* New York: Plenum.

Charmaz, K. (1991). *Good days, bad days: The self in chronic illness and time.* New Brunswick, NJ: Rutgers University Press.

Helgeson, V. S., & Mickelson, K. D. (2000). Coping with chronic illness among the elderly. In S. B. Manuck, R. Jennings, B. S. Rabin, & A. Baum (Eds.), *Behavior, health, and aging* (pp. 153–178). Mahwah, NJ: Erlbaum.

Leary, M. R., Tambor, E. S., Terdal, S. K., & Downs, D. L. (1995). Self-esteem as an interpersonal monitor: The sociometer hypothesis. *Journal of Personality and Social Psychology, 68,* 518–530.

Taylor, S. E. (1989). *Positive illusions: Creative self-deception and the healthy mind.* New York: Basic Books.

VICKI S. HELGESON

Self-Monitoring

Self-monitoring is a technique used for health behavior assessment and intervention, which involves observing and recording information regarding one or more health behaviors. Self-monitoring is often initially used as an assessment strategy to gather information about a behavior prior to any intervention. However, individuals may be reactive to the task of self-monitoring and begin making behavioral changes simply in response to observing and recording their own behavior. Self-monitoring is considered to be useful for improving self-awareness and understanding of circumstances that elicit, maintain, and encourage further instances of a target behavior. Self-monitoring may also promote change by increasing a person's perceived control over his or her behavior, assisting with reasonable goal setting, and helping to monitor progress toward goals.

Self-monitoring has been used to assess and help change specific health-related behaviors, such as smoking, alcohol consumption, fluid intake for patients with kidney disease, diet, exercise, and sleep. Self-monitoring has also been used to gather information about physiological states, such as blood pressure or glucose levels, and subjective internal states, such as degree of subjective pain or fatigue. Some self-monitoring methods use equipment, such as specialized instruments to measure blood pressure or glucose levels. A counter might be used to track the frequency of a specific behavior, such as cigarette smoking or exercise. However, self-monitoring often only requires a paper and pencil to chart specific information.

The amount and type of information recorded vary depending on the needs of the patient, but often include a target behavior, contextual information, and internal states that may be related to the behavior. Target behaviors may be recorded in various ways, including duration (e.g., minutes of exercise), amount (e.g., calories), or frequency (e.g., how often a person smokes). Contextual factors surrounding the target behavior are often recorded, such as the time it occurred, the setting, antecedents (e.g., what happened prior to the behavior), and consequences of the behavior, suggesting when a behavior is likely to occur and possible strategies for intervention. For example, a person attempting to lose weight might learn that he or she eats larger amounts of food in front of the television compared to other settings. In response, the person might start eating only in a separate room from the television to decrease food intake. Subjective information, such as mood or thoughts, might be recorded to help understand its relationship to a particular behavior. For example, a person might eat larger amounts when feeling anxious, which would suggest that alternate methods of coping with anxiety might help reduce food intake.

Self-monitoring is an assessment and intervention strategy for a wide range of health-related behaviors. Although it has been shown to facilitate short-term changes, longer-term changes are more likely when self-monitoring is combined with additional behavioral modification strategies. For example, interventions based on Frederick Kanfer's self-regulatory framework include self-monitoring as a first step, followed by self-evaluation using specific goals, and self-reinforcement for reaching goals. By helping people develop greater awareness, understanding, and control of their behavior, self-monitoring is an important strategy for assessing and changing health behaviors.

BIBLIOGRAPHY

Barton, K. A., Blanchard, E. B., & Veazey, C. (1999). Self-monitoring as an assessment strategy in behavioral medicine. *Psychological Assessment, 11,* 490–497.

Kanfer, F. (1991). *Helping people change: A textbook of methods* (4th ed.). New York: Pergamon.

Meichenbaum, D., & Turk, D. C. (1987). Behavioral modification approaches. *Facilitating treatment adherence: A practitioner's guidebook.* New York: Plenum.

ERICA L. JOHNSEN

Self-Regulation

Self-regulation refers to the processes by which individuals control or direct their thoughts, emotions, and actions to achieve their goals. According to self-regulation theory, behavior is guided by a motivational system of setting goals, developing and enacting strategies to achieve those goals, evaluating progress, and revising goals and actions accordingly. Increasingly, self-regulation models are being used to explain health behaviors taken to achieve goals of improving health, such as through changes in exercise or diet behaviors, and goals of avoiding illnesses and their consequences, such as through seeking medical care for unusual symptoms or adhering to medical treatments.

Fundamental to self-regulation models is the concept of feedback. When individuals perform behaviors, they search for and appraise information about the outcomes of the behaviors in terms of their success in moving them toward their desired states. This feedback process helps individuals keep on track in their efforts to attain their goals. Another aspect of self-regulation models is an emphasis on the role of emotions in motivating and guiding behavior. These models focus on how fear, joy, and other emotions influence the selection of goals and behaviors.

The concepts of self-control and will power are also important. Many health behaviors such as regular exercise, smoking cessation, and medication adherence require individuals to refrain from indulging in gratifying substances and activities or, alternatively, to engage in uncomfortable or inconvenient activities. According to self-regulation models, it is necessary to pay consistent attention to behavior and goals to maintain the self-control and will power needed to sustain these behaviors over time. Self-monitoring techniques, which involve recording behaviors in a log or diary, can help individuals keep their attention focused on the behaviors and their progress. For example, use of a daily log of food intake can improve individuals' success in losing weight.

Two models frequently used in health psychology research are Charles Carver's and Michael Scheier's self-regulation model and Howard Leventhal's commonsense model. The former is a model of general behavior that has been used to guide research on health and illness behaviors and outcomes, whereas the latter model focuses specifically on illness-related behaviors.

CARVER AND SCHEIER'S MODEL OF SELF-REGULATION

Carver and Scheier's model of self-regulation focuses on how people go through their daily activities by selecting goals and then choosing behaviors accordingly. According to this model, health behaviors can best be understood by considering how they relate to the individual's life goals. An individual can have many related goals (see Figure 1); for example, an individual can have a relatively abstract goal to "stay healthy," a more specific goal to "eat five fruits or vegetables each day," and an even more specific goal to "buy a salad at lunchtime." These goals have a hierarchical organization, with goals about the type of person one would like to "be" on top. These goals link with goals involving the kinds of actions one needs to "do," which in turn connect with more specific goals concerning motor behavior sequences involved in the action. Goals can also vary in terms of whether they involve approach or avoidance behaviors, that is, whether they involve moving a person toward a desired state (e.g., physical fitness) or away from an undesired state (e.g., getting HIV/AIDS).

The model also identifies how different emotional experiences occur during efforts to achieve goals. When individuals believe they are making good progress toward a desired goal (approach behavior), then they will experience positive affect such as pleasure or happiness. When they believe they are not making progress toward desired states, then negative affect such as depression will arise. Different kinds of positive and negative emotions are associated with avoidance goals and behaviors. When individuals believe they are doing well in avoiding undesirable states, they experience relief; when they feel their avoidance attempts are unsuccessful, they experience anxiety.

Expectancies as Determinants of Behavior

According to the Carver and Scheier model, expectancies play a critical role in self-regulation. Individuals typically encounter problems and challenges as they work toward their goals. Whether they continue to pursue those goals depends on their expectancies about their potential success (see Figure 2). If they feel confident that they can achieve their goals, they continue their efforts. If they have doubts, they are likely to give up. When beginning an exercise program, for example, efforts to maintain the program will depend on whether one has confidence that the exercise goal can be achieved.

Research has shown that individuals vary in their generalized expectancies, that is, their tendencies to expect positive or negative outcomes when facing uncertain conditions. Dispositional optimism is a personality characteristic involving the tendency to expect positive outcomes and to feel confident that one's goals will be attained. Compared to individuals who are low in dispositional optimism, those high in dispositional optimism tend to experience more positive emotions and show more persistence in goal-related efforts. These tendencies appear to have beneficial health effects. In studies conducted by Scheier and colleagues in 1989 and 1999 of individuals undergoing coronary artery bypass surgery, patients with high (versus low) dispositional optimism had faster recovery rates and a reduced likelihood of being rehospitalized in the months following surgery.

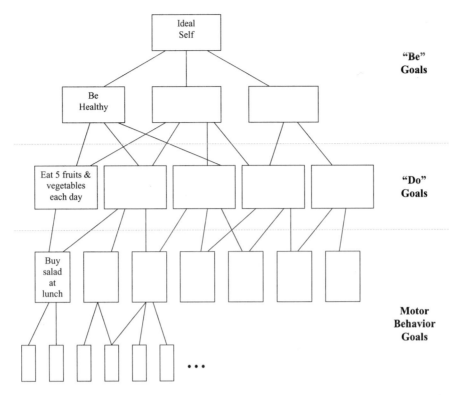

Figure 1. A hierarchical organization of goals. (Adapted from *On the self-regulation of behavior*, p. 000, by C. S. Carver & M. F. Scheier, 1998, New York: Cambridge University Press. Copyright 1998 by Cambridge University Press. Used with permission.)

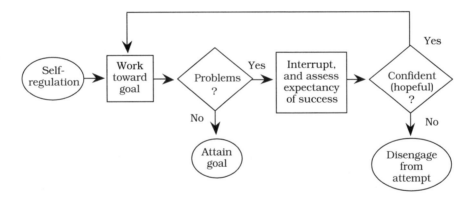

Figure 2. A depiction of the behavior decision process illustrating how expectancy assessments influence decisions to continue or disengage from further effort. (From goals and confidence as self-regulatory elements underlying health and illness behavior, by M. F. Scheier & C. S. Carver, in *The self-regulation of health and illness behavior* (pp. 17–41), edited by L. D. Cameron & H. Leventhal, 2003, London: Routledge. Copyright 2003 Routledge. Reprinted with permission.)

LEVENTHAL'S COMMONSENSE MODEL OF SELF-REGULATION

The commonsense model focuses on cognitions, emotions, and actions elicited in response to health threats. It gives particular emphasis to individuals' personal beliefs about illnesses and their commonsense rules for making health-related decisions. According to this model (see Figure 3), the perception of health threat cues simultaneously activates problem-focused self-regulation (efforts to control the health threat itself) and emotion-focused self-regulation (efforts to manage emotional distress).

At the problem-focused level, threatening cues (e.g., symptoms such as wheezing and difficulty breathing) elicit the activation and development of a cognitive representation of the health threat. This representation includes beliefs about five

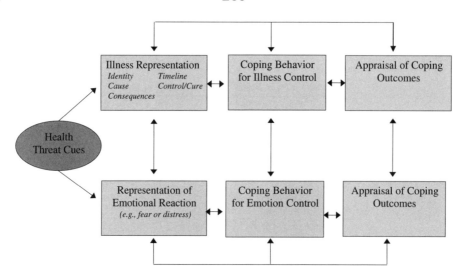

Figure 3.   The commonsense model of health and illness self-regulation.

attributes: (1) the identity of the condition, including its label (e.g., asthma) and associated symptoms (e.g., wheezing, shortness of breath, and dizziness); (2) the cause of the condition (e.g., heredity or exposure to dust mites); (3) its timeline or duration, which may be acute (short term), cyclical (it comes and goes over time), or chronic; (4) its consequences (e.g., asthma interferes with one's ability to play sports); and (5) the potential for its control or cure (e.g., it can be controlled using inhalers and medication). This representation guides the selection of coping behaviors for controlling the health threat (e.g., seeking medical care or using an inhaler), and the outcomes are appraised in terms of their success in doing so (e.g., whether the wheezing has subsided). The representation and coping behaviors are then revised accordingly.

At the same time that the health threat cues activate the problem-focused self-regulation process, they trigger emotional responses such as fear and distress. The experience of wheezing and breathing difficulties can evoke feelings of panic, for example, and activation of representational beliefs about asthma can further enhance distress and worry. Awareness of these emotions (the emotional representation) motivates the use of actions to alleviate them (e.g., seeking support from a friend). The outcomes of these behaviors are then appraised for their success in reducing distress, and these appraisals feed back to revise the emotional representation and coping efforts.

Illness representations and emotional distress often motivate the same coping behaviors (e.g., use of an inhaler). At times, however, they can motivate conflicting actions. For example, fear arousal can lead to avoidance of disease detection behaviors even when the individuals' beliefs motivate the use of these techniques. In a 1966 study of cigarette smokers conducted by Leventhal and Jean Watts, for example, those who viewed a fear-arousing program about lung cancer were less

likely than those viewing an alternative program to agree to undergo a chest x-ray.

Empirical Evidence for the Commonsense Model

Numerous studies provide evidence that the five representational beliefs identified by the commonsense model predict a wide variety of illness behaviors and outcomes. In patients with chronic illnesses, beliefs of a chronic timeline and serious consequences tend to be associated with avoidance tendencies and poor psychological adjustment, whereas beliefs that an illness is controllable predict greater use of active, problem-focused coping strategies and greater psychological well-being. Research also demonstrates that emotional distress influences health-protective behaviors in ways that are predicted by the self-regulation model. For example, distress has been found to promote protective behaviors such as performing breast self-examinations and seeking medical care for unusual symptoms. However, distress may promote protective behavior only when an individual has a specific plan for engaging in that behavior. In one illustrative study conducted by Leventhal, Robert Singer, and Susan Jones in 1965, individuals who received fear-arousing messages about the dangers of tetanus reported strong intentions to get a tetanus shot, but only those who received assistance in developing action plans for obtaining the vaccinations were likely to do so in the subsequent weeks.

CONCLUSION

Self-regulation models provide frameworks for understanding goal-directed health behavior, whether the goals involve improving health or avoiding illness. Carver and Scheier's model proposes that goals have a hierarchical organization, moving from more abstract goals down to more specific action goals. Emotions provide important feedback about one's progress in achieving goals, and expectancies critically influence decisions to continue efforts or to give up. Dispositional optimism, a tendency to have positive outcome expectancies, has been found to be associated with favorable health outcomes. Leventhal's commonsense model proposes that health threats activate both problem-focused and emotion-focused self-regulation. At the problem-focused level, behavior is guided by representational beliefs about the health threat's identity, cause, timeline, consequences, and potential for control or cure. The use of self-regulation models to address behavioral health issues is yielding new insights into how cognitions, emotions, and feedback processes influence health-related behaviors and outcomes.

BIBLIOGRAPHY

Baker, R. C., & Kirschenbaum, D. S. (1993). Self-monitoring may be necessary for successful weight control. *Behavior Therapy, 24*, 337–394.

Brownlee, S., Leventhal, H., & Leventhal, E. A. (2000). Regulation, self-regulation, and construction of the self in the maintenance of physical health. In M. Boekarts, P. R. Pintrich, & M. Zeidner (Eds.), *Handbook of self-regulation* (pp. 369–416). San Diego, CA: Academic.

Cameron, L. D., & Leventhal, H. (2003). *The self-regulation of health and illness behaviour*. London: Routledge.

Carver, C. S., & Scheier, M. F. (1998). *On the self-regulation of behavior*. New York: Cambridge University Press.

Hagger, M. S., & Orbell, S. (2003). A meta-analytic review of the commonsense model of illness representations. *Psychology and Health, 18*, 141–184.

Leventhal, H., Leventhal, E. A., & Cameron, L. D. (2001). Representations, proecedures, and affect in illness self-regulation: A perceptual–cognitive model. In A. Baum, T. Revenson, & J. E. Singer (eds.), *Handbook of health psychology* (pp. 19–47). Hillsdale, NJ: Erlbaum.

Leventhal, H., Singer, R., & Jones, S. (1965). Effects of fear and specificity of recommendations upon attitudes and behavior. *Journal of Personality and Social Psychology, 2*, 20–29.

Leventhal, H., & Watts, J. C. (1966). Sources of resistance to fear-arousing communications on smoking and lung cancer. *Journal of Personality, 36*, 154–168.

Scheier, M. F., & Carver, C. S. (2003). Goals and confidence as self-regulatory elements underlying health and illness behavior. In L. D. Cameron & H. Leventhal (Eds.), *The self-regulation of health and illness behaviour* (pp. 17–41). London: Routledge.

Scheier, M. F., Matthews, K. A., Owens, J. F., Magovern, G. J., Lefebvre, R. C., Abbott, R. A., & Carver, C. S. (1989). Dispositional optimism and recovery from coronary artery bypass surgery: The beneficial effects on physical and psychological well-being. *Journal of Personality and Social Psychology, 57*, 1024–1040.

Scheier, M. F., Matthews, K. A., Owens, J. F., Schulz, R., Bridges, M. W., Magovern, G. J., Sr., & Carver, C. S. (1999). Optimism and rehospitalization following coronary artery bypass graft surgery. *Archives of Internal Medicine, 159*, 829–835.

LINDA D. CAMERON
SHELEIGH LAWLER

Self-Report Methods

Self-report assessments are ubiquitous in the behavioral and social sciences (Stone et al., 2000). The methodology used to collect self-report information is based on asking people to report their experiences, feeling, or actions. Information about private states, such as mood and pain, can only be obtained through self-report. Paper-and-pencil questionnaires are the most common way of collecting self-report data, but structured interviews are also used.

The following are several examples of self-report assessments. Depression inventories ask individuals to indicate the presence and intensity of depressive symptoms currently or over the last few weeks. Food consumption inventories ask about recent meals, including the type and quantity of food consumed. Assessments of affect and mood often comprise a series of adjectives describing mood states, which are rated according to their intensity. Life event inventories ask people to check events from a list of serious occurrences (e.g., divorce, death of a loved one) that happened over the last year. Finally, personality inventories are intended to characterize relatively stable individual characteristics or traits and usually comprise a series of descriptive statements about patterns of thought, feeling, and behavior, which respondents rate in reference to themselves.

Although self-report instruments are used in most health psychology studies—as predictor, outcome, or mediator variables—concerns have been raised about their validity. One concern is that people do not use rating scales in the same way: Some tend to use the high end of the scale and others the low end. When examining associations between two or more scales (e.g., depression and pain), this type of reporting bias can create false relationships. Another concern has been that self-reports can be influenced by circumstances and mood at the time of reporting (Schwartz, 1999); people in a transient negative mood will tend to assess the overall quality of life negatively compared to times when they are feeling better. Similarly, the limited capacity of memory and other dynamic processes affecting recall (Gorin & Stone, 2001) affect the validity of self-report. For example, the recall of pain over several days is overly influenced by peak pain experiences and the level of recent pain. Likewise, when people are asked to recall the number of times they engaged in a behavior over a period of time (e.g., number of cigarettes smoke or exercised in the last week), they often use estimation strategies because they are unable to remember the discrete instances of the events. Estimations are prone to be biased by a person's beliefs about his or her health behavior, for example, "I exercise several times a week," rather than being veridical reports of the person's behavior over the exact time period being assessed. Momentary recording methods have been developed, in part, to overcome these recall biases.

Self-report is an essential tool for behavioral scientists to measure constructs that are not observable by others. There are, however, many limitations to peoples' ability to make accurate and valid self-reports, and these need to be kept in mind for the design of experiments and when interpreting self-reports.

Related Entry: Momentary Assessment

BIBLIOGRAPHY

Gorin, A. A., & Stone, A. A. (2001). Recall biases and cognitive errors in retrospective self-reports: A call for momentary assessments. In A. Baum, T. Revenson, & J. Singer (Eds.), *Handbook of health psychology* (pp. 405–413). Hillsdale, NJ: Erlbaum.

Schwarz, N. (1999). Self-reports. How the questions shape the answers. *American Psychologist, 54,* 93–105.

Stone, A. A., Turkkan, J., Jobe, J., Bachrach, C., Kurtzman, H., & Cain, V. (2000). *The science of self report.* Hillsdale, NJ: Erlbaum.

ARTHUR A. STONE
JOAN E. BRODERICK

Seligman, Martin E. P. (1942–)

Martin Seligman was born on August 12, 1942. He graduated summa cum laude in 1964 from Princeton University, and received his PhD in psychology from the University of Pennsylvania in 1967. He began his academic career at Cornell University and returned to the University of Pennsylvania in 1970, where has continued to teach. He is the Robert A. Fox Leadership Professor of Psychology at the University of Pennsylvania. Among his many accomplishments, Seligman has served as the director of the Positive Psychology Network since 2000. He served as president of the American Psychological Association (APA) in 1998 and serves on the APA Board of Trustees. In addition, Seligman serves on several advisory committees, including the National Association for Gifted Children, the National Interfaith Coalition for Spiritual Healthcare and Counseling, and the Board of Advisors for *Parents Magazine.* He is on the editorial boards of several scholarly journals, including *Applied Psychology: An International Review, Behaviour Research and Therapy,* and the *Journal of Preventative Psychology and Allied Disciplines.* He is a recipient of the Arthur Staats award for Unification of Psychology and the Psi Chi Frederick Howell Distinguished Lecturer award. He has also been an APA Master Lecturer and a National Academy of Practice in Psychology Distinguished Practitioner.

Seligman's work focuses on positive psychology, learned helplessness, depression, and optimism and pessimism. His re-

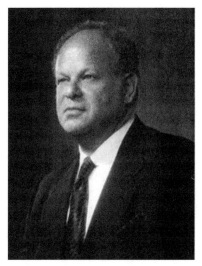

Seligman, Martin E. P.

search on learned helplessness as presented in his book *Learned Helplessness* (1975) presented the implications of learned helplessness in child development, physical health, and mental illness. This book included research that had dramatic implications for understanding, treating, and preventing depression. This research has been prominent in both the scientific and the popular literature. His work on learned optimism addressed why some people respond to negative events with depression and others learn to effectively cope. Along with others, Seligman presented the notion that the difference is based on attributional style. Pessimists attribute events to stable, global, and internal causes, which often leads to depression. He published two books, *Learned Optimism* (1991) and *The Optimistic Child* (1996), on this research. As president of the APA, Seligman was involved in the development of a new field of psychology called positive psychology. This field was designed to prompt researchers to embrace a more humanistic model to psychology as opposed to the disease model. Positive psychology focuses on the study of subjective experience, positive individual traits, and positive institutions. Seligman's work has had a profound influence on the treatment and prevention of depression in both clinical psychology and clinical health psychology.

JAMIE A. CVENGROS

Set-Point Theory

The set-point theory is an effort to understand why both laboratory rats and humans seem to resist substantial body weight change, even when their caloric intake is raised or lowered substantially. The body weight that a given organism maintains is referred to in this theory as the set point. The theory specifies that an individual's set point is physiologically regulated and that an area of the brain called the lateral hypothalamus plays a primary role in determining body weight set point.

The concept of set point evolved out of a series of observations that various mammals tend to return to a preexisting weight after periods of significant weight loss or weight gain. For example, during periods of significant famine or food shortages, people clearly tend to lose weight, but their weights generally returned to preexisting levels once adequate food is available. Similarly, it has been shown that humans who increase their food intake considerably may increase their weight by 15%–25%, but when the experimental increased food intake terminates, their weight typically returns to preexisting levels. It is believed that this is due to a tendency for the body to decrease the rate of calories utilized by the body when an individual loses weight and to increase calorie utilization when an individual has gained weight. Thus, extreme deviations from the set point become more difficult as the body attempts to counteract weight-related deviations through metabolic adjustments.

The observation that the human body tends to decrease metabolic rate when weight is lost has been used to explain why dieting in humans becomes increasingly difficult and weight loss is unlikely to be maintained. For example, obese individuals who show a 3% weight loss demonstrate a 17% decrease in rate of oxygen consumption, an indication of their metabolic rate. The fact that their metabolic rate decreased much more than their weight loss suggests that a physiological process related to metabolism is actively resisting further weight change. If set-point theory is correct, short-term diets or simple increases in exercise are unlikely to result in long-term weight change. Instead, set-point theory implies that lifetime commitments to low-calorie diets are essential for obese individuals to lose weight. However, set-point theory continues to be studied scientifically and although some predictions from the theory have been supported, others have not. For example, set-point theory predicts that individuals with substantial weight loss should display more psychological distress because they are "resisting" their set point. However, studies of individuals who have successfully lost weight and maintained the loss fail to reveal more psychological disturbance than unsuccessful dieters. Further scientific study of set-point theory is needed to better understand whether the body truly adjusts metabolic rates to preserve a predetermined set point for a given individual's weight.

Related Entries: Eating Disorders; Exercise, Effects and Benefits; Nutrition

BIBLIOGRAPHY

Keesey, R. (1989). Physiological regulation of body, weight and the issue of obesity. *Medical Clinics of North America, 73*, 15–28.

STEPHEN A. WONDERLICH
PATRICIA FREIBURGER

Shaping

The principles of operant conditioning give rise to a gradual learning process known as shaping. In shaping, an organism learns how to execute a more complex behavior by first learning how to execute smaller, simpler behaviors. Reinforcing these successive approximations leads to the ultimate goal of learning the complex behavior.

For example, scientists may teach laboratory rats how to walk across a cage and press a bar via shaping. This complex task will be broken down into smaller, more manageable behaviors for the rat, such as walking near the bar, standing on hind legs, making contact with the bar, and so on. At first, when the rat nears the bar, this behavior will be reinforced. After the rat has come to associate a reward with proximity to the bar, it will only be reinforced when it stands on its hind legs near the bar. The process continues in this fashion until the rat can walk over and press the bar without reinforcement at each step of the process.

Related Entry: Operant Conditioning

BIBLIOGRAPHY

The B. F. Skinner Foundation. Available at www.bfskinner.org.

ANDREW BEER

Skin Cancer

Skin cancer is the most common form of cancer in the United States, and it accounts for an estimated 1.3 million new cases of cancer each year. The incidence rate of *melanoma*, the most deadly form of skin cancer, has more than doubled since the early 1970s and continues to rise. The other, more common types of skin cancer are the nonmelanomas, mainly *basal cell carcinoma* and *squamous cell carcinoma*. Skin cancer is most common in fair-skinned individuals, and persons who lived in tropical, sunny climates when they were young are at increased risk.

The greatest risk factor for skin cancer is exposure to ultraviolet (UV) radiation, which comes mainly from the sun. It is believed that lifelong protection from the sun's rays would prevent most skin cancers. Because sun exposure during childhood accounts for an estimated 80% of the total lifetime exposure, children in particular can benefit substantially from preventive actions.

Whereas skin cancer is the most common cancer, it is also one of the most preventable. Behavioral recommendations for primary prevention of skin cancer include limiting time spent in the sun, avoiding the sun during peak hours (10 a.m. to 4 p.m.), using sunscreen with a sun protection factor (SPF) of 15 or higher when outside, wearing protective clothing (hats, shirts, pants) and sunglasses, seeking shade when outdoors, and avoiding sunburn. These behaviors, if consistently practiced, can help prevent all forms of skin cancer. There is some concern that using sunscreen will lead people who are trying to get a suntan to stay in the sun for a longer time, so another recommendation for prevention is not to intentionally bake in the sun or seek a tan.

An understanding of patterns of behavior can help to guide efforts to prevent skin cancer. More people take precautions at the beach or on vacation than when taking outdoor recreation. Parents are more likely to protect their children than themselves. Children are more often protected from UV radiation if their parents also protect themselves. Adolescents seem especially resistant to advice about skin cancer prevention and minimizing sun exposure.

Preventive interventions have demonstrated modest success, with the majority of programs being conducted in school settings. It is believed that the ideal intervention strategies for reducing exposure to ultraviolet radiation exposure are coordinated, sustained, community-wide approaches that combine education, mass media, and environmental and structural changes. Interventions within specific organizational settings such as schools, health care, recreation programs, and workplaces provide useful ways to reach important audiences like children, and are suitable venues for structural supports such as environmental and policy changes that complement educational efforts. It is generally agreed that environmental and structural changes also need to be part of successful skin cancer prevention efforts.

Skin cancer is an international problem and is now receiving increasing attention in the United States. It is hoped that models used in countries like Australia, where skin cancer rates are very high, can be successfully transferred to the United States, where skin cancer is a less prominent public health concern and the population also includes a higher proportion of dark-skinned individuals.

Related Entries: Cancer: Biopsychosocial Aspects, Health Belief Model, Risk Factor Screening, Theory of Reasoned Action and Planned Behavior

BIBLIOGRAPHY

American Cancer Society. (2000). *Cancer facts and figures—2000.* Atlanta; GA: American Cancer Society.

Arthey, S., & Clarke, V. A. (1995). Suntanning and sun protection: A review of the psychological literature. *Social Science and Medicine, 40,* 265–274.

Buller, D. B., & Borland, R. (1999). Skin cancer prevention for children: A critical review. *Health Education and Behavior, 26,* 317–343.

Glanz, K., Saraiya, M., & Briss, P. (2002). The impact of intervention strategies to reduce UVR exposure. In: D. Hill, D. English, & M. Elwood (Eds.), *Prevention of skin cancer* (pp. 00–00). New York: Kluwer.

Montague, B. R., & Sinclair, C. (2001). Slip! Slap! Slop! and SunSmart, 1980–2000: Skin cancer control and 20 years of population-based campaigning. *Health Education and Behavior, 28,* 290–305.

KAREN GLANZ

Smith, Timothy W. (1955–)

Timothy W. Smith was born July 6, 1955, in Buffalo, New York. He completed his BA degree at Gettysburg College in 1977 and his PhD in clinical psychology at the University of Kansas followed by a post-doctoral fellowship at the Brown University Program in Medicine. He is professor of psychology at the University of Utah, where he has been since completing his doctoral degree. Smith has published well more than 100 articles related to health psychology and has received numerous past awards for his scholarship. His primary research program addresses personality and social risk factors for cardiovascular disease. He has made seminal contributions in virtually every corner of this broad area of inquiry. Smith's work throughout the 1980s and into the mid-1990s involving behavioral, social, cognitive, and psychophysiologic correlates of trait hostility had a tremendous impact on shaping the way personality and health researchers throughout the world conceptualize, measure, and incorporate the hostility construct into biobehavioral models of disease risk. The series of social psychophysiologic experiments Smith conducted and published during this period demonstrated in a novel and compelling fashion the interactive and transactional influence that certain social contexts and trait hostility differences have on cardiovascular health risk.

Throughout the 1990s and into the new century the influence of Smith's scholarship on the field of health psychology medicine further intensified. He published a series of important empirical papers on social cognitive mediators of chronic disease

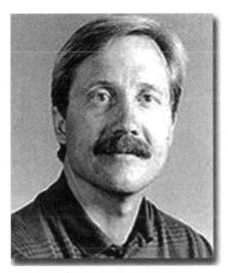

Smith, Timothy W.

adaptation (depression and regimen adherence) and began to shift his social psychophysiologic focus to marital and other dyadic contexts. In this most recent body of work, he has effectively applied broader theory and methods involving the interpersonal analysis of social behavior to the conceptualization and assessment of psychosocial risk factors for physical disease. His ongoing work involving studies on marital interaction, cardiovascular reactivity, and cardiovascular risk in both younger couples and elderly couples is poised to have the same degree of seminal and lasting impact on the field as did his earlier scholarship.

ALAN J. CHRISTENSEN

Smoking Cessation

Cigarette smoking is the leading preventable cause of disease and death in the United States, and results in enormous medical costs. The health benefits of quitting are substantial, even if smoking-related health problems already exist (U.S. Department of Health and Human Services [USDHHS], 1990). As the dangers associated with smoking and the benefits of quitting became more widely known, the prevalence of smoking among adults in the United States dropped from 40% in 1965 to 29% in 1987; most recent data indicate that approximately 23.3% of U.S. adults are current smokers (Centers for Disease Control [CDC], 1996; CDC, 2002; USDHHS, 1990). Smoking prevalence continues to decline, but not quickly enough to reach the target of 12% set in the *Healthy People 2010* objectives (USDHHS, 2000). Interest in quitting remains high among

the majority of regular smokers: 70% of current smokers report that they want to quit smoking, and 41% have made an attempt to quit in the preceding year (CDC, 2002). Despite the high level of interest in quitting smoking, long-term abstinence is extremely difficult to achieve.

FACTORS CONTRIBUTING TO CONTINUED SMOKING

Smoking cigarettes is extremely reinforcing. This is the result of both the physical addiction to nicotine and the habitual/psychological component of smoking. The physical addiction begins with the repeated administration of nicotine in cigarettes. Nicotine addiction follows the typical developmental pattern of any addiction: with repeated exposure to nicotine, tolerance develops, requiring increased levels of nicotine to achieve the physical effects experienced during early administrations. If nicotine is withheld, a set of negative physical effects known as withdrawal begins, and the person experiences increasingly stronger urges for the substance. Withdrawal symptoms and cravings can be relieved by administering more of the substance. Although dependence can develop to nicotine in any form, nicotine is delivered to the brain quickly when administered through cigarettes, which results in a particularly strong pattern of addiction.

There is also an extremely strong habitual component to smoking cigarettes, which creates a pattern of behavior that can be difficult to alter. Individuals tend to smoke in predictable settings associated with specific events, times of day, feelings, places, and other persons. When smoking is frequently repeated in a particular set of circumstances, smokers experience cravings and urges when presented with those contextual cues despite their physiological state. For example, smoking cigarettes is commonly paired with drinking alcohol and coffee. These events or settings become strongly associated with smoking, which results in a conditioned habit that can be difficult to change.

Another substantial influence on the addictive nature of cigarette smoking is the strong social influence on urges and cravings to smoke. One factor that adds difficulty to a quit attempt is the number of smokers in the environment. The more a person is exposed to cigarette smoking, the greater the difficulty that person will have with quitting. There may be many reasons this is true, including additional exposure to smoking cures, greater availability of cigarettes (increasing the probability of slips and relapse), less pressure to quit smoking, and less support for quitting efforts.

In addition, there is ample evidence to suggest that cigarette smoking has a host of positive psychological effects including mood regulation (smokers might smoke to help manage depression and anxiety) and increased attention and concentration. Given the strong physical addiction to nicotine, the habitual component of smoking cigarettes, and the psychological/social reasons for continued smoking, treatments used to stop smoking have been developed targeting these specific influences.

METHODS USED TO STOP SMOKING

Most smokers who have quit smoking have done so on their own or with minimal assistance. There are several types of minimal interventions that can be effective for quitting smoking. Brief cessation advice and counseling by health professionals during routine and other health care visits is an effective method of motivating smokers to quit and facilitating cessation. Success can be enhanced if health care professionals arrange for follow-up support. The largest problem with this type of cessation strategy is with health care providers consistently implementing the recommended treatment guidelines in real-world facilities.

There are many self-help cessation interventions aimed at reaching large populations of smokers. The formats of these programs include workbooks, pamphlets, video- or audiotapes, Internet sites, and hotlines that can provide assistance in planning and coping with a quit effort. Most smokers who wish to quit are not interested in attending formal treatment groups and would prefer to make their quit attempt on their own. Most self-help programs take the successful components from intensive cessation interventions and modify them for a minimal treatment paradigm. Recent research indicates that the success rates from these types of programs have been relatively modest, between 5% and 15% 12 months after the intervention; however, because these types of programs can be easily distributed to a large proportion of the population of smokers at a low cost, they can potentially result in a substantial number of individuals quitting.

Behavioral and cognitive skill building can enhance quit rates substantially. These types of programs are typically intensive, multisession interventions led by a health professional and presented to small groups of smokers who have voluntarily enrolled themselves in the program. These programs focus on teaching smokers the skills they need to prepare for quitting and cope with withdrawal and temptations to smoke. Formal programs typically include many different components including relaxation training, stress and mood management, strategies for harnessing social support, and addressing concerns regarding weight gain. Intensive clinical interventions result in relatively high quit rates, ranging from 20% to 40% 12 months after the end of the intervention. Whereas these types of interventions are very successful, relatively few smokers make use of these programs and prefer trying to quit smoking on their own.

There are a variety of pharmacologic aids to quit smoking. The most popular are the nicotine replacement therapies (NRT), which can be administered in many forms including patch, gum, spray, and inhaler. In the United States, patch and gum are sold over the counter, whereas spray and inhaler require a physician's prescription. NRT theoretically works by providing the smoker with stable levels of nicotine in the blood and therefore minimizing withdrawal symptoms and cravings for cigarettes. There is data to suggest that adding NRT to a more intensive behavioral cessation program roughly doubles quit rates; however, other data suggest that use of NRT products alone does not increase quit rates. There is one non-nicotine pharmacotherapy approved by the Federal Drug Administration for smoking cessation: bupropion SR, an atypical antidepressant. The mechanism of action of this medication is unknown, but the research evidence does not support the hypothesis that its effectiveness in smoking cessation is related to reducing depressive symptomatology. The data on the pharmacotherapies clearly illustrate that there is no silver bullet when it comes to quitting smoking.

MAINTENANCE AND RELAPSE ISSUES

Regardless of the type of intervention utilized, the majority of initial cessation successes result in a relapse back to smoking within the first 3 months after quitting. Although high relapse rates after an intensive and expensive intervention can be disappointing, some individuals are able to recycle their efforts into another quit attempt. For most smokers, it will take multiple serious efforts to achieve a period of prolonged abstinence. Given the high rates of relapse, many of the formal clinical interventions for smoking cessation include a treatment component to teach people how to recover from a slip during a quit attempt in order to avoid a relapse.

HEALTH BENEFITS OF QUITTING SMOKING

Smoking contributes to death from cardiovascular and respiratory diseases as well as a number of different types of cancers. The health benefits of quitting smoking are enormous and cover most of the major systems in the body. Some of the health benefits that occur rather quickly after quitting include increased lung function and improved circulation. The most important long-term health improvement resulting from cessation is that individuals who quit smoking live longer than those who continue to smoke. Other important health benefits of cessation include a decreased risk of developing lung cancer and a number of other types of cancer and a lowered risk of experiencing heart attacks, strokes, and other respiratory ailments. For women who quit smoking before getting pregnant or early in their pregnancy, their risk of having a low-birth-weight infant is significantly reduced (USDHHS, 1990). It is important to note that individuals who have already developed smoking-related health problems benefit from quitting smoking. Research indicates that for some conditions, quitting may improve the course of the physical ailment and in some cases increase overall survival.

In conclusion, although quitting smoking for prolonged periods of time is frequently difficult for individuals to accomplish, there are many effective intervention options to select from. The health benefits from quitting are substantial; thus, smokers should be strongly encouraged to continue putting forth strong efforts to quit smoking.

Related Entries: Addiction, Smoking Prevention

BIBLIOGRAPHY

Centers for Disease Control. (1996, July 12). Cigarette smoking among adults—United States, 1994. *Morbidity and Mortality Weekly Report, 45*, 588–590.

Centers for Disease Control. (2002, July 26). Cigarette smoking among adults—United States, 2000. *Morbidity and Mortality Weekly Report, 51*, 642–645.

Fiore, M. C., Bailey, W. C., Cohen, S. J., et al. (2000). *Treating tobacco use and dependence: Clinical practice guidelines.* Rockville, MD: Public Health Service.

Fiore, M. C., Novotny, T. E., Pierce, J. P., Giovino, G. A., Hatziandreu, E. J., Newcomb, P. A., et al. (1990). Methods used to quit smoking in the United States: Do cessation programs help? *Journal of the American Medical Association, 263*, 2760–2765.

Lichtenstein, E., & Glasgow, R. E. (1992). Smoking cessation: What have we learned over the past decade? *Journal of Consulting and Clinical Psychology, 60*, 318–527.

Marlatt, G. A., & Gordon, J. R. (Eds.). (1985). *Relapse prevention: Maintenance strategies in the treatment of addictive behaviors.* New York: Guilford.

Mermelstein, R. J., Karnatz, T., & Reichmann, S. (1992). Smoking. In Peter H. Wilson (Ed.), *Principles and practice of relapse prevention* (pp. 43–68). New York: Guilford.

Piasecki, T. M., & Baker, T. B. (2001). Any further progress in smoking cessation treatment? *Nicotine and Tobacco Research, 3*, 311–323.

U.S. Department of Health and Human Services. (1990). *The health benefits of smoking cessation: A report of the surgeon general.* Washington, DC: U.S. Government Printing Office.

U.S. Department of Health and Human Services. (2000). *Reducing tobacco use: A report of the surgeon general.* Washington, DC: U.S. Government Printing Office.

U.S. Department of Health and Human Services. (2000). *Healthy people 2010: Understanding and improving health* (2nd ed.) Washington, DC: U.S. Government Printing Office.

KATHLEEN R. DIVIAK

Smoking Prevention

There are more than one billion smokers worldwide. If current trends continue, 8.4 million smokers are estimated to die annually of smoking-related deaths by the year 2020. Tobacco use remains the single major preventable behavioral cause of death and disease in the United States. Despite the adverse health outcomes and enormous costs associated with smoking, nearly one-fourth of adult Americans—an estimated 50 million people—continue to smoke cigarettes. In addition, it has been estimated that more than 3,000 children and adolescents begin smoking each day. At least 70% of these young smokers want to quit smoking, but only approximately 5% succeed.

Since the 1964 report to the surgeon general on the health consequences of smoking, the public health community has played a key role in focusing efforts to reduce the continuing toll of tobacco use by discouraging smoking initiation and promoting smoking cessation. Universal interventions, that is, prevention programming delivered to an entire population regardless of risk status, have been utilized most often. Targeted interventions, which are designed to tailor programming to those groups at higher psychosocial-based risk (selective) or individuals who have demonstrated to be at greatest risk of continued smoking behavior (indicated), have also been implemented, but relatively few such programs exist.

Preventive interventions that have provided evidence of effectiveness include school-based educational programs, family-based informational programs, mass media campaigns, regulatory efforts, tobacco excise taxes, and comprehensive community-based activities. Although much more research is necessary, a comprehensive approach that combines these educational, social, regulatory, and economic aspects through multiple intervention modalities may be most effective in controlling and preventing tobacco uptake.

SCHOOL-BASED EDUCATIONAL PROGRAMS

The most widespread prevention approaches are those implemented through the school system and designed to counteract the psychosocial influences that promote tobacco use initiation. The two major psychosocial approaches that have been adopted by schools are the social influences approach and the more comprehensive personal and social skills enhancement approach. Social influences programs are designed to increase the awareness of social influences promoting drug use, alter norms regarding the prevalence and acceptability of drug use, and build drug resistance skills. Skills enhancement programs incorporate aspects of the social influence approach and also include general self-management and social competence skills. Literature reviews and meta-analyses of modern tobacco use prevention programs have indicated short-term (less than 24 months) reductions in the rate of initiation of tobacco use generally ranging from 30% to 50% or more in students exposed to social influences programs compared to control students. A few targeted programs implemented with older teens have found 27% prevalence reductions in tobacco use lasting up to 2 years post-program. These programs utilize a skill enhancement approach and also incorporate motivation enhancement material to effect changes in personal attitudes that may impede skill development and behavior change. In both universal and targeted programs, effective educational strategies are those that are implemented interactively rather than with a didactic lecture style. Although much less evidence exists for the long-term follow-up success of these tobacco use interventions, current empirical data indicate reductions ranging from approximately 10% to 15%, lasting for up to 15 years after programming.

Empirically validated programs are available for dissemination. These programs have been promoted for use through federal and state policies that require schools that receive funds from Safe and Drug-Free Schools and Communities and Tobacco Use Prevention Education (TUPE) programs to implement research-based programming. However, it appears that these "proven" programs still have not been widely adopted by the nation's schools. Instead, a large majority of schools are implementing tobacco prevention programs that are aggressively marketed and relatively easy to implement, but have not shown evidence of effectiveness or have not been properly evaluated.

FAMILY-BASED INFORMATIONAL PROGRAMS

Family involvement is a relevant means of providing prevention material outside of school. Various public health organizations have launched informational campaigns aimed at getting parents and teens to talk about tobacco use prevention. These family-based programs typically offer parent-based booklets and websites. Program contents typically stress the importance of teaching open communication and parents serving as good role models by not smoking, and discuss peer pressure, the role of the parent in prevention, responsible decision making, health consequences of smoking, and costs of smoking. One shortcoming of parent-based programming is that some efforts are directed at parents, not children. Thus, it is not clear whether their children will receive any relevant information. Furthermore, youth at highest risk for tobacco use are relatively unlikely to have parents who will take on the responsibility of teaching prevention material to their children or serve as support persons for other programming. One promising family-directed program utilized mailed booklets and telephone contacts by health educators. This program provided some evidence that

universal, family-based programming may prevent adolescent tobacco use.

MASS MEDIA CAMPAIGNS

Mass media (television, radio, film, and print) play an important role in smoking control activities, particularly among youth, who are heavily exposed and susceptible to media influences. Media-based campaigns have been used to communicate factual information about tobacco use, influence public perceptions of appropriate behavior, and directly counteract pro-tobacco advertising. Results from empirical studies that examine the impact of media campaigns have varied. Advertisements that graphically, dramatically, and emotionally portray the serious negative consequences of smoking are consistently ranked as the best among youth in terms of getting them to stop and think about not smoking. Furthermore, research on long-term preventive effects has indicated that an intervention combining mass media and school-based programming was more effective than the school-only program in preventing adolescent cigarette use across a follow-up period of 6 years.

REGULATORY EFFORTS

Since 1964, various legislation, policies, and litigation initiated by federal, state, and local governments have regulated tobacco product distribution, and may lead to prevention or cessation outcomes. Regulatory attempts include various restrictions on tobacco industry advertising and promotion, restrictions on access to tobacco by minors, and implementation of clean indoor-air policies. However, due to the powerful lobbying forces representing the tobacco industry, attempts to regulate tobacco industry activity in the United States have had only modest success compared to some other countries, including Canada and New Zealand. U.S. regulations include requirements for health-warning labels on all cigarette packages. In addition, these regulations include prohibition of broadcast media (television and radio) advertisements, prohibition of the purchase of tobacco products by individuals under the age of 18 years (in all but two states and Puerto Rico), and creation of a smoke-free environment in various settings. Smoke-free settings include government offices, eating and drinking establishments, and workplaces, and are quickly expanding in type and number across the United States. Unfortunately, tobacco control regulations are not always aggressively enforced due to lack of both funding and infrastructural support. Moreover, it is unclear whether regulatory efforts have induced changes in social norms regarding smoking, or, conversely, whether the passage of legislation and policies are a reflection of a social environment that discourages smoking. Regulatory approaches that restrict smoking across a range of environments (e.g., home, school, and public places) do show some real promise in reducing levels of smoking among adolescents.

TOBACCO EXCISE TAXES

Federal, state, and many local governments have imposed excise (per unit) taxes on tobacco products as a means of preventing or reducing tobacco consumption. Increased tobacco prices due to taxation may lead cost-conscious youth to refrain from starting smoking, reduce the amount that they smoke, or quit smoking. Research studies examining the effects of the price of tobacco products on youth smoking have shown mixed results, requiring further evaluation. However, the general consensus is that higher cigarette taxes would lead to significantly reduced smoking rates among youth. As another benefit, in addition to its potential to discourage smoking by youth, this strategy generates revenue (from tobacco users) that has helped to fund smoking control activities.

COMMUNITY-BASED ACTIVITIES

Many community-based programs take advantage of multiple channels of program delivery, and are the most comprehensive prevention services available. Community-wide efforts, including coalitions, campaigns, programs, and policies, have been increasingly used to prevent tobacco use within local communities. These projects typically involve multiple public and private organizations and agencies, such as law enforcement, social services, education, private businesses, and community- and faith-based organizations, which collaborate in support of strengthening, expanding, and coordinating existing smoking prevention initiatives. As a result, community interventions have the capability of coordinating and utilizing multiple systems, channels, and strategies to influence individual behavior, community-wide norms, and local policies related to youth tobacco use. Although community-based programs achieve some of the strongest preventive effects, they tend to be weaker in methodological design. In addition, community institutionalization of effective programming may be particularly difficult.

THE NEED FOR MULTIPLE MODALITIES OF DELIVERY—NATIONALLY AND INTERNATIONALLY

Studies of comprehensive community prevention initiatives suggest that smoking prevention programs that utilize multiple delivery modalities, whereby youth receive a consistent message across various contexts and over time, are most likely to yield and maintain positive program effects. Future system-wide approaches that include demand reduction efforts such as school-based, family-based, and mass media strategies, along with strong supply reduction approaches (e.g., restrictions on tobacco industry advertising and promotion, prohibition of minors' access to tobacco, environmental bans on smoking, and higher cigarette prices), may combine synergistically to maximize smoking prevention efforts across the nation.

Tobacco control efforts should be coordinated internationally. International tobacco control efforts should include the promotion of legislation on smoke-free venues and policies that follow international standards and are organized by national governments. These efforts should involve a sharing of research and technical expertise, funding of international tobacco control activities, and cooperation of organizations such as the World Health Organization and the World Bank, and discouragement of favorable tobacco trade export policies that undermine tobacco control efforts. By working together, the international tobacco control community will have the ability to help eradicate the culture of smoking created by the tobacco industry, moving another step forward in halting the worldwide epidemic of tobacco related death and disease.

Related Entries: Addiction, Smoking Cessation

BIBLIOGRAPHY

Bauman, K. E., Ennett, S. T., Foshee, V. A., Pemberton, M., King, T. S., & Koch, G. G. (2002). Influence of a family program on adolescent smoking and drinking prevalence. *Prevention Science, 3,* 35–42.

Chaloupka, F. J., & Warner, K. E. (2000). The economics of smoking. In A. J. Cuyler & J. P. Newhouse (Eds.), *Handbook of health economics* (pp. 00–00). New York: Elsevier Science.

Farrelly, M. C., Healton, C. G., Davis, K. C., Messeri, P., Hersey, J. C., & Haviland M. L. (2002). Getting to the truth: Evaluating national tobacco countermarketing campaigns. *American Journal of Public Health, 92,* 901–907.

Flynn, B. S., Worden, J. K., Secker-Walker, R. H., Pirie, P. L., Badger, G. J., Carpenter, J. H., et al. (1994). Mass media and school interventions for cigarette smoking prevention: Effects 2 years after completion. *American Journal of Public Health, 84,* 1148–1150.

Kaufman, N., & Yach, D. (2000). Tobacco control—Challenges and prospects. *Bulletin of the World Health Organization, 78,* 867.

National Cancer Policy Board. Institute of Medicine and National Research Council. (1998). *Taking action to reduce tobacco use.* Washington, DC: National Academy Press.

Ringwalt, C. L., Ennett, S., Vincus, A., Thorne, J., Rohrbach, L. A., & Simons-Rudolph, A. (2002). The prevalence of effective substance use prevention curricula in U.S. middle schools. *Prevention Science, 3,* 257–265.

Skara, S. N., & Sussman, S. (*in press*). A review of 25 long-term adolescent tobacco and other drug use prevention program evaluations. *Preventive Medicine.*

Sussman, S. (2002). Effects of sixty-six adolescent tobacco use cessation trials and seventeen prospective studies of self-initiated quitting. *Tobacco Induced Diseases, 1,* 35–81.

Tobler, N. S., Roona, M. R., Ochshorn, P., Marshall, D. G., Streke, A. V., & Stackpole, K. M. (2000). School-based adolescent drug prevention programs: 1998 meta-analysis. *Journal of Primary Prevention, 20,* 275–336.

U.S. Department of Health and Human Services. (2000). *Reducing tobacco use: A report of the Surgeon General.* Atlanta, GA: U.S. Department of Health and Human Services, Public Health Service, CDC, National Center for Chronic Disease Prevention and Health Promotion, Office on Smoking and Health.

Wakefield, M. A., Chaloupka, F. J., Kaufman, N. J., Orleans, C. T., Barker, D. C., & Ruel, E. E. (2000). Effect of restrictions on smoking at home, at school, and in public places on teenage smoking: Cross sectional study. *British Medical Journal, 321,* 333–337.

STEVE SUSSMAN
SILVANA SKARA

Social Comparison Theory

Social comparison, a pervasive aspect of daily life, consists in comparing oneself to others in order to evaluate or enhance some aspect of the self. The first systematic theory of social comparison was proposed by Leon Festinger, who was interested in the effects of social comparisons on self-appraisals of abilities and opinions. Since the 1980s, there has been the recognition that comparisons also influence the thoughts, feelings, and behaviors that affect physical health and illness. For example, if a teenager who surreptitiously smokes marijuana learns that most of his or her peers also smoke marijuana, he or she is more likely to think it is appropriate and continue to smoke. A surgery patient recovering in the hospital may feel better after comparing with patient in the next bed who is experiencing more pain and adversity after experiencing the same surgery. Researchers have devoted considerable effort to understanding what motivations prompt social comparison and its effects in health domains.

SELF-EVALUATION

Festinger proposed that people make social comparisons when they need to know when their opinions are correct and what their abilities allow them to do. When persons are trying to make accurate assessments about their abilities and opinions, their comparisons are motivated by self-evaluation. In some circumstances, certain opinions or abilities cannot be directly tested in the environment because of the costs involved or because objective standards are unavailable. To reduce uncertainty, people compare themselves with others. The general reasoning is that observing similar others, that is, people with similar personal attributes, allows them to learn about their own

possibilities for action and performance. For opinions, finding agreement with others should make one hold the view more confidently.

Stanley Schachter subsequently showed that social comparison also is important for the interpretation of ambiguous emotional states. When people anticipate a novel situation involving a noxious stimulus, such as a potentially painful medical procedure, they may be uncertain about the level of fear that is appropriate. Comparing with another patient also awaiting the same procedure provides a helpful index. In this regard, the recent introduction of Internet chatlines for specific patient groups may be popular because they provide users with the opportunity to compare opinions regarding the appropriateness and interpretation of symptoms, feelings, and expectations about the course of recovery.

Social comparison also may be involved in the interpretation of physical symptoms and decision to seek medical treatment. Access and awareness of internal symptoms are indirect and often ambiguous, leading to uncertainty. For example, whether people label diffuse symptoms such as body aches and feverishness as illness and consequently refer themselves for medical attention may depend on whether their friends are experiencing or have experienced the same symptoms. Extreme cases of symptom labeling via comparison occurs in mass psychogenic illness. These situations involve widespread symptom perception and feelings of being ill among groups of individuals in places like factories, schools, and military bases, even though there is no objective evidence of physical illness. Typically, such episodes occur when people who work closely together or know each other personally are already fatigued or anxious and experiencing ambiguous symptoms, which may only be due to stress. If someone in the group, however, thinks he or she contracted a flu or was bitten by a bug, this becomes a plausible illness label for the ambiguous symptoms, and soon, via social comparison, large numbers of people think they are ill, stay home from work, and seek medical care.

Social comparison also is integrally involved in people's evaluations of the appropriateness of health-relevant attitudes and beliefs. For matters of personal preference, such as deciding whether to select a family physician with a particular bedside manner, people compare views with others who share their personal tastes. In matters of fact, a person seeks someone with more knowledge and expertise, although even in matters of fact, the expert should share the person's basic values to be seen as credible.

SELF-ENHANCEMENT AND SELF-IMPROVEMENT

In some situations, people are more motivated to generate positive evaluations of themselves than to obtain an accurate assessment. Thomas Wills was interested in the kinds of comparisons people make when they feel threats to their subjective well-being. Such cases may arise when people experience a medical threat of some kind, such as learning to adjust to a chronic illness (e.g., cancer or kidney disease). According to Wills's downward comparison theory, people tend to selectively compare with other persons who are worse off than themselves to boost their sense of well-being. For example, in an early study that provided support for this idea, breast cancer patients seemed to benefit from strategic downward comparisons; nearly 80% of those interviewed, even though by available evidence they were not doing well, reported adjusting somewhat better or much better than other cancer patients. Positive contrastive effects are emphasized by downward comparison theory (e.g., "I only had a lumpectomy, but those other women lost a breast"). Because many medical patients experience threatening feelings as a result of their symptoms, pain, and uncertainty associated with their illnesses, downward comparisons might serve as a coping strategy to protect their self-esteem and improve psychological recovery. Much research has been done on the use of social comparison as a coping strategy in persons diagnosed with cancer, infertility, cardiac disease, arthritis, and other diseases.

All evidence gathered in the last two decades, however, does not show that downward comparisons are consistently beneficial for medical patients. Although victims of serious illness may think about or imagine there are others whose medical predicament are even worse, rarely do they prefer to affiliate with more debilitated patients, and such exposure does not necessarily produce positive reactions. Conversely, comparing with someone better off does not necessarily lead to negative feelings. This is because people also may experience a self-improvement motive, which directs comparison in the interest of improving the self. In particular, upward targets (superior role models) may provide hope and inspiration. For example, one experimental study found that exposing breast cancer patients to an audiotape of an interview with a very well-adjusted patient made them feel better about their own prognosis and treatment.

The affective effects of comparison apparently are not determined merely by whether the comparison is with a better versus a worse-off person because, as just noted, upward comparisons can produce positive feelings and downward comparisons can produce negative feelings in some instances. This is because exposure to a better-adjusted person can suggest to the patient that he or she is relatively disadvantaged or alternatively that he or she might be able to improve. Similarly, exposure to a worse-adjusted person can imply that the patient is relatively advantaged, or alternatively he or she might decline to a lower level in the future. The patient's reaction depends on which implication of the comparison is salient. As a result, social comparison sometimes produces assimilation (i.e., when the patient feels he or she is more like the comparison target) rather than contrast (i.e., when the patient feels that he or she is less like the target).

ASSIMILATION AND CONTRAST

Researchers have identified several factors that determine whether assimilation or contrast with a target occurs after comparison. If patients believe that they can obtain the same status as the comparison target or perceive an identification or connection to the target person, then assimilation is more likely. Contrast is maximized when the target is very distinctive or little connection to the target is perceived. More generally, factors that suggest the patient and the comparison target are similar in some way should facilitate seeing even more similarities with the target. On the other hand, factors that imply the patient and the target are different should increase perceived dissimilarity and consequently produce contrast. In addition, the degree to which the patient's self-concept is unclear and there is room for inclusion of additional information, then assimilation is encouraged, assuming there is some psychological connection perceived with the target.

People who differ in personality also respond differently to upward and downward comparisons in terms of assimilation and contrast. For example, cancer patients who are highly neurotic tend to react more negatively to both upward and downward comparison than do more emotionally stable patients. One explanation is that the neurotic individuals can more easily identify (and assimilate themselves) with patients who are worse off and feel less connection (and therefore contrast themselves) with those who are coping better.

Theory and research has shown how social comparisons provide information to reduce uncertainty regarding health-relevant opinions, behaviors, and symptoms. Comparisons also make people who are adjusting to serious health threats feel better about themselves, although whether their spirits will be lifted or lowered by being exposed to a better or worse-off comparison is determined by several factors. Health psychologists are actively researching the effects of social comparisons to develop interventions that promote the adoption of positive health behaviors and adjustment to serious medical threats.

Related Entries: Coping, Symptom Perception, Treatment Delay

BIBLIOGRAPHY

Festinger, L. (1954). A theory of social comparison processes. *Human Relations, 7*, 117–140.
Mechanic, D. (1972). Social psychological factors affecting the presentation of bodily complaints. *New England Journal of Medicine, 286*, 1132–1139.
Stanton, A., Danoff-Burg, S., Cameron, C., Snider, P., & Kirk, S. (1999). Social comparison and adjustment to breast cancer: An experimental

examination of upward affiliation and downward evaluation. *Health Psychology, 18*, 151–158.

Suls, J., Martin, R., & Wheeler, L. (2000). Three kinds of opinion comparison: The Triadic Model. *Personality and Social Psychology Review, 4*, 219–237.

Van der Zee, K., Buunk, B., & Sandersman, R. (1998). Neuroticism and reactions to social comparison information among cancer patients. *Journal of Personality, 66*, 175–194.

Wills, T. A. (1981). Downward comparison principles in social psychology. *Psychological Bulletin, 90*, 245–271.

Wood, J. V., Taylor, S. E., & Lichtman, R. (1985). Social comparison in adjustment to breast cancer. *Journal of Personality and Social Psychology, 49*, 1169–1183.

JERRY SULS

Social Psychology

The idea that social behavior can affect physical as well as mental health seems self-evident, and examples of such types of influence come to mind readily. People who enjoy supportive relationships with friends and family, for example, are less likely to get sick and are quicker to recover when they do; consequently, they tend to live longer. Conversely, the loss of significant social relationships due to death or divorce can have serious health consequences. Adults who are quick to anger or generally wary of others are more likely to develop coronary heart disease than those who are more easygoing; similarly, hostile children are more likely to develop weight problems and other health complications. All of these relations have been documented in research conducted over the last 30 years. Prior to 1970, however, the belief that health status and social behavior are closely (and reciprocally) related was not universally accepted by medical researchers, and it was not an issue for more than a handful of psychologists. Today, social psychology and health psychology are inextricably linked.

Health–social psychology is the study of the relation between social behavior and health. More specifically, it involves applying social psychological theories and principles to the study of health status and health behavior. Historically, social psychology has played a major role in the origin and the development of the area of health psychology. In fact, much of the early work in the 1970s that was instrumental in bringing health psychology to the attention of the broader psychology community was conducted in social psychology labs. These early studies indicated that perceived loss of control (including control of one's social life) can lead eventually to a myriad of health problems. This work was typical of future research in the area because it suggested that the relation between social factors and health outcomes is both direct and indirect.

INDIRECT SOCIAL EFFECTS

The indirect effect involves a mediator or intervening psychological factor. For example, minorities who make internal attributions for the discrimination they encounter (i.e., "They treated me that way because I am Black") are likely to experience frustration and anger, and this cognitive/affective response can, in turn, lead to cardiovascular problems or immune system deficiencies, which can result in increases in susceptibility to illness and disease. Conversely, perceiving that others are genuinely invested in one's well-being is associated with immunocompetence. In fact, this type of perception is a goal of most support groups and is a primary reason why they often succeed. There are numerous other ways in which social interactions can affect mental states (any parent of a teenager can attest to this relation), and that effect can then influence physical health status, through its link with the immune system. This basic, linked model, part of a biopsychosocial approach, has guided the efforts of researchers interested in studying stress reactions for some time.

DIRECT SOCIAL EFFECTS

Physical Attractiveness

The most direct way in which social behavior affects health status is through what could be called psychosocial motives. A primary example involves appearance. The desire to look attractive to others is a very fundamental motive—with evolutionary significance—that is manifested in many different behaviors. Some of those behaviors can be quite beneficial—exercise and watching one's diet, for example. The quest for the perfect body or a healthy complexion can put a person at risk for health problems, however, and, ironically, may end up actually harming appearance. Such is the case with exposure to ultraviolet (UV) light. Sun exposure is a known cancer risk, and there is accumulating evidence that exposure to UV rays from tanning lamps has similar effects. Moreover, UV exposure from either source has been shown to accelerate photoaging (it is estimated that >90% of skin aging is due to UV exposure); nonetheless, the popularity of tanning booths increased almost linearly over the last decade. The desire to look good encourages other behaviors that can endanger health, including eating disorders and fad diets, and having breast implants or cosmetic surgery. Although people often underestimate the risks associated with these behaviors, they are not ignorant of the dangers, and yet many appear to be willing to trade short-term gain for the possibility of long-term pain.

Competitiveness

Another psychosocial motive with possible health consequences is competitiveness. The desire to outperform others reflects a very basic social psychological process, called social comparison, which involves evaluating the self (including behavior) via comparison with others. As Leon Festinger (who created social comparison theory) suggested, one reason why people socially compare is to facilitate self-improvement: They want to learn more about themselves, but they also want to improve, and that often involves competing with others. Once again, competitiveness certainly can be functional and healthy, but examples of health risks and health problems due to irrational (overly enthusiastic) competition abound, from sports injuries, automobile racing accidents, and steroid use, to exhaustion from overwork.

SOCIAL INFLUENCE

Modeling

Most studies of social effects on health have examined social influence of one kind or another. For example, Bandura's social cognitive theory describes ways in which others within adolescents' social worlds can directly influence their health and health behavior. In addition to providing substances (or "risk opportunity"), friends, siblings, and even parents also model substance use, just as TV or sports stars sometimes do. Alternatively, models may demonstrate abstinence or a variety of healthy behaviors, including exercise, regular dental care, or physician visits. In fact, adolescents acquire most of their knowledge about health behavior from observation of others around them; the more they identify with these models, the more they learn from them. Studies of family dynamics and health consistently find that adolescents' healthy and unhealthy behaviors can be predicted accurately by examining the same behaviors of their family members. Moreover, as social cognitive theory suggests, it is the adolescents' perceptions of what others are doing that ultimately affect their behavior; some version of this subjective norm construct can be found in virtually all models of health behavior.

Misperceptions

Often perceptions of what others are doing are biased or distorted. For example, adolescents routinely overestimate the extent to which their peers are engaging in such unhealthy behaviors as smoking, binge drinking, or drug use. Several cognitive explanations for this tendency have been proposed. One is simply that people are more likely to notice and remember actions than inactions—smoking is more memorable than not smoking—and estimates of prevalence are usually based on ease of recall. Another cognitive explanation has to do with a social phenomenon known as pluralistic ignorance. Consider drinking: Nondrinkers are less likely to discuss their abstinence with their peers than drinkers are to discuss their consumption. As a result, nondrinkers (and drinkers as well) do not realize that a majority of their peers actually do not drink. Moreover, the overestimations that result from these misperceptions are important: The more adolescents exaggerate estimates of use among their peers, the more likely they are to start using or to escalate their current use.

SOCIAL COMPARISON

The desire to learn more about the self through comparison with others applies to physical states as well as behavior. For example, research by Suls and his colleagues has shown that people engage in a kind of social comparison of symptom interpretation. When experiencing a new symptom, they will look to others to get a sense of the seriousness of the symptom and what it means. How their experience compares with that of others may determine whether they decide to seek medical attention. Along the same lines, studies by social psychologists have shown that reactions to (bogus) information about illness susceptibility are determined partly by social factors, such as perceived prevalence: People worry less about an illness or genetic predisposition to a particular disease if they believe that either is common. Similarly, Klein and his colleagues have shown that people sometimes respond more to information about their relative risk of disease or injury than their absolute risk. Telling students that their likelihood of having a car accident is high in absolute terms (e.g., 60%), but lower than that of their peers, leads to less concern on their part than telling them that their absolute risk is low (30%), but higher than average. Clearly, social comparison in these kinds of situations can have an important impact on health behavior.

CHANGING HEALTH BEHAVIOR

In an effort to shape and/or modify health behavior, Public Service Announcements and education and intervention programs have borrowed extensively from social psychology. The idea of using attractive actors or sports figures in health messages, for example, comes directly from early research on persuasion, including studies of communicator characteristics. DARE and other refusal efficacy programs ("Just say no!") are based partly on studies of "inoculation" techniques, showing that resistance to persuasion can be bolstered by giving people samples of the types of arguments they are likely to encounter and teaching them how to refute these arguments. Evaluations of these programs indicate they are most effective when they adhere to principles discovered in social psychology labs: For example, keep fear at a reasonable level, provide explicit information as to what behavior is expected and why that behavior will help, and avoid demanding change, so as not to arouse psychological reactance. Finally, presenting accurate information about peers' risk behavior can be effective. Disabusing adolescents (and adults) of the prevalence overestimation described earlier has been shown to reduce participation in the behavior: The less common people believe a risk behavior is, the less willing they will be to do it.

CONCLUSIONS

It has often been suggested that the primary lesson learned from the first 50 years of social psychology research is that people consistently underestimate the extent to which their behavior and that of others is influenced by social factors; indeed, this tendency has been labeled the fundamental attribution error. This applies to health behavior as well—both health-promoting and health-impairing. Susceptibility to social pressure can lead to significant health problems, especially for young people. Nonetheless, this same susceptibility, when used judiciously and appropriately, can be very effective at bringing about health change and thereby improving quality of life.

Related Entries: Social Comparison Theory, Unrealistic Optimism

BIBLIOGRAPHY

Bandura, A. (1997). *Self-efficacy: The exercise of control.* New York: Freeman.

Buunk, B., & Gibbons, F. X. (Eds.). (1997). *Health, coping, and well-being: Perspectives from social comparison theory.* Mahwah, NJ: Erlbaum.

Gerrard, M., Gibbons, F. X., Benthin A., & Hessling, R. M. (1996). A longitudinal study of the reciprocal nature of risk behaviors and cognitions in adolescents: What you do shapes what you think and vice versa. *Health Psychology, 15,* 344–354.

Gibbons, F. X., & Eggleston, T. J. (1996). Smoker networks and the "typical smoker": A prospective analysis of smoking cessation. *Health Psychology, 15,* 469–477.

Gibbons, F. X., Gerrard, M., Blanton, H., & Russell, D. W. (1998). Reasoned action and social reaction: Willingness and intention as independent predictors of health risk. *Journal of Personality and Social Psychology, 74,* 1164–1181.

Salovey, P., Rothman, A. J., & Rodin, J. (1998). Health behavior. In D. T. Gilbert, S. T. Fiske, & G. Lindzey, *The handbook of social psychology* (4th ed., Vol. 2, pp. 633–683). New York: McGraw-Hill.

Stroebe, W. (2000). *Social psychology and health* (2nd ed.). Buckingham, UK: Open University Press.

Suls, J. M., & Wallston, K. (Eds.). (*in press*). *Social psychological foundations of health and illness.* Oxford: Blackwell.

FREDERICK GIBBONS
MEG GERRARD
ELIZABETH POMERY

Social Support

Social support refers to assistance provided by friends, family, and others to an individual who is facing stressful circumstances or problems. This assistance may be aimed at helping the stressed individual solve the problem or at easing the painful emotions caused by the problem. Social support can take many forms, including reassurance, encouragement, a new perspective on the problem, advice, needed resources, or physical assistance with tasks. People who report high levels of social support are less likely to become depressed or ill following stressful life events. There is evidence that their health is better overall and that they are more resistant to infection and recover more quickly from illness than people who report low levels of social support.

This entry covers specific types of social support, aspects of interpersonal relationships that are related to social support, measurement of social support, scientific evidence that social support affects health, and theories about how social support exerts its beneficial health effects.

TYPES OF SOCIAL SUPPORT

Although researchers use somewhat different terms, there is wide agreement on the most important types of social support. Some types of social support are directed at solving the problem or changing the circumstances that are causing the individual distress. These include information support and tangible support. Information support includes advice, guidance, and factual input on the problem situation. Tangible support includes needed resources, such as money or the loan of equipment. It also includes assistance with tasks, such as providing transportation or helping with child care. Support that is directed at problem solution is often termed instrumental support.

People who face difficult situations experience a wide range of emotions, which are often painful and may interfere with effective problem solving. Frequently, these emotions stem from specific beliefs about the self, other people, and the situation. Some types of social support are directed at diminishing the intensity of unpleasant emotions and altering the beliefs that cause them. The first such type is emotional support, which consists of expressions of caring, empathy, and concern. Emotional support reassures the stressed individual that he or she is not alone and that others care about his or her distress. The second is esteem support, which consists of encouragement and expressions of belief in the individual's skills, competence, and value. Esteem support combats beliefs in personal helplessness and fosters self-efficacy. Appraisal support, input on the nature or severity of the problem situation, also addresses beliefs that affect emotional reactions. When people are under stress, they often exaggerate the severity of their problems. Another person can often help the stressed individual put the problem in perspective and evaluate it as less catastrophic or unsolvable.

RELATED ASPECTS OF INTERPERSONAL RELATIONSHIPS

Social support is provided in the context of relationships with other people. Thus, a person who is completely socially isolated lacks social support. Most people have relationships with others, although the number and quality of relationships vary widely. A concept that is closely related to social support is that of the social network. A person's social network consists of the people with whom he or she interacts and who influence his or her life. Many different qualities of social networks have been studied, and some are related to social support. Number of persons in the social network is weakly related to social support. Those with more relationships report somewhat higher social support. However, there is evidence, especially among low-income women, that large networks can be a burden by demanding time, energy, and resources. Frequency of contact with other people is also modestly related to social support. Those who have more frequent contact with others report somewhat higher social support. Those who have networks in which most people know each other report somewhat higher social support, although there is evidence that for some kinds of stressful life events, a network with more diverse people from more diverse settings is most helpful.

Relationships with others are defined by social roles, such as parent, child, sibling, spouse, lover, friend, co-worker, committee member, and acquaintance. Number of roles relates to what is called social integration. There is evidence that people who play multiple social roles have better mental and physical health. It is not clear whether people who play multiple social roles have more social support or whether social integration enhances health in other ways, such as giving structure and predictability to daily life.

People who are experiencing difficult events in their lives are not always treated with warmth and concern. Especially when the person's problems persist over a long period of time, members of the social network may behave in negative or hurtful ways, such as criticizing the stressed person for failing to recover faster. Although this behavior is sometimes termed negative support, a better way to label criticism, complaints, and expressions of blame is negative behavior. Negative behavior has a strong harmful harmful effect on well-being. Most studies find that negative behavior has a larger impact than supportive behavior on well-being.

Actual attempts at assistance that have an unintended negative impact, such as undermining the stressed person's self-confidence, should be termed failed support attempts.

There is evidence that failed support attempts cause resentment in close relationships and can have negative effects on mental and physical health. Failed support attempts are not as damaging as negative behaviors.

MEASURING SOCIAL SUPPORT

Three different approaches to measuring the quantity and quality of social support in people's lives have been developed. These approaches are described well in a book edited by Sheldon Cohen, Lynn Underwood, and Benjamin Gottlieb. The first approach measures perceived social support. Measures of perceived social support assess people's subjective judgments about the extent to which members of their social network provide social support in times of need. Perceived social support measures incorporate judgments of the quality of the support that is available, sometimes through questions about how satisfied the individual is with the support he or she typically receives. A different approach measures received social support. Measures of received social support assess how frequently specific types of social support were provided by members of the social network, usually in the last month. Both perceived and received social support are measured with questionnaires. The third approach to measuring social support does not rely on questionnaires, but on observations of actual conversations. Observational coding systems to quantify observed social support typically yield frequency counts of different types of social support during a 10- to 20-min interaction in which one person is asked to disclose a personal problem or concern to another person. The emotional tone (e.g., warmth or hostility) of each social support behavior may also be evaluated. Observed social support measures were first developed in the early 1990s, so much less research has been published on their association with health than on measures of perceived and received social support, which have been used since the early 1970s.

There are advantages and disadvantages of each approach to measuring social support. Measures of perceived social support tap the recipient's subjective evaluations of the quality of support he or she believes is available from the social network. These evaluations may reflect subtle differences in the sensitivity and reliability of the person's support resources that are not captured by other kinds of support measures. Perceived support measures allow the individual to express the extent to which the support provided by the social network reflects his or her specific preferences and needs. However, measures of perceived social support have been criticized because of their subjectivity. People's personalities affect the way they evaluate others. Thus, it has been argued that measures of perceived social support reflect peoples' personalities more than the actual social support resources available to them. How much people like another person and feel they have in common with another person also affect judgments about that person's supportiveness. Perceived support may also be colored by relationship beliefs. Individuals who believe that others are generally responsive to their needs may perceive high levels of support in relationships that are not actually supportive. Some research shows that when an actual crisis occurs in peoples' lives, they receive less social support than they expected. Thus, estimates of type and quality of support that would be available if needed are biased in ways that decrease their accuracy. Despite these inaccuracies, an important point is that measures of perceived social support show by far the strongest associations with mental and physical health. Although peoples' perceptions of social support may be somewhat inaccurate, they appear to be very important to well-being.

Measures of received social support involve less subjectivity and are viewed as somewhat more accurate reflections of the support resources available to the individual because they are based on actual experiences in a specified time period. However, the circumstances of the time period when received support is measured may affect the nature of the person's responses. If received support is assessed during a period of relative calm, the results may not generalize to times of extreme crisis. Thus, actual support resources in times of extreme duress may be greater or less than would be expected based on one measurement of received support. Another issue is that received social support measures do not tap the quality of support received to the same degree as measures of perceived social support. Thus, many instances of support may be reported, but if none of them meet the specific needs or preferences of the stressed person, a high score may not reflect high-quality support. Measures of perceived and received support do not correlate very highly. Research shows that received social support scores are not as strongly associated with mental and physical health as are perceived support scores. In fact, some studies show that people who report higher levels of received support are actually more distressed. This may reflect the fact that when people face more severe stressful events, the people in their social network provide more support. Thus, level of received support may be an index of the severity of the stressor or the distress of the stress victim.

Measures of observed social support are useful for understanding exactly how people communicate support to one another. Not all social support attempts are successful. Observing actual support transactions provides information on verbal and nonverbal components of effective social support. This information is needed to develop interventions that help people become more effective support providers. Observational measures are not biased by the personality or relationship beliefs of the individual. However, like measures of received support, observational methods do not tap the subtle nuances of interactions that enter into people's subjective evaluations of the support they receive. Observational assessments of social support are also limited because they are based on a single brief interaction between two people. This small sample of behavior may or may not be representative of how the individuals typically interact. A related method for assessing social support that addresses this problem is the daily diary. Individuals are asked to keep daily records on their interactions with other people over a 1- to 2-week period. In a sense, people serve as their own observers. They complete ratings of how supportive interactions were and report on the content of the interactions they have with other people. Although the objectivity of a trained observer is lost, the advantage of the daily diary approach is the longer time frame over which support interactions are recorded. Most studies using observational and daily diary techniques to assess social support have focused on the relation between social support and the quality of specific relationships, such as marital satisfaction. Few studies have tested links between observed support and health. A small literature suggests that support measured in daily diary studies is associated with better mood and lower anxiety.

MEASUREMENT OF SOCIAL NETWORK VARIABLES AND SOCIAL INTEGRATION

Social network variables, such as number in the network and frequency of contact with network members, are typically assessed by asking individuals to generate a list of the people with whom they interact on a regular basis. Frequency of contact with each person is assessed, as well as other characteristics of the relationship with that person. Social integration is assessed by a series of questions about participation in social roles, such as marital status, contact with friends and relatives, church membership, and participation in organized and informal groups.

ASSOCIATIONS BETWEEN SOCIAL RELATIONSHIPS AND HEALTH

The relation between social support and health is not simple, and many questions remain about the aspects of social relationships that are most important to health. Some associations between social relationships and health are supported by strong and consistent evidence, but others are found less consistently. Research on ties between social integration and health began in the 1960s. In the mid-1970s, researchers began to investigate links between social support and health. The best known study of social integration and health was conducted in the 1960s and 1970s in Alameda County, California. Lisa Berkman and S. Leonard Syme studied the health and social integration of approximately 5,000 men and women over a 9-year period. They discovered that people were significantly less likely to die during that 9-year period if they were actively involved with family, friends, church, and civic organizations. This association between social integration and mortality was significant regardless of gender, income, or physical health at the beginning of the study. In fact, the researchers found that social isolation posed about the same degree of risk to health as cigarette smoking, high blood pressure, and obesity. The relation between social integration and mortality has been replicated in several studies. In addition, social integration has been associated with lower rates of mental and physical illness, better adjustment to chronic illness, and recovery following heart attack, stroke, and cancer. Sheldon Cohen and his colleagues conducted an experiment in which people were intentionally exposed to a cold virus. They found that people who were high on social integration were less likely to develop an upper respiratory illness than those who were low on social integration. In sum, there is abundant evidence that active involvement with other people is associated with better health. One question that remains concerning the effects of social integration on health is whether relationships are actually beneficial or whether social isolation is harmful.

Relatively few studies have examined links between perceived or received social support and mortality. However, in Sweden, Bertil Hanson found that elderly men with high social support were less likely to die over a 5-year period than men with low support, and Kristina Orth-Gomer found that middle-aged men with high levels of emotional social support were less likely to develop coronary artery disease than those with low levels. In the United States, Lisa Berkman and colleagues found that men with high levels of emotional support were more likely to survive a heart attack than men with low emotional support, and Alan Christensen and colleagues found that hemodialysis patients survived longer if they had high rather than low levels of support from their families. There is evidence from two additional studies that social support prevents stressful life events from increasing one's risk for mortality.

The most consistent health-related finding is that people who have high levels of perceived social support are less likely to become depressed following negative life events. Sheldon Cohen and Thomas Wills reviewed a large number of studies and concluded that perceived availability of social support protects or buffers people from emotional distress following a wide range of stressful life events, such as job loss, death of a loved one, and criminal victimization. A second consistent finding is that people with high perceived social support report that they are in better physical health than people who have low perceived support. This association must be interpreted with caution because psychological factors strongly influence self-assessments of health. People who are demoralized or depressed evaluate their physical health more negatively than people who are in good spirits. There is considerable evidence that people who have higher perceived support engage in healthful behaviors

more than people who perceive little social support from their network. For example, people with high perceived support tend to exercise, take their medication, and eat healthy foods more than people with low perceived social support. They are also less likely to abuse alcohol. People who perceive their spouse to be supportive are more successful when they try to lose weight or stop smoking.

The evidence that perceived and received social support influence objective measures of physical health is somewhat mixed. Bert Uchino and colleagues summarized the results of numerous studies and concluded that social support has a small but consistent association with blood pressure and a somewhat stronger association with healthy functioning of the immune system. They found that cardiovascular reactivity (increased heart rate) in response to a laboratory-induced stressor was significantly lower among people with high social support than among those with low social support. Mixed results have been found regarding the effect of social support on recovery from illnesses. Perceived support was significantly related to greater mobility, lower pain, less use of pain medication, and shorter hospital stay in some studies, but it was not related to pain, functional status, or health status in other studies.

Some studies have shown that negative behaviors have a greater influence on mental and physical health than supportive behaviors. In addition, not all support attempts are successful. For example, James Coyne and colleagues found that among heart attack survivors, spouse overprotectiveness undermined self-efficacy. Overly protective spouse behavior is associated with poorer functional status among patients with chronic back pain as well.

HOW DO SOCIAL RELATIONSHIPS INFLUENCE HEALTH?

There are two major theories regarding the influence of social relationships on health. The first is the direct effects model and the second is the buffering model. An excellent discussion of these theories is contained in a book edited by Sheldon Cohen, Lynn Underwood, and Benjamin Gottlieb.

The direct effects model states that relationships with other people can confer health benefits in good times and bad times through their influence on emotions, thoughts, and behaviors. It is most useful as an explanation for the link between social integration and health. The direct effects approach is rooted in ideas expressed over 100 years ago by Emile Durkheim. He believed that modern industrial society was harmful to people's well-being because it disrupted traditional social ties. People suffer in the absence of clear social roles and strong ties to family and community. Integration into a social network provides resources that are needed for healthy functioning. These include predictability, stability, clear role expectations, and a sense of belonging and purpose. All of these resources contribute to emotional well-being. Emotional well-being is known to influence physical health. People who are embedded in a social network also benefit from the resources they may obtain from members of their social network, such as advice on how to deal with health problems. Because they serve needed functions within their network, people may feel obligated to guard their health by engaging in healthful behaviors, such as exercise and regular physical examinations. It is also possible that social isolation is inherently damaging to people's health. Social integration may simply prevent the deleterious effects of isolation.

The buffering model states that relationships with other people primarily confer health benefits in times of duress by protecting or buffering the individual from the harmful effects of stressful life events on health. It is most useful as an explanation for the links between social support and health. John Cassel and Sidney Cobb were early and influential proponents of the buffering model of social support. In the 1980s, Sheldon Cohen and Thomas Wills wrote an influential scientific article about this model.

Both perceived and received social support play a role in the buffering model of social support. In the early stages of confronting a problem, the perception that support is available may allow people to appraise the problem as less severe because they believe that others are available to help them deal with the problem. Potentially harmful emotions of fear and despair may be averted. Actual support received may facilitate effective problem solving. Network members may provide input that helps the individual put the problem in perspective, further dampening dysfunctional emotional reactions. They may offer emotional and esteem support, which prevent feelings of isolation and helplessness. They may provide advice about how to solve the problem, and even offer to take direct action that will contribute to problem solution. Thus, the stressed individual may benefit from perceptions that others care about his or her dilemma and the belief that others are available to provide assistance and encouragement, and from input that allows him or her to appraise the problem realistically and take appropriate actions to remove or cope with the cause of his or her distress.

Both the direct effects model and the buffering model provide good explanations for how social support prevents negative attitudes, emotions, and behaviors. Researchers are striving to better understand how these factors influence the physiological processes involved in physical health and illness. There is evidence that psychological states influence neuroendocrine responses (the brain's regulatory activities), the immune system, and the cardiovascular system. When the physiology of stress and well-being is better understood, we will have a more complete picture of the mechanisms through which social integration and social support influence health.

In conclusion, multiple components of interpersonal relationships appear to have consequences for health. There is evidence that both social integration and social support decrease risk for mortality and predict better health outcomes; however, some studies have not found a significant link between these variables and health. Both social integration and social support appear to improve psychological well-being, but it is not clear under what circumstances or through what mechanisms psychological well-being translates into physical health. Research is progressing rapidly in this area and will shed light on the precise links among interpersonal relationships, social support, and health.

Related Entry: Social Support Questionnaire

BIBLIOGRAPHY

Berkman, L. F., Leo-Summers, L., & Horwitz, R. I. (1992). Emotional support and survival after myocardial infarction. *Annals of Internal Medicine, 117,* 1003–1009.

Berkman, L., & Syme, S. L. (1979). Social networks, host resistance and mortality: A nine-year follow-up study of Alameda County residents. *American Journal of Epidemiology, 109,* 186–204.

Cassel, J. (1976). The contribution of the social environment to host resistance. *American Journal of Epidemiology, 107,* 107–123.

Christensen, A. J., Wiebe, J. S., Smith, T. W., & Turner, C. W. (1994). Predictors of survival among hemodialysis patients: Effect of perceived family support. *Health Psychology, 13,* 521–525.

Cobb, S. (1976). Social support as a moderator of life stress. *Psychosomatic Medicine, 38,* 300–314.

Cohen, S., Doyle, W. J., Skoner, D. P., Rabin, B. S., & Gwaltney, Jr., J. M. (1997). Social ties and susceptibility to the common cold. *Journal of the American Medical Association, 277,* 1940–1944.

Cohen, S., Underwood, L. G., & Gottlieb, B. H. (2000). *Social support measurement and intervention: A guide for health and social scientists.* New York: Oxford University Press.

Cohen, S., & Wills, T. A. (1985). Stress, social support, and the buffering hypothesis. *Psychological Bulletin, 98,* 310–357.

Coyne, J. C., & Smith, D. A. F. (1994). Couples coping with myocardial infarction: Contextual perspective on patient self-efficacy. *Journal of Family Psychology, 8,* 43–54.

Durkheim, E. (1897/1951). *Suicide.* New York: Free Press.

Hanson, B. S., Isacsson, S.-O., Janzon, L., & Lindell, S.-E. (1989). Social network and social support influence mortality in elderly men: Prospective population study of men born in 1914 in Malmo, Sweden. *American Journal of Epidemiology, 130,* 100–111.

Orth-Gomer, K., Rosengren, A., & Wilhelmsen, L. (1993). Lack of social support and incidence of coronary heart disease in middle-aged Swedish men. *Psychosomatic Medicine, 55,* 37–43.

Uchino, B. N., Cacioppo, J. T., & Kiecolt-Glaser, J. K. (1996). The relationship between social support and physiological processes: A review with emphasis on underlying mechanisms and implications for health. *Psychological Bulletin, 119,* 488–531.

CAROLYN E. CUTRONA
KELLI A. GARDNER

Social Support Questionniare

Social support is generally defined as the role played by social relationships in individuals' psychological and physical health. It had long been observed that some people are better able than others to avoid negative effects from stress. One answer to why this is so came in 1976 when John C. Cassel provided evidence that the presence of others promoted disease resistance and prevention of pathological states in people and animals that were experiencing stress, and Sidney Cobb documented the clinical importance of feelings of belonging and being esteemed and valued. Because social support had many practical implications, defining and measuring it precisely became very important. Questionnaires were developed to assess such aspects of a person's life as the receipt of help in stressful situations, the perception of being cared about by others and their availability of help if needed, and the characteristics of the person's social network. Later research has shown that there is little agreement among these types of measures of social support. Measures of perceptions of support have been most useful as predictors of health outcomes.

The Social Support Questionnaire (SSQ), a measure of perceived available support, was one of the earliest measures and is still one of the most widely used. It assesses the social support that a person perceives to be available. The SSQ measures both the number of supporters available and the satisfaction with the support they may be expected to provide. A sample item reads, "Whom can you really count on to care about you regardless of what is happening to you?" The test taker is asked to list the initials and relationship of up to nine people under each item or to circle the words "No One" and then to indicate "How Satisfied" on a 6-point scale. Two scores, for number and for satisfaction, are recorded.

Although the majority of social support measures in use fit under the perceived support category, they differ in specifics that affect their use as predictors. Some, like the SSQ, sum across situations, others sum across individuals. Some measures consider perceived social support to be a general factor, which might be called a "sense of support." Others divide available social support into its various functions. The idea behind this approach is that the type of support perceived to be available must match the specific need created by a stressor in order to be effective.

As more research was carried out on social support, it became clear that support or lack of it from specific close relationships was also important. A measure of support and conflict in specific relationships, together with a general measure of social support, adds to prediction of health outcome.

The beneficial effects of social support and its role in health promotion, recovery from illness, and mortality risk are substantial, although the processes that link support and health are not well understood. Support has effects on the neuroendocrine and immune systems, presumably because of an increased level of physiological excitation. One of the strongest linkages between social support and health is in the area of coronary heart disease. Support can serve as a buffer against cardiac risk factors including physiological changes such as hypertension and cholesterol level and behavioral risk factors such as smoking and overweight. Perception of support availability is also important in depression, which itself is a mortality risk.

Related Entry: Social Support

BIBLIOGRAPHY

Cassel, J. (1976). The contribution of the social environment to host resistance. *American Journal of Epidemiology, 104*, 107–123.

Cobb, S. (1976). Social support as a moderator of life stress. *Psychosomatic Medicine, 38*, 300–314.

Sarason, B. R., Sarason, I. G., & Gurung, R. A. R. (2001). Close personal relationships and health outcomes: A key to the role of social support. In B. R. Sarason & S. W. Duck (Eds.), *Personal relationships: Implications for clinical and community psychology* (pp. 00–00). Chichester, UK: Wiley.

Sarason, I. G., Levine, H. M., Basham, R. B., & Sarason, B. R. (1983). Assessing social support: The Social Support Questionnaire. *Journal of Personality and Social Psychology, 44*, 127–139.

BARBARA R. SARASON

Society of Behavioral Medicine

The Society of Behavioral Medicine's mission is to foster the advancement of scientific knowledge surrounding behavioral, biological, and social determinants of health and disease, and to promote the application of this knowledge to assure optimal individual and population health outcomes.

The Society of Behavioral Medicine (SBM) was founded in 1978 as a multidisciplinary, nonprofit organization to advance the science and practice of behavioral medicine. Behavioral medicine is the multidisciplinary field concerned with the behavioral and social aspects of medical conditions. Consumers and a wide variety of health professionals are involved in behavioral medicine research and practice, including cardiologists, counselors, epidemiologists, exercise physiologists, family physicians, health educators, internists, nurses, nutritionists, pediatricians, psychiatrists, and psychologists. Behavioral medicine takes a life-span approach to health and health care, working with children, teens, adults, and seniors individually and in groups, and working with racially and ethnically diverse communities in the United States and abroad.

Today, SBM is the nation's premiere multidisciplinary organization dedicated to advancing the service and practice of behavioral medicine. The society represents over 2,500 behavioral and biomedical researchers and clinicians from more than 18 disciplines (e.g., psychophysiology, psychology, medicine, epidemiology, genetics, psychoneuroimmunology, nursing, health education, medical sociology, biostatistics, health policy). SBM's membership spans from student members (23%) and new investigators to the nation's leading experts in behavioral medicine research, practice, and policy, many of whom are fellows in the society. SBM provides the many disciplines represented with an interactive network for education and collaboration on common research, clinical, and public policy concerns related to prevention, diagnosis and treatment, rehabilitation, and health promotion. The vast majority of SBM members include one or more of the following health behavior change areas as their primary specialty or area of interest: physical activity/fitness, nutrition, obesity, tobacco cessation, addictive behaviors, HIV/AIDS prevention, compliance, public health, health communication, health promotion, and disease prevention.

SBM's current goals include integrating evidence-based behavioral medicine protocols into mainstream medicine; building public, practitioner, and policy-maker understanding of and demand for proven behavioral medicine interventions; increasing policy support for expanded behavioral medicine research and practice; maintaining and improving the quality of support and professional networking provided to members through its journal (*Annals of Behavioral Medicine*), newsletter (*Outlook*), website, annual meetings, and professional education and mentorship activities; and establishing collaborative working relationships with related professional and research organizations.

ANNALS OF BEHAVIORAL MEDICINE

Annals of Behavioral Medicine, the official journal of SBM, fosters the exchange of knowledge derived from the disciplines involved in the field of behavioral medicine and the integration of applicable basic and applied research. The journal, which is listed in *Index Medicus*, publishes empirical research articles, reviews, and special series of interest to researchers, clinicians, students, and trainees in health professions. Each year, the journal also publishes detailed proceedings and abstracts of SBM's annual meeting. A subscription is included as a member benefit of belonging to SBM. Individual and institutional subscriptions are also available through Lawrence Erlbaum and Associates (www.erlbaum.com). The journal is available in electronic and hard-copy formats.

OUTLOOK

Outlook, SBM's quarterly newsletter, keeps members abreast of recent advances in behavioral medicine through articles about the society's committee activities and news about members. The newsletter also includes classified advertising for positions available in behavioral medicine programs.

WEBSITE

The Society's website (www.sbm.org) offers members easy access to a variety of information including SBM's newsletter, a directory of training opportunities, behavioral medicine course syllabi, links to behavioral medicine-related websites, information about upcoming meetings, and programs and job announcements.

ANNUAL MEETINGS AND SCIENTIFIC SESSIONS

SBM's annual scientific meetings are held in the spring. Attendance is open to members as well as nonmembers. Information about locations, dates, and themes for upcoming meetings is available at the SBM website. Research presented at SBM's meeting is solicited through a general call for abstracts and reflects the multidisciplinary makeup of SBM's membership. Presentation formats for the meeting include paper, poster, seminar, and symposium. Invited lectures and workshops are also part of the program. A variety of continuing education credits are available to meeting attendees.

MEMBERSHIP INFORMATION

Membership in SBM is open to individuals with an interest in the field of behavioral medicine. Full membership in SBM requires completion of a terminal degree in behavioral medicine or a related field. Discounted rates are available for student members. The SBM website provides application information.

Related Entries: American Psychological Association, American Psychosomatic Society

BIBLIOGRAPHY

Society of Behavioral Medicine. Available at http://www.sbm.org

BETH KLIPPING

Socioeconomic Status and Health

Socioeconomic status (SES), traditionally assessed by income, education, and occupation, reflects individuals' material and social resources. Various theories of social stratification emphasize different aspects of SES and suggest different types of measurement. However, virtually all measures of SES are related to morbidity and mortality, suggesting that SES is a pervasive and robust influence on health.

WHAT IS THE ASSOCIATION OF SES AND HEALTH?

In industrialized countries, SES is related to health at all levels of the socioeconomic hierarchy. It is not simply that those in poverty experience poorer health than those with more income; even individuals well above the poverty level have poorer health than those who are relatively more affluent. At an individual level, the health burden of socioeconomic disadvantage is most acute for the very poorest. At a population level, because a far greater proportion of people are in the middle of the SES distribution than at the extremes, a substantial proportion of health effects related to socioeconomic factors occur to those who are not in extreme poverty. Although the association of SES and health extends to the top of the SES hierarchy, for some health outcomes (e.g., infant mortality), the association is stronger at the bottom than at the top. Thus, although health benefits still accrue as SES improves to the very top, the marginal benefits of higher SES may diminish at upper levels.

The monotonic relationship of SES and health has been demonstrated with each of the main components of SES. With regard to occupation, the Whitehall Studies of British civil servants found that higher occupational grade was associated with lower mortality, not only when comparing the lowest grade civil servants to the highest, but also when comparing midlevel civil servants to those at the highest levels. As noted, studies of income also reveal lower mortality as income increases, although there is a steeper drop in mortality associated with increasing income among those with the least income. Benefits of education also accrue to health not simply from high school graduation, but also from college graduation and from graduate degrees, although these benefits may not be equally enjoyed by men and women and by all racial/ethnic groups.

Given the association of SES with mortality, it is not surprising that SES is also related to morbidity. Incidence and prevalence of most diseases increase as SES decreases. The association is especially strong for cardiovascular disease, arthritis, diabetes, chronic respiratory diseases, and cervical cancer.

Incidence of mental diseases is also greater among lower-SES populations. Among the mental diseases, SES is most closely associated with schizophrenia, substance use, and anxiety disorders. There are a few diseases that show the opposite pattern and are more common among higher-SES individuals. Most notable are breast cancer and malignant melanoma. These associations are partially accounted for by SES-related differences in risk-related behaviors: delayed childbearing with regard to breast cancer and recreational tanning with regard to melanoma.

WHAT ACCOUNTS FOR THE ASSOCIATION OF SES AND HEALTH?

There is no single factor accounting for the association of SES and health. Several pathways have been identified, and are summarized in the following subsections.

Physical Conditions

Lower-SES individuals are subject to a range of health-damaging conditions. Less affluent populations have greater exposure to adverse living conditions including crowding, poor sanitation, peeling paint, substandard housing, proximity to dump sites, and greater air pollution. The environmental justice movement has raised awareness of such differential exposure. Environmental justice has been adopted by governmental agencies, including the Environmental Protection Agency, and has led to policy and zoning reform to assure a more equal burden of environmental risk.

Physical exposures also occur in the workplace. Lower-SES occupations more often involve manual labor, which may place workers at risk for injury and involve greater exposure to toxins. Material conditions, such as car and house ownership, have also been linked to better health, and appear to make an independent contribution to morbidity and mortality above and beyond the standard SES measures.

Access to Health Care

Those who are poorer, unemployed, and less educated are less likely to have access to high-quality health care. In the United States, private health insurance is tied to employment, and a substantial segment of the population is uninsured. The uninsured have less access to preventive services, screening and early diagnosis, and high-quality care. Even among those who have access to the same system of health care (e.g., members of health maintenance organizations), lower SES continues to be linked to poorer health outcomes. Knowledge of how to utilize the health system to get higher-quality care (which is likely to be greater among those with more education) may play a role in this association. However, it may also be due to conditions outside of the health care system linked to SES that are affecting outcomes.

Health Behaviors

Health behaviors are estimated to be responsible for more than 40% of premature mortality. Behaviors that are most responsible for premature mortality are smoking, sedentary lifestyle, poor diet, sexual risk behaviors, and substance use. Rates of these health-risking behaviors increase the lower one's income, education, and/or occupational status. For example, 52% of men with less than a high school education smoke cigarettes, compared to 43% of high school graduates and 29% of college graduates.

In addition to behavioral contributions to the onset of disease, SES-related behaviors may affect the course of disease. Treatment for many diseases and conditions requires close adherence to prescribed regimens. For example, the course of diabetes is greatly affected by dietary intake and monitoring of blood glucose. Diabetics with less education have been found to show poorer adherence, and differences in adherence largely account for the association of education and course of disease. Similar findings emerge with regard to adherence to antiretroviral therapy among HIV-positive patients.

Psychosocial Responses

Higher SES is associated with greater protection from adverse health effects of stress. Both acute and chronic stress are reported more frequently among those lower on the SES hierarchy. Possessing more resources, whether from higher education, income, or occupational status, may help people avoid situations that are stressful and also help them cope more effectively with those that they do encounter. It is easier to engage in active coping strategies, which are generally associated with better health, when one has more resources with which to address threatening situations. The wear and tear on the body of responding to more frequent and chronic exposures to stress heightens the risk of dysregulation of the hypothalamic–pituitary–adrenal axis, which is central to the stress response and to the development of disease.

More-threatening and adverse environments associated with lower SES may engender psychological responses that increase the risk of disease. Hostility, anger, optimism/pessimism, sense of control, and social support, all of which are associated with disease risk, are also related to SES. Though few studies have directly tested whether these psychological variables mediate the impact of SES on disease, there are numerous studies showing that they are related on one hand to SES and on the other hand to disease risk.

Health Affects SES

Although the predominant causal direction appears to be from SES to health, health may also affect SES. Individuals who are in poorer health may be less likely to achieve higher SES status. Children from poorer families are reported by their parents to have worse health. Poorer health in childhood can contribute to missed school and lower achievement. The impact of health on educational attainment is likely to be greatest from diseases that have their onset during childhood and adolescence (e.g., asthma, schizophrenia). In later life, those who become ill may be less likely to be able to work, which affects their income and occupational status.

HOW DOES SES RELATE TO RACE/ETHNICITY AND GENDER?

People of color in the United States generally have poorer health status than do White Americans. For example, compared to Whites, African-Americans have poorer overall health and higher rates of HIV/AIDS, diabetes, heart disease, cancer, and stroke For some conditions, racial/ethnic group differences become nonsignificant once socioeconomic factors (e.g., income) is controlled for. For other conditions, racial/ethnic group differences remain even after controlling for SES. These findings suggest that to some extent racial/ethnic health disparities are due to socioeconomic disadvantage, but that unique experiences associated with minority status (e.g., experiences of discrimination, residential segregation) also play a role. Associations of SES with health differ by gender as well as by race and ethnicity. The meaning of a given SES indicator may vary for men versus women and for Whites versus people of color, which suggests the importance of looking at SES influences on health within each group.

BIBLIOGRAPHY

Adler, N., Boyce, T., Chesney, M., Cohen, S., Folkman, S., Kahn, R., et al. (1994). Socioeconomic status and health: The challenge of the gradient. *American Psychologist, 49,* 15–24.

Case, A., & Paxson, C. (2002). Parental behavior and child health. *Health Affairs, 21,* 164–178.

Elo, I. T., & Preston, S. H. (1996). Educational differentials in mortality: United States, 1979–85. *Social Science and Medicine, 42,* 47–57.

Evans, G. W., & Kantrowitz, E. (2002). Socioeconomic status and health: The potential role of environmental risk exposure. *Annual Review of Public Health, 23,* 303–331.

Gallo, L. C., & Matthews, K. A. (2003). Understanding the association between socioeconomic status and physical health: Do negative emotions play a role? *Psychological Bulletin, 129,* 10–51.

Goldman, D. P., & Smith, J. P. (2002). Can patient self-management help explain the SES health gradient? *Proceedings of the National Academy of Sciences of the USA, America, 99,* 10929–10934.

Health, United States, 1998. National Center for Health Statistics. Website: www1.oecd.org/std/others1.html.

IOM Report: Committee on the Consequences of Uninsurance, Board on Health Care Services. (2002). *Care without courage: too little, too late.* Washington, DC: National Academy Press.

Kessler, R. C., McGonagle, K. A., Zhao, S., Nelson, C. B., Hughes, M., Eshelman, S., et al. (1994). Lifetime and 12-month prevalence of DSM-III-R. Psychiatric disorders in the United States. *Archives of General Psychiatry, 51,* 8–19.

Macintyre, S., Ellaway, A., Der, G., Ford, G., & Hunt, K. (1998). Do housing tenure and car access predict health because they are simply markers of income or self-esteem? A Scottish study. *Journal of Epidemiology and Community Health, 52,* 657–664.

Marmot, M. G., Davey, Smith, G., Stansfeld, S., Patel, C., North, F., Head, J., et al. (1991). Health inequalities among British civil servants: The Whitehall II study. *Lancet, 337,* 1387–1393.

McEwen, B. S. (2002). Research to understand the mechanisms through which social and behavioral factors influence health. In L. F. Berkman (Ed.), *Through the kaleidoscope: Viewing the contributions of the behavioral and social sciences to health* (pp. 31–35). Washington, DC: National Academy Press.

McGinnis, J. M., Williams-Russo, P., & Knickman, J. R. (2002). The case for more active policy attention to health promotion. *Health Affairs, 21,* 78–93.

Ostrove, J. M., & Adler, N. E. (1998). Socioeconomic status and health. *Current Opinion in Psychiatry, 11,* 649–653.

Smith, J. (1999). Healthy bodies and thick wallets: The dual relationship between health and socioeconomic status. *Journal of Economic Perspectives,* 145–166.

Williams, D. R. (1999). Race, socioeconomic status, and health: The added effects of racism and discrimination. *Annals of the New York Academy of Sciences, 896,* 173–188.

NANCY E. ADLER

Somatization

Somatization is the general tendency to experience or communicate emotional distress in the form of physiological symptoms. In a somatized clinical presentation, a patient may complain of bodily symptoms that have no organic explanation; bodily symptoms that are judged to be in excess of what might be expected on the basis of objective medical findings (with the assumption that "psychological overlay" complicates the physical disorder); or bodily symptoms that are observable, are not the result of detectable damage to an organ, but are presumed to be related to psychological factors (i.e., a functional somatic syndrome). Laurence Kirmayer and James Robbins noted that somatizing patients vary widely in the level of medically unexplained symptoms and illness worry they report, and this may create further distinctions in the subtypes present in primary care medical settings.

In all subtypes, if a medical professional attempts to convince the patient that the somatic symptoms are manifestations of stress or anxiety, the patient often feels that his or her condition has been misunderstood. Somatizing patients are reluctant to accept psychosocial explanations for their suffering. They persistently seek medical diagnoses and treatments despite reassurances that they are not seriously ill. In addition, they tend to use medical services in inefficient or maladaptive ways, such as consulting multiple providers for the same complaint.

The general concept of somatization is different from Somatization Disorder, which is a psychiatric condition defined by the *Diagnostic and Statistical Manual of Mental Disorders* (*DSM-IV*; American Psychiatric Association, 1994). Individuals who are diagnosed with Somatization Disorder display impaired functioning and a complex pattern of somatic complaints that involves multiple bodily sites and functions. Both forms are common in patients seen by general medical practitioners. The prevalence of somatization is rising with the progressive medicalization of our society. Accurate understanding and detection of this condition might help to reduce the somatizing patients' disproportionately high number of medical visits, drug prescriptions, and surgical procedures.

Several models have been proposed to explain the phenomenon of somatization. The defense model holds that patients unconsciously substitute physical symptoms for psychological symptoms to keep their emotional distress out of awareness. This model is based on the classic ideas of conversion and defense that were common in the early history of psychosomatic medicine. Unfortunately, this model does not fit with the empirical evidence that anxiety and depressive symptoms are typically presented along with somatization symptoms.

As an alternative to the defense model, somatization may be explained as the result of amplification of nonspecific distress. In this model, underlying distress gives rise to both physical and psychological symptoms in individuals who possess a neurotic personality style, or a perceptual style inclined to make negative interpretations of ambiguous signals. This would help account for the fact that some of the most common somatization symptoms seen in medicine, such as dizziness, shortness of breath, and chest pain, are also known to be the core symptoms of anxiety.

Related Entries: Neuroticism, Psychosomatic Medicine

BIBLIOGRAPHY

American Psychiatric Association. (1994). *The diagnostic and statistical manual of mental disorders* (4th ed.). Washington, DC: American Psychiatric Association.

Barsky, A. J., & Borus, J. F. (1995). Somatization and medicalization in the era of managed care. *Journal of the American Medical Association, 274,* 1931–1938.

Kirmayer, L. J., & Robbins, J. M. (1991). Three forms of somatization in primary care: Prevalence, co-occurrence, and sociodemographic characteristics. *Journal of Nervous and Mental Disease, 179,* 647–655.

Kirmayer, L. J., & Robbins, J. M. (Eds.). (1991). *Current concepts of somatization: Research and clinical perspectives.* Washington, DC: American Psychiatric Press.
Lipowski, Z. J. (1988). Somatization: The concept and its clinical application. *American Journal of Psychiatry, 145,* 1358–1368.

HEIDI T. BECKMAN

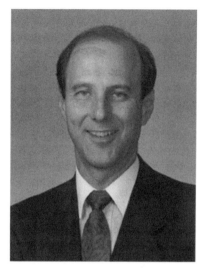

Spiegel, David

Spiegel, David (1945–)

David Spiegel was born on December 11, 1945. He is Willson Professor in the School of Medicine, associate chair of psychiatry and behavioral sciences, and medical director of the Center for Integrative Medicine at Stanford University School of Medicine. Spiegel is known for his long-term studies of the psychological and physiological benefits of support groups for women with metastatic breast cancer. He was the first to demonstrate that group support results in significantly enhanced survival time for cancer patients. His widely cited 10-year randomized clinical trial, which was published in the *Lancet* in 1989, demonstrated that women with metastatic breast cancer who received weekly structured emotional and social support along with traditional medical care exhibited less anxiety, depression, and pain than women who did not receive such support. Moreover, the women assigned to participate in support groups lived on average 18 months longer than did their counterparts who did not receive such support. He also showed that such support groups actually alter patients' coping styles, causing them to be less inclined to suppress their own emotional responses to stress. This survival study was referred to in *Newsweek* (August 14, 2000) as a "classic," and was the subject of Bill Moyers' Emmy Award-winning "Healing and the Mind" Public Broadcasting Service series. This research has contributed to increased acceptance of support groups as an important complement to traditional cancer care, and has stimulated the development of a new field of research on mind–body interactions for people with cancer, HIV disease, and other illnesses.

Spiegel has also explored mind–body mechanisms that link the psychosocial and physical components of illness. In an article in the *Journal of the National Cancer Institute*, he demonstrated that abnormal daily patterns of cortisol, a stress hormone, predict shorter survival time for women with breast cancer. These and similar studies are demonstrating how stress and support can affect endocrine and immune functioning of cancer patients, with important health consequences.

Spiegel has also examined the physiological mechanisms underlying mind–body interactions. Using brain imaging techniques, including brain electrical activity mapping and positron emission tomography (PET), he has demonstrated how hypnosis reduces pain and refocuses attention through specific effects on the parts of the brain that process sensory input. In a PET study featured on the cover of the *American Journal of Psychiatry*, Spiegel and colleagues at Harvard showed that hypnotic alteration of color vision is associated with specific changes in blood flow in the parts of the brain that process color vision. Thus, the subjective changes induced by hypnosis in perception were associated with measurable physiological changes in the brain's perceptual processing: Believing is seeing.

Spiegel earned a bachelor's degree with a major in philosophy at Yale, and completed his medical and psychiatric training at Harvard. His career at Stanford has been devoted to examining the connection between feeling and healing.

DAVID SPIEGEL

Stanford Heart Disease Prevention Program

By the late 1960s, epidemiologic studies showed that elevated blood pressure, cholesterol, and smoking increased the risk of dying from heart disease. The Stanford Heart Disease Prevention Program (SHDPP) was founded by John W. Farquhar in 1971. This program comprised a multidisciplinary group of researchers based at the Stanford University Medical Center, who worked to determine whether changing these risk factors at the community level could prevent cardiovascular disease. The Stanford Five City Project (Stanford FCP), which addressed this problem, was the largest research effort ever undertaken by the

SHDPP, receiving two decades of National Heart, Lung, and Blood Institute support (1978–1998).

The Stanford FCP built on findings from the Three Community Study, conducted in the mid-1970s, which involved three geographically separated small towns in northern California. Two of these towns received an extensive mass media campaign over a 2-year period. The third community served as a control. People from each community were interviewed and examined before the campaigns began and 1 and 2 years afterward to assess their knowledge and behavior related to cardiovascular disease (e.g., diet and smoking) and to measure physiological indicators of risk (e.g., blood pressure, plasma cholesterol). In contrast to the control community, in which an increase in the risk of cardiovascular disease was observed, the treatment communities experienced a substantial and sustained decrease in risk over the 2-year study period. These results strongly suggest that mass media education campaigns designed to target entire communities may be very effective at reducing the risk of cardiovascular disease.

Encouraged by these results, the researchers at the SHDPP undertook an even bolder experiment, the Stanford FCP, designed to test whether community-wide health education could reduce stroke and coronary heart disease. Two treatment cities ($N = 122,800$) and two control cities ($N = 197,500$) were compared for changes in knowledge of risk factors, blood pressure, plasma cholesterol level, smoking rate, body weight, and resting pulse rate. A fifth city was used to also assess cardiovascular morbidity and mortality. Treatment cities received a 5-year, low-cost, comprehensive program that employed social learning theory, a communication-behavior change model, community organization principles, and social marketing methods, resulting in approximately 26 hr of exposure to education via various media channels. Risk factors were assessed in a cohort of the same individuals followed longitudinally and in cross-sectional surveys at baseline and three later assessment points. After 30–64 months of education, significant net reductions in community averages favoring treatment occurred in plasma cholesterol level, blood pressure, resting heart rate, pulse rate, and smoking. At the follow-up assessment in 1989–1990, blood pressure improvements that were observed in all cities from baseline to the end of the intervention were maintained in treatment, but not in control cities.

Cholesterol levels continued to decline in all cities at follow-up. There were no longer differences in smoking rates between the cities. Over the entire 14 years of the study, the combined cardiovascular disease event rate declined about 3.0% per year. However, the change in trends between periods was slightly, but not significantly, greater in the treatment cities. Two other large, community-wide intervention projects occurred at the same time as the Stanford FCP: the Minnesota Heart Health Project and the Pawtucket Heart Health Project. These projects reported similar results and influenced a number of other studies that attempted to improve health through community interventions.

In 1984, to expand the scope of studies to a broader range of problems, issues, and methods, the SHDPP evolved into the Stanford Center for Research in Disease Prevention (SCRDP), whose mission is to conduct interdisciplinary research into the prevention and control of chronic disease. The SCRDP conducts problem-focused research, using mainly experimental methods, to test and disseminate disease prevention and control programs. The SCRDP involves collaboration among a broad array of health professionals and social and behavioral scientists who share public health and population perspectives in planning and conducting research.

Related Entries: Cardiovascular System, Coronary Heart Disease

BIBLIOGRAPHY

Farquhar, J. W., Fortmann, S. P., Flora, J. A., Taylor, C. B., Haskell, W. L., Williams, P. T., et al. (1990). Effects of community-wide education on cardiovascular disease risk factors. The Stanford Five-City Project. *Journal of the American Medical Association, 264,* 359–365.

Fortmann, S. P., & Varady, A. N. (2000). Effects of a community-wide health education program on cardiovascular disease morbidity and mortality: the Stanford Five-City Project. *American Journal of Epidemiology, 152,* 316–323.

Winkleby, M. A., Taylor, C. B., Jatulis, D., & Fortmann, S. P. (1996). The long-term effects of a cardiovascular disease prevention trial: The Stanford Five-City Project. *American Journal of Public Health, 86,* 1773–1779.

C. BARR TAYLOR

STD Prevention

INTRODUCTION

Sexually transmitted diseases (STDs) are an underrecognized public health concern among sexually active youth and adults in the United States. Among the major STDs, HIV (human immunodeficiency virus) poses the greatest threat to public health, having caused nearly 500,000 deaths in the United States and more than 20 million deaths worldwide since the beginning of the epidemic. Other commonly occurring STDs, when left untreated, can also lead to severe, long-term health problems, including infertility, complications during pregnancy, and several forms of life-threatening cancer. Health psychologists play an important role in STD prevention and treatment efforts by

Table 1. Common Sexually Transmitted Diseases (STDs) in the United States[a]

STD	Type of pathogen	Incidence in the U.S. (estimated number of new infections each year)	Medical complications (partial listing)
Chlamydia	Bacterial	3 million	In women: pelvic inflammatory disease; reproductive health difficulties, including increased risk for sterility, ectopic pregnancy, and miscarriage; chronic pelvic pain In men: Inflammation of the prostate gland and testes; urethral scarring; fertility problems Both women and men: increased HIV transmission risks; abnormal genital discharge; pain with urination
Gonorrhea	Bacterial	650,000	In women: pelvic inflammatory disease; reproductive health difficulties, including increased risk for sterility, ectopic pregnancy and miscarriage; chronic pelvic pain For men: Inflammation of the testicles; prostrate and urethral scarring; infertility In both women and men: increased HIV transmission risks; abnormal genital discharge; pain with urination
Hepatitis B	Viral	120,000	In both women and men: inflammation of the liver, liver failure, and liver cancer
Herpes	Viral	1 million	In both women and men: painful genital sores and blisters; increased HIV transmission risk
HIV/AIDS	Viral	40,000	In both women and men: severe immunodeficiency; increased risk for a variety of life-threatening opportunistic infections and certain forms of cancer
Human papillomavirus	Viral	5.5 million	In women: increased risk of cervical cancer In both women and men: external warts; anal cancer
Syphilis	Bacterial	70,000	In both women and men: genital chancre sore (primary stage); transient rash (secondary stage); serious damage to internal organs, including the heart, eyes, brain, nervous system, bones, and joints (late syphilis); syphilis infection is also associated with increased HIV transmission risk
Trichomoniasis	Bacterial	5 million	In women: increased risk for preterm delivery among pregnant women In men: inflammation of the prostate and bladder In both women and men: increased HIV transmission risk

[a] Incidence data from Cates (1999).

developing interventions to promote sexual behavior change, and by assisting already infected individuals with mental health adaptation, medication adherence, and health behavior change efforts.

SCOPE OF THE PROBLEM

In the United States, STDs constitute a major epidemic, with approximately 15 million people becoming infected with an STD each year. The Centers for Disease Control and Prevention report that chlamydia and gonorrhea are the first and second leading reported infectious illness in the United States, respectively, and together constitute 80% of the notifiable cases reported to the agency. Although the incidence of one STD—syphilis—has declined substantially in recent years, other prominent STDs continue to spread through the population, with little evidence of abatement (see Table 1 for common STDs).

All sexually active people, regardless of gender, race, sexual orientation, and economic status, are affected by STDs. Teenagers and young adults under the age of 25 years are among those who are most vulnerable to STDs, accounting for nearly two-thirds of all identified cases. Young people are at increased risk because they are more likely than older adults to have multiple sexual partners and to engage in unprotected sex. Other people who are at increased risk for contracting an STD include those living in poverty, people who lack access to adequate health care resources, and members of disenfranchised populations (e.g., sex workers, homeless persons, persons with mental illness).

STDs are often referred to as a hidden epidemic, and many people are unaware of their broad impact and serious health consequences. At least two factors contribute to the lack of public awareness concerning STDs. First, many people who contract an STD do not experience symptoms, or, in some cases, experience symptoms only after a long lag time following initial infection. Thus, STDs, including HIV, are often transmitted by individuals who are free of symptoms and unaware of their infection. Second, stigmatizing attitudes directed toward those who contract an STD contribute to the hidden nature of the STD epidemic. Because of stigma and shame, many people delay seeking STD testing and medical care, and avoid disclosing their infection to others.

IMPACT ON HEALTH

Among the major STDs, HIV disease clearly poses the greatest health risks. Improved treatments for HIV, which include the use of protease inhibitors and other antiretroviral therapies, have led to a decline in AIDS-related deaths in the United States and other nations with access to modern medicine. However, there is still no cure for HIV, and AIDS-related illnesses continue to claim many lives in the United States. Indeed, AIDS was the fifth-leading cause of death among young adults in the United States in 2000.

Women experience far greater burden in terms of health problems stemming from non–HIV-related STDs. Sexually transmitted human papillomavirus (HPV) is the leading risk factor for the development of cervical cancer. Although preventable through early detection, cervical cancer remains the most common cause of death attributable to sexually transmitted infections other than HIV. Reproductive health difficulties are also a major concern among women who contract an STD. Infections of the upper genital tract in women, referred to as pelvic inflammatory disease (PID), are a common consequence of gonorrhea and chlamydia infections. Women who develop PID are at increased risk for infertility because of damage to the fallopian tubes. PID also increases the likelihood of ectopic pregnancy, a serious and potentially fatal condition in which a fetus develops outside of the uterus. Because STDs can be transmitted to the fetus (through the placenta) and to a developing infant through breast-feeding, STDs that occur during pregnancy can result in a number of complications, including miscarriage, still birth, and premature delivery. STD acquisition in newborns often results in severe health consequences, including damage to the brain, spinal chord, and major organs.

Among men, health-related consequences stemming from STDs include increased risk for cancer of the penis and anus, liver disease, and increased occurrence of epididymitis, a treatable condition involving inflammation around the testicle. Other difficulties, including penile discharge, pain during urination, and testicular swelling and pain, are generally responsive to treatment and do not, in and of themselves, lead to serious medical complications. Although men experience far fewer health-related consequences stemming from STDs, early detection and treatment remains critical because new infections are commonly spread by infected men to their female partners.

Many prevalent STDs also increase a person's susceptibility to HIV. Furthermore, among individuals who are already infected with HIV, STD coinfections can increase the likelihood that HIV is transmitted to sexual partners. Thus, STD treatment and prevention programs not only can minimize health risks stemming from specific STDs, but can also serve to reduce the likelihood of HIV infection. The health impact of STDs could be greatly reduced through STD screening programs, which promote early STD detection and treatment. Most bacterial STDs can be cured through the use of antibiotic treatments. For viral STDs, potent antiretroviral treatments are available that can suppress symptoms and reduce the likelihood that the virus will be spread to other sexual partners. However, STDs typically go undetected, often until serious symptoms emerge.

PREVENTION OF STDs

STDs are most commonly transmitted to an uninfected partner through vaginal, anal, or oral sex. Some STDs (e.g., HIV and hepatitis) are also transmitted through needle sharing among intravenous drug users. In general, sexual transmission occurs less efficiently through oral sexual contact relative to anal or vaginal sex. Latex condoms, when used correctly, reduce the risks of transmitting most major STDs (including HIV).

Efforts to prevent the spread of STDs include both behavioral and biomedical approaches. Behavioral approaches to STD prevention emphasize efforts to promote adoption of safer sex strategies, including consistent use of condoms during sexual intercourse, avoiding sex with multiple partners (monogamy), or abstinence. Biomedical approaches to STD prevention emphasize the identification and treatment of those who are already infected with an STD. Prompt treatment of both viral and bacterial infections can dramatically reduce or eliminate the possibility of further STD transmission. Biomedical approaches also include vaccination programs, although effective vaccines are only widely available to prevent several forms of hepatitis.

A central challenge for STD prevention efforts is to develop interventions that promote modification of a pleasurable, albeit risky behavior (i.e., sex without a condom). As such, interventions based on psychological theory have proven to be instrumental in efforts to reduce such risky behaviors. For STDs other than HIV, many people are simply unaware of or misinformed about the risks and health consequences. However, even people who are well informed about STDs are often unmotivated to change their sexual behavior. For example, most people are aware of HIV and its severe health consequences, but often underestimate the degree to which they are personally vulnerable to HIV infection. Thus, a major emphasis for STD/HIV prevention programs is to increase awareness of personal vulnerability to STDs, increase the social acceptability of sexual behavior change, and provide training that enhances interpersonal skills needed to initiate condom use with a reluctant partner.

Historically, efforts to promote safer sex have focused on HIV prevention, with relatively little emphasis on prevention of other STDs. However, health psychologists and other specialists are increasingly aware of the importance of combining HIV and STD prevention efforts. Combining HIV and general STD prevention is advantageous both because non–HIV-related STDs cause serious health complications and because prevalent STDs increase a person's susceptibility to HIV infection.

Project RESPECT, a large-scale study involving men and women recruited through STD clinics, provides an example of an ambitious program to reduce the spread of both HIV and other STDs. Compared with patients receiving standard care, participants who received one of two counseling interventions emphasizing formulation of personalized risk reduction plans reported more condom use at 3- and 6-month follow-up assessments, and fewer new STDs at both 6- and 12-month follow-ups. These findings highlight the potential for using clinic-based interventions as an efficient means of reducing the occurrence of STDs.

MENTAL HEALTH ADAPTATION AND ADHERENCE

Persons diagnosed with an STD often face formidable challenges and stressors. STD-related stigma, shame, and discrimination often prevent individuals from seeking social support and disclosing their illness to others. Furthermore, an STD diagnosis often puts a strain on existing intimate relationships, raising concerns about partner fidelity and further transmission of the STD. Finally, treatments and medical complications can themselves be a source of considerable distress. Such illness-related coping challenges are most apparent among persons living with HIV disease, where long-term survival is by no means assured, and day-to-day existence involves coping with demanding treatment regimens, recurrent side effects, and worry over possible disease progression. Clinical health psychologists play an important role in the development and implementation of interventions to reduce stress, depression, and other mental health difficulties among persons with an STD. For example, cognitive–behavioral stress management programs have shown promise as an approach to reducing distress and improving health among persons living with HIV.

Medication adherence is an additional challenge faced by many STD patients. Adherence in the context of STD care refers to the act of closely following or sticking to a recommended drug regimen. In the case of HIV disease, patients who report even modest deviations from a regimen often experience more rapid disease progression. For this reason, behavioral scientists are developing intervention approaches designed to improve medication adherence among patients with HIV. Behavioral strategies, including multiple reminders (e.g., daily pill boxes, daily checklists, watch alarms), self-management skills training, and problem solving to facilitate integration of medication regimens into daily activities, are components that are likely to be useful when developing individually tailored adherence interventions. Poor adherence can also be problematic in the context of non–HIV-related STD care. For example, persons with PID are sometimes hospitalized solely for the purpose of assuring adequate adherence to a complete round of antibiotic treatment. Fortunately, several common STDs are now treatable through the use of single-dose therapies, which can be directly observed by a treatment provider.

CONCLUSIONS

STDs will remain a major public health concern for the foreseeable future. HIV disease has served to raise awareness of the importance of safer sex, but has often overshadowed efforts to promote awareness of other, more prevalent STDs, which also carry significant health risks. Health psychologists will continue to play an important role in developing interventions to prevent STD transmission and promote improved adaptation among those who contract STDs. In the future, behavioral interventions will likely feature greater integration of STD and HIV treatment and prevention.

Related Entries: Contraception, HIV/AIDS, Human Sexuality, Pregnancy

BIBLIOGRAPHY

Antoni, M. H., Cruess, D. G., Cruess, S., Lutgendorf, S., Kumar, M., Ironson, G., et al. (2000). Cognitive–behavioral stress management intervention effects on anxiety, 24-hr urinary norepinephrine output, and T-cytotoxic/suppressor cells over time among symptomatic HIV-infected gay men. *Journal of Consulting and Clinical Psychology, 68*, 31–45.

Bartlett, J. A. (2002). Addressing the challenges of adherence. *Journal of Acquired Immune Deficiency Syndromes, 29* (Supplement 1), S2–S10.

Cates, W., Jr. (1999). Estimates of the incidence and prevalence of sexually transmitted diseases in the United States. American Social Health Association Panel. *Sexually Transmitted Diseases, 26*, (Supplement), S2–S7.

Centers for Disease Control and Prevention. (2000). Summary of notifiable diseases: United States, 2000. *Morbidity and Mortality Weekly Report, 49*(53).

Institute of Medicine. (1997). *The hidden epidemic: Confronting sexually transmitted diseases.* Washington, DC: National Academy Press.

Kamb, M. L., Fishbein, M., Douglas, J. M., Jr., Rhodes, F., Rogers, J., Bolan, G., et al. (1998). Efficacy of risk-reduction counseling to prevent human immunodeficiency virus and sexually transmitted diseases: A randomized controlled trial. Project RESPECT Study Group. *Journal of the American Medical Association, 280*, 1161–1167.

Kelly, J. A., & Kalichman, S. C. (2002). Behavioral research on HIV/AIDS primary and secondary prevention: Recent advances and future directions. *Journal of Consulting and Clinical Psychology, 70*, 626–639.

Workowski, K. A., & Berman, S. M. (2002). CDC sexually transmitted diseases treatment guidelines. *Clinical Infectious Diseases, 35* (Supplement 2), S135–S137.

PETER A. VANABLE

Stimulus Control

Stimulus control is a method of reducing negative or maladaptive behaviors based on the principles of respondent (or classical conditioning) learning. Briefly, by capitalizing on the conditioned relationship between a stimulus and a response and modifying the stimulus, it is possible to break the stimulus–response relationship. Stimulus control is best understood in the broader concept of respondent learning. In the theory of respondent learning, a stimulus becomes unconditionally connected to a response. For example, for a smoker, cigarettes become unconditionally connected to a craving for more cigarettes (i.e., the process of addiction). Eventually, that stimulus becomes paired with other conditioned stimuli that can bring about the same conditioned response. In the example of the smoker, the cigarettes are paired with certain smoking contexts (e.g., in a bar, with a meal, or during a work break), and these contexts become sufficient to elicit the craving response. Stimulus control would be used to break the connection between the unconditioned stimulus (cigarettes) and the conditioned stimulus (smoking context).

Stimulus control can be used to modify many health behaviors. For example, stimulus control can be used to treat insomnia. Normally, a bed is unconditionally connected to sleep. However, for insomniacs, the bed often becomes associated with wakefulness. This generally occurs through the pairing of bed (the unconditioned stimulus) with other "awake" behaviors like reading, watching television, or working on the computer. Thus, bed becomes conditionally connected to wakefulness. Stimulus control would be useful to break the connection between bed and other behaviors. For example, by prohibiting nonsleep behaviors in bed and promoting good sleep hygiene, bed will again become paired with sleep, and insomnia should improve.

Stimulus control can also be used to modify dieting behavior. As with nicotine eliciting cravings for more cigarettes, food can elicit cravings for more food. Often, eating is paired with other conditioned stimuli such as certain times of day, certain groups of people, and certain settings. For example, a woman may find that she always goes to the office lounge on her lunch break. While she is there, she talks with coworkers and eats a candy bar from the vending machine. Thus, the office lounge and the coworkers have been conditionally connected to a craving for sweets. Stimulus control would suggest that the woman disrupt the association of a break with eating. She could go to a different place, without vending machines, to spend her lunch break to disrupt the connection between the office lounge and snacks. Alternatively, she could take her lunch break at a different time than her coworkers, to separate the connection between her coworkers and the sweet snacks.

Just as stimulus–response connections can be quite powerful, stimulus control can be a powerful tool for modifying health behaviors. In addition to smoking, sleeping, and eating behaviors, it can be used to modify drinking behavior, exercise behavior, and pain behavior. Stimulus control is inexpensive and easily self-implemented; it does not require the aid of a therapist or a counselor. With a certain amount of insight, self-monitoring, and will power, a client can engage in stimulus control techniques.

Related Entry: Classical Conditioning

BIBLIOGRAPHY

Sternber, R. J. (1997). *Pathways to psychology.* Orlando, FL: Harcourt Brace.

JAMIE A. CVENGROS

Stone, Arthur A.

Arthur A. Stone completed his doctoral work in clinical psychology at the State University of New York at Stony Brook in 1978; he then joined the departments of psychiatry and psychology in the medical school at Stony Brook. He is professor and vice-chair of the psychiatry department and director of the Applied Behavioral Medicine Research Institute at the medical school. His early work grew out of dissatisfaction with major life event approaches to assessing environmental stress. This led to the development of a checklist of daily events and research on the influence of desirable and undesirable events and mood in the genesis of upper respiratory symptoms. His interest in understanding the dynamics of the stress and illness process also led to the development of a daily coping assessment and to other studies addressing issues in coping assessment. In order to explain the stress–illness associations observed in his and others' studies, Stone conducted several investigations on possible immunological mediation of these process; he was especially interested in the role of the secretory immune system. More recently, he has examined the hypothalamic–pituitary–adrenal (HPA) axis on an ambulatory basis using salivary cortisol techniques. He has also explored the effects of disclosure of traumatic experiences on rheumatoid arthritis and asthma.

Stone's recent interests have focused on an even finer-grained understanding of the interplay between environmental influences and physiological processes, especially the HPA axis. He has been involved with the development of ecological

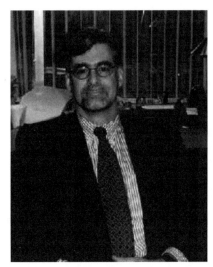

Stone, Arthur A.

momentary assessment, a technique for intensively monitoring individuals in their natural environments. A second current interest is applied behavioral medicine interventions. The programmatic goal of the institute he directs is the development of novel psychosocial assessments and interventions for medical illnesses. Institute projects have addressed issues in dermatology, rheumatology, neurology, pulmonology, oncology, and urology. He and his students have been especially interested in the role of written emotional expression about past traumas and its effect on chronic diseases. His interests in self-report research led to him chairing a National Institutes of Health conference called "Science of Self-Report: Implications for Researchers and Clinicians."

Stone is a fellow of several professional societies including the American Psychological Association, the Society of Behavioral Medicine, and the American Psychosomatic Society, and he is an elected member of the Academy of Behavioral Medicine Research. He has served on the boards of national behavioral medicine societies (American Psychosomatic Society and the Academy of Behavioral Medicine Research) and as the president of the Academy of Behavioral Medicine Research (2000–2001). An editorial board member of many scientific journals, he was also an associate editor of *Health Psychology* for 5 years, and editor-in-chief of the *Annals of Behavioral Medicine* from 1997 through 1999. Stone is the editor-in-chief of *Health Psychology*, the premier journal in this field. He has been a member of several National Institutes of Mental Health review panels and recently completed his tenure as the chair of the RPHB-3 review panel of the National Institutes of Health. In 1995, Stone received the American Psychological Association's Distinguished Health Psychologist—Senior Award.

ARTHUR A. STONE

Stress Appraisal

The concept of appraisal helps explain why people respond differently to a given stressful event, or, for that matter, why the same person might respond differently at different times to the same event. One student, for example, remains calm as he or she approaches an important exam, whereas another student becomes highly anxious. Getting caught in traffic will cause a person to get very anxious on one occasion, but not on another. Even an event that is universally regarded as severely stressful, such as the death of a spouse, will elicit a wide range of responses across individuals.

Two kinds of appraisal, primary appraisal and secondary appraisal, are involved in determining the degree to which a given event is stressful for an individual. Primary appraisal refers to the personal significance of a situation. It asks the question, "Am I in trouble?" The evaluation of personal significance has to do with the meaning of what is happening in relation to the person's values, beliefs, and goals. Rejection by a top medical school will be more stressful for a person who has always wanted to go to that medical school than for a person whose goal is to get into any one of several medical schools. Feedback that one does not write very well will be more stressful for a student who aspires to be a great writer than for a student who simply wants to get a passing grade.

Secondary appraisal has to do with the evaluation of options for coping. It asks the question, "What can I do?" Secondary appraisal is often cast in terms of personal control: Is there something the person can do to control the situation, or is it a situation the person has to accept? This appraisal is often complex. In some situations, nothing can be done to control the outcome of the situation, but the person can control his or her response to it. This is often referred to as secondary control. Alternatively, there may be something that can be done to change the outcome of a situation, but to exercise that option may cause conflict elsewhere. This is often the case when money is needed to solve a problem. The money may be needed for more than one purpose. To use it to deal with the immediate problem—say, pay a bill—may mean that another bill goes unpaid.

Together, primary and secondary appraisal determine whether the situation is perceived as stressful—as a harm or loss, a threat, or a challenge. The greater the personal significance and the less adequate the options for coping, the more intense is the stress appraisal. The appraisals of harm, loss, or threat are accompanied by negatively toned emotions such as fear, anger, worry, or sadness. Challenge refers to the possibility of mastery or gain. It is included as a stress appraisal because challenge always contains the possibility of failure. It is accompanied by positively toned emotions such as eagerness and excitement, as well as negatively toned emotions such as fear. Because appraisal is a process, the person's judgments regarding personal significance and options for coping are likely to be revised as the situation unfolds.

Related Entries: Coping, Stress Management

BIBLIOGRAPHY

Lazarus, R. S. (I991). *Emotion and adaptation.* New York: Oxford University Press.

Scherer, K. R., Schorr, A., & Johnstone, T. (Eds.). (2001). *Appraisal processes in emotion.* New York: Oxford University Press.

SUSAN FOLKMAN

Stress Inoculation

Stress inoculation training (SIT) is a form of cognitive–behavioral therapy based on the notion of inoculation or immunization. SIT was developed in the 1970s by Donald Meichenbaum and is built on the premise that exposing patients to milder forms of stress and teaching them to cope with these can actually inoculate them from the effects of more severe, future stressors. SIT comprises three phases: (1) conceptualization, (2) skills acquisition and rehearsal, and (3) application and followthrough. The conceptualization phase begins with the formation of a collaborative relationship between the therapist and patient and a discussion aimed at assisting the patient to better understand how his or her thoughts and attempts at coping influence life stress.

In the skills acquisition and rehearsal phase, specific coping skills are taught to the patient and then practiced primarily within session and eventually in actual situations. Patients are encouraged to use preexisting coping skills, modify maladaptive coping patterns, and develop additional coping strategies such as relaxation training, positive thinking, problem solving, communication skills, and attention diversion.

In the final phase, application and followthrough, the patient practices these newly learned coping skills in increasingly stressful situations, first by using anxiety-arousing imagery, behavioral rehearsal, modeling, and role playing, then in actual situations. This graduated exposure is meant to inoculate the patient against future stressful events. An additional key element of this phase is the use of relapse prevention techniques. Here, the patient identifies future, high-risk situations in which

lapses could occur and then rehearses coping strategies for these situations. The patient is also taught to view relapses as opportunities for learning versus catastrophic events. Booster and follow-up sessions may be necessary as well. Throughout these phases, efforts are made to ensure that the patient attributes positive changes to himself or herself.

SIT has been used in a variety of situations in which stress, anxiety, or fear is problematic. One example of the effectiveness of SIT is in assisting a person—call her EK—with her adjustment to stressful dental procedures. EK would become so anxious at the thought of her dental appointment that she would become physically ill prior to any such appointment. SIT helped her to identify specific thoughts (e.g., "This is going to be too painful") and images (e.g., excessive blood loss) that precipitated past anxiety attacks and eventual avoidance behavior as demonstrated by postponed or canceled appointments. Relaxation techniques and cognitive strategies (e.g., use of positive coping statements such as, "It's okay; I just have to take a deep breath and calm myself down") were taught and then practiced within the session. EK was then asked to list her fears from least to most fearful as it related to her dental appointments. Once she felt more comfortable in her imagined exposure to these events, role playing was employed to portray a dental office visit. Encouragement was provided throughout with emphasis placed on her taking credit for successful experiences. EK was then instructed to use these coping skills in the actual situation as she telephoned for an appointment, prepared for it, and visited the dentist without incident.

Several studies support the usefulness of SIT in reducing symptoms associated with posttraumatic stress disorder, dental pain, performance-related stress and anxiety, and a multitude of medical and psychological adjustment problems.

Related Entries: Stressful Medical Procedures

BIBLIOGRAPHY

Meichenbaum, D. (1985). *Stress inoculation training.* Elmsford, NY: Pergamon.

Meichenbaum, D. (1993). A constructivist narrative perspective on stress and coping: Stress inoculation applications. In L. Goldberger & S. Breznitz (Eds.), *Handbook of stress: Theoretical and clinical aspects* (2nd ed., pp. 00–00). New York: Free Press.

Meichenbaum, D. (1993). Stress inoculation training: A 20-year update. In Paul M. Lehrer & Robert L. Woolfolk (Eds.), *Principles and practice of stress management* (2nd ed., pp. 373–406). New York: Guilford.

Pierce, T. W. (1995). Skills training in stress management. In W. O'Donohue & L. Krasner (Eds.), *Handbook of psychological skills training: Clinical techniques and applications* (pp. 306–319). Needham Heights, MA: Allyn & Bacon.

MICHAEL G. KAVAN

Stress Management

Stress management is the use of psychological interventions to reduce physical reactions (such as muscle tension, high blood pressure, insomnia, and gastric discomfort) to demanding environmental situations. These uncomfortable reactions may be associated with negative states such as anxiety, depression, anger, pain, or illness. Reduction of discomfort may be achieved by directly counteracting the stress through relaxation, by changing one's view of the situation (reappraisal) or by changing the situation (e.g., increasing the use of available social support). In addition, where it is known that a stressful situation is forthcoming, such as surgery, advance training in stress management techniques (stress inoculation) may be very helpful. A combination of these techniques has been called the cognitive–behavioral approach to stress management. Stress management is the most fundamental psychological therapy in health psychology.

RELAXATION, MEDITATION, AND ATTEMPTS TO REDUCE AROUSAL

The use of relaxation to combat stress predates Hans Selye's brilliant analysis defining stress in 1950. In 1929, Edmund Jacobson proposed progressive relaxation to deal with muscle tension. The Jacobson technique relies heavily on the assessment of muscle tension and the reduction of activity in the muscles. He concluded that muscle tension was important in the formation of high blood pressure, ulcers, and other diseases. Relaxation has been demonstrated to be helpful in limiting acute stress effects as well. For example, Janice Kiecolt-Glazer and her colleagues at Ohio University found positive effects of relaxation in regulation of the immune system affected by acute stress.

Harvard's Herbert Benson noted that many cultures have developed meditative traditions that are very helpful in inducing muscle relaxation and other benefits. Benson observed that relaxation interventions in muscle tension have a long history dating back to antiquity.

Progressive relaxation, especially in an abbreviated 15- to 20-min form, has been a very popular technique in clinical practice. An individual tenses and relaxes each muscle group of the body progressively working from one area to the next and then concludes with general deep relaxation. Jacobson observed that perception of high muscle tension adapts so that one cannot feel tension after it is prolonged. The technique is a fairly active one. Muscles can relax more after tension or exercise than after not tensing. This may have something to do with the health benefits of exercise. For example, Kenneth Cooper and his colleagues in Texas found a significant relationship between death from all causes and low fitness. An additional benefit is that instructions for progressive relaxation can be tape recorded and one can achieve a degree of control over the time spent in relaxation. Variations on the progressive relaxation technique have been a cornerstone of stress management for decades.

A relaxation program may incorporate a variety of techniques to avoid boredom. A specific program may be tailored to the background of the individual. The Benson meditative technique promotes focusing on a slowly repeated sound image while in a comfortable position away from distractions. This is a very portable technique, which requires no equipment, and may be adapted to special conditions like walking for angina patients. Individuals with a religious orientation may gain the benefit of spirituality in repetitions of a certain sound or name. The mindfulness meditation promoted by Jon Kabat-Zinn has the advantage of concentrating on the "here and now" and is very consistent with some cognitive therapy approaches. The mental imagery approaches of Anees and Katherina Sheikh involve visualizing oneself in a safe, unstressed, desirable situation for a specified amount of time. This may logically appeal to people with high powers of imagination and offer a temporary distraction. The autogenic, or self-generated, relaxation described by Wolfgang Luthe is often incorporated into other approaches; for example, on a tape for progressive relaxation one might instruct a person to imagine their hands warming. Hypnosis (the use of suggestion) or biofeedback (the use of monitoring instrumentation) in assisting relaxation may be helpful, but individual differences in appeal and capability must be considered as well as expense. Breath control techniques have not been as useful as one might expect. Perhaps, as Stephen Porges and his colleagues at the University of Maryland found, some stress may be created in trying to control breathing. Whereas the techniques vary and the cognitive benefits may differ, the use of these techniques in stress management has the primary goal of reducing muscle tension and physiological arousal. Stanford's Richard Lazarus and Susan Folkman would classify these approaches as emotion-focused coping because relaxation diminishes the arousal and the emotional state.

REAPPRAISAL

Lazarus's early research indicated that individual interpretation of situations is very important with respect to the nature of the stress effects. He observed a paradoxically high arousal in measures associated with emotional sweating in Japanese students watching a control film that did not seem to stress American students. His questions, after the experiment, led to the observation that the Japanese students were more upset at the possibility of having their emotions revealed by the instruments than were the Americans. Lazarus and Folkman took this cultural difference and other observations to suggest that stressed individuals could reappraise their situation to view it as not as stressful.

Researchers have observed that certain approaches to reappraisal may be effective. The perception of helplessness seems to be particularly stressful, and anything that can be done to make the individual feel less hopeless and more in charge is beneficial. As noted, Lazarus and Folkman offered an analysis of coping techniques based on a focus on the problem versus a focus on the emotion to assist the stressed individuals in understanding how to reappraise the situation. Susan Kobasa concluded that those hardy individuals who feel more in control, are more committed, and accept situations as a challenge are less likely to report stress effects than their counterparts. These cognitive attitudes can be taught in stress management programs. Significantly, Rod Martin of the University of Western Ontario in Canada concluded that the relationship between humor, health, and longevity has not been consistently found, and studies that support this relationship may have been flawed methodologically. Thus it seems appropriate to work on a reappraisal of the situation rather than on humor as a distraction. In Lazarus and Folkman's terminology, this would be a problem-focused method of coping.

CHANGING THE STRESSOR

The stressed individual often has much more control of the stressful situation than is perceived. Barbara and Irwin Sarason and many others have noted that individuals who perceive high social support do better with stressors. Sheldon Cohen and Leonard Syme's anthology on social support and health also documents this relationship. Those with low social support may actually be under more stress than their counterparts, but these individuals may be counseled to increase social support by increasing contact with supportive relatives and friends and thus reduce the stress. People under stress can also seek to make new relationships in new environments through supportive counseling. Patients with the stress of a disease may excessively limit themselves socially and increase their stress due to loneliness. Education and counseling may reveal that limitations are not as severe as perceived. Support groups often serve this function. Vocational, financial, and interpersonal counseling may also be tools for effectively changing the environmental issues at hand. Therefore these interventions could also be described as problem focused.

STRESS INOCULATION

Donald Meichenbaum at the University of Waterloo in Canada has advocated the very logical concept of teaching man-

agement techniques before the stress as an inoculation against that stress. Stress effects include mental confusion and emotional responses that make it difficult for the stressed individual to effectively engage in appropriate interventions. Emmelkamp and his colleagues from the Netherlands concluded that short-term, after-the-fact, therapies like critical incident stress debriefing have not been as effective as hoped in reducing the risk of post traumatic stress syndrome. These quick interventions do provide some immediate comfort and contacts for further therapy when that is necessary, but unfortunately do not apparently meet the primary goal of preventing serious stress reactions. The stress inoculation methods have been adapted to after-the-fact situations because stress tends to cycle with memories of the traumatic event. However, Foa and her colleagues at the University of Pennsylvania found that exposure therapy, in which a patient gradually confronts stressful situations, has longer-lasting benefits than stress inoculation after the trauma. When individuals are relatively unstressed before surgery or predictable emergencies, it would be very prudent for them to understand the stress management techniques of conceptualization, skills acquisition, and rehearsal and to have practiced the skills involved as Meichenbaum has suggested. Perhaps these beneficial skills should be a standard part of the education system.

COGNITIVE–BEHAVIORAL MODIFICATION

Cognitive–behavioral approaches integrate stress management techniques and offer increased benefit over single techniques. Many cognitive–behavioral approaches integrate behavioral with medical interventions in a multidisciplinary approach. For example, Kenneth Holroyd and fellow researchers at Ohio University concluded that cognitive techniques and medication can be combined to treat tension headaches. The physician Dean Ornish has created a lifestyle change program, which includes stress management, exercise, and dietary control to regulate cardiovascular disease. When one emotional reaction or pain is evident, cognitive–behavioral interventions may focus on that condition as in anger, anxiety, depression, and pain management. Cognitive–behavioral interventions show the best promise in management of stress, probably because of their eclectic nature.

Stress management can involve interventions at every level of a stress model (Figure 1). These include the stress reaction (relaxation and exercise), the appraisal of the situation (reappraisal), the stressor itself (changing the situation), and even before the environmental demand (stress inoculation), A combination of techniques (cognitive–behavior modification) perhaps integrated with physical medicine (multidisciplinary approach) seems to offer advantages. Such techniques may focus

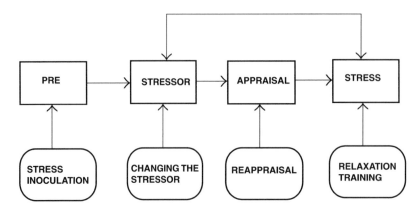

Figure 1. Stress management model.

on specific emotions or stresses as in anger, anxiety, depression, or pain management.

Related Entries: Stress Appraisal, Stress Inoculation

BIBLIOGRAPHY

Alden, A., Dale, J. A., & DeGood, D. E. (2001). Interaction effects of affective state and focus of mental imagery on pain analgesia. *Applied Psychophysiology and Biofeedback, 26,* 117–126.

Benson, H. (1975). *The relaxation response.* New York: Morrow.

Blair, S. N., Kohl III, H. W., Paffenbarger, R. S., Clark, D. G., Cooper, K. H., & Gibbons, L. W. (1989). Physical fitness and all-cause mortality: A prospective study of men and women. *Journal of the American Medical Association, 262,* 2395–2402.

Cohen, S., & Syme, S. L. (Eds.) (1985). *Social support and health.* Orlando, FLA: Academic.

Coyne, J. C., & Racioppo, M. W. (2000). Never the twain shall meet? Closing the gap between coping research and clinical intervention research. *American Psychologist, 55,* 655–675.

Dale, J. A., & DeGood, D. E. (1997–98). The emerging role of the psychologist in pain management. *Advances in Medical Psychotherapy, 9,* 1–20.

DeGood, D. E. (1997). *The headache and neck pain workbook.* Oakland, CA: New Harbinger.

DeGood, D. E., Crawford, A. L., & Jongsma, A. E., Jr. (1999). *The behavioral medicine treatment planner.* New York: Wiley.

Foa, E. B., Dancu, C. V., Hembree, E. A., Jaycox, L. H., Meadows, E. A., & Street, G. P. (1999). A comparison of exposure therapy, stress inoculation training, and their combination for reducing posttraumatic stress disorder in female assault victims. *Journal of Consulting and Clinical Psychology, 67,* 194–211.

Folkman, S., & Moskowitz, J. T. (2000). Positive affect and the other side of coping. *American Psychologist, 55,* 647–655.

Hermann, C., Blanchard, E. B., & Flor, H. (1997). Biofeedback treatment for pediatric migraine: Prediction of treatment outcome. *Journal of Consulting and Clinical Psychology, 65,* 611–617.

Holroyd, K. A., O'Donnell, F. J., Stensland, M., Lipchik, G. L., Cordingley, G. E., & Carlson, B. W. (2001). Management of chronic tension-type headache with tricyclic antidepressant medication, stress management therapy, and their combination: A randomized controlled trial. *Journal of the American Medical Association, 285,* 2208–2220.

Jacobson, E. (1929). *Progressive relaxation: A physiological and clinical investigation of muscular states and their significance in psychology and medical practice.* Chicago: University of Chicago Press.

Kabat-Zinn, J. (1995). *Wherever you go there you are: Mindfulness meditation in everyday life.* New York: Hyperion.

Kiecolt-Glaser, J. K., Marucha, P. T., Atkinson, C., & Glaser, R. (2001). Hypnosis as a modulator of cellular immune dysregulation during acute stress. *Journal of Consulting and Clinical Psychology, 69,* 674–682.

Kobasa, S. C. (1979). Stressful life events, personality, and health: An inquiry into hardiness. *Journal of Personality and Social Psychology, 37,* 1–11.

Lazarus, R. S. (1966). *Psychological stress and the coping process.* New York: McGraw-Hill.

Lazarus, R., & Folkman, S. (1984). *Stress, appraisal and coping.* New York: Springer.

Luthe, W. (1969). *Dynamics of autogenic neutralization.* New York: Grune & Stratton.

Martin, R. (2001). Humor, laughter, and physical health: Methodological issues and research findings. *Psychological Bulletin, 127,* 504–519.

Meichenbaum, D. (1977). *Cognitive–behavior modification: An integrative approach.* New York: Plenum.

Meichenbaum, D. (1985). *Stress inoculation training.* New York: Pergamon.

Meichenbaum, D. (1996). Stress inoculation training for coping with stressors. *Clinical Psychologist, 49,* 4–7.

Ornish, D., Scherwitz, L. W., Billings J. H., Gould, K. L., Merritt, T. A., Sparler, S., et al. (1998). Intensive lifestyle changes for reversal of coronary heart disease. *Journal of the American Medical Association, 280,* 2001.

Pierce, G. R., Sarason, B., & Sarason, I. (1992). General and specific support expectations and stress as predictors of perceived supportiveness: An experimental study. *Journal of Personality and Social Psychology, 63,* 297–307.

Sargunaraj, D., Lehrrer, P., Hochron, S. M., Raush, L., Edelberg, Robert, P., & Stephen, W. (1996). Cardiac rhythm effects of .125-hz paced breathing through a resistive load: Implications for paced breathing therapy and the polyvagal theory. *Biofeedback and Self-Regulation, 21,* 131–147.

Selye, H. (1950). *The physiology and pathology of exposure to stress; a treatise based on the concepts of the general-adaptation-syndrome and the diseases of adaptation.* Montreal: Acta.

Selye, H. (1956). *The stress of life.* New York: McGraw-Hill.

Seye, H. (Ed.). (1980). *Selye's guide to stress research.* New York: Van Nostrand Reinhold.

Sheikh, A., & Sheikh, K. (Eds.). (1989). *Eastern and Western approaches to healing: Ancient wisdom and modern knowledge.* New York: Wiley.

Suinn, R. (2001). The terrible twos—anger and anxiety: Hazardous to your health. *American Psychologist, 56,* 27–32.

van Emmerik, A. A. P., Kamphuis, J. H., Hulsbosch, A. M., & Emmelkamp, P. M. G. (2002). Single session debriefing after psychological trauma: A meta-analysis. *Lancet, 360,* 766–775.

J. ALEXANDER DALE

Stressful Life Events

Although the concept of stress has been difficult to define, most researchers agree that stress results when an organism is forced to make a substantial adjustment to environmental events that are appraised as threatening or harmful. Perhaps most important in the definition of stress is the relationship between external events and internal, or personal, reactions or responses. According to Richard Lazarus and Susan Folkman, stressful life events occur when individuals are confronted with life events (e.g., an exam) that they consider relevant to their well-being and that they believe challenges or exceeds their abilities and resources, leading to difficulty in meeting the demands of the environment. As a result, the individual experiences stress, which results in various behavioral, psychological, emotional, cognitive, and biochemical changes.

Measures of stressful life events differ widely in their time frame and specificity. One of the most widely used measures of stressful life events is the Social Readjustment Rating Scale. This scale consists of 43 items with preassigned values weighting the impact of each of the events on the inventory. Items include death of a spouse (100 points), fired from work (47 points), and change in sleep (16 points). High scores on this scale have been related to such diverse disorders as tuberculosis, arthritis, heart disease, schizophrenia, depression, and athletic injury. Similar scales have been developed for a variety of age and ethnic groups. The life events inventories focus on major life events; other measures have been developed which focus on less cataclysmic, but more frequent stressors. Examples include the Hassles Scale, the Daily Stress Inventory, and the Daily Stress Scale. These scales inquire about events like demands at work, interpersonal conflict, standing in line, and getting caught in traffic. Recently, ecological momentary assessment approaches have been used to obtain measures of stress at multiple points during the day. These measures randomly cue individuals to report on the level of stress they experience during several intervals of the day.

Research has shown that the experience of stressful life events is related to various health outcomes. Although leading researchers in this area generally conclude that not all types of stress are detrimental to one's health and well-being, experiencing severe and chronic distress can have detrimental effects on health. For example, chronic stress related to life events such as job demands has been linked to the development of cardiovascular disease. In addition, David Krantz and Shera Raisen report that financial stressors, as experienced by those low in socioeconomic status, are related to negative cardiovascular changes.

Stressful life events have been implicated in other health conditions as well. Anita DeLongis and her colleagues reported a significant relationship between the reported number and intensity of daily hassles and complaints of somatic illness. Molly McKenna and her colleagues have also linked cancer to the experience of stressful events. Their research shows that the source and chronicity of stress, in addition to coping ability and perceived severity of the stressor, are related to the development of cancer.

In summary, stress can negatively affect an individual in a variety of ways, including psychologically and physically. One way of assessing the stress an individual experiences is to measure the number, chronicity, and severity of stressful life events that are present. Given that stress has been shown to have such negative consequences for health, learning skills to cope with the effects of stress can be useful. Employing relaxation techniques, for example, is one such way to effectively cope with the effects of stressful life events.

Related Entries: Coping, General Adaptation Syndrome, Stress Appraisal

BIBLIOGRAPHY

Bolger, N., DeLongis, A., Keesler, R. C., & Schilling, E. A. (1989). Effects of daily stress on negative mood. *Journal of Personality and Social Psychology, 57,* 808–818.

Brantley, P. J., & Jones, G. N. (1989). *Daily Stress Inventory professional manual.* Odessa, FL: Psychological Assessment Resources.

DeLongis, A., Coyne, J. C., Dakof, G., Folkman, S., & Lazarus, R. S. (1982). Relationship of daily hassles, uplifts, and major life events to health status. *Health Psychology, 1,* 119–136.

Kanner, A. D., Coyne, J. C., Schaefer, C., & Lazarus, R. S. (1981). Comparison of two modes of stress measurement: Daily hassles and uplifts versus major life events. *Journal of Behavioral Medicine, 4,* 1–39.

Krantz, D. S., & Raisen, S. E. (1988). Environmental stress, reactivity and ischaemic heart disease. *British Journal of Medical Psychology, 61,* 3–16.

Lazarus, R. S., & Folkman, S. (1984). *Stress, appraisal, and coping.* New York: Springer-Verlag.

McKenna, M. C., Zevon, M. A., Corn, B., & Rounds, J. (1999). Psychosocial factors and the development of breast cancer: A meta-analysis. *Health Psychology, 18,* 520–531.

ROCHELLE L. BERGSTROM
DAVID A. WITTROCK

Stressful Medical Procedures

Technological advances in medicine and dentistry have led to an increase in stressful diagnostic and treatment procedures, presenting problems for health care providers. Agitated patients require more analgesia or sedation, and are more likely to encounter complications. Evidence also indicates that those who tolerate procedures poorly recover more slowly. Finally, those who experience greater distress during a medical or dental procedure may be less likely to return for additional diagnosis or treatment.

INVASIVE AND NONINVASIVE PROCEDURES

Stressful procedures are those that tax a patient's ability to adapt physically and emotionally. Many procedures invade the person's physical boundaries, often while the person is conscious or only minimally sedated. Invasive procedures include all types of surgery, many dental procedures, diagnostic procedures such as cardiac catheterization and colonoscopy, specimen collection, particularly the drawing of blood, and repetitive procedures such as burn debridement and cancer chemotherapy.

Procedures do not need to be invasive to be considered stressful. Noninvasive diagnostic procedures such as magnetic resonance imaging and computed tomography (CT) scan often require the patient to remain perfectly still for several minutes inside a narrow tunnel. Other procedures involve relatively minor bodily invasions, but may involve great psychological threat, such as genetic testing for breast cancer vulnerability.

There is great variability among people in how a procedure may affect them. For some, the experience of surgery is less challenging than lying inside a CT scanner for 45 min. According to Hans Selye, the Austrian physiologist and father of the concept of human stress, the stressfulness of a situation lies not in the situation itself, but in how the person reacts to it.

EMOTIONAL AND COGNITIVE RESPONSES TO STRESSFUL PROCEDURES

The emotional response to a stressful procedure is characterized by feelings of fear, anxiety, and panic. The accompanying physiological response to these emotions can include increased heart rate, sweating, increased blood pressure, and increased muscle tension. Selye referred to this initial response as the alarm reaction.

The cognitive reactions, the thoughts that accompany this experience, may include catastrophizing cognitions ("This is terrible!"), predictions of harm, and a perception of loss of control. The psychologist Richard Lazarus called this cognitive process the primary appraisal of the situation. Efforts to prepare patients to tolerate stressful medical and dental procedures have primarily been aimed at altering these initial emotional and cognitive responses.

EFFORTS AT INTERVENTION

The first study to systematically prepare patients for a stressful medical procedure was conducted by the physician Lawrence Egbert and his colleagues at the Massachusetts General Hospital in 1964. A group of patients scheduled for major surgery was given specific information about what they would experience before, during, and after the operation, and about how to best manage pain after the surgery. This group required less pain medication in the hospital and were ready for discharge sooner than a comparable group of patients that was not given the information and instructions. This study set the stage for more systematic studies of preparing patients for surgery. Since then, interventions have been tested in primarily two areas: the provision of information, intended to alter patients' stress-related cognitions, and variants of distraction and relaxation training, intended to alter the emotional and physical responses to stressful medical and dental procedures.

PROVISION OF INFORMATION

There are two types of information that may be given in preparing people for medical or dental procedures: procedural and sensory. Procedural information consists of a description of the procedures involved in the event: what actions will be taken, the timing of actions, and the likely outcomes. Sensory information consists of the sensations a person is likely to experience during and after the procedure.

Both types of information should help a patient develop accurate expectations and feel a sense of increased control in the situation. Some have argued, however, that sensory information should be more effective than procedural information because the foreknowledge of how something will feel can actually help alter the sensation. Procedural information only provides a view of what will occur. In the case of extensive or very invasive procedures, this type of information might actually be undesirable for some people.

To answer the question as to which type of information is more effective, psychologists Jerry Suls and Choi K. Wan reviewed studies in which procedural and sensory information was compared. Although sensory information yielded better outcomes than procedural information in some categories, the biggest effects were seen with a combination of procedural and sensory information. The recommendation for patients facing stressful procedures, then, would be that both sensory and procedural information should be provided.

DISTRACTION

Distraction interventions seek to draw the patient's attention away from the details of the stressful procedure. In this way the person is less apt to fully process the experiences as they occur, and the emotional impact should be less. Distraction procedures may involve having the patient listen to music, watch a video, or perform a cognitive task such as mental arithmetic. Intentional shifting of attention away from a stressful experience can increase pain tolerance and decrease physiological arousal and emotional distress.

Literature reviews by Mullen and Suls in 1982 and by McCaul and Malott in 1984 added to our knowledge about the utility of distraction. Distraction results in less distress in the short term, but attentional strategies that seek to change perception of the stressor may have better effects in the long-term. Additionally, the more attention the distraction strategy requires, the more effective it becomes. Distraction strategies are effective at low intensities of pain or distress, but are ineffective at higher intensities. At higher intensities of distress, people may no longer be able to distract themselves, and may be forced to employ a more attention-oriented coping strategy (e.g., trying to control the sensory aspects of the experience through relaxation). Distraction remains an attractive option for intervention in relatively low-stress procedures.

RELAXATION INTERVENTIONS

Relaxation has frequently been used to alter the emotional and physiological impact of stressful procedures. Relaxation accomplishes several goals at once. First, it directly dampens the physiological reactivity seen in stressful situations. It lowers heart rate and blood pressure, and helps to diminish muscle tension. Second, because systematic relaxation requires concentration, it acts as a distraction from the stressful experience. Finally, the availability of relaxation offers the person a way to have some control in the situation.

Relaxation training may consist in having the person alternately contract and release muscle groups, as in progressive muscle relaxation, or may simply involve asking the patient to breathe deeply and to concentrate on keeping the body relaxed. The training may consist of practice before the medical procedure, or of following taped relaxation instructions while undergoing the procedure. Relaxation training has demonstrated effectiveness in reducing patient distress in a number of settings, including abdominal surgery, oral surgery, and gastrointestinal endoscopy.

OTHER METHODS

Other methods have also been used to help prepare patients, particularly children, for stressful medical procedures. In systematic desensitization, the patient is exposed to anxiety-provoking stimuli (e.g., the dental drill, a syringe) while relaxed and calm, before the actual medical or dental procedure begins. The intent is to minimize the physical and emotional reactions of the patient when he or she encounters those stimuli during the actual procedure.

Modeling involves the patient watching another person, usually on film, go through the same stressful procedure that he or she will go through. The models provide sensory and procedural information, and set a standard of behavior to follow. Models tend to work best in those with no experience with the stressful procedure.

Combined techniques or programs have also been used to prepare patients. Stress inoculation, for example, occurs in three stages: client preparation (information), skills training, and application training. Stress inoculation has been conducted for patients undergoing orthopedic surgery, dental treatment, and open heart surgery. Most programs to prepare patients for stressful procedures have multiple components, combining information with coping skills training (e.g., relaxation, distraction).

Other techniques have been employed to help patients prepare for stressful procedures, including hypnosis, meditation, and imagery. Hypnosis has been used extensively in medicine and dentistry for acute pain control. The effectiveness reported for hypnosis, however, as for meditation and imagery interventions, may simply be the result of relaxation.

INTERACTIONS WITH COPING STYLE

It is generally assumed that any intervention that provides the patient with an increased sense of control will be helpful to that person. However, an intervention that is not congruent with a person's coping style may be ineffective, or even harmful.

Coping style refers to a person's preferred way of dealing with a stressful encounter. Several coping styles have been identified in the literature. Among these is the tendency to either avoid, ignore, or deny the details of a situation. Those who do this have been termed blunters by psychologist Suzanne Miller, and those who attend to those details are called monitors. Related coping-style types include repressors, who are similar to blunters, and sensitizers, who resemble monitors.

Providing detailed information to blunters has been found to actually increase patient distress in some cases. On the other hand, relaxation and distraction strategies tend to be most effective with those people who prefer to avoid or ignore the details of stressful situations.

CONCLUSIONS

As medicine continues to advance and access to care widens, exposure to stressful medical procedures will increase. The demand for high-quality care will increasingly require that patients facing stressful medical and dental procedures be prepared. Intervention programs that combine multiple modalities, including preparatory information, distraction, and relaxation, will probably prove to be the most useful. Delivery of these interventions, however, will have to be adjusted according to the coping preferences of the patient.

Related Entries: Stress Inoculation, Stress Management

BIBLIOGRAPHY

Egbert, L. D., Batit, G. E., Welch, C. E., & Bartlett, M. K. (1964). Reduction of postoperative pain by encouragement and instruction of patients: A study of doctor–patient rapport. *New England Journal of Medicine, 270,* 825–827.

Lazarus, R. S. (1966). *Psychological stress and the coping process.* New York: McGraw-Hill.

Litt, M. D., Nye, C., & Shafer, D. (1995). Preparing for oral surgery: Evaluating elements of coping. *Journal of Behavioral Medicine, 18,* 435–459.

Logan, H., Baron, R. S., Keeley, K., Law, A., & Stein, S. (1991). Desired and felt control as mediators of stress in a dental setting. *Health Psychology, 10,* 352–359.

Miller, S. M. (1988). The interacting effects of coping styles and situational variables in gynecologic settings: Implications for research and treatment. *Journal of Psychosomatic Obstetrics and Gynecology, 9,* 23–34.

McCaul, K. D., & Malott, J. M. (1984). Distraction and coping with pain. *Psychological Bulletin, 95,* 516–533.

Mullen, B., & Suls, J. (1982). The effectiveness of attention and rejection as coping styles: A meta-analysis of temporal differences. *Journal of Psychosomatic Research, 26,* 43–49.

Selye, H. (1956). *The stress of life.* New York: McGraw-Hill.

Suls, J., & Wan, C. K. (1989). Effects of sensory and procedural information on coping with stressful medical procedures and pain. A meta-analysis. *Journal of Consulting and Clinical Psychology, 57,* 372–379.

Turk, D. C., Meichenbaum, D., & Genest, M. (1983). *Pain and behavioral medicine: A cognitive–behavioral perspective.* New York: Guilford.

MARK D. LITT

Structured Interview for Assessment of Coronary-Prone Behavior

The Structured Interview (SI) provides a rich sample of behavior, which has been used to assess several attributes indicative of coronary-prone behavior. Ray Rosenman and Meyer Friedman devised the SI to assess the Type A behavior pattern (TABP). It has also proved to be a valuable method for the assessment of more specific characteristics of the TABP such as hostility and dominance.

The SI lasts approximately 15 min and consists of questions dealing with the major characteristics of the Type A individual: job involvement, competitiveness, impatience, and irritability. Trained assessors rate the respondent's behavior from recordings. Although content is taken into consideration, the assessors concentrate on the respondent's style of speaking. Explosive or rapid speech, interruptions, excessive loudness, and self-aggrandizing statements are taken to be indicative of the TABP. This emphasis on speech stylistics has also been an important part of systems for scoring hostility and other attributes. Friedman and Linda Powell have extended this emphasis on stylistics to cover nonverbal behaviors as well.

Soon after it was shown that TABP assessments predicted the development of coronary heart disease in Western Collaborative Group Study (WCGS) participants, researchers instituted more refined assessment procedures, which broke the TABP into its components. Reassessments of the WCGS interviews examined the individual contributions of the various behaviors that make up the TABP. A rating of Potential for Hostility emerged as a potent predictor of coronary events. Other research confirmed the importance of hostility, and recent studies have concentrated on its measurement. Several refinements in interview-based hostility assessment have followed. These have reduced the subjectivity of the ratings and more clearly defined the attributes being judged. Assessors are trained to be especially aware of indications of irritation or contempt for the interviewer or others.

There are numerous advantages to the interview approach to the assessment of hostility. It evokes a rich set of behaviors, which allow the raters to take into account the wide variety of expressions of hostility, whereas questionnaire measures tend to predefine hostility in a narrow way. In addition, respondents may be reluctant to verbally report their hostility, but these denials are often betrayed by their behavior during the interview. It is also likely that many respondents are not very introspective and are therefore unaware of their interaction style. These factors may account for the fact that SI-assessed hostility is weakly correlated with scores on self-report questionnaires. Test–retest reliabilities have been found to be high over periods of up to 4 years for hostility and 10 years for TABP, indicating that the measures reflect stable predispositions.

The advantages of SI-based measures have translated into demonstrations of associations with coronary heart disease in both prospective and cross-sectional data. Hostility ratings predicted coronary events in the Multiple Risk Factor Intervention Trial as well as the WCGS. They have also been shown to correlate with coronary artery disease severity in both patient and nonpatient samples.

Of course, SI-based assessment techniques have their drawbacks. Although high interrater reliabilities are common, training is necessary for this to be achieved. SI assessments are logistically and economically difficult to perform in large studies.

However, the many advantages of the SI and its excellent track record of success in studies of health make it a worthwhile tool to include in studies when at all possible.

Related Entries: Coronary Heart Disease, Type A Behavior Pattern

BIBLIOGRAPHY

Barefoot, J., & Lipkus, I. (1993). Assessment of anger–hostility. In A. Siegman & T. Smith (Eds.), *Anger, hostility and the heart* (pp. 43–66). Hillsdale, NJ: Erlbaum.

Rosenman, R. (1978). The interview method of assessment of the coronary-prone behavior pattern. In T. Dembroski, S. Weiss, J. Shields, S. Haynes, & M. Feinlieb (Eds.), *Coronary prone behavior* (pp. 55–69). New York: Springer-Verlag.

JOHN C. BAREFOOT
THOMAS L. HANEY

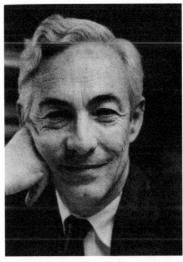
Stunkard, Albert

Stunkard, Albert

Albert Stunkard has been professor of psychiatry at the University of Pennsylvania since 1962. During this time he has had an active teaching career, chaired the department of psychiatry from 1962 to 1973, and served as interim chairman during 1996 and 1997. His major activities, however, have been in research, primarily on obesity and eating disorders. In 1955 he described the night eating syndrome characterized by morning anorexia, evening hyperphagia, insomnia, and eating after sleep onset. It appears to be a stress-related circadian disorder of eating, sleeping, and mood that involves a phase-onset delay. Successful treatment with a selective serotonin reuptake inhibitor has recently been reported. He was the first to describe binge eating, in 1959.

In 1985 Stunkard developed the Eating Inventory, which refined the concepts of dietary restraint, disinhibition, and hunger and has been reported in more than 400 publications. His research has advanced the medical profession's understanding of both environmental and genetic aspects of obesity. The effect of the environment was demonstrated in the strong association of social class and obesity and in the influence of social class of origin on the prevalence of obesity. The effect of both genetics and environment was demonstrated in a study using the Danish Adoption Register. His studies of twins, both identical and fraternal, both raised together and reared apart, provided the strongest early evidence for the influence of genetics in human obesity.

A major emphasis in Stunkard's research has been on treatment, including pharmacotherapy and the introduction for behavior therapy for obesity. He conducted the first studies showing the salutary effects of surgery on very severe obesity and the only study of psychoanalysis and obesity, which showed modest weight losses. He recently published what may be the most successful treatment of obesity yet reported. For the last 9 years he has conducted studies of the growth and development of children at high and low risk for obesity. These studies have shown that a decrease in energy expenditure does not contribute to the development of obesity, whereas overeating does. He is the author of more than 400 publications, mostly in the field of obesity and eating disorders, and his research has been supported for more than 40 years by the National Institutes of Health. He has served as president of five professional societies and is on the editorial boards of eight journals.

ALBERT STUNKARD

Suicide

Suicide is the act of intentionally taking one's own life. The study of suicide is essential because suicide is so pernicious and claims the lives of numerous people yearly. Those attempting suicide are experiencing a tremendous amount of psychological pain, and are likely to feel a great deal of hopelessness about their future.

EPIDEMIOLOGY

Even though suicide in the United States has dropped from the 9th-leading cause of death in 1996 to the 11-leading cause of death in 1999, it remains a persistent problem. More than 30,000 people die each year by suicide, and more than 84 people commit suicide each day. The national rate of suicide is 10.7/100,000, meaning that of every 100,000 people in the United States, 10.7 take their own lives. However, the number of suicides may be underestimated due to underreporting. Suicide is underreported for a number of reasons, including fear of stigma and of legal complications. It can also be difficult to distinguish a suicide from an accidental death.

Although women attempt suicide more often, more men die by suicide. The rate for women is 4.1/100,000 each year, and the rate for men is nearly four times as much, at 17.6/100,000. This gender difference involves the type of suicide method used. Men tend to use more lethal methods, whereas women are more likely to use less lethal methods, which provide more opportunity for rescue or resuscitation.

In general, the rate of suicide increases with age. The age group that commits the largest number of suicides is that of people 65 years of age and older, at a rate of 15.9/100,000. However, 15- to 24-year-olds are also at high risk; in this age group, suicide is the third-leading cause of death, following only to accidents and homicide. The suicide rate for 15- to 24-year-olds is 10.3/100,000, and every year 4,000 people between the age of 15 and 24 years die by suicide.

The rate of suicide varies among different ethnic groups. In the United States, Whites have substantially higher rates of suicide than African Americans, although the rate for African Americans has been increasing. White men older than 65 years have the highest rate of suicide (37/100,000), and African-American women tend to have the lowest rate (2/100,000). The rate for African-American men has been increasing over time and is 11.4/100,000. Hispanics have a lower rate of suicide than Whites, and the rate for Native Americans tends to vary, but is extremely high in some regions.

CAUSES AND CONTRIBUTORS

No single risk factor causes a person to commit suicide, and people who attempt suicide usually exhibit a number of risk factors. A strong predictor of future suicidal behavior is previous suicidal behavior. People who have attempted suicide before are up to eight times more likely to attempt suicide again. Individuals with a history of suicidal behavior in the family are also at greater risk for suicide, due, in part, to the influence of as-yet-unidentified genes.

There are a number of other risk factors to consider. One is the presence of one or more mental disorders. Many people who die by suicide meet the diagnostic criteria for at least one mental disorder. Disorders that are most associated with suicidal behavior are mood disorders and substance abuse disorders. Personality disorders are also related to an increased risk of suicide. A biological risk factor associated with suicidal behavior

is reduced serotonin levels. Serotonin has clearly established links to suicide and is the primary neurotransmitter implicated in suicide risk. Suicidal behavior is also often correlated with cognitive biases or distortions in which people are likely to hold a negative view of the self, the world, and the future. Some people who are suicidal also have deficits in their interpersonal problem-solving skills, impulse control problems, and impaired coping abilities.

Social factors also are related to suicidal behavior. A lack of social support, which may be related to poor social skills, isolation, and loss of relationships, may play a role in the suicidal process. Negative life events are related to suicidal behavior such that suicides are more likely to occur during stressful than nonstressful times. Having close relationships and a supportive environment can be a protective factor against suicide. It has been found that a history of child abuse is related to a greater number of suicide attempts, particularly in adolescence.

WARNING SIGNS AND PREDICTORS

The need for assessment of risk in suicide is crucial. By identifying individuals who are at risk for suicide, interventions can be conducted to help prevent a tragedy. As stated previously, a strong predictor of future suicidal behavior is more than one previous suicide attempt. Other considerations that can be easily assessed are whether the person thinks about and desires suicide, and has a plan and has prepared to actually attempt suicide. Individuals who have thought about suicide, but do not have a plan, and have at least two other risk factors as described should be considered at least at moderate risk for suicide. Individuals who have had multiple suicide attempts in the past, or who have a plan and are prepared to attempt suicide, should be considered to be at least at moderate risk in the presence of any additional risk factor. Therefore, when trying to establish an individual's risk for suicide, it is important to evaluate his or her current suicidal thoughts and plans in addition to all risk factors that may be present.

PREVENTATIVE STEPS AND TREATMENT

With regard to treatment, a solid empirical base does not exist in the suicidality literature. A common treatment approach for a person who is suicidal is hospitalization. However, there is not strong empirical support for the effectiveness of hospitalization. Psychotropic medications are used with some suicidal patients to help stabilize their moods. Many studies indicate that techniques involving cognitive–behavioral therapy and problem solving are safe and effective for suicidal people. Sometimes therapists also work with suicidal clients on skill building and personality development.

SUICIDE AND CHRONIC PHYSICAL ILLNESS

Although it is true that physical illness increases the risk of suicidal behavior, and is in fact a risk factor for suicide, it would be incorrect to assume that having a terminal illness causes suicidality. The majority of people diagnosed with a terminal illness do not attempt suicide. The risk for suicide is elevated among people with particular illnesses. Cancer patients and those with neurological disorders commit the largest number of suicides among the physically ill.

It is not the physical illness that increases people's inclinations to suicidal behavior per se. What is more likely is that the factors associated with a physical illness lead to increased suicidal behavior. These factors can include a number of stressful issues that a patient experiences through the course of an illness. Many people have difficulties before they are diagnosed because they are worried about the possibility of having a disease. Once people are diagnosed, they have to confront the reality that they have a disease and are faced with anxiety about cures, prognosis, and financial issues. After their diagnostic period, many people worry about the success of their treatment and have social problems such as loss of income. These new doubts, fears, and worries could lead to a crisis reaction, possibly precipitating suicidal behavior.

There are a number of other factors associated with an increased risk of suicide among the physically ill. Often it is possible for physical illness to contribute to other physical, psychological, and social problems. Included in these problems are pain, the loss of ability to work, social limitations, and pressure for payment from financial support agencies. When people are ill, they often experience changes in their perceptions of their self and relationships with significant others. These perceptions of changes, as well as actual changes, can also contribute to suicidal behavior.

Suicide kills many every year. In the United States nearly 30,000 people die every year by suicide, with the most at-risk people being White men older than 65 years. Although no single risk factor causes a person to commit suicide, there are a number of risk factors associated with suicidal behavior. These risk factors include age, sex, psychiatric diagnosis, a history of a previous suicide attempt, a history of child abuse, stressful life events, lack of social support, impulsivity, cognitive distortions, and active suicidal thoughts and behaviors. Although some treatments have been found to be helpful for people with suicidal ideations, there is no one reliable treatment that has been proven to be effective. Though the research is limited, cognitive–behavioral therapy is building a reputation as a treatment of choice for suicidal symptoms. Most people with physical illnesses do not commit suicide. However, suicidal behavior is strongly related to physical illness, and is related in particular to cancer and neurological illnesses. The correlation between suicide and physical illness is likely due to the stressors associated with a physical illness as opposed to the physical illness itself.

Related Entries: Depression, Euthanasia and Physician-Assisted Suicide

BIBLIOGRAPHY

American Association of Suicidology. *Suicide data page: 1999.* Modified November 16, 2001. Available at www.suicidology.com

Golblatt, M. J. (2000). Physical illness and suicide. In R. W. Marris, A. L. Berman, & M. M. Silverman (Eds.), *Comprehensive textbook of suicidology* (pp. 00–00). New York: Guilford.

Joiner, T., & Rudd, D. M. (Eds.). (2000). *Suicide science: expanding the boundaries.* Norwell, MA: Kluwer Academic.

Joiner, T., Walker, R., Rudd, D. M., et al. (1999). Scientizing and routinizing the assessment of suicidality in outpatient practice. *Professional Psychology: Research and Practice, 30,* 447–453.

Lester, D. (2001). The epidemiology of suicide. In D. Lester (Ed.), *Suicide prevention* (pp. 3–16). Philadelphia: Brunner-Routledge.

McIntosh, J. L. (2000). Epidemiology of adolescent suicide in the United States. In R. W. Marris, S. Canetto, J. McIntosh, & M. Silverman, (Eds.), *Review of suicidology* (pp. 3–33). New York: Guilford.

Overholser, J. C., Spirito, A., & Adams, D. (1999). Suicide attempts and completion during adolescence: A biopsychosocial perspective. In A. J. Goreczny & M. Hersen (Eds.), *Handbook of pediatric and adolescent health psychology* (pp. 413–428). Needham Heights, MA: Allyn & Bacon.

Rudd, M. D., Joiner, T., & Rajab, H. M. (2001). *Treating suicidal behavior: An effective, time-limited approach* New York: Guilford.

Stenager, E. N., & Stenager, E. (2000). Physical illness and suicidal behaviour. In K. Hawton & K. van Heeringen (Eds.), *The international handbook of suicide and attempted suicide* (pp. 405–417). Chichester, UK: Wiley.

LaRicka R. Wingate
Jessica S. Brown
Thomas E. Joiner, Jr.

Sudden Infant Death Syndrome (SIDS)

Sudden infant death syndrome (SIDS) is a classification by exclusion. It is identified as the cause of death in infants less than 1 year of age when no other cause of death has been identified after thoroughly examining the case, the autopsy, the death scene, and the history of the infant. It has been suggested that SIDS claims the lives of 3,000 to 4,000 infants in the United States annually, accounting for more than one-third of all infant deaths. The peak incidence of SIDS falls between 2 and 4 months of age. The rate of SIDS had dropped steadily since 1992, but began to level off in 2000.

The precise cause of SIDS is not known; however, a variety of proposed mechanisms have been suggested, including asphyxia, hyperthermia or overheating, and the rebreathing of air leading to hypoxia. Other research has suggested that it may result from abnormal sleep/wake, temperature, or cardiorespiratory regulation. Recent research has focused on long QT syndrome (LQTS), a genetic disorder associated with cardiac arrhythmia, as playing a role in some SIDS deaths.

A variety of factors have been implicated in increasing risk for SIDS. Among the leading factors are placing an infant on his or her stomach while he or she is sleeping, placing the infant in soft bedding, dressing the infant too warmly for sleeping, and the presence of a smoker in the home. Other risk factors include low socioeconomic status, young maternal age, unwed mothers, less formal maternal education, maternal depression, late or no prenatal care, and low birth weight. Less commonly identified risk factors are parental drug use, infants sharing a bed with adults, infants sleeping alone in a room, and bottle feeding. More SIDS deaths occur during the winter months, among male infants, and among non-White infants. African-American and Native American infants are at two to three times higher risk for SIDS than the national average.

A variety of risk reduction strategies have been suggested. Among the best known is lying the infant on his or her back for sleep. The rate of SIDS has decreased by approximately 40% since the introduction of the Back to Sleep campaign by the National Institute of Child Health and Human Development in 1994. Other risk reduction strategies include a drug- and smoke-free environment before and after birth, keeping infants warm but not overheated (especially in the winter), encouraging breast feeding, and not placing the infant in or around soft surfaces, such as pillows, quilts, and soft mattresses.

In light of the literature suggesting a link between LQTS and SIDS, it has been suggested that an electrocardiogram should be done during the second or third week of life to identify LQTS. If the test indicates the presence of LQTS, implementation of appropriate treatment could reduce the risk.

Related Entry: Public Health

BIBLIOGRAPHY

Guntheroth, W. G., & Spiers, P. S. (2001). Thermal stress in sudden infant death syndrome: Is there an ambiguity with the rebreathing hypothesis. *Pediatrics, 107,* 693–698.

Kum-Nji, P., Mangrem, C. L., & Wells, P. J. (2001). Reducing the incidence of sudden infant death syndrome in the Delta region of Mississippi: A three-pronged approach. *Southern Medical Journal, 94,* 704–710.

Sullivan, F. M., & Barlow, S. M. (2001). Review of risk factors for sudden infant death syndrome. *Paediatric and Perinatal Epidemiology, 15,* 144–200.

Task Force on Infant Sleep Position and Sudden Infant Death Syndrome. (2000). Changing concepts of sudden infant death syndrome: Implications for infant sleeping environment and sleep position. *Pediatrics, 105,* 650–656.

W. Hobart Davies
Jennifer L. Specht

Symptom Perception

Rather than passively receiving information about the body, individuals perceive physical symptoms through an active and constructive process. Physical symptoms are thought to arise from a process in which changes in the functioning of the body are detected, attended to by the individual, and given meaning through their labeling as symptomatic of a given physical condition. As will be seen, there are numerous points at which this process can be influenced by physical, psychological, and social circumstances. For example, changes in the body can be missed, sensations that are not symptoms of disease can be mislabeled as symptomatic and acted on inappropriately, and actual symptoms of disease can be detected and attended to, but mislabeled as nonsymptomatic, delaying treatment and affecting medical outcomes.

Physical symptoms provide subjective information about the state and well-being of the body. The relationship between physical symptoms and objective measures of health, however, is modest at best. There is ample evidence that even when physical functioning can be measured objectively, many people with conditions such as asthma, hypertension, and diabetes base their daily medical management on their perception of physical symptoms. For example, although blood pressure can be measured easily, and research suggests that people are not very accurate in estimating blood pressure from their symptoms, many people with hypertension use their perception of symptoms to guide the level of their physical activity and the taking of medication.

SYMPTOM PERCEPTION ACCURACY

When an individual reports that she or he is experiencing a physical symptom, such as headache, she or he is reporting what is essentially a personal and private experience. The experience is observable only to the individual with the headache, and others gain knowledge of it only through observable illness behavior, that is, what the individual says or how she or he behaves. Some physical symptoms can be assessed for how accurately they map onto physical functioning, such as an individual reporting that his or her headaches relate to high blood pressure, which itself can be measured objectively. Most perceptions, however, have no such measurable referent. Regardless of the ability to validate accuracy (e.g., measurement of blood pressure), the sensations that an individual perceives (e.g., headache), and the way in which these perceptions are processed remain unobservable to others. These experiences are subjective and influenced by a number of environmental and psychological factors. Given this, it is not surprising that there is only a modest relationship between the symptoms people report and objective indicators of their physical functioning.

Further complicating this process is evidence not only that individuals differ in the accuracy with which they can identify physical symptoms related to their body's functioning, but that an individual's accuracy can change over time, as in James Pennebaker's study of people with diabetes. In this study, people with poorly controlled diabetes were more accurate in identifying the physical symptoms related to blood glucose fluctuations than people with well-controlled diabetes. This may be understandable, as poorly controlled diabetes results in more changes in glucose level and greater opportunity to learn which physical sensations relate to these changes. Later, when their diabetes was better controlled and changes in glucose level less pronounced, people's beliefs about which sensations related to glucose level did not change even though the actual symptoms related to glucose did, and they became less accurate. Thus, experience, expectation, and learning affect the perception of physical symptoms as well as physical factors. The main factors influencing the perception of symptoms that have been studied are those related to the symptoms themselves, demographic factors, attentional factors, and personality and mood factors. As will be seen, the distinctions made among these factors are at times arbitrary, and factors often overlap.

SYMPTOM FACTORS

Physical symptoms can be characterized along a number of different dimensions, such as duration, frequency, and quality, and these dimensions affect the likelihood that symptoms will be recognized. Sensations that are more intense and appear suddenly, such as pain, are more likely to be noticed and labeled as symptomatic than sensations that are indistinct and longstanding, such as tiredness. Sensations in different parts of the body may also be more likely to be noticed. For example, sensations in the chest may be more likely to be noticed and labeled as symptoms than sensations in the arm. Differences in symptom perception dimensions such as these can present difficulties for individuals, as some very serious conditions (e.g., heart attack) may be experienced along dimensions that are less likely to be noticed (e.g., numbness in arm), delaying identification and treatment.

PHYSICAL FACTORS

The ability to detect and report physical symptoms may also be affected by the state of the body itself. An area that has been studied extensively is the ability of individuals to detect and report on their cardiac activity, with the consistent finding that individuals differ in this ability. One factor that may

account for differences is an individual's physical conditioning. Individuals with a lower proportion of body fat are better discriminators of cardiac activity than others, and individuals with larger, more efficient hearts, like athletes, tend to be better at reporting cardiac activity than less conditioned individuals. In these cases, body fat may act as an insulator, dampening the vibrations made by cardiac activity, and decreasing the ability of individuals to perceive cardiac activity.

In other cases, alterations in the functioning of nerves may influence symptom perception. One complication of diabetes, neuropathy, damages nerves, often of the feet and legs. Individuals with this condition may experience symptoms due to the nerve damage (e.g., pain, numbness, tingling, loss of balance). However, they also lose sensation in the extremities, which may lead them to miss physical symptoms associated with minor injuries. This missed perception can lead to delays in treatment and result in serious infection, which sometimes requires amputation.

DEMOGRAPHIC FACTORS

Older age and lower economic status have been shown to relate to an increase in symptom reporting. It is unclear whether this results from greater variability in health status, cultural factors, or some other cause. A large number of studies have been performed examining gender differences in the reporting of physical symptoms. Whether gender differences exist in symptom reporting is unclear, with some studies demonstrating that women report more physical symptoms than men, and other studies showing no difference between the groups. What is clear is that men and women use different types of information to understand their physical functioning.

Studies that bring people into the laboratory to examine accuracy of symptom reporting suggest that men are more accurate perceivers of cardiovascular, gastrointestinal, and blood glucose activity than women. However, field studies, which occur in natural environments, have suggested that women are equal to and perhaps more accurate than men in this ability. These strikingly different findings appear to result from gender-based differences in the information men and women use to understand their symptom experiences. In making decisions about physical sensations, men tend to relay more heavily on internal, physiological cues, whereas women are more likely to rely on external, environmental cues, such as time since last meal or level of physical activity. Laboratory-based studies usually put great effort into controlling both the environment in which the experiment takes place and the availability of external information by having all participants equated on such things as time of day of the experiment, time since last meal, and level of activity. This places greater emphasis on internal cues and may favor the informational style more common in men. Field studies, which are more naturalistic, allow participants to use both internal and external cues to inform their judgments about their physical state. Thus, differences in accuracy are diminished.

ATTENTIONAL FACTORS

Individuals are limited in the amount of information that they can attend to and process at any given time. Thus, they must strike some balance between attending to internal and external information, and their ability to recognize internal, physical symptoms will depend on the ratio of internal to external information. James Pennebaker has suggested that when the environment is stimulating and exciting, attention tends to focus externally, and there is less capacity to attend to internal information, such as physical sensations. Conversely, an unstimulating and boring environment tends to increase the focus on internal states, which may lead people to notice more physical sensations. This competition-of-cues theory has been repeatedly upheld in research demonstrating that individuals report more physical symptoms in unstimulating environments than in challenging and exciting ones, even when the physical tasks they are performing are equal. It may also help explain why distraction is a useful short-term means of coping with physical discomfort.

MOOD AND PERSONALITY FACTORS

Personality and mood have also been linked to symptom perception and reporting. Individuals experiencing negative mood states (e.g., sadness) report more physical symptoms than individuals experiencing positive mood states (e.g., happiness). These findings hold for both laboratory studies in which negative mood is manipulated and field studies in which negative mood occurs naturally.

The aspect of personality that has been examined most in relation to symptom perception is neuroticism or negative affectivity (NA). NA is best thought of as a dimension of normal personality that encompasses susceptibility to negative moods, introspection, and a tendency to interpret the world and the self in negative terms. NA has been reliably linked to increased reports of physical symptoms across a wide range of populations and symptoms. However, although high-NA individuals report more physical symptoms than low-NA individuals, they do not appear to differ in objective health status. Thus, NA relates to symptom reporting, but not health.

David Watson and James Pennebaker suggested that the introspection and emotional distress that underlie NA influence the labeling of physical sensations, and may account for differences in symptom reporting. This symptom perception

hypothesis suggests that an internal focus of attention coupled with distress leads individuals to scan their bodies more frequently, leading them to notice more physical sensations. Because they are anxious and see things negatively, these sensations are more likely to be labeled as signs of physical pathology, and to be reported as symptoms. This increase in the reporting of symptoms regardless of disease explains the results of studies finding no relationship between NA and illness.

Symptom perception is a constructive process in which individuals make meaning of sensory information by detecting, attending to, labeling, and making attributions about its cause and significance. This process is influenced simultaneously by multiple factors, including psychological, physical, and environmental conditions. Although people vary widely in their ability to accurately perceive and report on physical symptoms, and use symptoms to guide their health care behavior, the relationship between reports of physical symptoms and objective indices of health and disease is modest.

Related Entries: Neuroticism, Treatment Delay

BIBLIOGRAPHY

Costa, P. T., & McCrae, R. R. (1987). Neuroticism, somatic complaints and disease: Is the bark worse than the bite? *Journal of Personality, 55,* 299–316.

Croyle, R. T., & Uretsky, M. B. (1987). Effects of mood on self-appraisal of health status. *Health Psychology, 6,* 239–253.

Fillingim, R. B., & Fine, M. A. (1986). The effects of internal versus external information processing on symptom perception in an exercise setting. *Health Psychology, 5,* 115–123.

Friedman, H. S., & Booth-Kewley, S. (1987). The "disease-prone personality": A meta-analytic view of the construct. *American Psychologist, 42,* 539–555.

Larsen, R. J., & Kasimatis, M. (1991). Day-to-day physical symptoms: Individual differences in the occurrence, duration, and emotional concomitants of minor daily illnesses. *Journal of Personality, 59,* 387–423.

Leventhal, H., Diefenbach, M., & Leventhal, E. A. (1992). Illness cognition: Using common sense to understand treatment adherence and affect cognition interactions. *Cognitive Therapy and Research, 16,* 143–163.

Pennebaker, J. W. (1982). *The psychology of physical symptoms.* New York: Springer-Verlag.

Pennebaker, J. W. (2000). Psychological factors impacting the reporting of physical symptoms. In A. Stone (Ed.), *The Science of self-report: Implications for research and practice* (pp. 523–570). Mahwah, NJ: Erlbaum.

Smith, G. R., Monson, R. A., & Ray, D. C. (1986). Patients with multiple unexplained symptoms. Their characteristics, functional health, and health care utilization. *Archives of Internal Medicine, 146,* 69–72.

Watson, D., & Pennebaker, J. W. (1989). Health complaints, stress, and distress: Exploring the central role of negative affectivity. *Psychological Review, 96,* 234–254.

Watson, D., & Pennebaker, J. W. (1992). Situational, dispositional, and genetic bases of symptom reporting. In J. A. Skelton & R. T. Croyle (Eds.), *Mental representations in health and illness* (pp. 60–84). New York: Springer-Verlag.

STEVEN C. PALMER

Tt

Taylor, Shelley E. (1946–)

Shelley Taylor is professor of psychology at UCLA and a leading researcher on stress, coping, and disease processes. Taylor's early research in health psychology focused on psychosocial issues surrounding cancer and its treatment. From this work, she developed cognitive adaptation theory, which maintains that people actively strive to achieve a positive sense of the self, the world, and the future following an intense personal threat, through the processes of finding meaning, regaining a sense of personal control, and engaging in motivated social comparisons with others. This work continues to guide current thinking about adjustment to trauma.

In this research, Taylor uncovered a curious trend, namely that adjustment to chronic illness often depended on "positive illusions," that is, seeing the self, the world, and the future in a somewhat falsely positive way. This work subsequently became a highly influential model for understanding not only health-related threats, but threats to the self more generally. Recently, Taylor and her colleagues extended these ideas to illness progression and have shown that falsely positive beliefs about one's vulnerability to AIDS and its complications among HIV-seropositive people are associated with a slower course of HIV infection.

Taylor's research has also focused on social support. With colleagues, she developed the stress theory tend-and-befriend, a complimentary model to fight-or-flight, which maintains that people cope with threat not merely by fighting or fleeing from it, but also by tending to their young and affiliating with the social group in order to protect against stress. This tend-and-befriend process may be biologically rooted in oxytocin and endorphins and be particularly characteristic of females' stress

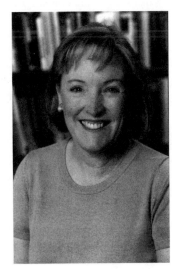

Taylor, Shelley E.

responses. This work has extended into an analysis of risky families, which identifies pathways by which conflict-ridden, cold, and unsupportive families may erode the health of offspring long into adulthood.

Taylor has been active in the profession. She helped to found one of the earliest health psychology programs at UCLA. When interest among psychologists in health-related issues grew, Taylor wrote the first textbook for the field, *Health Psychology*, which continues to be a primary source for training students in the field. Taylor's work has led to many awards including the Distinguished Scientific Contribution Award from the American Psychological Association, Yale University's Wilbur Lucius Cross Medal, the Donald Campbell Award in Social Psychology, and the Outstanding Scientific Contribution Award in Health Psychology.

BIBLIOGRAPHY

Taylor, S. E., & Brown, J. (1988). Illusion and well-being: A social psychological perspective on mental health. *Psychological Bulletin, 103*, 193–210.

Taylor, S. E., Klein, L. C., Lewis, B. P., Gruenewald, T. L., Gurung, R. A. R., & Updegraff, J. A. (2000). Biobehavioral responses to stress in females: Tend-and-befriend, not fight-or-flight. *Psychological Review, 107*, 411–429.

Shelley E. Taylor

Technology and Health

Over the past four decades, computer technology has improved exponentially while cost has decreased. Personal computers (PCs) are more sophisticated, and PC-based programming languages are powerful yet relatively easy to use. Technological applications to health psychology practice are considerable in number and scope. As managed care places new demands on health care service provision, it is essential for health psychologists to capitalize on emerging technologies to facilitate efficient practice. However, these new developments require sensitivity to emerging ethical issues as new ethical guidelines and principles are developed, and as new state and federal policies affect health psychology practice.

This overview considers how recent technological developments affect the practice of health psychology with respect to administration, clinical practice, and training. First addressed is the use of developing technology (such as electronic media) for administrative activities. Then the clinical application of computers to therapy (e.g., online forums of counseling via the Internet, telehealth) and computer-assisted assessment (administration, scoring, and interpreting tests with computers and computer software) are reviewed. Finally, computer-assisted training of health psychologists (e-learning, online supervision, virtual practicum using the Internet or satellite technology) is addressed, concluding with a review of professional organization responses to emerging technologies.

A BRIEF HISTORY

Computer-based applications in psychology-related professions began in the 1960s, with computer-based test interpretation. During the 1970s, researchers expanded computer-assisted testing capabilities to include administration, scoring, and interpretation of psychological tests, and their use increased over time. With less success than its assessment-based counterparts, computer-assisted psychotherapy also began in the 1960s, evolving into various types of computer-assisted therapies including professional consultation programs, client ther-

apeutic learning programs, and online therapy. New and powerful PC technology increases efficiency and productivity and can replace mundane pencil-and-paper tasks in health psychology practice. However, health psychologists need to consider the assets and limitations of technological applications before implementing them.

ADMINISTRATION

As computer technology is infused into health psychology practice, the use of paper, typewriter, and pen may be replaced by fax machines, Internet capabilities, wireless satellite networks, and personal digital assistants (also available in cellular phone combinations). Cell phones, e-mail, and fax technologies are commonplace.

Health psychologists are cautioned not to send confidential data through these technologies without appropriate precautions, if at all. To implement these technologies, health psychologists need to carefully apply existing standards of ethical practice to these emerging technologies, as well as consider emerging issues unique to these new tools. The American Psychological Association's (APA) *Ethical Principles of Psychologists and Code of Conduct* (1992; revised 2002) requires that psychologists "maintain appropriate confidentiality in creating, storing, accessing, transferring, and disposing of records under their control, whether these are written, automated, or in any other medium" (Section 5.04).

Personal computer systems comprise hardware and software. Hardware is electrical and mechanical equipment, such as the central processing unit in the chassis of the computer, monitors, printers, and various peripheral devices. Software is programming code that directs the hardware to run various applications, such as word processors for creating text documents, spreadsheets for numerical record keeping, databases for file records, combinations or suites of similar applications, and previously mentioned assessment and therapeutic programs.

Hardware that stores electronic media includes internal hard drives; floppy disk drives; compact disk drives; ZIP and JAZ drives, which are similar to floppy disk technology; and servers with large data storage drives for a network of computers. Hardware can be safeguarded with mechanical lock and key, but once turned on, such systems are vulnerable unless protected by security software that requires a password to access to the system. Health psychologists can use a server to manage a network of computers (e.g., a local area network), which can be accessed by others over telephone lines. Systems can be designed with the appropriate safeguards and security protocols to maintain confidentiality.

The Health Insurance Portability and Accountability Act is a federal statute related to the management of electronic data in health psychology and allied health settings. Signed into law in August 1996, it was designed to protect Americans from losing their health insurance when they changed jobs or residences. The act also set up consistent standards for transmitting electronic health care claims, storing information, and protecting an individual's privacy. The Department of Health and Human Services set up a deadline of April 14, 2003, for professionals to standardize their practices in line with the privacy rule requirements of the act. As with all new legislation, regulatory standards are evolving as the new law is implemented, so health psychologists need to check with their professional associations for updates.

COMPUTER-ASSISTED THERAPY

Virtual psychotherapy programs are therapeutic software products marketed to operate without therapist assistance. In general, such technology has yet to be widely implemented; further research is needed to evaluate its effectiveness. Educational programs have experienced the most success. Career counseling often involves information provision, which is ideal for computer-assisted venues. Computerized career counseling benefits clients who are highly motivated and goal directed. However, clients with less-clear goals and less motivation for independence may benefit less.

Cognitive retraining therapy occurs in rehabilitation settings, where computer programs can implement repetitive exercises to enhance cognitive functioning, including alertness, attention, concentration, fine-motor skills, memory, and certain language abilities (e.g., spelling, reading, and word finding). Therapeutic computer programs have also been developed to assist people dealing with AIDS, drug and alcohol abuse, obesity, burn pain, personal distress, sexual dysfunction, smoking cessation, depression, phobias, violent offenders, and stress (Peterson, 2003).

As computer technology progresses, so will computer-assisted therapies. Researchers will need to compare the outcomes of real-life service modalities and computer-assisted ones, determine what factors contribute to effective therapy, and evaluate client safety issues (e.g., the tendency to accept computer-generated data at face value). Although cost savings, convenience, and independent use are benefits associated with such technology, health psychologists need to be aware of potential negligence in its use. As malpractice suits are litigated, resulting laws, codes, and standards will evolve.

ONLINE FORUMS OF THERAPY

Online forums of psychology-related service provision use the Internet, a product of computer networks originally used by the U.S. military to communicate with education, government, and business institutions working on military projects. The World Wide Web (WWW) consists of computer servers and graphical interfaces connected to the Internet, which exchange audio, visual, and text-based information. Online forums have been described a number of ways in the psychological literature: psychotherapy in cyberspace, counseling on the information highway, behavioral telehealth, cybercounseling, telepsychology, WebCounseling, and, simply, counseling over the Internet.

Online forums in counseling and psychology have taken several forms. Intranet, or closed Internet systems, permit virtual psychotherapy with a controlled audience. Therapeutic consultants can provide services through Internet chat rooms. Bulletin board systems can be organized around a topic of interest, moderated or unmoderated, where people can read postings or add their own. Internet relay chat allows two people to correspond in real time. Computer conferencing allows groups of individuals to converse simultaneously through text.

Telehealth services provide access to health information and services remotely. Such services have recently gained government support. Health care providers are eligible for Medicare reimbursements equal to coverage for office visits for telehealth services to rural areas determined by the federal government to have shortage of health professionals. The APA's Board of Professional Affairs has allocated resources since 1997 to consider the ethical implications of telepsychology, and articulated and disseminated information regarding its relationship to telehealth and telemedicine.

Many states have developed legislation related to online counseling-related services. One issue of concern is how credentialing is managed across jurisdictions (e.g., someone in New York providing services to Illinois). Outcomes of malpractice lawsuits involving behavioral telehealth will dictate case law. Koocher and Morray (2000) provided some useful precautions in using this new technology.

Sampson and his associates (1997) accurately predicted the development of an information highway where cable service carriers will combine efforts with telephone services, allowing access to the Internet and the WWW through television cable networks. They predicted such technology could be used to advertise online counseling services and provide real-time video conferencing for clients to shop for potential therapists and for therapists to screen clients. Their predictions were accurate, as psychology services increasingly occur over Web and other telehealth modalities, providing access to consumers in remote areas or who are unable to travel.

COMPUTER-ASSISTED ASSESSMENT

Computer-assisted assessment includes automated administration, scoring, and interpreting of personality tests, cognitive tests, and structured interviews. Such technology has experienced widespread use. Computer-assisted testing also advanced the use of adaptive or tailored testing, which allows

Table 1. Websites and Sources with Developing Standards

National Career Development Association Guidelines for the Use of the Internet for Provision of Career Information and Planning Services (1997)	www.ncda.org/about/polnet.html
American Counseling Association (ACA), in collaboration with ERIC/Counseling and Student Services Clearinghouse	Cybercounseling and Cyberlearning: Strategies and Resources for the Millenium (Bloom & Walz, 2000)
ACA Ethical Standards for Internet Counseling (1999)	www.counseling.org
American Psychological Association (APA), Commonsense in a 'Dot Com' World (1986)	http://www.apa.org/practice/dotcom.html
APA Ethics Committee, discussion of services by telephone, teleconferencing, and Internet	http://www.apa.org/ethics/stmnt01.html
National Board of Certified Counselors, suggestions to guide the practice of WebCounseling (1997)	www.nbcc.org/ethics/wcstandards.htm
Center for the Study of Technology in Counseling and Career Development	www.career.fsu.edu/techcenter/
Federal Communications Commission, grants for public, nonprofit entities wishing to develop their potential in these areas	www.fcc.gov/healthnet

the examinee's responses to determine which subsequent items are to be administered, reducing the number of items necessary, providing more difficult items for higher-ability examinees, and more achievable, less discouraging items for lower-ability examinees.

Storing and retrieving test data can be more reliable with computer applications than traditional means, minimizing human error. However, as with computer-assisted therapy applications, reliability of computer-assisted assessment relies on the health psychologist using it. A computer cannot observe the examinee during testing, nor interpret a test score in light of environmental stimuli, distracters, or arousal level of the client during assessment. Neuropsychological testing in particular relies on a stimulus–response complexity that is difficult to duplicate with current computer technology.

The *Standards for Educational and Psychological Testing* (American Education Research Association, American Psychological Association, National Council on Measurement in Education, 1999) address computer-based testing in general, the development of computer-administered tests, the use of computer-generated test interpretations, and the implementation of computer adaptive testing. To use test norms established on paper-and-pencil versions, the computerized version must be psychometrically equivalent.

TRAINING

The Internet can be used to train psychologists through distance learning and remote supervision. In supervision, e-mail can be used to share professional ideas and information with supervisees in remote and distant areas. Removing the face-to-face interaction between supervisor and supervisee may limit the data to which supervisors may respond (e.g., body language, reaction to constructive criticism). However, with the development of satellite and computer technology that allows

real-time video and audio interaction, these limitations can be minimized.

Distance learning can use television, radio, and satellite broadcasting in place of *in vivo* course instruction. HTML programming (a programming language for Web pages) capabilities and multimedia presentation of written material and high-quality graphics can be used by educators to make learning interactive and interesting. Curriculum can be delivered in a synchronous (real-time) scheduled presentation of on-line streaming video or in an asynchronous mode (e.g., the Blackboard or WebCT systems), where students can interact with the system as time allows. Combinations of the two modalities can be used for multimodal interactive curriculum. As with remote supervision, distance learning is useful to persons in remote areas, for students with limited mobility, and for professionals with busy schedules or economic limitations.

Health psychologists involved with distance learning initiatives need to be concerned about program integrity and continuity. An *in vivo* course may not translate well to a distance-learning format. Research is necessary to compare the effects of technology on traditional learning paradigms.

RESPONSE TO EMERGING TECHNOLOGIES

In response to the emerging technologies reviewed, counseling and psychology-related professional organizations have begun to address new standards of practice, and legislators have developed new statutes as case law presents. Practicing health psychologists should remain aware of developing information as they employ new technologies. Useful sources of such information are listed in Table 1.

This entry addressed emerging technologies in health psychology service provision and the ethical issues related to their implementation. The human element in health psychology remains essential to effective practice, with technology facilitating psychologists' efforts to provide efficient and effective interventions to the people whom they serve.

BIBLIOGRAPHY

American Counseling Association. (1995). American Counseling Association code of ethics and standards of practice. *Counseling Today, 37,* 33–40.

American Counseling Association. (1999). *Ethical standards for Internet online counseling.* Available at www.counseling.org

American Educational Research Association, American Psychological Association, National Council on Measurement in Education. (1999). *Standards for educational and psychological testing.* Washington, DC: American Educational Research Association.

American Psychological Association. (1986). *Guidelines for computer-based tests and interpretations.* Washington DC: Author.

American Psychological Association. (1992). *Ethical principles of psychologists and code of conduct.* Washington, DC: Author. Available at http://www.apa.org/ethics

American Psychological Association. (1997, November 5). *Services by telephone, teleconferencing, and Internet: A statement by the ethics committee of the American Psychological Association.* Available at http://www.apa.org.ethics/stmnt01.html

Bloom, J. W., & Walz, G. R. (Eds.). (2000). *Cybercounseling and cyberlearning: Strategies and resources for the millennium.* Alexandria, VA: American Counseling Association.

Commission on Rehabilitation Counselor Certification. (June 2001). *Code of professional ethics for certified rehabilitation counselors and CRCC guidelines and procedures for processing complaints.* Rolling Meadows, IL: Author.

Council for Accreditation of Counseling and Related Education Programs. (1996). *CACREP accreditation standards and procedures manual* (*rev. ed.*). Alexandria, VA: Author.

Council on Rehabilitation Education. (2000). *Re-accreditation manual for rehabilitation counselor education programs.* Rolling Meadows, IL: Author.

Glueckauf, R. L., Whitton, J. D., & Nickelson, D. W. (2002). Telehealth: The new frontier in rehabilitation and health care. In M. J. Scherer, (Ed.), *Assistive technology: Matching device and consumer for successful rehabilitation* (pp. 197–213). Washington, DC: American Psychological Association.

Hufford, B. J., Glueckauf, R. L., & Webb, P. M. (1999). Home-based, interactive videoconferencing for adolescents with epilepsy and their families. *Rehabilitation Psychology, 44,* 176–193.

Kilvingham, Jr., F. M., Johnston, J. A., Hogan, R. S., & Mauer, E. (1994). Who benefits from computerized career counseling? *Journal of Counseling and Development, 72,* 289–292.

Koocher, G. P., & Morray, E. (2000). Regulation in telepsychology: A survey of state attorneys general. *Professional Psychology: Research and Practice, 31,* 503–508.

National Board of Certified Counselors. (1997). *Code of ethics.* Charlotte, NC: Author.

National Board of Certified Counselors. (1997). *Standards for the ethical practice of WebCounseling.* Available at http://www.nbcc.org/ethics/wcstandards.htm

Peterson, D. B. (2003). Ethics and technology. In R. Rocco Cottone & Vilia, M. Tarvydas, *Ethical and professional issues in counseling* (2nd ed., pp. 00–00). Upper Saddle River, NJ: Merrill Prentice Hall.

Sampson, J. P., Jr., Kolodinsky, R. W., & Greeno, B. P. (1997). Counseling on the information highway: Future possibilities and potential problems. *Journal of Counseling and Development, 75,* 203–212.

Sampson, J. P., Jr., Reardon, R. C., Wilde, C. K., Norris, D. S., Peterson, G. W., Strausberger, S. J., et al. (1994). Comparison of the assessment components of 15 computer-assisted career guidance systems. In J. T. Kapes, M. Moran-Mastie, & E. A. Whitfield (Eds.), *A counselor's guide to career assessment instruments* (pp. 373–379). Alexandria, VA: National Career Development Association.

DAVID B. PETERSON

Testicular Self-Examination

Testicular cancer is the most common tumor found in men between 15 and 35 years of age. International incidence rates of testicular cancer more than doubled over the course of the 20th century. In 2002, 7,500 new cases and 400 deaths from testicular cancer were estimated to occur in the United States. Risk factors for this malignancy include White race, history of undescended testicle, and family history.

The typical presentation of testicular cancer is a painless lump or mass on the testicle. However, many patients also report aching, discomfort, firmness, or swelling within the scrotum. Early detection of malignancy is essential because testis tumors can double in size within a few weeks. Ten-year survival rates for patients at all stages is 95% or higher, but patients with earlier-stage cancers at diagnosis have a better long-term prognosis. For these reasons, many physicians recommend teaching testicular self-examination (TSE) to young men. However, large-scale routine screening for testicular cancer is a more controversial issue. Formal routine screening may not be justifiable because testicular cancer is relatively rare and has a high cure rate, and studies do not show declines in mortality following large-scale screening efforts.

Men are advised to conduct TSE while standing under a warm shower to relax muscles that allow the scrotum to lengthen. Then, a single testicle is held between the thumb and the first two fingers. With the two fingers, the surface of the testicle is gently felt for a hard lump that is clearly different from the rubbery, uniform surface of the testicle. Men are taught that the structure at the back of the testicle is the epididymis, not a tumor.

Researchers have primarily focused on knowledge as a determinant of the practice of TSE among young males. Medical professionals rarely teach TSE to their young male patients. Therefore, it is not surprising that very few young men know about testicular cancer or how to perform proper TSE (0%–25%) and even fewer perform TSE regularly (0%–5%). Interventions designed to educate young men about testicular cancer and TSE have been shown to increase knowledge and intentions to practice TSE. However, educational interventions have shown small effects on reported practice of TSE, and some research shows low correlations between the practice of TSE and the level of TSE knowledge. Other studies suggest that effects of educational interventions may be enhanced by providing TSE reminders to participants such as posters or prompts from medical personnel.

The few studies examining psychological predictors of TSE practices have also yielded mixed results. For example, fear of cancer and intent to practice TSE have shown modest or insignificant associations with reported TSE practices in cross-sectional studies. An intervention based on the theory of planned behavior showed improved TSE adherence as compared to atheoretical interventions. However, measured variables associated with planned behavior theory could not adequately explain study results. In sum, the small number of studies examining potential influences of TSE practices have not offered convincing explanations for low rates of TSE practice.

Related Entry: Breast Self-Examination

BIBLIOGRAPHY

Brubaker, R. G., & Wickersham, D. (1990). Encouraging the practice of testicular self-examination: A field application of the theory of reasoned action. *Health Psychology, 9*(2), 154–163.

Kinkade, S. (2000). Testicular cancer. *American Family Physician, 59*(9), 25–39.

Friman, P. C., & Finney, J. W. (1990). Health education for testicular cancer. *Health Education Quarterly, 17*(4), 443–453.

Murphy, W. G., & Brubaker, R. G. (1990). Effects of a brief theory-based intervention on the practice of testicular self-examination by high school males. *Journal of School Health, 60*(9), 459–462.

PHIL ULLRICH

Theory of Reasoned Action and Theory of Planned Behavior

INTRODUCTION

The theory of reasoned action and the theory of planned behavior are two of the most widely used social cognition models. They have been extensively used to predict and deepen our understanding of a wide variety of behaviors, including health behaviors. This entry describes the models, defines the various components within the models, and summarizes how these models have been used to predict and explain intentions and behavior.

THE THEORY OF REASONED ACTION

Martin Fishbein and Icek Ajzen first outlined the theory of reasoned action (TRA) in their book *Belief, Attitude, Intention, and Behavior: An Introduction to Theory and Research*, published in 1975. The theory built on their considerable previous work on how attitudes were related to behavior. The TRA was concerned only with behaviors that were voluntary and under an individual's control. According to the TRA, voluntary behaviors can be predicted by intentions, which represent how motivated a person is to perform that behavior. Intentions can be predicted from attitudes and subjective norms. Attitudes are the overall evaluations of the behavior by the individual, and subjective norms consist of a person's beliefs about whether other people who are important to them think they should engage in the behavior.

In the same way that intentions are held to have determinants, attitude and subjective norm are also held to have determinants. According to the TRA, attitudes are a function of an individual's most important outcome beliefs and outcome evaluations. An outcome belief is a person's belief about how likely a certain outcome will be if a particular behavior is performed. A person believing that jogging every morning is very likely to result in him or her losing weight is an example of an outcome belief. Outcome evaluations are a person's evaluation of these beliefs. For example, thinking that losing weight is a good thing is an example of an outcome evaluation. The model suggests that a belief-based measure of attitude can be calculated by multiplying each outcome belief by its corresponding outcome evaluation and then summing the resulting scores across all the salient outcome beliefs.

Subjective norm is thought to be a function of normative beliefs and motivation to comply with referent groups. Normative beliefs are measured by asking individuals to rate how likely it is that specific salient groups or individuals (referents) think they should or should not perform the behavior. Motivation to comply is measured by asking individuals to rate how strongly motivated they are to comply with that referent. A belief-based subjective norm measure can be calculated by multiplying each normative belief with its corresponding motivation to comply and then summing the resulting scores across the salient referents. Alice Eagly and Shelly Chaiken (1993) noted that Fishbein and Ajzen were not suggesting that an individual performs such calculations each time he or she is faced with a decision about whether to perform a behavior. Instead, the results of such considerations are maintained in memory and retrieved and used when necessary. However, it is also possible for the individual to retrieve the relevant beliefs and evaluations when necessary.

Fishbein and Ajzen also included what they termed external variables in the TRA. These included such demographic variables as age, gender, occupation, socioeconomic status, religion, and education. Other external variables included personality traits, attitudes toward people, and attitudes toward institutions. In the TRA none of these variables directly influences intentions or behavior, they but exert their influence through the other variables in the model.

Applications of the TRA

The TRA has been used to explain and predict a wide range of social behaviors. Eagly and Chaiken reviewed the tests of the TRA and found that it has been applied to behaviors such as blood donation, church attendance, family planning, eating at fast food restaurants, smoking marijuana, mothers' infant-feeding practices, dental hygiene behaviors, and having an abortion. In 1988 Blair Sheppard and colleagues carried out a meta-analysis of 87 studies that had been based on the TRA and found that, on average, the TRA accounted for 66% of the variance in intentions, and the mean correlation between intention and behavior was 0.53.

Criticisms of the TRA

Despite the number of studies showing support for the TRA, it has also received some criticism. Much of the criticism directed at the TRA focused on the issue of control and on environmental factors that are related to this issue. Sheppard and colleagues (1988) noted that researchers are often interested in understanding and predicting behaviors that are not completely under a subject's volitional control. Allen Liska (1984) pointed out that by limiting the model to volitional behaviors, Ajzen and Fishbein were excluding a wide range of behaviors, including those that required "skills, abilities, opportunities and the co-operation of others" (p. 63).

Several studies using the TRA found that by adding a measure of self-efficacy (i.e., an individual's belief that he or she is capable of performing a specific behavior to attain a desired outcome), the predictive value of the model is increased. For example Lisa Tedesco and colleagues (1991) found that adding self-efficacy to the TRA significantly increased the explained variance in self-reported teeth brushing and teeth flossing.

In their description of the boundary conditions of the TRA, Ajzen and Fishbein (1980) clearly stated that the model applied to behaviors that were under volitional control and defended their position by stating that most behaviors of social relevance were under volitional control. They also stated that behaviors that were not under volitional control might better be thought of as goals with different stages, and that each stage of the process involved in achieving a goal might be predicted by the TRA. However, it became apparent that many activities that at first appear to be under volitional control are in fact often influenced by factors outside one's control. Eagly and Chaiken

(1993) noted that there are many behaviors that are not under volitional control, but are very socially relevant, such as drug use, seat belt use, and class attendance.

In 1985 Ajzen contended that most behaviors could be treated as goals, which may not necessarily be attained. Ajzen and Thomas Madden (1986) later gave the example of mechanical problems when trying to drive a car as an example of how some behaviors are not completely under volitional control. It was an acknowledgment of the importance of considering behaviors that are not completely under volitional control, which paved the way for the theory of planned behavior (TPB).

THE THEORY OF PLANNED BEHAVIOR

In 1986 Ajzen and Madden published a paper describing the TPB. The theory is identical to the TRA except that an additional component is added to the model (see Figure 1). In addition to attitude and subjective norm, the TPB argues that intentions can also be predicted by perceived behavioral control (PBC). In addition, when PBC reflects actual control, it is predicted to directly influence behavior. PBC is a person's expectancy that performance of a behavior is within his or her control. The concept is similar to Albert Bandura's (1982) concept of self-efficacy. Control is seen as a continuum with easily executed behaviors at one end and behavioral goals demanding resources, opportunities, and specialized skills at the other.

Perceived behavioral control is held to have determinants in the same way as the attitude and subjective norm components of the model. Ajzen (1991) suggested that a belief-based measure of control can be calculated by multiplying corresponding control beliefs and power items together and then summing the resulting scores. Control beliefs are perceptions of factors likely to facilitate (facilitators) or inhibit (inhibitors) the performance of a behavior. These factors include both internal control factors (information, personal deficiencies, skills, abilities, emotions) and external control factors (opportunities, dependence on others, barriers). For example, a control belief could be measured by asking an individual to rate how likely it is that a facilitator will be present in a certain situation. Power items are measured by asking participants how each of the facilitators or inhibitors would influence the likelihood of them performing the behavior.

So, according to the TPB, individuals are likely to follow a particular health action if they believe that the behavior will lead to particular outcomes that they value, if they believe that people whose views they value think they should carry out the behavior, and if they feel that they have the necessary resources and opportunities to perform the behavior.

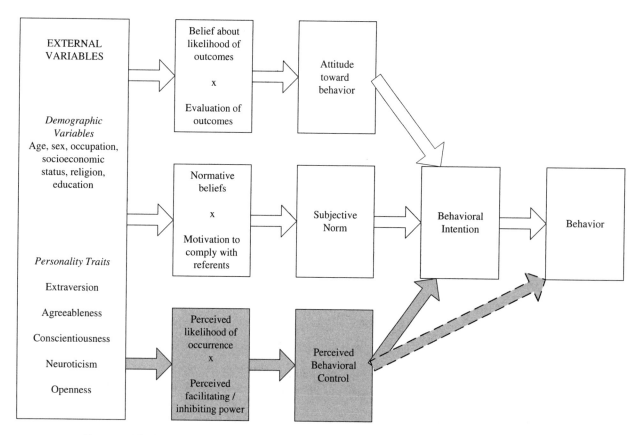

Figure 1.   The theory of planned behavior (the model without the gray components is the theory of reasoned action).

Applications of the TPB

Mark Conner and Paul Sparks (1996) noted that the TPB has been used to study a wide range of behaviors, including health behaviors such as smoking, alcohol consumption, sexual behaviors, health screening attendance, exercise, food choice, and breast or testicle self-examination. Several studies have provided evidence supporting the addition of PBC to the model. For example, a study by Ronald Schlegel and colleagues (1992) found that PBC contributed to the predictions of intentions and frequency of getting drunk in problem drinkers. A meta-analysis by Christopher Armitage and Mark Conner (2001) of 154 applications of the TPB revealed that intentions are normally well predicted by attitude, subjective norm, and PBC (39% variance explained), whereas behavior is well explained by intentions and PBC (27% variance explained).

The TRA and TPB have been widely tested and successfully applied to the understanding of a variety of behaviors. The TRA incorporates a number of important cognitive variables that appear to determine health behaviors, such as intentions, attitudes, and subjective norms. In addition to these variables, the TPB also includes a perceived behavioral control

component, which has been shown to improve the model's predictive power. Both theories state a clear causal ordering among variables in how they relate to behavior, allowing sophisticated analysis techniques to be applied to assessing the model. In addition, researchers are also starting to use the TPB to inform health interventions.

Related Entries: Health Belief Model, Self-Efficacy, Transtheoretical Model

BIBLIOGRAPHY

Ajzen, I. (1985). From intentions to actions: A theory of planned behavior. In J. Kuhl & J. Beckman (Eds.), *Action–control: From cognition to behavior* (pp. 11–39). Heidelberg: Springer.

Ajzen, I. (1991). The theory of planned behavior. *Organizational Behavior and Human Decision Processes, 50*, 179–211.

Ajzen, I., & Fishbein, M. (1980). *Understanding attitudes and predicting social behavior.* Englewood, NJ: Prentice-Hall.

Ajzen, I., & Madden, T. J. (1986). Prediction of goal-directed behavior: Attitudes, intentions, and perceived behavioral control. *Journal of Experimental Social Psychology, 22*, 453–474.

Armitage, C. J., & Conner, M. (2001). Efficacy of the theory of planned behavior: A meta-analytic review. *British Journal of Social Psychology, 40*, 471–499.

Bandura, A. (1982). Self-efficacy mechanism in human agency. *American Psychologist, 37*, 122–147.

Conner, M., & Sparks, P. (1996). The theory of planned behavior and health behaviors. In M. Conner & P. Norman (Eds.), *Predicting health behavior* (pp. 121–162), Buckingham, UK· Open University Press.

Eagly, A. H., & Chaiken, S. (1993). *The psychology of attitudes.* Fort Worth, TX: Harcourt Brace Jovanovich.

Fishbein, M., & Ajzen, I. (1975). *Belief, attitude, intention, and behavior: An introduction to theory and research.* Reading, MA: Addison-Wesley.

Liska, A. E. (1984). A critical examination of the causal structure of the Fishbein/Ajzen attitude–behavior model. *Social Psychology Quarterly, 47*, 61–74.

Schlegel, R. P., D'Avernas, J. R., Zanna, M. P., DeCourville, N. H., & Manske, S. R. (1992). Problem drinking: A problem for the theory of reasoned action? *Journal of Applied Social Psychology, 22*, 358–385.

Sheppard, B. H., Hartwick, J., & Warshaw, P. R. (1988). The theory of reasoned action: A meta-analysis of past research with recommendations for modifications and future research. *Journal of Consumer Research, 15*, 325–343.

Tedesco, L. A., Keffer, M. A., & Fleck-Kandath, C. (1991). Self-efficacy, reasoned action, and oral health behavior reports: A social cognitive approach to compliance. *Journal of Behavioral Medicine, 14*, 341–355.

Mark Conner
Brian McMillan

Transtheoretical Model

The transtheoretical model (TTM), also known informally as the stages-of- change model, has been influential in the field of health psychology. The TTM has most frequently been applied to smoking cessation, but has also been applied to many other health-related behaviors. The core of the TTM is the stages-of-change construct, which is a set of five classifications. The first three stages describe people currently engaged in a problem behavior, for example, smoking cigarettes. The precontemplation stage comprises people who are least ready change the problem behavior, the contemplation stage represents an intermediate level of readiness to change, and the preparation stage represents the highest level of readiness to change. There are also two stages defining people who have already changed the problem behavior. The action stage is defined as the first 6 months postchange, and maintenance is defined as sustained change beyond 6 months. The stages-of-change are best understood as intermediate outcomes in the process of long-term behavior change. Stage progression is conceptualized as progress toward behavior change, and ultimately to long-term maintenance of behavior change.

STAGES OF CHANGE AND THE TTM

The stages-of-change construct is only one component of the TTM. Other variables associated with the TTM have been hypothesized as mediators for stage progressions. These variables are known as the processes of change and the pros and cons of smoking. Much research has focused on the relationships between the stages-of-change and these process variables.

THE APPEAL OF THE TTM

The intuitive appeal of the TTM is similar to the appeal of stage models generally. To illustrate, consider the example of smoking cessation. If smokers could be arranged in an ordered set of categories leading to cessation, then interventions could be designed for each category to foster progressive stage movements leading ultimately to cessation and sustained abstinence. In other words, interventions could be matched to stage.

MEASURING THE STAGES

There has been little consistency regarding the measurement of the stages-of-change. Part of this lack of standardization is the inevitable result of defining stages for different problem behaviors. However, even within a specific behavior, such as smoking cessation, many different staging schemes have been employed. Despite the heterogeneity of staging methods, some generalizations can be made. There are essentially two classes of methods for measuring stages. The most common method is a staging algorithm. Staging algorithms rely largely on questionnaire items that require yes-or-no answers to questions regarding intention to change a behavior within fixed time frames. For example, the most recent smoking cessation algorithm defines the precontemplation-stage smokers as those who indicate that they do not intend to quit smoking in the next 6 months. Contemplators, according to the same algorithm, intend to quit in the next 6 months, and either are not seriously thinking about quitting within the next 30 days, had not made at least one 24-hr quit attempt in the last year, or both. Preparation-stage smokers are seriously thinking about quitting in the next 30 days and had at least one 24-hr quit attempt during the last year.

The second method of measuring stages involves continuous scales. Based on this method, each individual receives a "stage score" for each of the stages in the model. Thus, based on this method, an individual can have high stage scores for multiple stages simultaneously.

EMPIRICAL EVALUATIONS OF TTM

The TTM is a multifaceted model with a voluminous research literature. Weinstein et al. (1998) propounded four principles by which all stage models, including the TTM, can be evaluated. Next, the TTM is evaluated for each of these four principles.

Principle 1. Stages should consist of qualitatively different and mutually exclusive categories. The stages-of-change, at the conceptual level, comprise a sequence of qualitatively distinct categories. Precontemplators, in theory, are not yet contemplating cessation. Contemplators, in theory, are contemplating cessation, and preparers are, in theory, preparing for a quit attempt. However, theory and measurement cannot be separated. Substantial evidence suggests that the stages-of-change algorithm does not classify smokers into qualitatively different categories. One group of studies pointing to this conclusion is made up of studies employing both the stages-of-change algorithm and alternative measures of readiness to quit within the same sample of smokers. For example, several studies have indicated that large percentages of smokers classified as precontemplators are, in fact, contemplating a quit attempt. Discrepancies were also observed for the contemplation and preparation stages. In addition, researchers have noted the arbitrary distinction between the action and maintenance stages.

Continuous scales for each stage clearly does not conform to Principle 1. This method allows for individuals to have relatively high scores for multiple stages simultaneously. This approach contradicts the idea that stages are mutually exclusive categories.

Principle 2. There should be an ordering of the stage categories. The second principle presented by Weinstein et al. is that stages should follow an ordered sequence. Within the context of smoking cessation, this means that stages should follow a progressive series leading to cessation and maintained abstinence. The stages-of-change algorithm satisfies this requirement. It should be noted, however, that stages are not an invariant sequence. Individuals can skip stages, and regress to earlier stages. Some authors consider the skipping and regressing of stages to be inconsistent with a true stage theory, whereas others do not see this as an important contradiction of stage principles.

Principle 3. There should be similar barriers to change for individuals within each stage. If members of stage are qualitatively similar to one another, then group members should also face similar barriers for making progressive stage movements. This is the rationale underlying the idea of stage-matched interventions. There are two ways to evaluate the TTM with regard to Principle 3: (1) prospective studies of stage transitions and (2) stage-matched intervention studies.

Prospective Studies of Stage Transitions

First, reliable predictors of specific stage transitions should be identified. There have been very few studies addressing this issue. To complicate matters, there are several studies that appear to evaluate the prediction of progressive stage movements, but in fact do not. The first smoking study to use processes of change and pros and cons as predictor variables for stage movements was that of Prochaska et al. (1985). The results of this study were inconsistent, with approximately half of results for individual processes and pros and cons pointing in the hypothesized direction and half pointing in the opposite direction. Surprisingly, only one smoking study since 1985 has tested the capacity of processes of change and pros and cons to predict stage transitions. This study, by Herzog et al. (1999), found processes of change and pros and cons to be ineffective predictors of stage movements.

Stage-Matched Intervention Studies

The record of interventions based on the TTM has been modest. For instance, one prominent smoking cessation study, by Prochaska et al. (1993), compared four interventions: stage-based manuals alone, American Lung Association (ALA) manuals alone, stage-based manuals plus counseling, and stage-based manuals plus individualized computer feedback. Not surprisingly, the multicomponent interventions outperformed the two manuals-only conditions. The two manuals-only conditions (ALA vs. stage) produced comparable results, but the action-oriented ALA manuals produced greater cessation rates for baseline precontemplators than the stage-based manuals. This result runs counter to TTM theorizing, which agues that a major strength of the model lies in its recognition of the particular needs of precontemplators, who are said to be poorly served by standard action-oriented interventions.

Another study, by Quinlan and McCaul (2000), compared stage-matched and stage-mismatched interventions in a sample of precontemplation-stage smokers. The results revealed no advantage for the stage-matched intervention, and moreover revealed a nonsignificant trend in favor of the stage-mismatched condition. Another prominent smoking study, by Aveyard et al. (2001), employed a stage-based intervention for adolescents in Great Britain. The results showed no advantage for the stage-based intervention compared to a control condition.

The TTM has been used to design interventions of a variety of health behaviors (e.g., diet, exercise, and alcohol abuse). Several scholars have conducted reviews of TTM-based interventions for various behaviors. These reviews have come to the same general conclusion: Evidence supporting TTM-based interventions is mixed at best.

Principle 4. There should be different barriers to stage transitions among people in the different stages: If stages are qualitatively different categories, then what helps smokers in one stage should be different than what helps smokers in other stages. Principle 4 would also require that different predictors were significant for different stage transitions. However, no variables have reliably predicted progressive movements out of any of the stages. Likewise, the modest record of stage-matched interventions further indicates that Principle 4 is not satisfied.

CONCLUSION

The TTM has influenced many researchers and clinicians in their thinking regarding addictions and other health behaviors. At the conceptual and heuristic level, the model has been successful. At the scientific level, however, the TTM has been less of a success.

Related Entries: Health Belief Model, Theory of Reasoned Action and Theory of Planned Behavior

BIBLIOGRAPHY

Aveyard, P., Sherratt, E., Almond, J., Lawrence, T., Lancashire, R., Griffin, C., et al. (2001). The change-in-stage and updated smoking status results from a cluster-randomized trial of smoking prevention and cessation using the transtheoretical model among British adolescents. *Preventive Medicine, 33*, 313–324.

Bandura, A. (1997). Editorial: The anatomy of stages-of-change. *American Journal of Health Promotion, 12*, 8–10.

Davidson R. 1998. The transtheoretical model: A critical overview. In W. R. Miller & N. Heather (Eds.), *Treating addictive behaviors* (pp. 22–45). New York: Plenum.

Farkas, A. J., Pierce, J. P., Gilpin, E. A., Zhu, S. H., Rosbrook, B., Berry, C., et al. (1996). Is stage of change a useful measure of the likelihood of smoking cessation? *Annals of Behavioral Medicine, 18*, 79–86.

Herzog, T. A., Abrams, D. B., Emmons, K. A., & Linnan, L. (2000). Predicting increases in readiness to quit smoking; a prospective analysis using the contemplation ladder. *Psychology and Health, 15*, 369–381.

Herzog, T. A., Abrams, D. B., Emmons, K. A., Linnan, L., & Shadel, W. G. (1999). Do processes of change predict smoking stage movements? A prospective analysis of the transtheoretical model. *Health Psychology, 18*, 369–375.

Prochaska, J. O., DiClemente, C. C. & Norcross, J. C. (1992). In search of how people change: Applications to addictive behaviors. *American Psychologist, 47*, 1102–1114.

Prochaska, J. O., DiClemente, C. C., Velicer, W. F., Ginpil, S. E., & Norcross, J. C. (1985). Predicting change in smoking status for self-changers. *Addictive Behaviors, 10*, 396–406.

Prochaska, J. O., DiClemente, C. C., Velicer, W. F., & Rosi, J. S. (1993). Standardized, individualized, interactive, and personalized, self-help programs for smoking cessation. *Heath Psychology, 12*, 399–405.

Quinlan, K. B., & McCaul, K. D. (2000). Matched and mismatched interventions with young adult smokers: Testing a stage theory. *Health Psychology, 19*, 165–171.

Sutton, S. R. (2001). Back to the drawing board? A review of applications of the transtheoretical model to substance use. *Addiction, 96*, 175–186.

Weinstein, N. D., Rothman, A. J., & Sutton, S. R. (1998). Stage theories of health behavior: Conceptual and methodological issues. *Health Psychology, 17*, 290–299.

THADDEUS A. HERZOG

Treatment Delay

DEFINITION OF TREATMENT DELAY

Treatment delay is defined as the time that elapses from when a person first notices or recognizes a symptom or potential health problem until the time she or he receives definitive treatment by a health care provider. Treatment delay is an important phenomenon in health care because it affects the ability of clinicians to deliver appropriate treatment in a timely manner. Delay in treatment can result in increased morbidity and mortality. For example, if a person is experiencing symptoms of a heart attack, delay in seeking care prevents the application of proven treatments such as thrombolysis or angioplasty that minimize or prevent the heart attack. Delay results in greater destruction of heart muscle, leading to a poorer prognosis and reduced quality of life.

From a temporal standpoint, delay time is divided into patient delay and system or structural delay (e.g., transport, diagnostic, appointment, treatment, and hospital delays). System delays are relatively controllable, that is, amenable to structural changes in the health care system The result is improved efficiency in diagnosis and treatment. However, reduction of patient delay has proven much more challenging. Persons experiencing symptoms for diseases such as heart attacks, breast cancer, asthma, and others continue to delay unacceptably long periods of time despite massive patient education and early detection efforts.

One of the more notable examples of public education efforts has been in the area of patients experiencing heart attacks. Efforts to reduce delay in patients experiencing symptoms of a heart attack originally concentrated on reducing transport and hospital delay. These efforts were relatively successful, and it is generally felt that these times have been reduced as much as logistically possible. In the largest study to date, the Rapid Early Action for Coronary Treatment investigators reported that transport and hospital delay accounted for 3% to 8% and 22% to 33% of the total delay time, respectively. However, patient delay accounts for 50% to 75% of delay time. This time has not been reduced over the last two decades despite major efforts to educate the public.

Patient delay also comprises a substantial proportion of total delay time for women who experience symptoms of breast cancer. These times also have not been reduced despite aggressive education campaigns. Finally, asthma patients (adults and children) delay despite experiencing severe symptoms and patient education efforts.

STAGES OF TREATMENT DELAY

Patient delay is a complex, multifaceted problem, and the time between symptom onset and seeking definitive treatment is often divided into phases to gain a better understanding of the issue. The process of evaluating an illness may be different based on a number of factors, including timing of the symptoms (i.e., early or late in the process), their potential seriousness, and the amount of discomfort experienced. Researchers have labeled the stages of patient delay slightly differently; however, there is general agreement that it is helpful to divide them into the following three stages.

1. *Appraisal delay* is the period of time in which the person first notices that something is different or wrong and performs an appraisal of the situation. In other words, the person must decide if what she or he is experiencing is an illness or something out of the ordinary. If the answer to the question is "No," the result is appraisal delay. If the answer is "Yes, there is something wrong," she or he proceeds to the next stage, that of illness delay. Appraisal delay involves a mental representation of the health threat and is affected by the patient's subjective experience, the sense of vulnerability to illness, and general knowledge about that illness.

2. *Illness delay* is the period of time in which the person decides whether the symptoms are serious enough to require attention by a health care professional. If the individual judges the symptoms important enough to require action, then various alternatives are considered. Recently, illness delay has been categorized as the time taken to determine the coping or action plan. These coping and action plans operate on both emotional and cognitive levels.

3. *Utilization delay* is the period of time where the person assesses the costs and benefits of seeking care as well as the barriers to seeking care. If patients do not perceive that seeking care is worth the effort or that the barriers are too great, they continue to delay.

4. *Total patient delay time* is the sum of appraisal, illness, and utilization delay time.

INFLUENCE OF PSYCHOSOCIAL FACTORS ON TREATMENT-SEEKING BEHAVIOR

There are a number of psychosocial factors that influence treatment-seeking behavior. These factors may change somewhat depending on different disease states. People vary greatly in how they experience or perceive symptoms. Delay may increase if symptoms do not match a patient's expectation or are different than what she or he experienced previously in the same illness. Delay time can be increased if symptoms are vague, confusing, intermittent, or come on gradually. In the case of heart attack symptoms, patients often delay if they believe that the symptoms are not cardiac related. Severity of pain or other symptoms has not been shown to consistently affect delay time.

Patients delay longer when they hope that the symptoms will subside on their own, or if they try self-medication before seeking help. Delay is also increased if patients fail to recognize or understand the importance of symptoms. Patients are often worried about being embarrassed if their symptoms turn out to be nothing, and therefore delay longer. Interestingly, the presence of a family member or spouse increases delay in cardiac patients, but the presence of friends or coworkers *decreases* delay, presumably because they can evaluate the situation objectively and make more accurate assessments of appropriate courses of action than family members. On the other hand, telling a family member or friend *decreases* delay time in breast cancer patients.

Often, individuals are hesitant to bother the physician, hospital staff, family, and/or friends and will delay telling anyone. Asthma patients are known to delay seeking care because of previous negative experiences with emergency departments. Some asthma patients even fear that seeking medical care will somehow worsen their condition, which leads to a desire to "tough it out alone." Asthma patients also fear systemic corticosteriods because of side effects they experienced during prior treatments.

Some patients feel that if they enter the health care system by calling their physician or going to the hospital, they will lose control over their lives or that their lives will be disrupted. However, some research has shown that if patients believe that their condition can be treated effectively, they will seek help more quickly. This belief speaks to cost/benefit issues, with individuals more likely to seek immediate treatment if the treatment is known to have a positive impact on morbidity and mortality. A sense of fatalism, various self-care behaviors, perceived constraints, and in appropriate problem-solving style increase delay in breast cancer patients.

Sociodemographic factors also can influence patient delay. In breast cancer patients, it has been found that lower income and education levels affect delay. Older age, ethnic minority, lower income, and public payer insurance tend to be associated with delay in myocardial infarction patients. Economic considerations such as the expense of medication or hospitalization have also been shown to delay care seeking in asthma patients.

SUMMARY

Because delay in providing care causes increased morbidity and mortality, health care providers must understand the reasons for delay so that they can intervene in an appropriate and effective manner. For example, if patients state that they delay seeking treatment for symptoms because they will be embarrassed if the symptoms are nothing, then an appropriate intervention might be for the health care provider to focus on this issue, acknowledging that embarrassment is a normal response. A cost/benefit argument might be made that given the benefit of early treatment, being wrong on occasion is less important than avoiding the potential disability and loss of personal productive capacity. Lastly, it is important to note that most factors influencing patient delay are often modifiable, and therefore and efforts to reduce patient delay have direct benefits to patients in terms of decreased morbidity and mortality.

Related Entry: Cognitive Representations of Illness

BIBLIOGRAPHY

Alonzo, A. A. (1986). The impact of the family and lay others on care-seeking during life-threatening episodes of suspected coronary artery disease. *Social Science and Medicine, 22*, 1297–1311.

Burgess, C., Hunter, M. S., & Ramirez, A. J. (2001). A qualitative study of delay among women reporting symptoms of breast cancer. *British Journal of General Practice, 51*, 967–971.

Burgess, C. C., Ramirez, A. J., Richards, M. A., & Love, S. B. (1998). Who and what influences delayed presentation in breast cancer? *British Journal of Cancer, 77*, 1343–1348.

Caldwell, M. A., & Miaskowski, C. (2002). Mass media interventions to reduce help-seeking delay in people with symptoms of acute myocardial infarction: Time for a new approach? *Patient Education and Counseling, 46*, 1–9.

Caplan, L. S., Helzlsouer, K. J., Shapiro, S., Wesley, M. N., & Edwards, B. K. (1996). Reasons for delay in breast cancer diagnosis. *Preventive Medicine, 25*, 218–224.

Clark, L. T., Bellam, S. V., Shah, A. H., & Feldman, J. G. (1992). Analysis of prehospital delay among inner-city patients with symptoms of myocardial infarction: Implications for therapeutic intervention. *Journal of the National Medical Association, 84*, 931–937.

Dempsey, S. J., Dracup, K., & Moser, D. K. (1995). Women's decision to seek care for symptoms of acute myocardial infarction. *Heart and Lung, 24*, 444–456.

Dracup, K., McKinley, S. M., & Moser, D. K. (1997). Australian patients' delay in response to heart attack symptoms. *Medical Journal of Australia, 166*, 233–236.

Dracup, K., & Moser, D. K. (1997). Beyond sociodemographics: Factors influencing the decision to seek treatment for symptoms of acute myocardial infarction. *Heart and Lung, 26*, 253–262.

Facione, N. C. (1993). Delay versus help seeking for breast cancer symptoms: A critical review of the literature on patient and provider delay. *Social Science and Medicine, 36*, 1521–1534.

Facione, N. C., Miaskowski, C., Dodd, M. J., & Paul, S. M. (2002). The self-reported likelihood of patient delay in breast cancer: New thoughts for early detection. *Preventive Medicine, 34*, 397–407.

GISSI. (1995). Epidemiology of avoidable delay in the care of patients with acute myocardial infarction in Italy. A GISSI-generated study. GISSI—Avoidable Delay Study Group. *Archives of Internal Medicine, 155*, 1481–1488.

Janson, S., & Becker, G. (1998). Reasons for delay in seeking treatment for acute asthma: The patient's perspective. *Journal of Asthma, 35*, 427–435.

Johnson, J. A., & King, K. B. (1995). Influence of expectations about symptoms on delay in seeking treatment during myocardial infarction. *American Journal of Critical Care, 4*, 29–35.

Kenyon, L., Ketterer, M., Gheorghiade, M., & Goldstein, S. (1991). Psychological factors related to prehospital delay during acute myocardial infarction. *Circulation, 84*, 1969–1976.

Leventhal, H., Nerenz, D. R., & Steele, D. J. (1984). Illness representations and coping with health threats. In A. Baum, S. E. Taylor, & J. E. Singer (Eds.) *Handbook of psychology and health* (pp. 219–252). Hillsdale, NJ: Erlbaum.

Newby, L. K., Rutsch, W. R., Califf, R. M., et al. (1996). Time from symptom onset to treatment and outcomes after thrombolytic therapy. GUSTO-1 Investigators. *Journal of the American College of Cardiology, 27*, 1646–1655.

Ottesen, M. M., Kober, L., Jorgensen, S., & Torp-Pedersen, C. (1996). Determinants of delay between symptoms and hospital admission in 5978 patients with acute myocardial infarction. The TRACE Study Group. Trandolapril Cardiac Evaluation. *European Heart Journal, 17*, 429–437.

Reilly, A., Dracup, K., & Dattolo, J. (1994). Factors influencing prehospital delay in patients experiencing chest pain. *American Journal of Crit Care, 3*, 300–306.

Safer, M. A., Tharps, Q. J., Jackson, T. C., & Leventhal, H. (1979). Determinants of three stages of delay in seeking care at a medical clinic. *Medical Care, 17*, 11–29.

Schmidt, S. B., & Borsch, M. A. (1990). The prehospital phase of acute myocardial infarction in the era of thrombolysis. *American Journal of Cardiology, 65*, 1411–1415.

Simons-Morton, D. G., Goff, D. C., Osganian, S., et al. (1998). Rapid early action for coronary treatment: Rationale, design, and baseline characteristics. REACT Research Group. *Academic Emergency Medicine, 5*, 726–738.

KATHLEEN DRACUP

Treatment Efficacy Versus Effectiveness

The concepts of efficacy and effectiveness play distinct, yet complementary, roles in treatment outcome research. In general, efficacy research is the more traditional approach in health psychology, whereas effectiveness research is a more recent focus. Efficacy research demonstrates that a treatment or intervention promotes change in a controlled setting, whereas effectiveness research is focused toward demonstrating that a particular treatment promotes change under a wide array of settings (or in "real life").

A treatment can be said to efficacious when it has been documented that the treatment, and no other cause, is responsible for differential change between a control (often untreated) group and an experimental (treated) group. Such a demonstration, which is akin to the concept of internal validity, is imperative to demonstrate that a treatment or intervention can reliably produce expected changes. Perhaps the most common and scientifically valid method for documenting efficacy is the randomized, double-blind, placebo control study, wherein carefully selected participants are randomly assigned to either receive the treatment or not. Randomization of a homogeneous sample into a treatment or a control group allows for the inference that treatment, and nothing else, is producing change. Although the demonstration of efficacy is a vital process, the efficacy demonstrated in research studies may not be present in clinical practice. Because highly controlled conditions are often needed to test treatment efficacy, these studies are typically conducted in laboratory or clinical settings that may be quite different from what a typical patient would see in normal practice. Furthermore, patients enrolled in clinical efficacy trials may be somewhat dissimilar to the "typical" patient seen in practice (e.g., efficacy trials may exclude individuals with certain comorbid conditions). To take the important step of showing that a treatment that works in the controlled scientific setting also works in clinical practice or community settings, a different approach is required.

Effectiveness is a much more diffuse concept, not based in any one particular research methodology, and is interested in demonstrating that a particular treatment produces meaningful change within a typical applied or clinical setting (e.g., a mental health facility or a primary care hospital). It is not uncommon for efficacious treatments to be ineffective in the real world. Because real-world settings are typically less structured, have more heterogeneous treatment populations, and integrate many different forms of treatment, previously documented efficacious treatments may lose their effectiveness when applied in the real world. In particular, these differences can decrease the effectiveness of a treatment by obscuring the effects of the efficacious treatment. Therefore, in many ways, effectiveness research is interested in showing external validity, that is, that the results of the laboratory-based efficacy research can be generalized to larger and more diverse populations. Effectiveness research is more likely to demonstrate that the previously documented efficacious study can be used in a typical setting, where conditions are necessarily much less structured than in the laboratory. This is often a much more complicated and difficult process than efficacy trials.

It is widely recognized that effectiveness research should play a much larger role than it previously has in treatment outcome studies. This particularly true for treatments that have been shown to be efficacious; the next step should be to demonstrate that the treatment can be useful in the real world. There-fore, recent internal changes in the National Institute of Mental Health have promoted the development and funding for effectiveness studies. This focus on the public health model should have the effect of increasing the frequency and importance of effectiveness studies, which may serve to promote the transfer of new technology from the laboratory to applied settings.

BIBLIOGRAPHY

Clarke, G. N. (1995). Improving the transition from basic efficacy research to effectiveness studies: Methodological issues and procedures. *Journal of Consulting and Clinical Psychology, 63,* 718–725.

Niederehe, G., Street, L. L., & Lebowitz, B. D. (1999). NIMH support for psychotherapy research: Opportunities and questions. *Prevention and Treatment, 2.*

DAN J. NEAL
JOSHUA SMYTH

Turk, Dennis C. (1946 –)

Dennis C. Turk, PhD, born March 15, 1946, is John and Emma Bonica Professor of Anesthesiology and Pain Research, University of Washington. His research has focused on the assessment and treatment of patients with diverse pain syndromes. He has (1) developed a comprehensive assessment instrument to assess a range of psychosocial and behavioral factors believed to be important in the chronic pain experience; (2) investigated the importance of appraisal, beliefs, expectations in the experience of pain, depression, and behavioral responses; (3) developed a classification of pain patients based on psychosocial and behavioral characteristics; (4) evaluated the efficacy of integrated cognitive–behavioral interventions in treating pain sufferers; and (5) studied the potential of matching treatments to patient subgroup characteristics.

Studies have demonstrated that patients' appraisals affect their experience of pain. For example, patients' beliefs about their ability to control and cope with problems influenced their perceptions of pain severity, disability, and health care consumption. These variables accounted for greater amounts of variance in perceived pain, activities, and physician visits than did demographics or disease status. Other studies demonstrated that patients' perceptions of control over symptoms were associated with pain, interference with activity, and adaptive responses. Furthermore, the association between pain and depression was mediated by the patients' perceptions of how pain affected their lives, and their beliefs in their ability to control their pain.

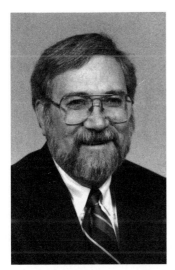

Turk, Dennis C.

Turk developed an empirically derived taxonomy of pain patients based on responses to an instrument that he and his colleagues developed, the West Haven–Yale Multidimensional Pain Inventory (MPI). Three subgroups were identified: (1) dysfunctional—high levels of pain, life interference, emotional distress, and low levels of perceived control and activity; (2) interpersonally distressed—low levels of social support and high levels of negative responses from significant others; and (3) adaptive copers—relatively low pain severity, life interference, and emotional distress, and high levels of perceived control. Turk has shown that these subgroups are independent of medical diagnosis. These subgroups have been replicated in studies with different pain disorders and in different countries.

Turk's studies have demonstrated that patients who report that symptoms began following a trauma differ in physical disability, psychologic distress, and functional activities compared to patients for whom the symptoms had an insidious onset. These differences are independent of physical findings and disability status. These results suggest that treatment of chronic pain patients should address physical factors and their beliefs and attributions.

Studies conducted by Turk demonstrated that a treatment that combined cognitive and behavioral with nonpharmacolgic modalities (e.g., physical therapy, intraoral devices) reduced pain, depression, and disability for pain patients. Studies demonstrated differential response of patients to treatments tailored to the psychosocial classification, supporting the validity of the classification and the importance of addressing subgroup characteristics in treatment planning.

DENNIS C. TURK

Type A Behavior Pattern

INTRODUCTION

Initially, Type A behavior (TAB) was considered as characterizing a hurried workaholic with an abundance of impatience and free-floating hostility who was at high risk for a heart attack. Free-floating hostility was characterized as frequent, outwardly expressed anger, which could directed toward anyone or anything at anytime. In more recent years, the description of TAB has been expanded and refined to include constant attempts to dominate others and prove oneself (e.g., attempts to "win" every interpersonal encounter), superficial goal and status seeking (e.g., obsessive job involvement), a chronic sense of time urgency, a deep-seated lack of self-esteem and fear of failure, perfectionism, narcissism, free-floating hostility, facial displays of disgust and glaring in response to mild annoyances, harsh and forceful voice mannerisms, motorized body movements suggestive of extreme stress or anxiety (e.g., hand clenching, restlessness, motor tenseness, and hyperalertness), physical signs of extreme stress (e.g., constant perspiration) and an inability to play, relax, or fantasize. A Type A person (TA) need not display all of the characteristics.

People who do not display TAB are referred to as Type Bs—the absence of TAB. Type Bs are assumed to be more secure and have more flexible coping skills. They have a greater ability to give and receive love, and can derive pleasure from relaxing, recalling past experiences, and listening to others. In contrast, a TA's hostility and attempts to dominate others may leave him or her isolated and without social support.

DISCOVERY OF TAB

From the late 1700s through the 1940s, many physicians and psychologists suggested that heart attacks are more likely to occur in people who are hurried, hard driving, overly ambitious, and hostile. Most myocardial infarctions (MIs, "heart attacks") are caused by coronary artery disease (CAD). CAD is the narrowing of the coronary arteries as a result of fibrous tissue formation and calcification around the arteries. If the artery becomes sufficiently narrow, the heart will not receive enough oxygen and the result will be an MI. CAD can begin as early as childhood, and usually slowly develops over many years so, that most MIs do not occur until middle or old age. Coronary heart disease (CHD) refers to MIs and other symptoms and conditions that result from CAD such as recurrent chest pains, or angina.

In the 1700s, CHD was a rare disease. However, an epidemic increase occurred in densely populated and industrialized urban areas. Today, CHD is the most common cause of death and disease in the United States. CHD accounts for 450,000 deaths every year, and currently 12,000,000 Americans live with CHD.

As CHD became more common, the general public became aware of the alleged connection between behavior and CHD as early as the 1920s. For example, the president of the Metropolitan Life Insurance Company stated, "Physicians, statisticians and others who are studying heart disease suspect that much of it is induced by the hurrying mode of life so general in this country."

In the 1950s, two cardiologists, Meyer Friedman and Ray Rosenman, began a lifelong investigation into what they referred to as TAB and its relationship to MIs and the underlying disease that causes MIs—coronary artery disease. Friedman and Rosenman defined TAB as a personality type characterized by an excessive competitive drive, a constant and very intense sense of time urgency, and free-floating hostility. Their book describing their research was a bestseller in the mid 1970s. Largely due to the popularity of their book and subsequent reports in the media, TAB has found its way into the American lexicon and its consciousness. The alleged damaging effects of many aspects of TAB are frequently found in popular fiction such as Harlan Ellison's short story "Repent Harlequin, Said the Tick-Tock Man" and songs such as "I'm in a hurry (and don't know why)."

DIAGNOSING TAB

Most methods for diagnosing TAB do not tap all of its aspects. Initially, TAB was primarily diagnosed by vigorous voice stylistics and subtle indications of hostility (e.g., interrupting the interviewer) during a structured interview. The most widely used questionnaire that assesses TAB is the Jenkins Activity Survey. This questionnaire assesses three qualities of TAB: time urgency, hard-driving competitiveness, and achievement striving. In recent years, new structured interviews and questionnaires have been developed. In addition, many methods have been developed to assess particular aspects of TAB. For example, there are many ways to assess hostility, although most are not specifically designed to diagnose so-called free-floating hostility.

Many of the methods for detecting TAB are believed to be inadequate. For example, individuals who are active, fast moving, dominant, and vigorous are not necessarily Type A. These characteristics can simply be the result of an active temperament. Similarly, people who have a strong but not overly obsessive desire to achieve are not necessarily TA. No methods are available for assessing positive Type B behaviors.

Depressed TAs may be diagnosed as Type Bs because the depression masks their underlying vigorous and aggressive temperament. Other aspects of TA can also be difficult to assess. For example, TAs are frequently stoic and may report being insecure or having greater levels stress or anxiety. Structured interview assessments for TAB look for physical signs and behaviors associated with TAB that TAs may not be aware of. In contrast, questionnaires assume TAs can accurately report their own behavior. Perhaps the assumption that TAs can accurately report their behavior is false, given that self-report measures appear to be less predictive of CHD.

CAUSES OF TAB

Although relatively little research has attempted to identify the causes of TAB, several hypotheses have been forwarded. Meyer Friedman suggested that TAB is caused by a deep-seated sense of self-esteem that is brought about by a discrepancy between TAs' achievements and their aspirations. That is, TAs' aspirations are so high that they can never meet their own expectations. This type of perfectionism causes TAs to struggle to achieve more. The consequences of this struggle result in other aspects of TAB such a chronic sense of time urgency, free-floating hostility, and obsessive achievement striving.

Houston and Vavak suggested that an obsessive need to prove one's self may begin in childhood as feelings of insecurity and negative attitudes toward others. These negative attitudes are a consequence of parental behavior that lacks genuine acceptance, is overly strict, critical, and demanding of conformity, and is inconsistent with regard to disciplinary treatment. This type of upbringing may give TAs an overly self-critical nature. Their self-criticism may cause them to feel greater responsibility for accomplishing work and more self-directed anger.

Another way to understand what causes TAB is to examine the coping skills that TAs lack. TAs appear to lack the skills necessary to enjoy life. They also tend to use active coping strategies (i.e., attempts to control their situation) to the exclusion of other strategies (e.g., emotional control or conflict resolution, or avoidance). When faced with an uncontrollable situation, TAs are more likely to feel helpless and depressed.

Some research suggests that TAB increases as a result of job stress. However, it is unclear whether obsessive job involvement is the problem or whether stressors at work cause obsessive job involvement.

TAB AS A RISK FACTOR FOR CHD

A prospective study is the best scientific method for identifying things that put people at greater risk for disease. A prospective study surveys an initially healthy group of people and follows them over time to determine whether those with an alleged risk factor (e.g., TAB) are at greater risk for incurring a particular disease (e.g., CHD). The prospective Western Collaborative Group Study assessed TAB in 3,154 healthy men

Number of Studies

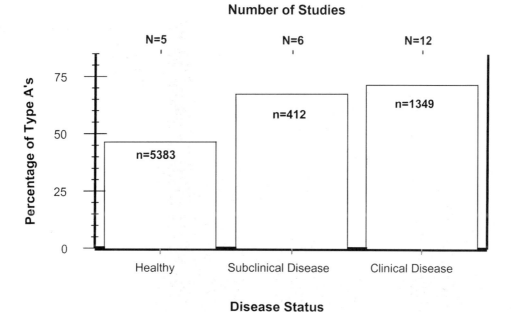

Figure 1. Relationship between Prevalence of Type A Behavior and Disease Status

and followed them for 8½ years. TAs were more than twice as likely to incur an MI as Type Bs. Encouraged by the results of this study, other researchers also began investigating the possible health-damaging effects of TAB. By 1981, there was sufficient evidence to convene a special National Institutes of Health review panel. The review panel concluded that TAB was a risk factor for CHD and that the magnitude of risk was equal to or greater than other well-known risk factors for CHD including elevated total serum cholesterol, elevated blood pressure, and smoking.

The national review panel's conclusions spurred more research. However, a new type of methodology was used, referred to as a "high-risk" study design. It was believe that high-risk studies had the advantages of requiring fewer research subjects to find statistically reliable effects over a shorter period of time. High-risk studies examine whether a risk factor is associated with disease among people who already have the disease or are at high risk for incurring the disease. The advantage of the high-risk study is that many new cases of CHD occur over a much shorter period of time. Although the original Western Collaborative Group Study included more than 3,000 men, new high-risk studies often used fewer than 100 people.

An unfortunate side effect of this high-risk thinking is that research on women was largely ignored. High-risk studies attempted to obtain research subjects who were at the highest risk for disease. Women were often excluded from studies because men are at higher risk for CHD. Perhaps for this reason, most of the TA research through the 1990s was primarily conducted on men.

Many high-risk studies relied on a medical procedure that is referred to as an angiography. An angiography can be used to determine a person's level of CAD. TAB was assessed among patients who had undergone an angiography. Although the first two high-risk studies found the expected relationship between TAB and CHD, subsequent angiography studies found no relationship.

Other researchers began to investigate whether TAB was a risk factor for CHD among people with other risk factors for CHD (e.g., people who smoke). This type of high-risk study also found no relationship between TAB and CHD. Finally, several high-risk studies examined whether TAs who had already had one MI were more likely to have a second MI. Again, the answer was no. Even a 22-year follow-up of the participants of the original Western Collaborative Group Study found that TAs with a prior MI were no more likely to have a second fatal MI than Type Bs. In addition, the 22-year follow-up found that as many Type Bs as TAs had incurred a fatal MI.

Despite the initially promising results, many became convinced that TAB was not a risk factor for CHD. At the 1987 annual meeting of the Psychosomatic Society, the question arose as to whether further research on TAB was warranted. However, the story of TAB was far from over.

In the early 1990s, the discrepancy between the high-risk studies conducted in the 1980s and earlier studies was explained. Figure 1 shows the percentages of TAs found among the types of participants used in research on TAB: people who (1) have no CHD, (2) have suspected or subclinical levels of CAD, and (3) have substantial CAD, or clinical disease. The

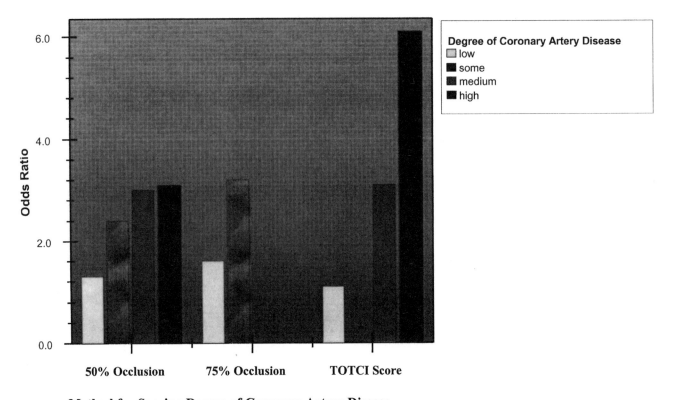

Method for Scoring Degree of Coronary Artery Disease

Figure 2.   Relationship between Type A behavior and severity of coronary artery disease. Based on angiography studies from meta-analysis (Miller et al., 1991). TOTCI, Total coronary index.

average percentage of TAs found in each category is presented in Figure 1. The data are based on research conducted in the United States. Studies outside the United States had to be excluded from Figure 1 because, as had been suspected by earlier researchers, TAB is more prevalent in the United States. Figure 1 only includes those studies that assess TAB by the original structured interview method. At the top of the Figure 1, *N* indicates the number of studies that had data representing one of the three groups. For example, *N* = 5 studies assessed the percentage of TAs among healthy people. The total number of people included in all studies associated with one of the three bars in Figure 1 is reported inside the bar, where *n* gives the total number of people. For example, the five studies that examined TAB among healthy people included a total of 5,383 people. The total number of people who volunteered for this research is substantials, so that fairly firm conclusions can be drawn from these data.

In Figure 1, about 47% of healthy people were diagnosed as TA. The percentages of TAs are roughly equal in the groups with subclinical and clinical disease—around 70%. The bar chart suggests that TAs are more likely to develop CHD because a higher percentage of TAs are found among people with clinical or subclinical (evolving) CHD.

The high-risk studies could not detect a relationship because the difference in percentages of TAs is very small or nonexistent between the subclinical and clinical groups. Healthy people are excluded from high-risk studies, and so no comparisons can be made between healthy people the subclinical and clinical groups. These results are not surprising because if TAB causes CAD, one would assume that higher numbers of TAs would be found both in people with initial signs of CAD and those with confirmed CHD. Although this sort of nonrelationship is found for other risk factors for CHD such as smoking, only TAB was discounted on the basis of these high-risk studies.

Prior data from high-risk studies can also illustrate that TAs are more likely to have more severe CAD. Several different criteria have been used to decide whether a person has clinically significant CAD that may require medical intervention. These criteria include (1) having one coronary artery that is at least 50% occluded, (2) having one artery that is at least 75% occluded, and (3) scoring at an appropriate level on a more complex scoring system referred to as the Total Coronary Index (TOTCI). Higher scores on these indices reflect greater levels of CAD.

In Figure 2, the odds ratio on the abscissa refers to the increased odds of being a TA, given a certain level of CAD.

This odds ratio assumes that among healthy people, only about half are TA (as suggested in Figure 1). For example, Figure 2 shows that the odds of being a TA among people who had the highest TOTCI scores is six times greater than for Type Bs. That is, TAs are six times more likely to have severe TOTCI-diagnosed CAD than Type Bs. Regardless of the scoring method, as the degree of CAD increases, the probability of being TA increases. Therefore, TAs are more likely to have severe CAD.

In recent years, the varied descriptions of what comprises TAB and research suggesting that TAB actually may be a combination of different aspects of a person's coping skills, mental health, environment, and personality have led to a refocusing of research on attempts to identify specific toxic elements of TAB. In particular, substantial research indicates that hostility increases one's chances of developing CHD, and cynicism is predictive of longevity in general. At the 22-year follow-up of the participants in the Western Collaborative Group Study, social dominance and hostility were associated with an increased risk for developing CHD.

Although research in recent years has moved away from attempting to demonstrate that all aspects of TAB increase a person's chance of developing CHD, the psychosocial risk factors that have been identified are as a whole surprisingly consistent with the characteristics or consequences of TAB. In particular, research indicates that social dominance, hostility, job stress, depression, and social isolation all place one at greater risk for CHD.

CHANGING TAB TO REDUCE THE RISK FOR CHD

In the Recurrent Coronary Intervention Project, 1,013 post-MI patients were assigned to one of three groups for $4\frac{1}{2}$ years. One group received thirty-three 90-min cardiac counseling sessions from cardiologists, who gave traditional advice to people with a recent MI (e.g., advice about exercising, quitting smoking, lowering cholesterol, surgical recommendations, etc.). A second group received sixty-six 90-min cardiac and TAB-reducing counseling sessions. A third group received no counseling.

The TAB counseling sessions appeared to be successful in that 35% of those in the TAB counseling group were able to reduce their TAB, whereas less than 10% in the other groups reduced theirs. After $4\frac{1}{2}$ years, a second MI occurred in 28.2% of those assigned to the no-counseling group and 21.2% in the cardiac counseling group. In contrast, only 12.9% of patients had recurrent MIs in the TAB counseling group. The TAB counseling substantially reduced both the number of recurrent MIs and the number of fatalities. A study conducted in Italy using counseling sessions based on the Recurrent Coronary Intervention

Project's counseling sessions also successfully reduced recurrent CHD. The TAB counseling stressed anger management, developing coping skills, and other qualities associated with Type B behavior.

TA RISK FOR HEALTH PROBLEMS BESIDES CHD

There is considerable evidence that TAs are at higher risk for other physical and emotional problems. In particular, TAB has been associated with accidents, violent deaths, stroke, artery disease other than coronary artery disease, minor illnesses, absenteeism, nightmares, reprimands at work, increased health problems when older, depression, anxiety, neuroticism, infections, migraines, and reports of stress. Perhaps because not all methods of diagnosing TAB tap the same aspects, not all assessment devices relate to all of the aforementioned outcomes.

POSSIBLE MECHANISM(S) BY WHICH TAB CAUSES CHD

Research has failed to determine why TAB increases a person's chances for developing CHD. However, several explanations have been proposed.

Job stress is a risk factor for CHD, and research suggests that TAs give themselves more stress, particularly in their work environments.

TA tendencies toward hostility and attempts to dominate others can rob them of their social support structure and leave them socially isolated. A lack of social support and/or social isolation are risk factors for CHD.

When faced with failure or a loss of control, TAs are at higher risk for depression. Depression is also a risk factor for CHD. Furthermore, poor coping mechanisms and fewer healing resources can leave TAs vulnerable to the effects of stress life events.

Another possible linkage between TAB and CHD is lifestyle. TAs incessant struggle to control their environment may cause them to ignore their health in ways that put them at higher risk for CHD (e.g., taking insufficient time for physical activity, smoking, and having a poor diet). The hostility component of TAB appears to have this effect.

The self-induced stress associated with TAB may cause CHD. Stress activates the sympathetic nervous system, which causes short-term cardiovascular responses (e.g., elevated blood pressure and heart rate). TAs exhibit stronger cardiovascular responses in response to stress. Chronic activation of the sympathetic nervous system can produce pathophysiological processes that can in the long run can produce CHD. A review of these processes can be found elsewhere in this encyclopedia.

An explanation of one possible method through which TAB may produce pathophysiological processes that result in CAD can serve to illustrate the complexity and difficulty associated with this area of research. Recently, it has been discovered that infectious or inflammatory processes are involved in the development of CHD. Recent research has also revealed that stress and depression have a substantial effect on the immune system, which controls the body's reaction to diseases associated with infection or inflammation. Therefore, TAB may cause stress and depression, which results in impaired immune function, which in turn causes CHD. The Recurrent Coronary Intervention Project reduced rates of depression in the TAB counseling group. Therefore, TAB counseling may reduce the chance of a recurrent MI because it keeps TAs from getting depressed or allows them to recover from depression after an initial MI. However, there are many plausible rival explanations for these findings. For example, depression and TAB are also associated with sleep problems, which are risk factors for CHD. The stress produced by TAB may aggravate existing sleep problems, which may increase the likelihood of an MI. Given that there are many risk factors for CHD and many possible biological routes through which risk factors may exert an effect on CHD, it is difficult to determine which routes are the most important in producing CHD and in determining which are caused by TAB. In sum, the path or paths that link TA stress to CHD may be very complex.

SUMMARY

In April 2001, Meyer Friedman died at the age of 90. He described himself as a recovering TA. His belief was that having TAB is like being an alcoholic. A TA must always struggle to keep things in perspective. Friedman's charisma and persistence have made TAB the subject of a substantial body of research on the influence of personality and emotions on physical health. This research can be found in many other entries of this encyclopedia. His popular book made TAB a part of the American lexicon and its consciousness. His legacy will not easily be forgotten.

TAB is a set of personal characteristics that include social dominance, free-floating hostility, overly zealous job involvement, an inability to enjoy life, physical tenseness and stress, harsh and forceful voice mannerisms, and unrealistically high aspirations. TAB increases a person's risk for CHD. However, research has moved away from attempting to demonstrate that TAB increases a person's chances for developing CHD and instead has attempted to identify toxic subcomponents of TAB. Interventions to reduce TAB among people with prior MIs

appear to reduce the chance of a second MI. TAB also increases a person's risk for many other health problems.

Related Entry: Jenkins Activity Survey

BIBLIOGRAPHY

Akashiba, T., Kawahara, S., Akahoshi, T., Omori, C., Saito, O., Majima, T., et al. (2002). Relationship between quality of life and mood or depression in patients with severe obstructive sleep apnea syndrome. *Chest, 22*, 861–865.

American Heart Association. (2001). *2001 Heart and stroke statistical update.* Dallas, TX: Author.

Bananian, S., Lehrman, S. G., & Maguire, G. P. (2002). Cardiovascular consequences of sleep-related breathing disorders. *Heart Disease, 4*, 296–305.

Bluen, S. D., Barling, J., & Burns, W. (1990). Predicting sales performance, job satisfaction and depression by using achievement–strivings and impatience–irritability dimensions of Type A behavior. *Journal of Applied Social Psychology, 35*, 307–311.

Blumenthal, J. A., Herman, S., O'Toole, L. C., Haney, T. L., Williams, R. B., & Barefoot, J. C. (1985). Development of a brief self-report measure of the Type A (coronary-prone) behavior pattern. *Journal of Psychosomatic Research, 29*, 265–274.

Blumenthal, J. A., Williams, R. B., Kong, Y., Schanburg, S. M., & Thompson, L. W. (1978). Type A behavior pattern and coronary atherosclerosis. *Circulation, 58*, 634–639.

Booth-Kewley, S., & Friedman, H. S. (1987). Psychological predictors of heart disease: A quantitative review. *Psychological Bulletin, 101*, 343–362.

Brunson, B. I., & Matthews, K. (1981). The Type A coronary-prone behavior pattern and reactions to uncontrollable stress: An analysis of performance strategies, affect and attributions during failure. *Journal of Personality and Social Psychology, 40*, 906–918.

Burke, R. J., & Deszca, E. (1984). What makes Sammy run—so fast and aggressively? Beliefs and fears underlying Type 'A' behavior. *Journal of Occupational Behavior, 5*, 219–227.

Chesney, M. A., Elkman, P., Friesen, W. V., Black, G. W., & Hecker, M. H. L. (1997). Type A behavior pattern: Facial behavior and speech components. In P. Ekman & E. L. Rosenberg (Eds.), *What the face reveals: Basic and applied studies of spontaneous expression using the Facial Action Coding System (FACS). Series in affective science,* (pp. 453–468). New York: Oxford University Press.

Cooper, C. L., Kirkcaldy, B. D., & Brown, J. (1994). A model of job stress and physical health: The role of individual differences. *Personality and Individual Differencs, 16*, 653–655.

DiMatteo, M. R., Lepper, H. S., & Croghan, T. W. (2000). Depression is a risk factor for noncompliance with medical treatment: Meta-analysis of the effects of anxiety and depression on patient adherence. *Archives of Internal Medicine, 160*, 2101–2107.

Ellison, Harlan. (1991) "'Repent, Harlequin!' Said the Ticktockman." In T. Dowling (Ed.), *The Essential Ellison.* Morpheus International: Beverly HIlls, CA. (pp. 877–886).

Evans, G. W., Pasane, M. N., & Carrere, S. (1987). Type A behavior and occupational stress: A cross-cultural study of blue-collar workers. *Journal of Personality and Social Psychology, 52*, 1002–1007.

Frank, F. A., Heller, S. S., Kornfeld, D. S., Spron, A. A., & Weiss, M. B. (1978). Type A behavior pattern and coronary angiographic findings. *Journal of the American Medical Association, 240*, 761–763.

Friedman, H. (2000). *The self-healing Personality: Why some people achieve health and others succumb to illness* (2nd ed.). Lincoln, NE: iUniverse.com.

Friedman, H., & Booth-Kewley, S, (1987). Personality, Type A behavior coronary heart disease: The role of emotional expression. *Journal of Personality and Social Psychology, 53*, 783–792.

Friedman, M., Fleischmann N., & Price, V. (1996). Diagnosis of Type A behavior pattern. In R. Allan & S. Scheidt (Eds.), *Heart and mind: The practice of cardiac psychology* (pp. 179–196). Washington, DC: American Psychological Association.

Friedman, M., & Rosenman, R. H. (1974). *Type A behavior and your heart.* Greenwich, CT: Fawcett.

Friedman, M., Thoresen, C. E., Gill, J. J., Ulmer, D., Powell, L. H., Price, V. A., et al. (1986). Alteration of Type A behavior and its effect on cardiac recurrences in post myocardial infarction patients: Summary results of the Recurrent Coronary Prevention Project. *American Heart Journal, 112*, 653–665.

Friedman, M., & Ulmer, D. (1984). *Treating Type A behavior and your heart.* New York: Knopf.

Fukunishi, I., Moroji, T., & Okabe, S. (1995). Stress in middle-aged women: Influence of Type A behavior and narcissism. *Psychotherapy and Psychosomatics, 63*, 159–164.

Furnham, A., & Linfoot, J. (1987). The Type 'A' behavior pattern and the need to prove oneself: A correlation study. *Current Psychological Research Review, 6*, 125–135.

Hayano, J., Kimura, K., Hosaka, T., Shibata, N., Fukunishi, I., Yamasaki, K., et al. (1997). Coronary disease-prone behavior among Japanese men: Job-centered lifestyle and social dominance. Type A Behavior Pattern Conference. *American Heart Journal, 134*, 1029–1036.

Hemingway, H., & Marmot, H. (1999). Studies of Type A behavior, hostility and coronary heart disease. *British Medical Journal, 318*, 1460–1467.

Houston, B. K. (1988). Introduction. In B. K. Houston & C. R. Snyder (Eds.), *Type A behavior pattern* (pp. 212–253). New York: Wiley.

Houston, B. K., Babyak, M. A., Chesney, M. A., Black, G., & Ragland, D. R. (1997). Social dominance and 22-year all-cause mortality in men. *Psychosomatic Medicine, 59*, 5–12.

Houston, B. K., Chesney, M. A., Black, G. W., Cates, D. S., & Hecker, M. H. L. (1992). Behavioral clusters and coronary heart disease risk. *Psychosomatic Medicine, 54*, 447–461.

Houston, B. K., & Vavak, C. R. (1991). Hostility: Developmental factors, psychosocial correlates, and health behaviors. *Health Psychology, 10*, 9–17.

Iwanaga, M. (2000). Effects of personality responsibility and latitude for Type A and B individuals on psychological and physiological stress responses. *International Journal of Behavioral Medicine, 7*, 204–215.

Jamal, M. (1990). Relationship of job stress and Type A behavior to employee's job satisfaction, organization commitment, psychosomatic health problems and turnover motivation. *Health Relations, 42*, 727–738.

Jenkins, C. D. (1978). Behavioral risk factors in coronary disease. *Annual Review of Medicine, 29*, 543–562.

Jenkins, C. D., Zyzanski, S. J., & Rosenman, R. H. (1971). Progress toward validation of a computer-scored test for the Type A coronary-prone behavior pattern. *Psychosomatic Medicine, 33*, 193–202.

Kalpan, B. H. (1992). Social health and the forgiving heart. The Type B story. *Journal of Behavioral Medicine, 15*, 3–14.

Kawachi, I., Sparrow, D., Kubzansky, L. D., Spiro, A., 3rd, Vokonas, P. S., & Weiss, S. T. (1998). Prospective study of a self-report type A scale and risk of coronary heart disease: Test of the MMPI-2 type A scale. *Circulation, 98*, 405–412.

Kop, W. J., & Cohen, N. (2001). Psychological risk factors and immune system involvement in cardiovascular disease. In R. Ader, D. L. Felten, &

N. Cohen (Eds.), *Psychoneuroimmunology* (Vol. 2, 3rd ed., pp. 525–544). San Diego, CA: Academic.

Libby, P., Ridker, P. M., & Maseri, A. (2002). Inflammation and atherosclerosis. *Circulation, 105*, 1135–1143.

Lyness, S. A. (1993). Predictors of differences between Type A and B individuals in heart rate and blood pressure reactivity. *Psychological Bulletin, 114*, 266–295.

Miller, G. E., & Cohen, S. (2001). Psychological interventions and the immune system: A meta-analytic review and critique. *Health Psychology, 20*, 47–63.

Miller, T. (1994). High-risk studies are influenced by indirect range restriction. *Journal of Behavioral Medicine, 17*, 567–588.

Miller, T. Q., Smith, T. W., Turner, C. W., Guijarro, M. L., & Hallet, A. J. (1996). A Meta-analytic review of research on hostility and physical health. *Psychological Bulletin, 119*, 322–348.

Miller, T. Q., Turner, C. W., Tindale, R. S., Posavac, E. J., & Dugoni, B. L. (1991). Reasons for the trend toward null findings in research on Type A behavior. *Psychological Bulletin, 110*, 469–485.

Murrah, R. (1992). I'm in a hurry (and don't know why). Recorded by Alabama. On *American pride* [compact disk], New York: RCA.

Musante, L., MacDougall, J. M., & Dembroski, T. M. (1984). The Type 'A' behavior pattern and attributions for success and failure. *Personality and Social Psychology Bulletin, 10*, 544–553.

National Center for Health Statistics of the Centers for Disease Control and Prevention. (1999). Heart disease and stroke. In *Healthy People 2010 conference edition* (Chapter 12). Washington: U.S. Government Printing Office.

Niemczyk, S. J., Jenkins, C. D., Rose, R. M., & Hurst, M. W. (1987). The prospective impact of psychosocial variables on rates of illness and injury in professional employees. *Journal of Occupational Medicine, 29*, 645–652.

Ragland, D. R., & Brand, R. J. (1988a). Type A behavior and mortality from coronary heart disease. *New England Journal of Medicine, 318*, 65–69.

Ragland, D. R., & Brand, R. J. (1988b). Coronary heart disease mortality in the Western Collaborative Groups Study: Follow-up experience of 22 years. *American Journal of Epidemiology, 127*, 462–475.

Review Panel on Coronary-Prone Behavior and Coronary Heart Disease. (1981). Coronary-prone behavior and coronary heart disease: A critical review. *Circulation, 63*, 1199–1215.

Rosenman, R. H. (1978). The interview method of assessment of the coronary-prone behavior pattern. In T. M. Dembroski, S. M. Weiss, J. L. Shields, S. G. Haynes, & M. Feinleib (Eds.), *Coronary-prone behavior* (pp. 55–69). New York: Springer-Verlag.

Rosenman, R. H., (1986). Current and past history of the Type A behavior pattern. In T. H. Schmidt, T. M. Dembroski, and T. Blumchen (Eds.), *Biological and psychological factors in cardiovascular disease* (pp. 00–00). New York: Springer-Verlag.

Rosenman, R. H., Brand, R., Jenkins, D., Friedman, M., Straus, R., & Wurm, M. (1975). Coronary heart disease in the Western Collaborative Group Study: Final follow-up of 8.5 years. *Journal of the American Medical Association, 233*, 872–877.

Scherwitz, L. (2001). In Memoriam: Meyer Friedman, M. D. *Outlook: A Quarterly Newletter of the Society of Behavioral Medicine, 00:00*–00.

Siegman, A. W., & Smith, T. W. (Eds.). (1994). *Anger, hostility and the heart.* Hillsdale, NJ. Erlbaum.

Smith, T. W., & Christensen, A. J. (1992). Hostility, health and social contexts. In H. S. Friedman (Ed.), *Hostility, coping, and health* (pp. 33–48). Washington, DC: American Psychological Association.

Smith, T. W., & Ruiz, J. M. (2002). Psychosocial influences on the development and course of coronary heart disease current status and implications for research and practice. *Journal of Consulting and Clinical Psychology, 70*, 548–568.

Table 1. Summary of Studies of Type C, Cancer, and HIV/AIDS

Type C variable measured	Immune, physiological, or medical outcome variable associated/predicted	Study
Denial/minimization of health concerns	Delay in seeking medical attention associated with thicker melanoma lesions	Temoshok et al. (1984)
Dysynchrony between psychological self-reports and physiological stress responses to emotional stimuli	Lower self-report of perturbation combined with higher skin conductance distinguished melanoma patients from heart disease patients and controls	Kneier and Temoshok (1984)
Semantic differential ratings (by coders) of Type C vs. Type A characteristics	More unfavorable melanoma-prognostic indicators (tumor thickness)	Temoshok et al. (1985)
Emotionally inexpressive (as rated from videotaped interviews)	Fewer lymphocytes at site of primary melanoma lesion (poorer prognosis)	Temoshok (1985)
Nonassertiveness in complying with imposing requests by others	Unfavorable immune changes associated with HIV progression	Solomon et al. (1991)
Higher Type C scores on Vignette Similarity Rating Method	HIV progression from asymptomatic status to AIDS or more advanced disease at 6- and 12-month follow-ups	Solano et al. (1993, 2002)

Suls, J., & Sanders, G. S. (1988). Type A behavior as a general risk factor for physical disorder. *Journal of Behavioral Medicine, 11*, 201–226.

Suls, J., & Wan, C. K. (1989). The relation between Type A behavior and chronic emotional distress: A meta-analysis. *Journal of Personality and Social Psychology, 57*, 503–512.

Tan, V. L., & Hicks, R. A. (1995). Type A-B behavior and nightmare types among college students. *Perceptual and Motor Skills, 81*, 15–19.

Theorell, T., Tsutsumi, A., Hallqist, J., Reuterwall, C., Hogstedt, C., Fredlund, P., et al. (1998). Decision latitude, job strain, and myocardial infarction: A study of working men in Stockholm. *American Journal of Public Health, 88*, 68–74.

Woo, E. (2001). Meyer Friedman; Doctor identified 'Type A' behavior. *Los Angeles Times* (Sunday, May 6), p. 00.

TODD Q. MILLER

Type C Coping/Behavior Pattern

The Type C behavior pattern, hypothesized to be related to the progression of cancer, was first elaborated and operationally defined in a 1981 study of risk factors associated with malignant melanoma, the most lethal form of skin cancer. Independently, British researchers had posed the question of whether there might be a Type C for cancer in an abstract published the previous year. Although Type C has sometimes been referred to as the "cancer-prone personality," this is misleading on two accounts: (1) although studies have linked Type C to cancer progression, there is no research establishing its relationship to the *development* of cancer; and (2) Type C is conceived of, not as a particular personality, but as a learned pattern of behavior that emerges and becomes increasingly evident as a function of coping with stress.

In studies conducted at the University of California San Francisco (UCSF) School of Medicine, Type C was defined as a constellation of (1) cognitive proclivities (decreased awareness of needs, feelings, and bodily sensations while attending to perceived needs of others), (2) verbal and nonverbal expressive patterns (repressing emotions, particularly anger, and not asserting needs while presenting a pleasant facade), and (c) specific coping behaviors (minimizing problems, and appeasing and working hard for others) (see Table 1). As hypothesized, inattention to symptoms contributed to delay in seeking medical attention for suspicious lesions; delay was found to be significantly associated with tumor thickness, the strongest negative prognostic indicator for melanoma. The hypothesized dysynchrony in Type C individuals between a calm facade and repressed physiological arousal was captured using a method that contrasted self-report of perturbation with physiological stress response as measured by skin conductance response (SCR). Melanoma patients had significantly more dysynchronous responses (reporting little upset but with higher SCR), in contrast to cardiovascular disease patients, who displayed the opposite pattern; controls showed a more synchronized pattern.

In Temoshok's model, Type C and Type A are polar opposites, but equivalently maladaptive, and the adaptive Type B forms the third point in this conceptual triangle. In an early study at UCSF, raters used 17 semantic differential scales, which contrasted descriptors of Type A (e.g., impatient, hostile) or Type C (e.g., passive, appeasing) to assess videotaped patient interviews. Controlling for biological and demographic risk factors, higher Type C versus A ratings were significantly correlated with tumor thickness.

Another study tested the hypothesis that inappropriately dampened expression of emotion is the pathogenic core of the Type C pattern by examining its relationship with a significant immunologic mediator of melanoma outcomes. Ratings of patients' emotional expressiveness (*less* Type C) on videotape were strongly and significantly correlated with more lymphocytes infiltrating the tumor base.

More recently, the Type C coping pattern has been evaluated in the context of another immunologically mediated disease, HIV infection. A key aspect of Type C, nonassertiveness in complying with others' requests against one's own wishes, was associated with disease progression and unfavorable changes among immune parameters relevant to HIV progression. Using the Vignette Similarity Rating Method to assess Type C and other coping styles, an Italian study reported that originally asymptomatic HIV-infected individuals who were more Type C were more likely to develop symptoms of AIDS at 6- and 12-month follow-ups. A separate study of 200 asymptomatic men and women found that higher baseline Type C coping scores significantly predicted progression at the same follow-up intervals among participants classified at baseline as having more compromised immunity.

Related Entry: Cancer: Biopsychosocial Aspects

BIBLIOGRAPHY

Kneier, A. W., & Temoshok, L. (1984). Repressive coping reactions in patients with malignant melanoma as compared to cardiovascular disease patients. *Journal of Psychosomatic Research, 29*, 139–153.

Morris, T., & Greer, S. (1980). A 'Type C' for cancer? Low trait anxiety in the pathogenesis of breast cancer. *Cancer Detection and Prevention, 3*, 102.

Solano, L., Costa, M., Salvati, S., Coda, R., Aiuti, F., Mezzaroma, I., et al. (1993). Psychosocial factors and clinical evolution in HIV infection: A longitudinal study. *Journal of Psychosomatic Research, 37*, 39–51.

Solano, L., Costa, M., Temoshok, L., Salvati, S., Coda, R., Aiuti, F., et al. (2002). An emotionally inexpressive (Type C) coping style influences HIV disease progression at six and twelve month follow-ups. *Psychology and Health, 17*, 641–655.

Solomon, G. F., Kemeny, M. E., & Temoshok, L. (1991). Psychoneuroimmunologic aspects of human immunodeficiency virus infection. In R. Ader, D. L. Felten, & N. Cohen (Eds.), *Psychoneuroimmunology* (2nd ed., pp. 1081–1114). San Diego, CA: Academic.

Temoshok, L. (1985). Biopsychosocial studies on cutaneous malignant melanoma: Psychological factors associated with prognostic indicators, progression, psychophysiology, and tumor–host response. *Social Science and Medicine, 20*, 833–840.

Temoshok, L. (1987). Personality, coping style, emotion, and cancer: Toward an integrative model. *Cancer Surveys, 6*, 837–857.

Temoshok, L. (2000). Psychological response and survival in breast cancer. *Lancet, 355*, 404–405.

Temoshok, L. (2000). Complex coping patterns and their role in adaptation and neuroimmunomodulation: Theory, methodology, and research. *Annals of the New York Academy of Science, 917*, 446–455.

Temoshok, L. (2003). Type C: A proposed psychosocial risk factor for cancer. In R. Fernandez Ballesteros (Ed.), *The encyclopedia of psychological assessment* (Vol. 2, pp. 1052–1056). Thousand Oaks, CA: Sage.

Temoshok, L., DiClemente, R. J., Sweet, D. M., Blois, M. S., & Sagebiel, R. W. (1984). Factors related to patient delay in seeking medical attention for cutaneous malignant melanoma. *Cancer, 54*, 3048–3053.

Temoshok, L., & Dreher, H. (1992). *The Type C connection: The behavioral links to cancer and your health*. New York: Random House.

Temoshok, L., & Fox, B. H. (1984). Coping styles and other psychosocial factors related to medical status and to prognosis in patients with cutaneous malignant melanoma. In B. H. Fox and B. H. Newberry (Eds.), *Impact of psychoendocrine systems in cancer and immunity* (pp. 258–287). Lewiston, NY: Hogrefe.

Temoshok, L., & Heller, B. W. (1981). Stress and "Type C" versus epidemiological risk factors in melanoma. In *Proceedings of the 89th Annual Convention of the American Psychological Association (Los Angeles, August, 1981)* (pp. 155–156). Washington, DC: American Psychological Association.

Temoshok, L., Heller, B. W., Sagebiel, R. W., Blois, M. S., Sweet, D. M., DiClemente, R. J., et al. (1985). The relationship of psychosocial factors to prognostic indicators in cutaneous malignant melanoma. *Journal of Psychosomatic Research, 29*, 139–154.

LYDIA R. TEMOSHOK

Uu

Unrealistic Optimism

People are said to be unrealistically optimistic when they underestimate the chances of experiencing a negative event or overestimate the chances of experiencing a positive event. This bias was first defined by Neil Weinstein as a social comparison with others, namely, the mistaken belief that we are less likely than others to experience negative events and more likely to experience positive events. However, unrealistic optimism can also be established by comparing a prediction with an actual outcome or with a more objective prediction of that outcome. Other terms representing this bias are optimistic bias and illusion of unique invulnerability. Unrealistic optimism is one of several biases related to the self-concept, such as the better-than-average heuristic (whereby people believe they are better than others on a wide range of dimensions), the uniqueness bias (the belief that one's abilities and moral attributes are unique), and the self-serving bias (thinking that one's successes are due to internal causes and failures are due to external causes), and these various biases have similar causes, as enumerated in what follows.

Unrealistic optimism has been observed for a wide range of life events, particularly health and safety issues such as lung cancer, colorectal cancer, heart disease, stroke, fatal car accident, HIV infection, unplanned pregnancy, and alcoholism. The bias is most likely to exist for life events that are controllable and temporally distant, and is less likely to be displayed in people who are ill, depressed, or in a bad mood. Unrealistic optimism seems to pervade all age groups and both genders. In addition, people have similarly biased beliefs about their risk-related behaviors such as their diet, level of physical activity, and amount of alcohol consumption.

In their review of research on unrealistic optimism, James Shepperd and Marie Helweg-Larsen summarized the various factors thought to cause unrealistic optimism. Cognitive antecedents include failing to take into account what other people do to decrease their risks, applying stereotypes of the kinds of people who have a given health problem, believing that because a problem has yet to occur, the future likelihood is low, and being generally unaware of the risk factors for a given problem. Motivational factors include the desire to protect a positive sense of self, the need to feel that one's risks are lower than those of others, and the need to reduce anxiety and worry.

Whether unrealistic optimism promotes health is a matter of debate. Some studies (including several by Shelley Taylor and her colleagues) show that unrealistic optimism is adaptive because it reduces worry, increases attention to risk information, creates hope in difficult situations, and motivates one to take measures necessary to produce positive outcomes. However, other studies (including work by Neil Weinstein and his colleagues) show that unrealistically optimistic people are more likely to engage in risk-increasing behaviors, and are less likely to learn information about how to reduce their risk. Future research is likely to elucidate when and under what conditions unrealistic optimism is most health promoting.

Related Entry: Optimism and Health

BIBLIOGRAPHY

Helweg-Larsen, M., & Shepperd, J. A. (2001). Do moderators of the optimistic bias affect personal or target risk estimates? A review of the literature. *Personality and Social Psychology Review, 51*, 74–95.

Taylor, S. E., & Brown, J. D. (1988). Illusion and well-being: A social psychological perspective on mental health. *Psychological Bulletin, 103*, 193–210.

Weinstein, N. D. (1980). Unrealistic optimism about future life events. *Journal of Personality and Social Psychology, 39*, 806–820.

Weinstein, N. D., & Klein, W. M. (1996). Unrealistic optimism: Present and future. *Journal of Social and Clinical Psychology, 15*, 1–8.

WILLIAM M. P. KLEIN

$\mathrm{W_w}$

Wallston, Kenneth A. (1942–)

Kenneth A. Wallston was born in Stamford, Connecticut, on July 2, 1942. He is a professor of psychology in nursing at Vanderbilt University in Nashville, Tennessee, where he has served on the faculty since 1971. Before that, he was a research associate of Howard Leventhal's at the University of Wisconsin–Madison after completing his PhD in social psychology at the University of Connecticut in Storrs in 1968. One of the founders of the Division of Health Psychology (Division 38) of the American Psychological Association, Wallston has served the division as its treasurer, its president, and the editor of the division newsletter, *The Health Psychologist*. He is also the division's historian.

Wallston is best known within the field as one of the developers of the Multidimensional Health Locus of Control (MHLC) Scales, a set of health belief measures that has been used in numerous studies around the world since it was first introduced in the mid 1970s. In addition to the MHLC Scales, Wallston has been involved in the development of many other psychometric instruments, among which are measures of health value, desire for control, perceived health competence, arthritis helplessness, pain coping strategies, and trust.

In addition to his work developing and validating psychometric tools, Wallston has been the principal (or coprincipal) investigator on a number of research grants investigating such diverse topics as factors influencing information disclosure to nurses, effects of choice and predictability in health care settings, weight management specialist training, and smoking cessation in newly diagnosed cardiovascular patients. Since the early 1980s, he and his colleagues have been studying how persons with rheumatoid arthritis adjust to living with a chronic health condition. He also helped evaluate the

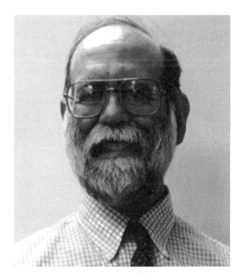

Wallston, Kenneth A.

effects of a nurse-run cognitive–behavioral intervention program for women with rheumatoid arthritis. Most recently, his research involves studying the effects of expressive writing on persons with chronic medical conditions such as diabetes and HIV/AIDS.

Wallston's entire career as a faculty member has been devoted to assisting nursing faculty and graduate students in both nursing and psychology to conduct health-related research. In addition to guiding students' dissertations, Wallston teaches quantitative research methods and statistics to nursing doctoral students. He has served as chair of the Vanderbilt University Faculty Senate and has been elected to membership in the Academy of Behavioral Medicine Research. He is also a fellow in the American Psychological Association and the Society of Behavioral Medicine.

KENNETH A. WALLSTON

Weiss, Stephen (1937–)

Stephen Weiss received his academic training from the University of Maryland (BA in psychology, 1959), Temple University (MA in psychology, 1961), the University of Arizona (PhD in psychology, 1965), and the Johns Hopkins School of Hygiene and Public Health (MPH in international health, 1993).

Weiss began his professional career as a predoctoral intern in the Department of Medical Psychology at the University of Oregon Medical School. Under the guidance of Dr. Joseph Matarazzo, he became interested in clinical medical psychology, completing his dissertation, "Psychological Adjustment Following Open Heart Surgery." He held academic appointments at the University of Arizona (1964–1967), the Johns Hopkins School of Medicine (1967–1970), the Uniformed Services University School of the Health Sciences (1978–1991), and the Johns Hopkins School of Hygiene and Public Health (1975–1994) prior to going to the University of Miami in 1993.

In addition to his academic positions, Weiss served with the U.S. Peace Corps as director of selection for Latin America (1969–1971) and director of training for Africa (1971–1974). Returning from 2 years in the Ivory Coast, West Africa, he accepted a position with the National Institutes of Health as chief of the Behavioral Medicine Branch of the National Heart, Lung and Blood Institute (1974–1992). It was during those years that he became involved in the formation of several national and international organizations devoted to the conceptual integration of knowledge and practices in the behavioral and biomedical sciences to further our understanding of the prevention of disease and the promotion of health. He was a founder of the Division of Health Psychology of the American Psychological Association, the Society of Behavioral Medicine, the Academy of Behavioral Medicine Research, and the International Society of Behavioral Medicine, serving as president of all four organizations in their early developmental years. He chaired numerous national and international working conferences related to health psychology and behavioral medicine, including the Arden House Conference on Education and Training in Health Psychology (1983). He also served as chair of numerous committees and task forces for professional and scientific organizations and was appointed to task forces under the auspices of the White House, the Institute of Medicine of the National Academy of Sciences, the Office of the Surgeon General, the Department of Health and Human Services, among others.

Weiss has authored or coauthored more than 100 papers, monographs, and scientific reviews, and has also edited

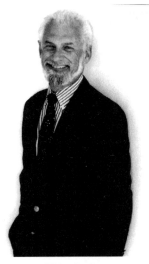

Weiss, Stephen

10 volumes on biobehavioral approaches to the prevention and control of chronic disease. Since completing his public health training in 1993, he has shifted his area of scientific concern from cardiovascular health and illness to the prevention and control of HIV/AIDS. He is the principal investigator and co-principal investigator of three U.S. and international National Institutes of Health-supported research grants concerning behavioral interventions for primary and secondary prevention of HIV/AIDS, and is the protocol co-chair for two large-scale international clinical trials related to HIV prevention.

STEPHEN WEISS

Women's Health

Virtually every woman can expect to experience at least one chronic illness or disorder in her lifetime, and the incidence of chronic health problems increases with age. By age 55 years, more than 80% of women experience at least one chronic health problem. Major attention to and support for women's health research has only emerged in the past dozen years, however, and the scientific pursuit of knowledge about women's health and gender differences in health has been legitimized in the same time period. Research on the psychology of women's health, a field in its infancy only a decade ago, is growing healthily into its adolescence, and the quality and quantity of work in the area have grown impressively.

The topic of women's health is a broad one, and is continually evolving. It covers the psychological, social, cultural, economic, and political processes that affect women's physical health as well as how gender influences the relation between behavior and health. Many people, particularly in medicine, equate women's health with reproductive health: menstruation, fertility, childbearing, and menopause. However, the study of women's health goes beyond this, to encompass those illnesses more common among (but not limited to) women or some subgroups of women, for example, breast cancer, arthritis, and eating disorders. It also involves health psychological phenomena as they apply to women and their health: stress; coping and adapting to illness; interpersonal processes in health, illness, and health care (e.g., social support, caregiving); behavioral, psychological, social, economic, and cultural risk factors for particular diseases; factors related to the promotion of good health (e.g., exercise, diet, screening); social problems (e.g., poverty, violence) and their related health consequences; and preventive interventions to enhance health and well-being.

This entry cannot cover all of these topics, and instead focuses on a few illness conditions that affect women disproportionately, and for which there exists a knowledge base regarding gender or gender differences. Heart disease and cancer are the two leading causes of mortality for women; arthritis and rheumatic diseases are the greatest cause of disability. The incidence of HIV/AIDS is increasing at an alarming rate for women, and is a public health priority.

Additional accounts of the excellent work in the psychology of women's health can be found in the references listed in the bibliography.

BRAIDING TOGETHER GENDER AND HEALTH

Why do we need a separate entry on women's health? After all, many of the topics just described are equally applicable to women and men. Unfortunately, for most of the last century, the results of research done only with men were considered to be applicable to both women and men. The idea that there might be meaningful differences between men and women in their experience of illness, or in the factors that lead to illness, was generally ignored unless a hormonal (biological) difference was suggested. Moreover, these hormonal differences, most often related to reproductive processes, were used to justify the exclusion of women from medical and even, in some cases, psychological research. That is, the restriction of medical research to men was the result of efforts to protect women, particular women in the childbearing years, from the risks of experimentation.

Medical doctors have actively promoted the notion of gender differences in health since the early 18th century. However, the differences they emphasized centered on reproductive health and often were used to establish that women's primary role was

that of mother and wife. Medicine, as any other human enterprise, is determined by political and social forces that shape the *social construction* of the phenomenon. Thus, the study of women's health has been determined by culturally held beliefs about women's roles. When the society constructs women's role as subordinate, the research topics and interpretations of the research confirm the need to protect, decide for, and even exclude women from certain activities.

In the early 19th century, Helmholtz's principle of energy conservation was used to justify limitations imposed on access to higher education for women. Higher education was considered to be too much of a burden for women's fragile physiology. Intellectual activities were believed to take too much energy away from reproductive activities. Fast-forward ahead a century: With the women's movement of the 1960s, the increase of women in higher education, and the fight for reproductive rights, there is a different social construction of women's roles. An outcome of this has been greater interest in women's health, including women's own choices regarding health.

We know now that it is important to understand biological, psychological, and social factors in health and health behavior among both women *and* men, and that the benefits of including women in health research outweigh the risks. Research guidelines instituted by the National Institutes of Health in the mid-1990s dictate that research studies must include women and men unless there is a very good reason for excluding women. This policy has been but one social structural factor that has increased the amount of research on women's health in the last decade.

Many studies examine the linkages between women's behavior and their health outcomes. This is part of a move within the behavioral sciences and within medicine to use a more comprehensive *biopsychosocial model* to understand health. The biopsychosocial model goes beyond a biomedical model, which emphasizes only biological causes of illness, to include psychological and social determinants as well. Thus, behavioral or psychosocial factors are pivotal in the prevention, development, and progression of disease.

Recently, the World Health Organization has recognized the existing gender inequities in health. These inequities are concentrated in the areas of health risks and opportunities to enjoy health, health needs, access to health resources, responsibility in the health sector, and power in the health sector. Women have a greater chance of having a health problem, but they have fewer opportunities to enjoy good health because they tend to have less education, employment, and income than men. Women make up the majority of the working population, yet do not have as much control over health policies and decision making as men because they tend to hold lower-status jobs.

GENDER DIFFERENCES IN HEALTH AND ILLNESS

Let's start with the big difference: Women live longer than men in almost all developed countries, and have lower death rates at virtually every age and for most causes of death, even when taking reproductive status and age into account. However, women consistently report worse health status and greater morbidity (symptoms) than men do. Health surveys repeatedly show that females have higher rates of illness, disability days, and use of health services. Intuitively, this seems contradictory. Why should the sex that has a health *dis*advantage end up with a mortality *ad*vantage?

One reason is that women's reports about their health are probably a combination of real morbidity and (less accurate) symptom perceptions. Data from both community surveys and interviews show higher rates of acute and chronic illnesses for females (although injury rates are higher for males). This difference remains stable even when reproductive health conditions are removed. However, these conditions are less severe and are often non–life-threatening diseases. Women do report more disability overall (limitations on daily activities) than men do. However, reports of disability depend not only on the type of illness and its severity, but also on social roles and obligations. Men report more limitations of their usual activities *when they are ill* than women do. One explanation is that women's caregiving roles—as mother, spouse, and household manager—leave them less time for not performing daily activities.

Many illnesses are linked to gender, either by genetics, physiology, or lifestyle factors. For example, many autoimmune disorders (such as rheumatoid arthritis), some gastrointestinal disorders (irritable bowel syndrome), some forms of cancer (e.g., breast cancer), and osteoporosis are more prevalent among women. Recent studies show that lifestyle factors such as stress and smoking not only differ in their prevalence between women and men, but may effect men and women differently at a physiological level

Cardiovascular Disease

Cardiovascular disease refers to all diseases related to the heart or blood vessels, including coronary heart disease (CHD), stroke, hypertension, and congestive heart failure. Coronary heart disease and other cardiovascular diseases are the leading causes of death in women in the United States despite the fact that they are considerably more common among men. Between the ages of 35 and 74 years of age, the death rate for CHD is 2.7 times higher among men than women, but this gender gap narrows with age. Although CHD is sometimes associated with menopause, there is not a sharp rise in CHD at this time; most heart disease occurs in both men and women after the age

of 65 years. Initial episodes of myocardial infarction (MI) are more often fatal in women than men, and women have more unrecognized MIs. What might be the cause of this?

More than 2.5 million U.S. women are hospitalized for cardiovascular-related diseases annually, yet little is known about cardiovascular diseases in women in terms of their course, differential diagnosis, treatment, and prognosis. This is due in part to the historical exclusion of women from clinical trials and in part because of differential medical care. We are also learning more about the protective role of estrogen in preventing heart disease.

Heart disease continues to be viewed as a disease of men, not women. Physicians are less likely to attribute the same symptoms to heart disease in women than they are in men. Women's symptoms are often attributed to noncardiac causes such as psychological issues or hormonal changes (e.g., during menopause). Women may seek care more slowly than men following onset of symptoms, so their condition is more likely to be more serious at the time of hospital admission.

In general, women are then treated less aggressively than men for CHD. Women are less likely to be referred than men for either coronary artery bypass surgery or angioplasty. Women may receive less benefit from bypass surgery than men; some studies suggest that women appear to have a higher mortality rate from bypass surgery, but one must consider that women entering cardiac surgery tend to have poorer health status, be older, and have fewer psychosocial resources than men who undergo similar surgical treatment.

There are known gender differences in risk factors associated with cardiac diseases. Physiological/biological factors include family history of heart disease, hypertension, diabetes, obesity, and older age. Behavioral risk factors include use of oral contraceptives, smoking, and lack of exercise and physical activity. Psychosocial factors include hostility and use of social resources. For example, hostility is risk factor for CHD and social support a protective factor. However, for women with high hostility levels, social support may be a less protective factor for women than it is for men with the same hostility levels. Recent studies also show that marital quality may be a stronger predictor of women's survival after heart attack than men's.

Smoking is a strong risk factor for CHD and a greater risk factor for women than for men. Moreover, women often perceive smoking as a reliable way of managing stress and controlling their weight. Advertising encourages smoking in women as a way of staying thin, attractive, and "cool."

Little is known about recovery from heart attack and bypass surgery because most studies have included only male patients. Women take longer to recuperate from their surgery, are more restricted in their activities, spend more days in bed, are less likely to return to work, and take longer to resume activities than men. Women are less likely to participate in cardiac rehabilitation and exercise programs, but when they participate at the same level, women gain the same health benefits as men do. In addition, several studies have shown women to be more anxious and depressed, and those women who retire from work after surgery have worse emotional adjustment than male patients do. Again, it is not clear whether these are true gender differences or attributable to the fact that women who undergo bypass surgery start out in poorer health, are older, and have fewer economic and social resources.

Breast Cancer

The disease women fear most is breast cancer. The incidence of breast cancer in North American women has increased steadily over the last 50 years, culminating in the present 1-in-8 lifetime risk for developing the disease. As scientists improve methods of prevention, early detection, and treatment, growing numbers of women are living with breast cancer for longer periods of time. In response to this trend, clinical researchers have increasingly focused on quality-of-life issues. Although 20% to 30% of women with breast cancer experience significant psychological distress, this distress is substantially reduced in the year following diagnosis, and the majority of women with breast cancer are well adjusted. One to 2 years after treatment, women with breast cancer do not differ from healthy women in psychological status.

Research has documented numerous psychosocial and physical effects of breast cancer, including emotional difficulties, problems associated with sexuality, negative changes in body image, pain and suffering, threats to one's self-esteem or self-concept, disruptions in daily activities, challenges to one's beliefs about the world, and problems with interpersonal relationships.

One difficulty that appears to be shared by many women with the disease is the fear of recurrence. Between 60% and 99% of women voice this fear. Moreover, fears about breast cancer recurrence, unlike overall psychological distress, do not necessarily dissipate over time. Although 57% of women survive to 15 years after diagnosis, approximately 70% of breast cancer survivors still fear the possibility of recurrence 5 years after diagnosis. These fears have been associated with psychological distress among both current cancer patients and cancer survivors. Younger women have stronger fears, a finding that may be due to the generally more aggressive nature of breast cancer among younger women, or a sense that a cancer diagnosis early in the life cycle is particularly unexpected.

A number of medical characteristics influence psychosocial adjustment to the initial breast cancer diagnosis. Treatment decision making (e.g., choosing mastectomy as opposed to breast-conserving surgery), undergoing treatment itself (e.g., chemotherapy, radiation, hormone therapy), and time since diagnosis have been associated with adjustment. Chemotherapy has been associated with decreased adjustment, varying with its toxicity and assaults on the body (nausea and vomiting, hair

loss, weight gain, fatigue). In some studies, however, psychological distress increases again after the termination of treatment because women no longer feel they are actively fighting the disease and have no concrete evidence of disease processes (e.g., a shrinking tumor).

Results regarding the type of surgery have been equivocal. A recent meta-analysis (a statistical technique for combining the results of many studies) suggests that there may be modest benefits to having breast-conserving surgery (BCS), in terms of psychological, marital–sexual, and social adjustment, body/self-image, and cancer-related fears. In contrast, a longitudinal study showed that women who had BCS were more distressed and perceived less social support than women who had mastectomies. In another study, women who had chosen BCS rated their physicians' support of their choice as more important than did women who chose mastectomy, perhaps because they needed reassurance that BCS was as likely to have a positive medical outcome.

Coping with breast cancer, or any cancer, means different things for different people at different points in the illness, in part because it occurs in the context of other life circumstances. Instead of producing global distress, cancer often produces what psychosocial cancer researcher Barbara Andersen has termed "islands" of psychosocial disruption that vary across the course of the illness. That is, not only are there many different aspects or adaptive tasks of breast cancer to cope with, but these islands rise above the water at different times. Thus, when women are asked to report how they cope with their breast cancer, it is impossible to know which aspects of breast cancer they are thinking about. Which aspects of having cancer are most salient for that woman *at that time*? For example, studies of women undergoing chemotherapy or taking tamoxifen suggest that adjustment may be disrupted with new treatments or even in the absence of treatment, which gives no cues of remission or recurrence. Even asking women how they cope with a more focused aspect of their cancer, such as chemotherapy or cancer-related pain, has a limitation. A woman undergoing chemotherapy may have to deal with excessive fatigue, fears about the long-term physical effects of this treatment, or sexual difficulties resulting from induced menopause. Likewise, the pain caused by a woman's cancer may prevent her from completing daily activities or may heighten fears about the progression of her illness.

As with other stressors, women with breast cancer use a wide range of coping techniques: cognitive, behavioral, problem-focused, and emotion-focused strategies, involving approach and avoidance of the stressor. The coping strategies of cognitive reappraisal, seeking social support, and avoidance consistently have been identified as among the most common strategies for coping with breast cancer. Overall the strategies of acceptance, positive reframing, and seeking and using social support have proved to be beneficial for women with breast cancer. Accepting the illness, or "learning to live with it" (as opposed to accepting responsibility for the illness), is conceptualized as a functional or beneficial coping response, and research with breast cancer patients has found it to be related to improved adjustment. Similarly, positive reframing involves a cognitive attempt to reappraise the stressor of illness, to change its meaning, in order to view it in a more positive light. For example, a woman undergoing chemotherapy may think of the accompanying nausea as evidence that the treatment is working, rather than evidence that the drugs are harming her body. Positive reframing has been identified as one of the most common strategies for coping with breast cancer and has been related to greater psychological adjustment.

Avoidant coping, including denial, behavioral or cognitive disengagement, and some tension-reduction strategies, such as using drugs or drinking, are consistently related to increased distress. Denial is the refusal or inability to acknowledge facts about the breast cancer. There is some controversy over whether denial is a beneficial coping strategy for women with breast cancer. Evidence suggests that it may be helpful at the time of diagnosis, when the woman is flooded with emotional reactions, and detrimental if it delays treatment decisions or is used continually or as a primary coping strategy. Avoidant coping has predicted greater distress after cancer diagnosis and after surgery, and in one study predicted cancer progression 1 year later.

Arthritis and Rheumatic Diseases

The rheumatic diseases, arthritis, and musculoskeletal conditions constitute more than 100 different illnesses and conditions, affecting nearly 40 million people in the United States. Arthritis and musculoskeletal disorders are the most common self-reported chronic conditions affecting women. *Rheumatoid arthritis* (RA) is a chronic, systemic illness whose cardinal manifestations of joint inflammation, swelling, and stiffness result in severe pain, joint destruction, fatigue, and physical disability. The course of RA is unpredictable and highly variable, with symptoms that flare and remit. The average age of onset of RA is between 25 and 50 years, although the incidence and prevalence of the disease increase with age. The prevalence of RA is much greater for women than for men: at different points in the lifespan, between two and six times as many more women than men have RA. *Systemic lupus erythematosus* (SLE) is an autoimmune disease that involves multiple systems of the body. Symptoms may include malaise; fever; weight loss; joint pain; renal, cardiac, neurological, and liver problems; and skin and mucous membrane problems. Almost 90% of patients with SLE are women, and it occurs more often among African-American women. *Osteoarthritis* (OA) is the most common form of arthritis, and is most prevalent among older people; it is marked by pain in an involved joint (or joints) that worsens with activity, joint stiffness and enlargement, and functional impairment. Women are twice as likely as men, and African-American

women are twice as likely as White women, to have OA of the knee, and OA of the knee is more likely to result in disability than OA in any other joint.

Most forms of arthritis pose a set of common stressors, including recurrent severe joint pain, potential disability, loss of role functioning, increased risk for developing depression, and frequent medical care. The treatment regimens, especially for RA and SLE, can involve medications with unpleasant side effects. Except for SLE, most forms of arthritis pose no immediate life threat, but the experience of symptoms and the course of the disease are unpredictable. Therefore successful adaptation requires that one cope with uncertainty as well as with concrete illness symptoms.

Women with RA report more symptoms than men, but when disease severity is taken into account, women actually have *fewer* symptoms than men. This finding suggests that women do not overreport symptoms, but have more severe disease and may in fact be less likely to complain about symptoms than men are.

The symptoms associated with arthritis often lead to functional limitations. As a result, women with arthritis have lower participation in the labor force, and it is generally reported that the economic impact of arthritis is much more severe for men than for women. The economic impact of women's work disability due to arthritis is underestimated, however, because arthritis and its disability significantly affect women's "home" work (nurturing, raising families, housework), which is economically undervalued for ill and nonill women alike.

Physical disability affects quality of life in other ways as well. In one study of women with rheumatoid arthritis, approximately 40% of the women reported limitations in such important role activities as making arrangements for others and taking them places, maintaining social ties by writing or calling, and visiting or taking care of sick people. In addition, women who experienced these types of limitations were less satisfied with their ability to provide support to family and friends compared to unimpaired women. The nurturing role—a very important role for women—has been neglected in most past research on adaptation to illness. The presence of chronic disease is a risk factor for depression when it involves the loss of the ability to perform valued social roles. Again, this suggests that to understand the impact of chronic disabling illness, we must examine not just physical limitations, but women's psychological interpretations of the meaning of those limitations.

The most frequently studied effect of arthritis on psychological functioning has been its impact on depression. Depressive disorders and depressive symptoms are more prevalent in people with rheumatic diseases than in people without any serious, chronic illness. Women not only are at greater risk than men for some of the more common and serious rheumatic diseases, but also are at greater risk for depression. If depression in women with rheumatic diseases is overlooked, then declines in functioning caused by depression could be mistakenly attributed to the rheumatic disease and result in overtreatment. Alternatively, if symptoms of depression are mistakenly assumed to be a natural part of the disease process that does not warrant treatment, women may suffer unnecessarily.

Wishful thinking, self-blame, and other avoidant coping strategies have been associated with poorer psychological functioning for both women and men with rheumatic disease. Active coping strategies, and strategies such as information seeking and cognitive restructuring, have been associated with better psychological functioning. However, in a study of daily coping processes in which RA patients were studied over 75 consecutive days, women and men differed in the use of only one of seven coping strategies: Women tended to seek social support to a greater degree. Women made a greater number of coping efforts overall and used a greater diversity of coping strategies than men. These findings suggest that women may be more flexible in their coping efforts.

HIV/AIDS

AIDS is the third-leading cause of death among women aged 15 to 24 years. The prevalence of AIDS among women continues to increase, although it has decreased among men (Centers for Disease Control and Prevention, 2001). The proportion of AIDS cases reported among women more than tripled between 1985 and 1999, going from 7% to 25% of the total cases. The statistics are even more tragic for minority women. African-American and Hispanic women together represent less than one-fourth of U.S. women, yet they account for more than three-fourths (78%) of AIDS cases reported to date among women in the United States. In 2000, African-American and Hispanic women represented 80% of HIV/AIDS cases reported in women.

Among the major routes of HIV/AIDS transmission for women are heterosexual intercourse and needle sharing among injection drug users. In 2000, 38% of women with AIDS were infected through heterosexual exposure to HIV, and injection drug use accounted for 25% of cases. Many women infected heterosexually were infected through sex with an injection drug user (CDC, 2002). To understand and combat the epidemic of AIDS/HIV among women, one needs to understand and combat substance abuse and risky sexual behaviors in women. Moreover, these two risk factors are interdependent: Use of alcohol has been implicated in spread of HIV/AIDS among women, particularly among adolescent girls, because it often impairs judgment, leading to more risky sexual behaviors. Studies suggest that use of alcohol during or before sex often leads to risky sexual practices, such as unprotected intercourse, multiple sexual partners, and partners whose HIV status is unknown (or not communicated).

Although condom use is the only contraceptive method that prevents both sexually transmitted diseases and pregnancy, it is also a method controlled by men. Psychosocial factors play a great role in the process of negotiation of condom use. Although women need to exercise a proactive stance to use condoms to avoid undesirable pregnancy and the transmission of HIV, they are rarely encouraged to be assertive in terms of sexual behavior, and may even suffer undesirable consequences such as loss of income, loss of sexual relationship, and even violence.

The Centers for Disease Control and Prevention (CDC, 2003) has identified several directions for preventive efforts to reduce the transmission of HIV among women: (1) target risky behaviors that are associated with HIV/AIDS, (2) increase preventive efforts among female adolescents and minority women, (3) focus more on drug use and HIV transmission among women, and (4) provide women with female-controlled contraception methods. It is hoped that research in the next decade will address these issues in depth.

GROWTH AND RESILIENCE

Recent trends in psychology have highlighted the importance of positive psychology, that is, looking at health and positive growth as well as illness and pathology. It is critical to acknowledge women's strengths in the face of adversity rather than focus solely on their weaknesses. Recognizing women's strengths means focusing on positive aspects of well-being, such as personal growth or strengthened social ties, as well as on distress. In many studies of women with cancer and other illnesses, women spontaneously describe positive outcomes of their experience.

The concept of resilience (alternatively called thriving, personal growth, and benefit finding) is a new way to look at the outcomes of facing health problems. Resilience refers to how some individuals are able to maintain strength and experience personal growth in the face of severe or prolonged adversity. Some researchers propose that there are resilient individuals, who have a definable set of characteristics that enable them to adapt successfully to stressful circumstances. Others suggest that resilience may be the coping process of fending off maladaptive responses to stress, thus leading to better mental health. Resilience can also be thought of as the long-term end product of facing a severe stressor or challenge, such as chronic illness. Whichever approach is used, the focus of a resilience perspective is one of positive adaptation, not simply the absence of pathology.

Resilience or thriving does not depend solely on physical health outcomes, but includes psychological, social, and spiritual growth. More to the point, thriving may be possible in the absence of physical recovery from disease, as in the case of an individual fighting an illness such as ovarian cancer or HIV/AIDS.

Resilience and thriving offer a new way to include gender in our definitions of health because it moves beyond viewing health issues solely in terms of vulnerability, deficits, or risk factors and refocuses on strengths and capabilities. Although women experience greater degrees and different types of stress than men, they also have a broader fund of stress-resistance resources. On the biological level, hormones provide a protective health advantage to women, at least until menopause, reducing risk of cardiovascular disease and osteoporosis. On the psychosocial level, social relationships may be a key to women's resilience. Research has found that women have stronger support networks and more ability to mobilize help in a crisis than men, both of which have been linked to better adaptation. Moreover, there is recent evidence that the expression of emotions, long considered a coping strategy linked to depression, may be an adaptive strategy for women and not for men. Clearly, in health psychology research, we need to adopt gendered approaches, not and define phenomena not simply relative to a male norm or in terms of gender differences, but as they vary within a heterogeneous population including women, with various strengths and competencies.

BIBLIOGRAPHY

Amaro, H. (1995). Love, sex and power: Considering women's realities in HIV prevention. *American Psychologist, 50,* 437–447.

Barrett-Connor, E. (1997). Sex differences in coronary heart disease: Why are women so superior? *Circulation, 95,* 252–264.

Baum, A., Revenson, T. A., & Singer, J. E. (Eds). (2001). *Handbook of health psychology.* Mahwah, NJ: Erlbaum.

Centers for Disease Control and Prevention. (2001).

Centers for Disease Control and Prevention. (2002).

Centers for Disease Control and Prevention. (2003).

Chesney, M. A., & Ozer, E. A. (1995). Women and health: In search of a paradigm. *Women's Health: Research on Gender, Behavior, and Policy, 1,* 3–26.

DeVellis, B. M., Revenson, T. A., & Blalock, S. (1997). Arthritis and autoimmune diseases. In S. Gallant, G. P. Keita, & R. Royak-Schaler (Eds). *Health care for women: Psychological, social and behavioral issues* (pp. 333–347). Washington, DC: American Psychological Association.

Gallant, S. J., Keita, G. P., & Royak-Schaler, R. (1995). *Health care for women: Psychological, social, and behavioral influences.* Washington, DC: American Psychological Association.

Ickovics, J. R., Thayaparan, B., & Ethier, K. A. (2001). Women and AIDS: A contextual analysis. In A. Baum, T. A. Revenson, & J. E. Singer (Eds.), *Handbook of health psychology* (pp. 817–839). Mahwah, NJ: Erlbaum.

Mays, V. M., & Cochran , S. E. (1988). Issues in the perception of AIDS risk and risk reduction activities by Black and Hispanic/Latina women. *American Psychologist, 43,* 949–957.

O'Leary, V. E., & Ickovics, J. R. (1995). Resilience and thriving in response to challenge: An opportunity for a paradigm shift in women's health. *Women's Health: Research on Gender, Behavior, and Policy, 1,* 121–142.

Stanton, A. L., & Gallant, S. J. (1995). *The psychology of women's health: Progress and challenges in research and application.* Washington, DC: American Psychological Association.

Stanton, A. L., Lobel, M., Sears, S., & DeLuca, R. S. (2002). Psychosocial aspects of selected issues in women's reproductive health: Current status and future directions. *Psychological Bulletin, 70,* 751–770.

Taylor, S. E., Klein, L. C., Lewis, B. P., Gruenewald, T. L., Gurung, R. A. R., & Updegraff, J. A. (2000). Biobehavioral responses to stress in females: Tend-and-befriend, not fight-or-flight. *Psychological Review, 107,* 411–429.

TRACEY A. REVENSON
IDA JELTOVA

Workplace Stress

Due to the increasing amount of time people spend in the paid labor force, there has been widespread interest in the impact that stress at work can have on health. This field identifies job stressors and their effects on individuals and families, investigates the processes that link job stress to health and the sources of individual and group differences in those processes, and designs programs to reduce workplace stress.

WHAT IS WORKPLACE STRESS?

Researchers have identified two main types of job stressors. The first type includes stressors inherent in the occupation or job, such as heavy workloads, repetitive and boring tasks, and a lack of control at work. A workload can be heavy in a number of different ways; it might require extended hours, a high degree of alertness, or a pressured pace. Repetitive or boring tasks, such as those associated with factory/assembly line work can also be stressful. In jobs with low decision latitude, the worker has little or no control over aspects such as scheduling, location, or the manner in which tasks are completed. Interpersonal relationships with coworkers or supervisors that are nonsupportive or actively hostile are a second main type of job stressor. Many individuals work in jobs that combine several of these stressors, and in these cases the effects of the different stressors are compounded. For example, a lack of control at work may exacerbate the impact of high demands or a lack of supervisor support.

Two individuals can experience the same job condition in different ways. A number of psychological variables, such as mood, values, attitudes, and expectations, color perceptions and descriptions of the workplace. This subjective aspect of job stressors poses a dilemma for researchers who are interested in conditions as they exist outside of the individual. That is why many studies rely on objective measures (e.g., number of calls handled by police radio dispatchers) or on independent ratings to assess workplace stressors. One common approach is to use an imputation technique in which an average score, derived from ratings made by a large group of people, is assigned to each person with that job title.

HEALTH OUTCOMES

Exposure to the workplace stressors just described is associated with a number of mental and physical health problems. For example, many researchers posit that positive and supportive social relationships at work enhance psychological well-being by helping to meet human needs for affiliation, approval, and a sense of belonging. Consistent with this point of view, more symptoms of anxiety and depression are reported by people who describe their social relationships at work, particularly supervisor relations, as nonsupportive. In addition, individuals who describe their jobs as involving heavy demands or constant time pressure also tend to report more emotional distress. One way to describe these problems is burnout, which refers to a combination of emotional exhaustion, physical fatigue, and cognitive weariness. The impact of workplace stress on psychological functioning is complicated by the fact that mental health can also shape some conditions at work. For instance, an individual's emotional distress can cause problems in his or her relationships with supervisors and coworkers. It is a continuing challenge for researchers in this field to study the mutual influence exerted by workplace stressors and emotional distress.

Stress interferes with the regulation of stress hormones, heart functioning, and the immune system. Workplace stress has been found to increase blood pressure not only during work hours, but also at home and even at rest. As a result, an increased risk of cardiovascular disease (CVD) is one of the primary health consequences of chronic exposure to workplace stress. Increased mortality rates have been associated with failure of a business, being fired or laid off, demotion, and personal troubles with coworkers. Studies of physical health outcomes have focused on job strain, the discrepancy between facing a high demand for performance and having little control over work tasks. It is estimated that about 15% to 25% of the working population falls into the high-strain-risk group. Job strain is associated with CVD risk factors, such as hypertension, as well as with CVD-related death. These types of health outcomes are not linked solely to job strain.

FAMILY OUTCOMES

The physical and emotional residues of stress are carried beyond the end of the workday, and they continue to influence social behavior. This is seen most prominently in the family.

Occupational stressors can result in marital and parent–child relationships that are less sensitive and responsive and more negative and conflictual. There are at least two ways by which stress can be imported into the family. First, feelings of frustration, anger, or disappointment at work can be expressed at home through greater irritability and impatience and more power assertion. Second, some individuals use social withdrawal as a way of coping with job stress. In this case, there is a pervasive reduction in both the amount of social interaction and emotional responsiveness. Over time, repeated instances of social withdrawal may corrode family members' feelings of closeness and lead to feelings of resentment and to more negative interactions. Whatever the particular mechanism, it appears that the transfer of stress from work to home is most likely to occur when workplace stressors are associated with the employed person feeling overwhelmed or having difficulty managing multiple work and family responsibilities.

JOB STRESS AS A PROCESS

Although research has mainly focused on the long-term health consequences of chronically stressful conditions at work, there has also been study of the short-term psychological and biological changes that accompany day-to-day fluctuations in occupational stressors. It is hoped that a better understanding of short-term responses to stress will clarify the processes that link stress in the workplace to long-term health. For example, most of the models in this field assume that immediate psychological or emotional responses to a stressor are an important part of the pathway leading to poor health. Researchers have taken the first step toward testing this assumption by showing that a temporary increase in distressed mood follows a day at work characterized by more negative social interactions or more pressures and demands than usual.

In addition to having an immediate psychological impact, high-job-strain situations are also hypothesized to result in acute biological arousal. There is evidence of heightened physiological arousal, such as increased blood pressure, heart rate, and excretion of certain stress hormones (such as epinephrine and cortisol) on high-stress days at work. Such systemic changes can ultimately contribute to the development of CVD. Behaviors are another important part of the pathway through which stress exerts an impact on health. Work stress can affect health-related behaviors by altering dietary patterns, disturbing restful sleep, and encouraging maladaptive coping responses, such as smoking and drinking. Ironically, these behaviors tend to increase physiological arousal on high-stress days. By studying these and other acute reactions, investigators hope to uncover the mechanisms that connect workplace stress with long-term mental and physical health outcomes.

INDIVIDUAL AND GROUP DIFFERENCES

Not all individuals react to workplace stress in the same way. For example, individual differences in coping strategies (how one reacts when faced with an occupational stressor), the quality of life outside of work (such as how much support an individual receives from his or her social network), and the previously mentioned differences in perception all help to shape an individual's vulnerability to occupational stressors. Two sources of group differences are gender and socioeconomic status (SES). Some research suggests that the physiological consequences of high job strain may be more significant for women than for men. The jobs available to people with low-SES backgrounds are often those that are the most demanding, allow the worker the least amount of control, and offer the fewest rewards. Thus, job strain may play an important role in linking low SES to poor health.

INTERVENTION

Stress-management interventions are sometimes implemented in the workplace to help employees deal more effectively with symptoms of stress, to modify employees' appraisal of stressful situations, or both. Techniques such as progressive muscle relaxation, biofeedback, meditation, and cognitive–behavioral skills training are commonly used in these programs,

and reports suggest they produce positive results, such as lowering anxiety, blood pressure, levels of stress hormones, muscle tension, and absenteeism. A less common approach is to alter the sources of stress at work through job redesign or organizational change strategies.

Related Entry: Stress Management

BIBLIOGRAPHY

Marmot, M. G., Bosma, H., Hemingway, H., Brunner, E., & Stansfeld, S. (1997). Contribution of job control and other risk factors to social variations in coronary heart disease incidence. *Lancet, 350,* 235–239.

Murphy, L. R. (1996). Stress management in work settings: A critical review of the health effects. *American Journal of Health Promotion, 11,* 112–135.

Perry-Jenkins, M., Repetti, R. L., & Crouter, A. C. (2000). Work and family in the 1990's. *Journal of Marriage and the Family, 62,* 981–998.

Quick, J. C., & Tetrick, L. E. (2003). *Handbook of occupational health psychology.* Washington, DC: American Psychological Association.

Repetti, R. L. (1993). The effects of workload and the social environment at work on health. In L. Goldberger & S. Breznitz (Eds.), *Handbook of stress* (2nd ed., pp. 368–385). New York: Free Press.

Schnall, P. L., Belkic, K., Landsbergis, P., & Baker, D. (2000). The workplace and cardiovascular disease. *Occupational Medicine: State of the Art Reviews, 15,* 00–00.

RENA L. REPETTI
ANGELA MITTMANN

Contributors

Ronald P. Abeles, PhD, Office of Behavioral and Social Sciences Research, National Institutes of Health

Nancy E. Adler, PhD, Department of Psychiatry, University of California, San Francisco

Melissa A. Alderfer, PhD, Department of Psychology, The Children's Hospital of Phildelphia

David G. Altman, PhD, Department of Public Health Sciences, Wake Forest University School of Medicine

Norman B. Anderson, PhD, American Psychological Association

Katherine L. Applegate, PhD, Weight Loss Surgery Center, Duke University Medical Center

William C. Bailey, PhD, Lung Health Center, University of Alabama at Birmingham

Albert Bandura, PhD, Department of Psychology, Stanford University

John C. Barefoot, PhD, Department of Behavioral Psychiatry, Duke University

Andrew Baum, PhD, Departments of Psychiatry and Psychology, University of Pittsburgh

Heidi T. Beckman, PhD, Prairie View at Newton Medical Office Plaza, Newton, Kansas

Andrew Beer, Department of Psychology, University of Iowa

S. Beth Bellman, Department of Psychology, University of Iowa

Rochelle L. Bergstrom, MS, Department of Psychology, North Dakota State University

Ali A. Berlin, MA, Department of Medical and Clinical Psychology, Uniformed Services University of the Health Sciences, Bethesda, Maryland

Jim Blascovich, PhD, Department of Psychology, University of California, Santa Barbara

George A. Bonanno, PhD, Department of Counseling and Clinical Psychology, Teachers College, Columbia University

Jack W. Brehm, PhD, Department of Psychology, University of Kansas

Joan E. Broderick, PhD, Department of Psychiatry, Stony Brook University, Stony Brook, New York

Jessica S. Brown, Department of Psychology, Florida State University

James Bunde, Department of Psychology, University of Iowa

Mali Bunde, Department of Psychology, University of Iowa

James Butler, PhD, Behavioral and Community Health Services, University of Pittsburgh

Lucie M. T. Byrne-Davis, MSc, Medical Research Council Health Services Research Collaboration, University of Bristol, Bristol, England

345

Linda D. Cameron, PhD, Department of Psychology, University of Auckland, Auckland, New Zealand

Kate B. Carey, PhD, Department of Psychology, Syracuse University

Michael P. Carey, PhD, Center for Health and Behavior, Syracuse University

Yolanda Cartwright, PhD, RD, School of Public Health, University of Minnesota

Delwyn Catley, PhD, Department of Psychology, University of Missouri–Kansas City

Heather Champion, Department of Public Health Sciences, Wake Forest University School of Medicine

Alan J. Christensen, PhD, Department of Psychology, University of Iowa

Karin Coifman, Department of Counseling and Clinical Psychology, Teachers College, Columbia University

Mark Conner, PhD, School of Psychology, University of Leeds, Leeds, England

Richard J. Contrada, PhD, Department of Psychology, Rutgers—The State University of New Jersey

Beth L. Cook, PhD, Department of Psychiatry, University of California, San Francisco

Matthew J. Cordova, PhD, Pacific Graduate School of Psychology, Palo Alto, California

Erin S. Costanzo, MA, Department of Psychology, University of Iowa

Julie K. Cremeans-Smith, MA, Department of Psychology, Kent State University

Carolyn E. Cutrona, PhD, Institute for Social and Behavioral Research and Department of Psychology, Iowa State University

Jamie A. Cvengros, Department of Psychology, University of Iowa

Ralph B. D'Agostino, PhD, Department of Mathematics and Statistics, Boston University

J. Alexander Dale, PhD, Department of Psychology, Allegheny College, Meadville, Pennsylvania

Judith C. Daniluk, PhD, Department of Counseling Psychology, University of British Columbia, Vancouver, Canada

Sharon Danoff-Burg, PhD, Department of Psychology, University at Albany, State University of New York

W. Hobart Davies, PhD, Department of Psychology, University of Wisconsin – Milwaukee

Gerald M. Devins, PhD, Department of Psychiatry, University Health Services and University of Toronto, Toronto, Canada

Mary Amanda Dew, PhD, Departments of Psychiatry, Psychology, and Epidemiology, University of Pittsburgh School of Medicine

Michael Diefenbach, PhD, Division of Population Science, Fox Chase Cancer Center, Philadelphia

Richard A. Dienstbier, PhD, Department of Psychology, University of Nebraska–Lincoln

Amanda J. Dillard, Department of Psychology, North Dakota State University

Andrea F. DiMartini, MD, Department of Psychiatry, University of Pittsburgh School of Medicine

Kathleen R. Diviak, PhD, Health Research and Policy Centers, University of Illinois at Chicago

Sara L. Dolan, Department of Psychology, University of Iowa

Kathleen Dracup, RN, DCSc, FAAN, School of Nursing, University of California, San Francisco

Paul R. Duberstein, PhD, Departments of Psychiatry and Oncology, University of Rochester Medical Center

Christopher L. Edwards, PhD, Department of Psychology, Duke University Medical Center

Shawna L. Ehlers, PhD, Department of Clinical and Health Psychology, University of Florida

Merrill F. Elias, PhD, Department of Mathematics and Statistics, Boston University

Scott Engel, MS, Department of Psychology, North Dakota State University

Jeanne L. Esler, PhD, Department of Psychiatry, Rhode Island Hospital, Providence

Susan A. Everson-Rose, MPH, PhD, Department of Preventative Medicine, Rush–Presbyterian–St. Luke's Medical Center, Chicago

Craig K. Ewart, PhD, Center for Health and Behavior, Syracuse University

Perry G. Fine, MD, School of Medicine, University of Utah

Susan Folkman, PhD, Osher Center for Integrative Medicine, University of California, San Francisco

Wilbert E. Fordyce, PhD, Department of Rehabilitation Medicine and Pain Service, University of Washington School of Medicine

Christopher R. France, PhD, Department of Psychology, Ohio University

Andrea J. Frank, Department of Psychology, University of Iowa

Christina L. Franklin, Department of Psychology, University of Iowa

Patricia Freiburger, Department of Neuroscience, Neuropsychiatric Research Institute, Fargo, North Dakota

Derek R. Freres, PhD, Department of Psychology, University of Pennsylvania

Gerald W. Friedland, MD, FRCPE, Stanford University School of Medicine

Michael A. Friedman, PhD, Department of Psychology, Rutgers—The State University of New Jersey

David B. Fruehstorfer, MEd, Department of Psychology, Kent State University

Judy Garber, PhD, Department of Psychology, Vanderbilt University

Kelli A. Gardner, Department of Psychology, Iowa State University

Marc Gellman, PhD, Department of Psychology, University of Miami

Meg Gerrard, PhD, Department of Psychology, Iowa State Univesity

Frederick Gibbons, PhD, Department of Psychology, Iowa State University

Mazy E. Gillis, PhD, Department of Psychology, Wayne State University, Detroit, Michigan

Karen Glanz, PhD, MPH, Social and Behavioral Sciences Program, University of Hawaii

Alan G. Glaros, PhD, School of Dentistry, University of Missouri–Kansas City

Janice Kiecolt-Glaser, PhD, Department of Psychiatry, Ohio State Univesity

Ronald Glaser, PhD, Department of Molecular Virology, Immunology, and Medical Genetics, Ohio State University

David C. Glass, PhD, State University of New York at Stony Brook

Deanna M. Golden-Kreutz, PhD, Department of Psychology, Ohio State University

Laura Gorman, PhD, Department of Psychology, University of Iowa

Elizabeth K. Gray, Department of Psychology, University of Iowa

Peter J. Green, PhD, Department of Psychology, Barton College, Wilson, North Carolina

Angela J. Grippo, Department of Psychology, University of Iowa

Perry N. Halkitis, PhD, Department of Applied Psychology, New York University

Thomas L. Haney, Department of Behavioral Psychiatry, Duke University

Vicki S. Helgeson, PhD, Department of Psychology, Carnegie Mellon University

Elise J. Herndon, MA, Department of Psychology, University of South Carolina

Thaddeus A. Herzog, PhD, University of South Florida, H. Lee Moffitt Cancer Center and Research Institute, Tampa, Florida

Jennifer Hoffman Goldberg, PhD, Stanford Center for Research in Disease Prevention, Stanford University School of Medicine

Steven D. Hollon, PhD, Department of Psychology, Vanderbilt University

Michael F. Hoyt, PhD, Department of Psychiatry, Kaiser Permanente Medical Center, San Rafael, California

L. K. George Hsu, MD, Department of Psychiatry, Tufts University School of Medicine

Jennifer S. Hunt, PhD, Department of Psychology, University of Nebraska–Lincoln

Barry E. Hurwitz, PhD, Department of Psychology, University of Miami

Ida Jeltova, PhD, School Psychology PsyD Program, Fairleigh Dickinson University, Teaneck, New Jersey

Erica L. Johnsen, MA, Department of Psychology, University of Iowa

Christopher J. Johnson, Department of Psychology, University of Texas at El Paso

Debra L. Johnson, PhD, Department of Psychology, University of Iowa

Thomas E. Joiner, Jr. PhD, Department of Psychology, Florida State University

R. D. Jones, PhD, Department of Clinical Neurology, University of Iowa

Randall S. Jorgensen, PhD, Center for Health and Behavior, Syracuse University

Robert M. Kaplan, PhD, Department of Family and Preventative Medicine, University of California, San Diego

Michael G. Kavan, PhD, Departments of Family Medicine and Psychiatry, Creighton University, Omaha, Nebraska

Barbara A. Keeton, Administrative Officer, American Psychological Association Division 38, Health Psychology

Abby C. King, PhD, Stanford Center for Research in Disease Prevention, Stanford University School of Medicine

William M. P. Klein, PhD, Department of Psychology, University of Pittsburgh

Beth Klipping, Executive Director, Society of Behavioral Medicine, Middleton, Wisconsin

Connie L. Kohler, PhD, Department of Health Behavior, University of Alabama at Birmingham

Willem J. Kop, PhD, Department of Medical and Clinical Psychology, Uniformed Services University of the Health Sciences, Bethesda, Maryland

David Krantz, PhD, Department of Medical and Clinical Psychology, Uniformed Services University of the Health Sciences, Bethesda, Maryland

Zlatan Krizan, Department of Psychology, University of Iowa

Edward Krupat, PhD, Department of Psychology, Massachusetts College of Pharmacy and Health Science, Boston

Kristin Kuntz, MA, Department of Psychology, Ohio State University

Jeffrey Lackner, PsyD, School of Medicine and Biomedical Sciences, University of Buffalo, The State University of New York

Sheleigh Lawler, Department of Psychology, University of Auckland, Auckland, New Zealand

William J. Lawton, MD, Department of Internal Medicine, University of Iowa Hospitals and Clinics

Richard S. Lazarus, PhD, University of California, Berkeley

Allen Lebovits, PhD, Departments of Anesthesiology and Psychiatry, New York University Medical Center

Suzanne C. Lechner, PhD, Department of Psychiatry, University of Miami

Jennifer E. Lee-Howard, Department of Psychology, University of Iowa

Kathleen C. Light, PhD, Department of Psychiatry, University of North Carolina School of Medicine

Mark D. Litt, PhD, Department of Behavioral Sciences and Community Health, University of Connecticut Health Center

Marci Lobel, PhD, Department of Psychology, State University of New York at Stony Brook

Patricia Lounsbury, RNC, MEd, CCRN, FAACVPR, Iowa CHAMPS (Cardiovascular Health, Assessment, Management, and Prevention Services), University of Iowa Heart Care

Mark A. Lumley, PhD, Department of Psychology, Wayne State University, Detroit, Michigan

Kenneth Mah, PhD, Department of Psychiatry, University Health Network and University of Toronto, Toronto, Canada

Stephen A. Maisto, PhD, Center for Health and Behavior, Syracuse University

Stephen B. Manuck, PhD, Department of Psychology, University of Pittsburgh

Christine A. Marco, PhD, Department of Psychology, Rhode Island College, Providence

G. Alan Marlatt, PhD, Addictive Behaviors Research Center, University of Washington

Leslie R. Martin, PhD, Department of Psychology, La Sierra University, Riverside, California

René Martin, PhD, College of Nursing, University of Iowa

Kevin S. Masters, PhD, Department of Psychology, Utah State University

Kevin D. McCaul, PhD, Department of Psychology, North Dakota State University

Elizabeth McDade-Montez, Department of Psychology, University of Iowa

Brian McMillan, PhD, School of Psychology, University of Leeds, Leeds, England

Mary W. Meagher, PhD, Department of Psychology, Texas A&M University

Ronald Melzack, PhD, Department of Psychology, McGill University, Montreal, Canada

Todd Q. Miller, PhD, Department of Psychology, University of St. Thomas, Houston, Texas

Anca Miron, Department of Psychology, University of Kansas

Angela Mittmann, Department of Psychology, University of California, Los Angeles

Doil D. Montgomery, PhD, Center for Psychological Studies, Nova Southeastern University, Fort Lauderdale, Florida

Tracy E. Moran, MA, Department of Psychology, University of Iowa

Larissa Myaskovsky, PhD, Department of Psychiatry, University of Pittsburgh School of Medicine

Nisha Nayak, Department of Psychology, University of Houston

Deborah Nazarian, PhD, Department of Psychology, Syracuse University

Dan J. Neal, Center for Health and Behavior, Syracuse University

Carissa Nehl, Department of Psychology, University of Iowa

Mary Lee Neuberger, RN, APN, Department of Internal Medicine, University of Iowa Hospitals and Clinics

Benjamin H. Newberry, PhD, Department of Psychology, Kent State University

Deborah L. Newberry, RPh, BCPS, Pharmacy Services, Summa Health System, Akron, Ohio

Michael T. Nietzel, PhD, Department of Psychology, University of Kentucky

Michael W. O'Hara, PhD, Department of Psychology, University of Iowa

Suzanne C. Ouellette, PhD, Graduate Center, City University of New York

Steven C. Palmer, PhD, Abramson Cancer Center, University of Pennsylvania

James W. Pennebaker, PhD, Department of Psychology, University of Texas in Austin

Christopher Peterson, PhD, Department of Psychology, University of Michigan

David B. Peterson, PhD, Institute of Psychology Rehabilitation Psychology Programs, Illinois Institute of Technology, Chicago

Jodie M. Plumert, PhD, Department of Psychology, University of Iowa

Elizabeth Pomery, Department of Psychology, Iowa State University

Katherine Raichle, MA, Department of Psychology, University of Iowa

Lynn P. Rehm, PhD, ABPP, Department of Psychology, University of Houston

Rena L. Repetti, PhD, Department of Psychology, University of California, Los Angeles

Tracey A. Revenson, PhD, Department of Psychology, Graduate Center, City University of New York

Michael A. Robbins, PhD, Department of Psychology, University of Maine

Elwood Robinson, PhD, Department of Psychology, North Carolina Central University

Barry Rosenfeld, PhD, ABPP, Department of Psychology, Fordham University

Alexander J. Rothman, PhD, Department of Psychology, University of Minnesota

Nan E. Rothrock, PhD, Department of Psychology, University of Iowa

John M. Ruiz, PhD, Western Psychiatric Institute and Clinic, University of Pittsburgh Medical Center

Josef I. Ruzek, PhD, Veterans Administration Palo Alto Health Care System, Palo Alto, California

Peter Salovey, PhD, Department of Psychology, Yale University

Edward P. Sarafino, PhD, Department of Psychology, The College of New Jersey, Ewing, New Jersey

Barbara R. Sarason, PhD, Department of Psychology, University of Washington

Derek D. Satre, PhD, Department of Psychiatry, University of California, San Francisco

Michael F. Scheier, PhD, Department of Psychology, Carnegie Mellon University

Margaret Schneider Jammer, PhD, School of Social Ecology, University of California, Irvine

Neil Schneiderman, PhD, Department of Psychology, University of Miami

Gary E. Schwartz, PhD, Department of Psychology, University of Arizona

Adele M. H. Seelke, Department of Psychology, University of Iowa

Ericka Nus Simms, Department of Psychology, University of Iowa

Silvana Skara, Institute for Health Promotion and Disease Prevention Research, University of Southern California

J. A. Skelton, PhD, Department of Psychology, Dickinson College, Carlisle, Pennsylvania

Martin Sliwinski, PhD, Department of Psychology, Syracuse University

Joshua Smyth, PhD, Department of Psychology, Syracuse University

Dominicus W. So, PhD, Department of Psychology, Howard University, Washington, D.C.

Laura J. Solomon, PhD, Department of Psychology, University of Vermont

Jennifer L. Specht, Department of Psychology, University of Wisconsin–Milwaukee

David Spiegel, PhD, Department of Psychiatry and Behavioral Sciences, Stanford University School of Medicine

Arthur A. Stone, PhD, Department of Psychiatry and Behavioral Science, Stony Brook University, Stony Brook, New York

Catherine M. Stoney, PhD, Department of Psychology, Ohio State University

Mary Story, PhD, RD, School of Public Health, University of Minnesota

Micah Stretch, MA, Department of Medical and Clinical Psychology, Uniformed Services University of the Health Sciences, Bethesda, Maryland

Albert Stunkard, PhD, Department of Psychiatry, University of Pennsylvania

Jerry Suls, PhD, Department of Psychology, University of Iowa

Steve Sussman, PhD, Institute for Health Promotion and Disease Prevention Research, University of Southern California

Galen E. Switzer, PhD, Departments of Medicine and Psychiatry, University of Pittsburgh School of Medicine, and Veterans Administration Center for Health Equity Research and Promotion

Nancy L. Talbot, PhD, Department of Psychiatry, University of Rochester Medical Center

C. Barr Taylor, MD, Department of Psychiatry and Behavioral Sciences, Stanford Medical Center

Shelley E. Taylor, PhD, Department of Psychology, University of California, Los Angeles

Lydia R. Temoshok, PhD, Behavioral Medicine Program, University of Maryland School of Medicine

Joe Tomaka, PhD, Health Science Department, University of Texas at El Paso

Paula M. Trief, PhD, Department of Psychiatry and Medicine, State University of New York Upstate Medical University, Syracuse

Dennis C. Turk, PhD, Department of Anesthesiology and Pain Research, University of Washington

Phil Ullrich, PhD, Department of Rehabilitation Medicine, University of Washington

John Urquhart, MD, FRCPE, FISPE, Department of Epidemiology, Maastricht University, Maastricht, Netherlands

Jatin G. Vaidya, Department of Psychology, University of Iowa

Peter A. Vanable, PhD, Center for Health and Behavior, Syracuse University

Brent Van Dorsten, PhD, Department of Rehabilitation Medicine, University of Colorado Health Sciences Center

K. Vedhara, PhD, Medical Research Council Health Services Research Collaboration, University of Bristol, Bristol, England

Heather Wade, School of Medicine, University of Iowa

Kenneth A. Wallston, PhD, School of Nursing, Vanderbilt University

Abraham Wandersman, PhD, Department of Psychology, University of South Carolina

Holly Wardlow, PhD, Department of Anthropology, University of Toronto

David Watson, PhD, Department of Psychology, University of Iowa

Lance S. Weinhardt, PhD, Center for AIDS Intervention Research (CAIR), Medical College of Wisconsin

Aliza Weinrib, Department of Psychology, University of Iowa

Stephen Weiss, PhD, MPH, Department of Psychology, University of Miami

DiGregorio Sharla Wells, PhD, Department of Psychology, Ohio State University

John S. Wiebe, PhD, Department of Psychology, University of Texas at El Paso

Paula G. Williams, PhD, Department of Psychology, Washington State University

Leo Wilton, PhD, Department of African Studies and Human Development, University of Binghamton, State University of New York

LaRicka R. Wingate, Department of Psychology, Florida State University

Katie M. A. Witkiewitz, PhD, Addictive Behaviors Research Center, University of Washington

David A. Wittrock, PhD, Department of Psychology, North Dakota State University

Philip A. Wolf, MD, Neurological Epidemiology and Genetics, Boston University School of Medicine

Stephen A. Wonderlich, PhD, Department of Neuroscience, Neuropsychiatric Institute, Fargo, North Dakota